Child and Adolescent Psychiatry

THE ESSENTIALS

Child and Adolescent Psychiatry

THE ESSENTIALS

Keith Cheng, MD

Adjunct Assistant Professor
Department of Psychiatry
Oregon Health & Science University
Portland, Oregon

Medical Director
Tirillium Family Services
Portland, Oregon

Kathleen M. Myers, MD, MPH, MS, FAACAP

Associate Professor
Department of Psychiatry & Behavioral Sciences
University of Washington School of Medicine
Seattle, Washington

Director
Consultation-Liaison Psychiatry
Department of Child Psychiatry & Behavioral Pediatrics
Children's Hospital & Regional Medical Center
Seattle, Washington

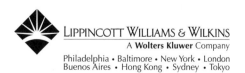

LIPPINCOTT WILLIAMS & WILKINS
A **Wolters Kluwer** Company
Philadelphia • Baltimore • New York • London
Buenos Aires • Hong Kong • Sydney • Tokyo

Acquisitions Editor: Charles W. Mitchell
Developmental Editors: Stacey Sebring and Lisa R. Kairis
Project Manager: Fran Gunning
Marketing Manager: Adam Glazer
Manufacturing Manager: Ben Rivera
Production Services: Laserwords Private Limited
Printer: Edwards Brothers

© 2005 by Lippincott Williams & Wilkins
530 Walnut Street
Philadelphia, PA 19106

Printed in the United States

Library of Congress Cataloging-in-Publication Data

Child and adolescent psychiatry : the essentials / [edited by] Keith
Cheng, Kathleen Myers.
     p. ; cm.
  Includes bibliographical references and index.
  ISBN-13: 978-0-7817-5187-2
  ISBN-10: 0-7817-5187-X
  1. Child psychiatry. 2. Adolescent psychiatry. I. Cheng, Keith.
II. Myers, Kathleen, MD. [DNLM: 1. Mental Disorders—therapy—Adolescent.
 2. Mental Disorders—therapy—Child. WS 350 C53504 2005]
RJ499.C48235 2005
618.92'89—dc22
                                                                    2005006352

Care has been taken to confirm the accuracy of the information presented and to describe generally accepted practices. However, the authors, editors, and publisher are not responsible for errors or omissions or for any consequences from application of the information in this book and make no warranty, expressed or implied, with respect to the currency, completeness, or accuracy of the contents of the publication. Application of this information in a particular situation remains the professional responsibility of the practitioner.

The authors, editors, and publisher have exerted every effort to ensure that drug selection and dosage set forth in this text are in accordance with current recommendations and practice at the time of publication. However, in view of ongoing research, changes in government regulations, and the constant flow of information relating to drug therapy and drug reactions, the reader is urged to check the package insert for each drug for any change in indications and dosage and for added warnings and precautions. This is particularly important when the recommended agent is a new or infrequently employed drug.

Some drugs and medical devices presented in this publication have Food and Drug Administration (FDA) clearance for limited use in restricted research settings. It is the responsibility of health care providers to ascertain the FDA status of each drug or device planned for use in their clinical practice.

The publishers have made every effort to trace copyright holders for borrowed material. If they have inadvertently overlooked any, they will be pleased to make the necessary arrangements at the first opportunity.

To purchase additional copies of this book, call our customer service department at (800) 638-3030 or fax orders to (301) 824-7390. Lippincott Williams & Wilkins customer service representatives are available from 8:30 am to 6:30 pm, EST, Monday through Friday, for telephone access. Visit Lippincott Williams & Wilkins on the Internet: http://www.lww.com.

10 9 8 7 6 5 4 3 2

Contributors

David Breiger, PhD
Acting Assistant Professor
Department of Psychiatry and Behavioral Sciences
University of Washington School of Medicine
Director
Neuropsychological Consultation Service
Department of Child Psychiatry and
    Behavioral Pediatrics
Children's Hospital & Regional Medical Center
Seattle, Washington

Beverly Jean Bryant, MD
Staff Psychiatrist
Child and Adolescent Psychiatry
Pine Grove Hospital
Hattiesburg, Mississippi

Tim Catlow, PsyD
Staff Psychologist
Children's Farm Home
Trillium Family Services
Corvallis, Oregon

Keith Cheng, MD
Adjunct Assistant Professor
Department of Psychiatry
Oregon Health & Science University
Medical Director
Trillium Family Services
Portland, Oregon

Ann M. Childers, MD
Staff Child Psychiatrist
Parry Center for Children
Trillium Family Services
Portland, Oregon

Brent Collett, PhD
Acting Assistant Professor
Department of Psychiatry and Behavioral Sciences
University of Washington School of Medicine
Attending Psychologist
Department of Child Psychiatry and
    Behavioral Pediatrics
Children's Hospital & Regional Medical Center
Seattle, Washington

Ann M. Hamer, PharmD
Clinical Pharmacy Specialist
College of Pharmacy
Oregon State University
Oregon Health & Science University
Portland, Oregon

Stefanie A. Hlastala, PhD
Acting Assistant Professor
Department of Psychiatry and Behavioral Sciences
University of Washington School of Medicine
Attending Psychologist
Department of Child Psychiatry and
    Behavioral Pediatrics
Children's Hospital & Regional Medical Center
Seattle, Washington

David A. Jeffery, MD, MAR
Adjunct Assistant Professor
Division of Child and Adolescent Psychiatry
Oregon Health & Science University
Chief
Secure Children's Inpatient Program
Trillium Family Services
Portland, Oregon

Jenise Jensen, PhD
Postdoctoral Fellow
Department of Psychology
University of Washington
Seattle, Washington
Postdoctoral Fellow
Department of Pediatric Psychology
Mary Bridge Children's Hospital
Tacoma, Washington

Ajit N. Jetmalani, MD
Clinical Assistant Professor
Department of Psychiatry
Oregon Health & Science University
Portland, Oregon

Kyle P. Johnson, MD
Assistant Professor
Division of Child and Adolescent Psychiatry
Department of Psychiatry
Department of Pediatrics
Oregon Health & Science University
Co-Director
Doernbecher Children's Hospital Sleep Program
Portland, Oregon

Alan E. Kazdin, PhD
Director
Yale University Child Study Center
John M. Musser Professor
Department of Psychology
Yale University School of Medicine
New Haven, Connecticut

Roy Lubit, MD, PhD
Assistant Professor
Department of Psychiatry
Mount Sinai School of Medicine
New York, New York

Lawrence A. Maayan, MD
Associate Research Scientist
Yale University Child Study Center
Associate Medical Director
Child Psychiatry Inpatient Service
Yale-New Haven Hospital
New Haven, Connecticut

Larry Marx, MD
Assistant Professor
Division of Child and Adolescent Psychiatry
Department of Psychiatry
Doernbecher Children's Hospital
Oregon Health & Science University
Portland, Oregon

Jon McClellan, MD
Associate Professor
Department of Psychiatry and Behavioral Sciences
University of Washington School of Medicine
Seattle, Washington
Medical Director
Department of Child Psychiatry
Child Study and Treatment Center
Lakewood, Washington

Kathleen M. Myers, MD, MPH, MS, FAACAP
Associate Professor
Department of Psychiatry and Behavioral Sciences
University of Washington School of Medicine
Director
Consultation-Liaison Psychiatry
Department of Child Psychiatry and
    Behavioral Pediatrics
Children's Hospital & Regional Medical Center
Seattle, Washington

Francheska Perepletchikova, MPhil
Graduate Student Clinician
Department of Psychology
Yale University
New Haven, Connecticut

Norman H. Reed, PhD
Director of Clinical Quality
Trillium Family Services
Portland, Oregon

Kay M. Reichlin, MD
Clinical Assistant Professor
Department of Psychiatry
Oregon Health & Science University
Portland, Oregon
Physician Specialist
Forensic Treatment Services
Oregon State Hospital
Salem, Oregon

Carol M. Rockhill, MD, PhD
Fellow, Child and Adolescent Psychiatry
Department of Psychiatry and Behavioral Sciences
Univeristy of Washington School of Medicine
Fellow, Child and Adolescent Psychiatry
Department of Child Psychiatry and
    Behavioral Pediatrics
Children's Hospital & Regional Medical Center
Seattle, Washington

D. Bianca Sava, MD
Postdoctoral Fellow, Child and
    Adolescent Psychiatry
Department of Child Psychiatry
Oregon Health & Science University
Portland, Oregon

Jamie L. Snyder, MD
Adjunct Assistant Professor
Department of Psychiatry
Creighton University
Omaha, Nebraska

Dorothy E. Stubbe, MD
Associate Professor
Yale University Child Study Center
Director
Residency Training Program in Child and
    Adolescent Psychiatry
Yale-New Haven Hospital
New Haven, Connecticut

E. Gene Stubbs, BA, MD
Associate Professor Emeritus
Department of Psychiatry
Department of Pediatrics
Oregon Health & Science University
Portland, Oregon

Jenny Tsai, MD
Assistant Professor
Division of Child and Adolescent Psychiatry
Department of Psychiatry
Oregon Health & Science University

Consulting Psychiatrist
Child Development and Retardation Center
Doernbecher Children's Hospital
Portland, Oregon

Nancy C. Winters, MD
Associate Professor
Department of Psychiatry
Oregon Health & Science University
Director
Residency Training Program in Child and
    Adolescent Psychiatry
Division of Child and Adolescent Psychiatry
Doernbecher Children's Hospital
Portland, Oregon

Joseph L. Woolston, MD
Albert Solnit Professor
Yale University Child Study Center
Chief
Department of Child Psychiatry
Yale-New Haven Hospital
New Haven, Connecticut

Acknowledgment

We would like to express our gratitude:

    To our patients who have taught us,

    To our colleagues who have provided sage advice, and

    To our family members (Karen, Will, and Allison) who have lent their support and patience with this endeavor.

Keith Cheng
Kathleen Myers

Since the inception of child and adolescent psychiatric training programs, there has been a shortage of child and adolescent psychiatrists. In 1993, the American Medical Association predicted that the number of youths needing psychiatric services would continue to increase and that the supply of child and adolescent psychiatrists would not keep up with the demand. This prediction has come true. Currently, there is a severe shortage of child and adolescent psychiatrists, and this shortage will extend many years into the future. The United States Bureau of Health Professions observes that at the current training and recruitment rate, the nation will have only two-thirds of the child and adolescent psychiatrists needed for the year 2020. To make matters worse for rural populations, child and adolescent psychiatrists tend to locate in metropolitan areas. This maldistribution is demonstrated nationally. For example, Massachusetts has 17.5 child and adolescent psychiatrists per 100,000 population, while West Virginia has only 1.75 per 100,000 population. On average, only 300 child and adolescent psychiatrists complete training each year. Unfortunately, the number of child and adolescent psychiatry training programs in the United States decreased from 120 to 113 between 1990 and 2003. Despite this decrease, the United States Surgeon General noted in 1999 that the rate of psychiatric illness in children and adolescents has been increasing.

Because of the shortage of child and adolescent psychiatrists, other clinicians are pressed to provide service for youths with mental health needs. It has been estimated that up to 20% of all children evaluated by primary care clinicians present with a behavioral or emotional disorder. Family practitioners, pediatricians, nurse practitioners, and even internists are providing psychiatric treatment for children or adolescents. General psychiatrists are also finding more youths in their practices. While these clinicians may have received some nominal training in child and adolescent psychiatry, they frequently note their need for a greater knowledge base in treating juvenile psychiatric disorders.

To meet this need, *Child and Adolescent Psychiatry: The Essentials* has been written. Comprehensive textbooks often contain too much information for nonspecialists who need to discern guidelines quickly for providing customary care to their young patients. This book is intended to provide succinct overviews of common child and adolescent psychiatric disorders and related issues that present in the outpatient setting.

The first section on assessment describes three basic modalities for evaluating children and adolescents with mental health complaints. The chapter on psychiatric assessment reviews the practical aspects of assessment, such as how to structure evaluation sessions and how to adapt to the developmental evaluation needs of children of various ages. The chapters on rating scales and psychological assessment describe how these ancillary evaluation modalities may enhance a psychiatric assessment. The second section on psychiatric disorders reviews the common psychiatric disorders likely to present in primary clinicians' or general psychiatrists' practice. The third section on special topics includes chapters on violence, suicide, trauma, maltreatment, and custody disputes. In the fourth and last section on treatment modalities, the major interventions are reviewed. The psychopharmacology chapter describes the psychotropic medications most frequently utilized to treat children and adolescents. This material should guide primary care providers and general psychiatrists to optimal, safe pharmacotherapy. The chapters on psychotherapy, family process, and behavioral interventions present basic information on these nonmedical interventions. They are presented to give the primary care clinician or general psychiatrist an idea of the psychotherapeutic interventions provided to the young patients that they share with mental health clinicians. The chapters on the Individuals with Disabilities Education Act and levels of care address educational and community structures that support the clinicians' work with youths to ensure the success of a comprehensive treatment plan.

Other professionals who may find this book useful include psychiatric social workers, psychologists, and child-care workers. For example, clinicians who work with child welfare or juvenile justice programs have many clients with mental illness who are either in treatment or in need of it. These chapters should provide background on the nature of these youths' illnesses and treatment needs to guide professionals to appropriate services for their young charges. Psychologists consulting with primary care practitioners will find useful clinical tidbits to help their medical colleagues provide appropriate medical interventions. Trainees in social work, psychology, and counseling may also find this text valuable as they work in their field placements. For trainees, the chapters on psychotherapy, family process, and psychopharmacology can provide a quick overview of information not concisely available in their training programs. Psychiatry residents and child and adolescent psychiatry fellows can use this text to prepare for specialty board examinations as a comprehensive textbook may be too esoteric or daunting to glean the most salient information needed for patient care. Finally, practicing child and adolescent psychiatrists may find selected chapters helpful, particularly for areas that are not in their usual daily practice. In particular, the chapters on rating scales, psychological assessment, the Individuals with Disabilities Education Act, and levels of care can update child and adolescent psychiatrists on important adjunctive issues. Our hope and the overall goal of this text is to effectively and efficiently share with other professionals the existing data in child and adolescent psychiatry so that we can all improve the lives of our young patients who are among the most needy, but underserved, youths.

Keith Cheng
Kathleen Myers

Contents

SECTION III Special Issues

SECTION IV Treatment

Evaluation

CHAPTER 1

Psychiatric Assessment of Children and Adolescents

NANCY C. WINTERS

JENNY TSAI

Introduction

The primary goal of psychiatric assessment of the child or adolescent is to determine whether psychopathology is present, and, if so, to establish a differential diagnosis, tentative diagnostic formulation, and treatment plan in collaboration with the family. In order to reach this goal, much information, clinical and historic, needs to be gathered. We describe here a comprehensive psychiatric assessment. There are, however, situations in which specialized or focused assessments occur (e.g., forensic evaluation or risk assessment), and we will briefly review some such situations. Since time for assessment may be limited by external constraints such as funding or resources, a cogent method of assessment and treatment planning is ever more pertinent.

A comprehensive psychiatric assessment should include the following elements: (a) important identifying information, for example, child's age, sex, grade in school; (b) the referral source and reason for referral; (c) sources of information; (d) history of the current problem(s); (e) past psychiatric history; (f) medical and developmental history including intrauterine experiences, and past and current medications; (g) educational history; (h) family social and psychiatric history; (i) social history including substance use, sexual behavior, peer relationships, and legal history; (j) history of trauma and/or stressors; (k) mental status evaluation; (l) clinical formulation and *Diagnostic and Statistical Manual of Mental Disorders,* Fourth Edition (DSM-IV) multiaxial diagnosis; (m) problem list; and (n) treatment plan keyed to the problem list (see Table 1.1).

In this chapter, we refer to children and adolescents as "children" except when discussing specific developmental variations. The term "parents" is used for the child's caregivers, who may include biologic, adoptive, or foster parents, or other family.

Special Considerations in Evaluating Children

There are a number of important differences between the psychiatric assessment of children and adults. The most pertinent issue is that an evaluation of a child is generally initiated by the child's parents or other adults involved in the child's care (as in the case of a school referral). An exception may be the older adolescent who independently seeks treatment. Children may thus be anxious or even shamed in the initial contacts, and it is important to establish a positive and safe climate for them.

The rapid pace of children's development, especially in early childhood, requires familiarity with the different competencies, vulnerabilities, and tasks of each stage of development. Different methods of collecting data and interviewing the child apply at different ages. For example, the infant or toddler is generally assessed with the parent, with special attention to the dyadic interactions, whereas adolescents are best able to furnish clinical information when interviewed alone. There are also differences in the way children at different ages are able to report their symptoms. The younger child has less ability to self-observe

TABLE 1.1. ESSENTIALS OF PSYCHIATRIC ASSESSMENT

- Identifying information (age, sex, grade in school, etc.)
- Sources of information
- Referral source
- Chief complaint or reason for referral (note that chief complaint may differ between parent and child)
- History of present situation
- Past psychiatric (mental health) history
- Current medications (and psychotropic medication history)
- Medical/developmental history
- Educational history (including special education services)
- Family history (both psychiatric and social aspects)
- Cultural context (migration history, ethnic identification, religious affiliation, etc.)
- Trauma history
- Social history (peer relationships, activities, sexual behavior, etc.)
- Use of electronic media, including Internet, video games, movies, etc.
- Substance use
- Legal history
- Mental status examination
- Clinical formulation (including strengths and prognosis)
- DSM-IV diagnosis
- Problem list
- Treatment plan, including patient and family's goals for treatment

and may not have the vocabulary to describe feeling states. Also, symptoms developed early, such as obsessions or compulsions, may be experienced by the child as part of himself and not be recognized as problems.

Because children are more dependent on their adult caretakers, it is not possible to conduct an adequate assessment without an understanding of important environmental characteristics and family relationships, as well as the child's response to them. Risk factors such as poverty, family violence, and parental substance abuse or mental health problems all increase the risk of a child developing a psychiatric disorder and may also impair the family's ability to adequately respond to the child's problem.

Development of a differential diagnosis also differs when evaluating children. First, those disorders not specific to childhood, such as depression or obsessive–compulsive disorder, may show developmental variations. For example, depressed children may present as more irritable than sad, and compulsions may be experienced as acceptable, or ego-syntonic. Additionally, a psychiatric disorder in evolution may have a different, possibly less "differentiated," earlier presentation. For example, young children with early oppositional behavior may later develop mood or anxiety disorders, and schizophrenia may be preceded by social abnormalities and neuropsychological deficits. Thus, the clinician must inform the parents that there can be some uncertainty about the eventual diagnosis. In practice, child psychiatric assessment is conceptualized as an ongoing process that occurs over time. The reality, however, is that children with mental health problems who are experiencing significant functional impairment cannot wait for intervention because of the negative impact on their development. Therefore, even in conditions of uncertainty, a preliminary diagnosis and treatment plan are important, as well as a plan for further data collection based on an initial hypothesis.

Sources of Information

The assessment of the child requires that information be obtained not only from the child, but also from the family, school, primary physician, and past mental health providers. Obtaining information from multiple sources allows the clinician to better gauge whether the problem is global (occurring across all settings) or circumscribed to a certain environment. For children in the juvenile justice, child welfare, special education, or developmental disabilities system, review of information from the agency records or caseworker is also essential. Past and current medical records are helpful in discerning possible medical issues that may contribute to behavioral or mood problems.

Clarifying the purpose of the referral at the outset is essential. Although the child's behavioral and mood problems may be the obvious reason for referral, other more covert intentions may be present. For example, a pending juvenile court decision may be motivating an adolescent to seek "treatment," rather than the condition itself propelling the desire for treatment. Parental custody conflicts and threats of school expulsion may be other motivating factors. These other intentions have implications for diagnosis and treatment planning, in addition to prognosis. For example, parental custody conflicts may influence a parent to overreport or underreport the child's symptoms. At times, the referral may have been requested by adults other than the parents, for example, by the school or court, in which case parental permission is needed unless the child is a ward of the state.

One informative question to ask at the beginning of an assessment is "why now?" Often, there is an acute stress incident that finally makes the parents realize their child needs help. Whether the parent recognizes the child's need for help soon after problems develop or after the child has become very disturbed provides information about the closeness of the parent–child relationship and how well the family functions in promoting the health of family members. Often, fear of stigma delays seeking help for mental health conditions, and understanding the parent or child's apprehensiveness facilitates forming a collaborative relationship. This may be especially important when there are cultural, ethnic, religious, or even social class differences between the patient and clinician.

Structuring the Interview

Structuring assessment interviews depends on the individual case. It may be appropriate to have one or two initial interviews with the parents alone, especially when the patient is a younger child. This allows the parents to share a history of the problem without concern about what the child may hear. It also allows the parents to communicate about their response to the child and their personal concerns that may impact the child's mental health. That is not to say this is the only approach. An advantage of an initial conjoint interview with the child and parents is the opportunity to observe family interactions, such as the family's manner of communicating with and about the child, whether the family exhibits aggression or affection, concern, or derision toward one another, who sets the rules, and whether the parents argue in front of the child.

With adolescents, however, it is usually preferable to include the adolescent in interviews with the parents, as not doing so may risk the teenager's feeling that the clinician is colluding with the parents, with the result that therapeutic alliance may be much more difficult to establish. In either case, the child or adolescent should be prepared for the evaluation. At times, when parents think their child may refuse to come to a psychiatric evaluation, they may deceive the child by saying he or she will be taken to a medical doctor or a special school. The clinician then has the extra challenge to overcome the child's sense of betrayal by the parents and to manage the child's displaced anger and annoyance. It is also helpful to advise the parents to communicate the purpose of the evaluation in a manner that is supportive and nonblaming of the child.

Once the family comes in, the primary task is to build a therapeutic alliance with the family and child. This means setting up an ambience of respect, warmth, and trustworthiness. Some means of doing this include having good eye contact, allowing ample time for all participants to describe their concerns, and speaking in a respectful, concerned way. Some adults and children may be intimidated by visiting a clinician. Asking the child simple questions such as his or her name or birthday, may help put the child at ease. Asking the child to spell his or her name or write down his or her birthday and other family members' birthdays on a piece of paper may lend valuable information regarding the child's cognitive abilities. With regard to teens, discussing hobbies, interests, and job responsibilities can create a sense of ease and convey that the clinician is interested in what they have to say.

Once a sense of mutual regard is established, the next stage of the interview involves exploring the reason for bringing the child in for evaluation, that is, the chief complaint. The goal is to ascertain the child's current difficulties and the impact of his symptoms on the parents and family. If there are several complaints, it is important to understand how disturbing each one is from the child's and parents' points of view, and which ones they would like to address first in treatment. As the assessment progresses, it is not uncommon for the prioritization of concerns to change. Elaborating on the chief complaint entails careful data gathering of the frequency and severity of the problem, as well as the where, when, and how of the situation. A detailed functional analysis of behavioral disturbance is helpful. Any triggering or alleviating factors should be explored. Does the behavior only occur at school, at home, or both? Is it in relation to only specific people, or does the child's behavior occur globally? What impact has this had on the child and the family? How long has the behavior or symptom been going on?

Exploring not only the present active issues is crucial; past psychiatric history, medical history, current medications, social history, school functioning, legal involvement, family psychiatric history, and the review of systems should also be explored. Reviewing each of these realms is important because each may provide a clue and/or have an influence on the present complaint and its manifestations. For example, if it is found that a teenager has abused illicit drugs in the past, it is possible that the parent's complaints that he is displaying agitated behaviors might be related to drug use. Similarly, in a child presenting with depressive symptoms, a review of the past medical history and current medications may yield clues regarding the etiology. Social history should also include a review of extracurricular activities and peer relationships, especially whether the child is being bullied at school. Also, clarifying the child's use of electronic media, including the Internet, video/computer games, and movies, may be important, as in the case of a teenager who has met with a stranger encountered on the Internet, or the child at risk for aggression whose behavior is exacerbated by violent content in movies or video games.

It is worth noting that each family member may have a different perspective about the child's problem. This is especially relevant in the case of the child's parents, who, whether living together or divorced, are likely to perceive the child differently. Each point of view is likely to contain some truth. Alternatively, they may disagree in a way that compromises their ability to function together as parents and thereby contributes to the presenting problem. Such differences may relate to the parents' family of origin issues, differences in parenting styles, psychiatric conditions, or current stressors.

An analysis of the child's environment is an integral part of the assessment. The child's functioning is highly influenced by his ecological context, which includes the "microsystem" of his family, school, and immediate neighborhood and the "macrosystem" of his larger community and culture. Exploring contributing factors within the home, school, community, and larger culture can yield clues for effective interventions. Culture is an integral aspect of family life that should be included in the child's assessment. Important aspects of the cultural interview include the family's ethnic identification, their relationship with a cultural community, the family's migration history, the structure of the extended family including languages spoken and roles of each family member, religious affiliations, child-rearing practices that may be related to culture, and the family's attitudes about illness and health care, including use of traditional healing. Of particular relevance to the presenting problem may be the child's attempts to live within both his family's traditional values and his new American culture. Such issues should be explicitly raised with the child and family so that they realize these are appropriate issues to discuss and that the clinician is interested in their circumstances (see Table 1.2).

Developmental Issues in the Evaluation of Children and Adolescents

One main goal during the history taking and mental status examination is to gauge the child's developmental stage to recommend appropriate interventions. This entails the evaluator's understanding both variations of normal and abnormal child development, including the expected range of behaviors at different ages and the typical manifestations of sundry forms of disturbances in each developmental phase. The evaluator ideally would be skilled in verbal and nonverbal techniques for assessing the child. In general, children are not silver-tongued historians who narrate their travails in a straightforward verbal fashion. Hence, in order to elicit information that may be helpful in evaluating the child's current

TABLE 1.2. ESSENTIALS OF HISTORY TAKING

- Clarify the chief complaint(s) and the goals for treatment
- Clarify who is requesting the assessment and for what purpose
- Find out in what contexts problems occur
- Incorporate information from school or child care, the other parent, health care or other mental health provider, and any other involved agencies, e.g., juvenile justice, child welfare
- Interview the child or adolescent alone, as well as the family

- Use open-ended questions; with young children, observing and describing play is more helpful
- Ask about sexuality, substance use, and self-harm behaviors or impulses
- Integrate information from parent(s) and child, especially in disruptive behavior disorders
- Observe and consider parent–child and family dynamics
- Consider discrepancies between different adults' perceptions of the child and between adults' and child's perceptions

mental status and developmental level, the evaluator should be familiar with a variety of techniques that may facilitate information sharing on the child's part, as summarized in Table 1.3.

Younger children, particularly preschool and early school-aged children, are more able to communicate their thoughts, fears, and perceptions of themselves and others through play. Techniques for engaging the child in evaluative play include: following the child's lead, using humor, exploring the child's interests, and matching the child's affect during the interview (see Table 1.4). For younger children, it is advisable to start out making observations about the child's play. Small children can easily become frustrated with too many questions and refuse to interact further. Other ways of engaging young children include reflecting the child's ideas and vocabulary, and using projective questions, for example, "If you had three wishes, what would they be?" "What animal would you choose to be if you could be one?" "Who would you take with you if you went on a trip to Mars?" One common nonverbal projective technique is children's drawings. The results of free drawing can yield insights into the child's present state and developmental level. An unstructured drawing allows the child to demonstrate his interests and

TABLE 1.3. DEVELOPMENTAL ASPECTS OF THE CHILD INTERVIEW

Preschool
- Use observational and play interaction as opposed to verbal assessment
- Assess motor functioning, language skills, and social relatedness
- Assess parent–child interaction
- Generally requires more time to complete evaluation

School-age
- Wide variation in ability to verbalize
- Integrate verbal techniques and play, encouraging imaginative themes
- Use of board games may facilitate verbal interaction, especially around rules
- Child can give history of both internalizing and externalizing symptoms, but need to integrate with parents' report, especially for internalizing symptoms
- Chronology and time frames difficult to comprehend
- Role of peers takes on increasing importance in child's life

Adolescence
- More able to think abstractly and make use of time frames, e.g., comparing current symptoms with usual baseline
- Able to give reliable history of symptoms, particularly internalizing symptoms
- Type of peer group reveals self-perception
- Increasing ability to self-reflect and show empathy for others, including parents

TABLE 1.4. ESSENTIALS FOR EVALUATION THROUGH PLAY

- Dollhouse with family of dolls (including mother, father, children), furniture, and toilet
- Set of play telephones
- Doctor kit
- Set of blocks or Legos for building
- Paper, pencils, and crayons for drawing and writing; clay or Play-Doh
- Puppets
- Animal, human figures, and motor vehicles for action-oriented play
- Board games (e.g., checkers, Candyland)

preoccupations. For example, as Pynoos and Eth have noted, children who have experienced trauma will frequently show the trauma event in their drawing when asked to draw whatever they wish. There are also several structured drawings with psychometric properties that may be used to ascertain the child's developmental level or internal processes. These include the Draw-A-Person, Kinetic Family Drawing, and House-Tree-Person Drawing. The child's sharing of his drawing also gives the clinician an experience of the child's interpersonal relatedness.

Toys can also facilitate the interaction with small children. A large number of toys is not needed. Ideally, the office would have toys that can allow a wide range of self-expression, fantasy, and role-play of child-relevant themes. Such toys include a set of play telephones; a family set of dolls; a dollhouse; action figures to allow for possible themes of dependency, avoidance, or aggression to be expressed; and materials such as modeling clay, which the child may shape into whatever he has on his mind. Having a few board games may be helpful for latency-aged children, who may enjoy competition with the interviewer. This provides an opportunity to assess the child's appreciation of the use of rules and ability to interact reciprocally and fairly.

In general, it is best to have toys available that are tailored to the child's developmental stage and issues, for example, toys that promote imaginative play; are not noisy, overly complex, or overstimulating; and, especially for the younger child, are simple to manipulate and safe. In an increasingly ethnically diverse population, it is helpful to have a variety of dolls of different ethnic appearances. This allows children of various cultures and ethnicity to express their family of origin issues as well as patterns of identification within the community. Furthermore, observation of the child drawing or playing not only yields information regarding the child's inner fantasy world and perceptions but also provides preliminary data regarding motor coordination, impulsivity, distractibility, ability to concentrate, or compulsivity.

When interviewing teens, it is important to offer some degree of confidentiality to allow them to openly discuss issues such as sexuality, substance use, illegal activity, or impulses to harm themselves. However, they should also be told that their parents need to be informed about any potential danger to them. It is best in that situation to help the teen to share the information with his parent. It is always important to spend some time in the assessment process interviewing the child or adolescent alone. Not only does this allow for direct assessment of his mental state, but it also gives him the opportunity to share his thoughts and concerns that he may be unable or unwilling to share with his parents (see Table 1.5).

Confidentiality Issues

Several aspects of confidentiality should be kept in mind during the evaluation. In the course of obtaining ancillary information, disclosing that a child is being evaluated

TABLE 1.5. ESSENTIALS OF INTERVIEWING ADOLESCENTS

1. Include the adolescent in the initial interview with his parents to allay concerns of collusion with the parents.
2. Interview the adolescent alone, providing him an ample opportunity to share his point of view, interests, and concerns, without judgment.
3. Inform the adolescent that what he shares will be confidential, with the exception of anything representing harm to him or others. Let him know that, should this information need to be shared with his parents, he will be informed, and if possible, present.
4. If the adolescent is not acknowledging there is a problem, pursue tactful questioning to collaboratively understand why his parents are concerned.
5. The interviewer should demonstrate an ability to empathize with the adolescent and show a willingness to see things from his point of view.
6. Positive feedback should be given to reinforce the adolescent's strengths and adaptive behaviors within his cultural context.
7. Address significant problems the adolescent is experiencing right away. Problem solve with the adolescent, supporting his ability to generate solutions within the constraints of his life circumstances, rather than giving advice.

psychiatrically requires consent by the child's legal guardian. Additional requirements as specified by the Health Insurance Portability and Accountability Act (HIPAA) concerning release of medical information, patients' review of records, and contacting patients also need to be observed. The clinician should also be aware of additional state laws relating to confidentiality and consent, particularly in relation to adolescents' rights with respect to releasing records to their parents. Confidentiality requirements do not absolve a clinician from the legal requirement to report suspected child abuse or neglect, although some states may have an exception for clinicians conducting psychotherapy.

THE MENTAL STATUS EXAMINATION

For the mental status examination portion of the assessment, the clinician assesses many aspects of the child; some of the following will already have been observed during history gathering.

The Child's Physical Appearance and Behavior: What is the child's general state of health? Is the child well nourished? Is the child small, average, or large for age? Are there dysmorphic features, bruises, or cuts? How is the child's grooming? Does the young child seem to be well cared for? What is the child's mode of dress (especially relevant in an adolescent) and is it appropriate to the child's gender, circumstances, and current fashion? Does the child look happy or sad in general, or anxious or angry?

Motor Function: Is the child hyperactive or does he show psychomotor retardation? Are there any abnormal movements such as tics, dystonias, or chorea? Are there motor asymmetries? How is the child's gait? Can the child do simple age-appropriate tasks such as hopping or drawing a circle? Subtle indices of neurologic dysfunction include pencil grasp, penmanship, smoothness of rapid alternating movements, and toe walking.

Affect and Mood: What is the range of affects displayed (full or constricted) and are they appropriate to the situation? What does the child say about his mood? Is this consistent with the child's affect? Young children may need prompts such as drawings of faces with different expressions to describe their emotions.

Speech and Language: How well does the child use language to communicate? Is the child's vocabulary and overall use of language developmentally appropriate? How is the child's verbal fluency? Does the child have articulation problems? Is the speech frenetic or pressured? Is the prosody normal? Does the child use nonverbal communication effectively? How does the child respond to "why" questions, for example, can the child express and embellish his ideas beyond answering "yes" or "no"? Is the child able to converse reciprocally?

Thought Process and Content: Is the thought process organized, logical, and goal-directed? Is the child's thinking idiosyncratic or delusional? Does the child have hallucinations? Does the child have suicidal thoughts/plans? Does the child engage in other self-injurious behavior? Does the child have aggressive or homicidal thoughts or plans? Does the child display any fears or worries? Are there specific themes to the child's play, such as repeated traumatic themes? How does the child describe himself or herself in play or words (and what does this suggest about his or her self-image)? What is the child's vision of his or her future? Who are the important people in the child's life? What are his attitudes toward family, school, and peers?

Social Relatedness: Does the child make eye contact? What is the parent–child interaction like? Is the child able to separate from his or her parents? When with the interviewer, what is the level of the child's engagement, relatedness, and ability to interact reciprocally? How does the child use verbal and nonverbal communication? Does the child appear to derive pleasure from the interaction? Does the child show expected curiosity and interest in the playroom, and does the child have an appropriate understanding of physical boundaries?

Intellectual Functioning: While considering where the child should be developmentally, intellectual functioning should be roughly gauged based on the following: vocabulary and language complexity, general fund of knowledge, level of play, complexity of drawings, and orientation to time, person, and place. A variety of standardized instruments also may be used, such as the Goodenough–Harris Draw-a-Person test.

Judgment and Insight: Judgment and insight vary with age and developmental level. Hypothetical questions that are keyed to the child's ability may be asked, for example, for a younger child, "What do you do when it's cold outside?" or for an adolescent, "What would you do if you were at a party and the friend who drove you was drinking alcohol?" Regarding insight, as adolescents are not initiating the evaluation, they may appear to have poor insight into their problems but may have the capacity to develop insight over time or recognize how others perceive their behavior. Young children may be able to relate that they feel sad or mad or may be aware that they get in trouble for certain behaviors.

RATING SCALES/ASSESSMENT INSTRUMENTS

Over the years, many adjunctive tools such as rating scales have been developed to assess psychiatric symptoms in children. The reader interested in a more thorough review of rating scales is referred to the following chapter in this text. Rating scales range from systematized questionnaires that assess psychiatric symptoms in general to those that probe specific areas of difficulty in depth. Advantages to using rating scales include their assisting the clinician in the systematic evaluation of the child, including detecting problems that are clinically significant but not part of the presenting problem. Some youths may reveal concerns in writing that they do not verbalize. Disadvantages of using rating scales include the time needed to complete them, the feeling of being "check-listed," and clinicians' tendency to overrely on rating scales for diagnosis (see Tables 1.6 and 1.7).

One must be aware of the limits of what the score on a rating scale might add to the clinical assessment. For example, one mental health worker had inquired of a psychiatrist why a patient was hospitalized when his Beck Depression Inventory (BDI) score was only a "3." As it turned out, the answer was that on the BDI the patient had endorsed that he wanted to kill himself, and on further clinical interview, this patient had endorsed enough intention that the psychiatrist felt that he warranted hospitalization, especially

TABLE 1.6. COMMONLY USED RATING SCALES

Broad band (covering a broad range of symptom areas)
Child Behavior Checklist (parent, teacher, youth self-report versions); Behavior Assessment System for Children (BASC)

Narrow band (for specific symptom areas)
ADHD: Conners' Rating Scales (parent, teacher, self-report versions)
Depression: Children's Depression Inventory (CDI);
Children's Epidemiological Scale for Depression (CES-D);
Beck Depression Inventory (BDI)
Obsessions/compulsions: Children's Yale-Brown Obsessive Compulsive Scale (CY-BOCS)
(a clinician-administered interview)
Anxiety: Multidimensional Anxiety Scale for Children (MASC); Screen for Child Anxiety Related Emotional Disorders (SCARED); Post-traumatic Stress Disorder-Reaction Index (PTSD-RI)
Level of functioning: Children's Global Assessment Scale (CGAS)

ADHD, attention deficit hyperactivity disorder.

when taking into account factors that were not in the scale, such as the patient's psychiatric history, substance use history, and current social support.

This being said, however, rating scales have numerous advantages that can contribute to efficient data gathering and improved clinical assessment. For example, the Conners' attention deficit hyperactivity disorder (ADHD) scale and the Child Behavior Checklist (CBCL) are straightforward questionnaires that can easily be given to the child's parents in the waiting room while the child is being assessed. Rating scales also play an important role in evidence-based interventions by providing an easy numeric score for monitoring response to treatment. Rating scales with demonstrated reliability and validity for the specific clinical issue being assessed will be most useful. Also important is the scale's sensitivity and specificity; whether the scale is suitable for the population, setting, and degree of training of the rater; and the scale's sensitivity to change during treatment. Ultimately, diagnosis and assessment are based on clinical judgment, with rating scales used as adjuncts to a competent history and examination.

At times, the clinician may refer the child for other specialized evaluations. Such evaluations may include formal psychological testing, including psychometric and projective evaluation and/or neuropsychological testing. These evaluations could be especially pertinent if the diagnosis continues to be unclear and the clinician needs further clarification of the child's cognitive abilities, personality and temperament, thought disturbances, and added information about symptoms. Medical consultation also would be appropriate

TABLE 1.7. ADVANTAGES AND LIMITATIONS OF RATING SCALES

Advantages
1. They are convenient, economical, and can be completed quickly.
2. Certain scales can be completed without specialized training. Parents, teachers, children, clinicians, and childcare workers can complete suitable versions to provide various contextual or ecological perspectives.
3. A wide range of data can be obtained.
4. They provide scores that are easy to analyze and follow in treatment.

Limitations
1. Rating scales do not yield a diagnosis.
2. Some scales require training to achieve good interrater agreement.
3. Rating scales compare individuals in terms of item and scale scores but may not provide individualized descriptions of persons apart from their specific pattern of scores.
4. Results are affected by the cooperation, knowledge, and candor of the rater, although gross distortions are clinically informative and can usually be detected by comparisons with other data.
5. Rating scales are subject to misuse when overinterpreted or interpreted too literally, in isolation from other relevant clinical data.

TABLE 1.8. MEDICAL FACTORS THAT MAY HAVE A PSYCHIATRIC PRESENTATION

Medications/drug-induced: Corticosteroids, benzodiazepines, amphetamines, anticholinergics, hallucinogens, antihypertensives
Endocrinologic: Cushing disease, adrenal insufficiency, diabetes, hypothyroidism, hyperthyroidism, hypopituitarism, androgenization
Infectious/immunologic: Infectious mononucleosis, HIV/AIDS, tuberculosis, neoplasms, lupus, erythematosis, chronic fatigue syndrome, PANDAS (pediatric autoimmune neuropsychiatric disorders associated with streptococcal infection)
Neurologic: Epilepsy, migraine headache, central nervous system tumor, traumatic brain injury (recent or old), anoxia, demyelinating processes
Genetic: Wilson disease, Prader–Willi syndrome, Klinefelter syndrome, Fragile X syndrome
Other: Uremia, hypoglycemia, electrolyte abnormalities

HIV/AIDS, human immunodeficiency virus/acquired immunodeficiency syndrome.

when there are questions concerning physical conditions and medications that may be influencing the child's psychiatric presentation. Such conditions can especially include conditions of a neurologic, metabolic, endocrinologic, or genetic nature as summarized in Table 1.8.

Clinical Formulation and Diagnosis

In this stage of the assessment, the clinician must formulate the most likely explanation of why the problem is occurring. This involves synthesizing the data that have been gathered and identifying the contributing factors that have brought the patient to assessment. As Barker notes, a comprehensive clinical formulation includes a summary of predisposing, precipitating, perpetuating, and protective factors contributing to the current problem. Each of these factors may be described along the following dimensions: (a) biologic/constitutional (including prenatal, birth, and early temperament), (b) psychological/personality/temperament, (c) family/interpersonal, and (d) socioenvironmental. For example, in a 10-year-old boy presenting with disruptive behavior, predisposing factors (i.e., vulnerabilities) can range from genetic loading for ADHD (constitutional factor) to a disrupted early attachment relationship (family/interpersonal factor). Precipitating factors (i.e., stressors) may include an acute medical illness (biologic factor) or loss of family housing (socioenvironmental factor). Perpetuating factors may include low self-esteem (psychological factor) or parental substance abuse (family factor). Protective factors (i.e., strengths) may include intelligence (constitutional factor) or a positive relationship with a warm, caring adult outside the family (family/interpersonal factor). Consideration of risk factors such as fetal drug exposure, poverty, abuse, low birth weight, difficult temperament, trauma exposure, and genetic factors is helpful in considering vulnerability to mental health disorders. The overall focus of the formulation is to understand what brings the youth to this point in life. In developing a formulation, it is helpful to consider the following:

- Why is the problem surfacing now?
- What is the interplay between constitution, personality, and environment?
- How are the parent(s)' and child's vulnerabilities interacting?
- How does the child's view compare with the parents' view of the problem?
- How have the child and family adapted to the problem? Might this explain some of the symptoms?
- How is the child's development being affected by the primary problem?
- What are the child and family's strengths that can support positive change?
- What social resources are available to support the child and family's strengths?

It should be remembered that just because a factor is present does not mean that it explains the problem. For example, a traumatic event may be less relevant to a child's disruptive behavior than mental retardation. Thus, the factors that appear most relevant to the presenting problems should be emphasized. With this caveat, the following components should be included in a comprehensive biopsychosocial formulation:

- Brief case summary (several sentences, including demographic information, chief complaint, presenting problems, major signs and symptoms, course of illness)
- Biologic characterization (genetic, medical, constitutional)
- Precipitating stressors
- Psychological characterization (personality, intrapsychic issues, defense mechanisms, cognitive style)
- Family and interpersonal factors
- Sociocultural factors (environment, larger ecological context)
- Integrative statement: how the factors above interact to lead to the current situation and the child's current level of functioning

This multifactorial synthesis need not comprise a major treatise. Rather, the various factors may be synthesized into a paragraph stated much as one clinician would do when referring a patient to a colleague. The clinician must then determine whether there is sufficient evidence of a diagnosable syndrome, as well as prognostic factors that may contribute to worsening or improvement of the condition. A multifactorial clinical formulation provides a useful springboard for generating a broad differential diagnosis. One should not forget to include in the differential diagnosis any relevant parent–child conditions, organic factors, and personality features, and address both internalizing and externalizing symptoms (which are often comorbid). It is essential that the full DSM-IV multiaxial diagnostic system be applied, as this system includes factors that may be contributing to the clinical picture as a whole and provides an overall assessment of how the child is functioning in the face of these psychiatric difficulties.

In many cases there are multiple factors to consider and/or comorbid conditions that complicate the diagnostic profile. A definitive diagnosis may not be appropriate initially. When the diagnostic picture is still unclear, it may be necessary to extend the evaluation period. The clinician should explain to the child and parents that ongoing assessment during treatment may be appropriate.

Special Situations

A number of special situations may lead to a request for psychiatric evaluation. Common among these are evaluations directly requested by another agency such as the school, juvenile justice, or child welfare agency. In these cases, it is important to clarify the specific reason for the referral and whether the custodial parent has given permission for the evaluation. Confidentiality issues differ in these specialized situations in that the parents and child need to understand that the evaluation report will be sent to the requesting agency. The specific question dictates the areas to be addressed in the evaluation. For example, a school may request evaluation of whether a child who has made a violent threat can safely return to school. Although this may appear to be a circumscribed question, a thorough evaluation must be done to assess the nature of the child's threat and risk of acting on the threat. The clinician should inquire about the event in some detail, including precipitating factors and chronic stressors in the environment in which the threat occurred, such as chronic bullying. A comprehensive evaluation is then conducted. In the written report, the clinician's recommendations should emphasize the most helpful and cautious approach that is in the best interest of the child. Recommendations should take into account the realities of the child's home life, as well as parental concerns and sensitivities.

Other assessments may focus on a particular clinical question, such as evaluation of suicidal risk to determine need for hospitalization. In this case, issues pertaining to safety must be emphasized. These include the presence of psychiatric disorder, severity of symptoms, history of suicide attempts, nature of the suicidal ideation and lethality of intent, access to means, personality variables (e.g., impulsivity), capacity for problem-solving, presence of social stressors, current substance abuse, availability of meaningful psychological support, and ability of the family to monitor the child at home.

When asked to do psychiatric evaluations in the midst of custody disputes, it is important to discern whether the evaluation is for legal purposes or for the purpose of helping the child with an emotional or behavioral problem. If the evaluation may be used in legal proceedings, Schetky and Benedek recommend that it should be done according to specific guidelines for forensic evaluation and should not be done by a treating clinician. Evaluations of physical or sexual abuse may require additional medical and specialized forensic methods, as described by the American Academy of Child and Adolescent Psychiatry. In preliminary assessments for the purpose of deciding whether to refer to a specialist, only open-ended, nonleading questions should be asked, for example, "Have you been touched in a way that made you uncomfortable?" rather than "Tell me what Mr. X did to you." In situations of suspected abuse, asking detailed questions about the abuse may prejudice a subsequent examination that may be used in legal proceedings.

Communicating Findings and Recommendations

Effectively communicating the clinician's findings to the parents and child is an essential part of the psychiatric assessment. Depending on the nature of the problem and the developmental level of the child, communicating the findings and recommendations may take place either with the child and family together or separately. Communicating information that is sensitive, such as discussing concerns that the child is mentally retarded or autistic, requires considerable tact, as well as education of the parents. Discussion of diagnoses such as schizophrenia or bipolar disorder that may be disconcerting or controversial requires time, sensitivity, and opportunity for open discussion and questions. It is important to emphasize the child's strengths, in addition to providing suggestions on what can assist with the child's difficulties. In situations when diagnostic clarity remains uncertain, this should be communicated to the family.

On the basis of the clinical formulation and diagnosis, the clinician's goal is to formulate a developmentally suitable approach to the treatment of the child's difficulties. Selection of appropriate treatment is based on multiple factors, including diagnosis and symptom severity, acute and ongoing risk of harm, capacity of the family to support treatment and provide a safe environment, capacity of the child to use interactive treatment approaches, and availability of treatment options in the community. A comprehensive biopsychosocial treatment plan should also include adjunctive interventions such as special education services for children with learning disorders or autism, or social skills training for children with problems in peer relationships.

The comprehensive psychiatric assessment of a child is a challenging task. Because of the variable capacity of the child to describe his symptoms, the interaction of the child's vulnerabilities and symptoms with his environment, and the evolving nature of childhood psychiatric disorders, assessment generally requires a longer time than assessment of adults. Thus, primary care physicians and general psychiatrists may want to collaborate with the child and adolescent psychiatrist or child psychologist to clarify complex diagnostic and treatment issues.

Ultimately, a comprehensive psychiatric assessment is well worth the time and resources involved. It holds the key to clarifying the causes of psychiatric disturbances and opens doors to future improvements. A comprehensive treatment plan based on an accurate clinical formulation and diagnosis can improve a child's functioning and make a difference in the lives of the child and family.

BIBLIOGRAPHY

American Academy of Child and Adolescent Psychiatry. Practice parameters for the psychiatric assessment of children and adolescents. *J Am Acad Child Adolesc Psychiatry* 1997;36(10 Suppl): 4S–20S.

American Academy of Child and Adolescent Psychiatry. Practice parameters for the forensic evaluation of children and adolescents who may have been physically or sexually abused. *J Am Acad Child Adolesc Psychiatry* 1997;36(10 Suppl): 37S–56S.

Barker P. Assessing children and their families. *Basic child psychiatry.* Oxford, UK: Blackwell Science, 1995:60.

Pynoos RS, Eth S. Witness to violence: the child interview. In Chess S, Thomas A, Hertzig M, eds. *Annual Progress in Child Psychiatry and Child Development.* New York: Brunner/Mazel, 1987:299–326.

Schetky DH, Benedek EP, eds. *Principles and practice of child and adolescent forensic psychiatry.* Washington, DC: American Psychiatric Press, 2002.

SUGGESTED READINGS AND RESOURCES FOR CLINICIANS AND FAMILIES

American Academy of Child and Adolescent Psychiatry, http://www.aacap.org/ On this web site, see in particular "Facts for Families and Other Resources", http://www.aacap.org/info_families/index.htm. Accessed 2005.
(A web site with offerings for clinicians and families; includes publications, policy statements, listings of resources.)

Barker P. Assessing children and their families. *Basic child psychiatry.* Oxford, UK: Blackwell Science, 1995.
(A concise and easy to read volume on assessment for clinicians.)

Cepeda C. *The psychiatric interview of children and adolescents.* Washington, DC: American Psychiatric Press, 2000.
(Well written and easy to read volume for clinicians on psychiatric interviewing of children.)

Koplewicz H. *It's nobody's fault: new hope and help for difficult children and their parents.* New York: Random House, 1996.
(Excellent book for parents on mental disorders in children, including etiology and how mental health treatments can help.)

National Institutes of Mental Health, http://www.nimh.nih.gov/publicat/index.cfm
(The most comprehensive web site on mental health for both clinicians and families; includes up-to-date research findings in all major areas of mental health; helpful links to other sites.)

CHAPTER 2

Psychiatric Rating Scales: Theory and Practice

KATHLEEN M. MYERS
BRENT COLLETT

Introduction

Rating scales gained popularity in the second half of the 20th century, largely as a response to the declining interest in projective measures, along with an increasing focus on scientific measurement, refinements in diagnostic nomenclature, development of new models of juvenile psychopathology, and the recognition that youths' own self-reports provide valuable information about their subjective experience and view of their problems. The term "rating scale" is broad and encompasses multiple types of measurement, including checklists, questionnaires, inventories, self-reports, others' reports about the youth, and other measures. In this chapter, we use the term "rating scale" to describe instruments that provide efficient assessment of a specific construct with an easily derived numeric score that is readily interpreted, whether completed by the youth or someone else, regardless of the response format, and irrespective of application.

Two broad categories of juvenile psychopathology that are typically assessed with rating scales are termed "externalizing disorders" and "internalizing disorders." "Externalizing disorders" refer to externally observable disruptive behaviors that generally cause distress to others leading to referral for mental health evaluation. Such disorders may or may not cause distress to the individual having the disorder. The *Diagnostic and Statistical Manual,* Fourth Edition (DSM-IV) categorizes these disorders as disruptive behavior disorders that include: attention deficit hyperactivity disorder (ADHD), oppositional defiant disorder (ODD), and conduct disorder (CD). "Internalizing disorders" refer to disorders that cause individuals subjective distress and may not be directly observable by others and/or do not cause others as much distress as they cause the individual suffering the disorder. Such disorders are categorized in DSM-IV as mood disorders and anxiety disorders. Examples include major depressive disorder, dysthymic disorder, bipolar disorder, panic disorder, generalized anxiety disorder, and social anxiety disorder. Traditionally, parent and teacher report methodology has been used to assess externalizing disorders and behaviors, while self-report methodology has been used to assess internalizing disorders and emotional functioning. However, there is increasing appreciation of the need to assess both of these broad dimensions using multiple informants, including parent/caregiver, teacher, and youths' own self report. Such an approach contributes to a better understanding of a youth's functioning across settings and from multiple perspectives.

This chapter discusses the use of rating scales in psychiatric assessment and treatment. Both theoretical issues affecting the functioning of rating scales and practical aspects of specific scales are reviewed. Emphasis is on scales that assess the externalizing and internalizing problems commonly treated in clinical practice. Most of these scales are widely used. They demonstrate *suitability* for youths, that is, they were either specifically constructed with children and adolescents or they represent modifications of adult scales that have then been appropriately studied with youths. A few scales are new and are still being examined but are presented because they fill a special niche. All of the scales presented here also have high *utility*, that is, they provide very useful information that could not be obtained in a more efficient manner. Therefore, these scales should benefit clinicians seeking inexpensive, informative, and psychometrically sound scales that are acceptable to youths and adults in daily clinical practice.

Advantages and Disadvantages of Rating Scales

The value of rating scales is indicated by their inclusion in the Practice Parameters of the American Academy of Child and Adolescent Psychiatry. These scales have multiple uses, including community screening, monitoring high-risk youths, selecting homogeneous groups for specific interventions, evaluating treatment, and determining outcome. They provide systematic coverage and quantification of behavior in order to compare the youth with self and peers over time, setting, and circumstances. When used to objectively document changes in behavior or symptom severity with treatment, rating scales offer clinicians a cost-effective method for making empirically sound treatment decisions consistent with evidence-based treatment.

Common difficulties with rating scales in clinical practice include users' unrealistic expectations and inadequate knowledge of scale functioning. Clinicians often inaccurately assume that an elevated score on these instruments equates to diagnosis, leading to the overreliance on rating scales to the detriment of other assessment procedures such as clinical interviews and direct behavioral observations. With their increasing popularity, an abundance of rating scales have been developed and commercially published. Although many of these scales have been well researched with child and adolescent populations, others are developmentally inappropriate, do not have adequate normative data, have not been used with clinical populations and/or demographic populations of interest, or have not been appropriately validated for their intended purpose. It is, therefore, incumbent on clinicians to take care in scale selection to ensure that these instruments (a) are used only for their intended purpose and the function(s) for which they have been validated; (b) are used in conjunction with other procedures, such as clinical interviews and behavioral observations; (c) are appropriate for their patient population; and (d) have established reliability and validity. Determining whether these criteria are met requires review of a scale's technical manual as well as the research literature. Users will want to determine with what populations the scale was standardized and with what other groups it has been investigated, what evidence exists of validity for the intended purpose, and how reliable the scale is over time and across different observers. Further, users should review a scale's specific item content and subscale labels. In many cases, subscale labels are relatively arbitrary and may not accurately describe the symptoms or behaviors covered by the individual items.

It is also important to consider the individual and situational factors that can affect a scale's performance. Youths who seek social acceptance may underreport symptoms ("denial" or "lying"), while those who feel overwhelmed may overreport ("faking"). Similarly, adult respondents who are exasperated by the youth's problems may convey their own distress and endorse many items, while others with a higher tolerance may portray the youth as relatively asymptomatic. As a result, different reporters may provide discrepant or "discordant" responses to behavioral rating scales. Indeed, agreement among reporters, even those who interact with a youth in the same setting, is often found to be modest at best. Further, not surprisingly, there is often little agreement between youths and their parents. This appears to be especially true for younger children, for those with externalizing disorders, and in cases of maternal depression or other parental psychopathology. The discordance among different respondents also reflects the considerable variability in a youth's behavior across settings, that is, contextual or ecologic factors. While a child with ODD may be very difficult to manage at home or in the community, he/she may show fewer behavioral problems in a highly structured classroom with a teacher skilled in behavioral management. By contrast, a highly anxious child may be able to function effectively in the familiar home setting, showing social withdrawal and behavioral inhibition only in the more anxiety-provoking school milieu. Overall, it is important to view the scale as a means of communication between respondent and clinician when interpreting scores, rather than considering the score as portraying some "truth." In order to adequately characterize and understand a youth's behavior, it is imperative to collect data from multiple sources and across multiple settings. The essential aspects of using rating scales are summarized in Table 2.1.

Psychometric Properties of Rating Scales

As with all forms of measurement, rating scales are subject to error. Psychometric data are used to estimate this error and help to determine whether a scale is appropriate for an intended application. Reliability refers to the consistency with which a scale's items measure the same construct, the stability of the scale's measurement over time, and consistency across respondents. Lack of reliability is referred to as "random error." Coefficients exceeding 0.80 support reliability, but also mean that up to 20% of the variability in scores is due to random error. There are different types of reliability to assess different aspects of a scale's functioning. *Internal reliability*, or *internal consistency*, represents the degree to which individual items comprising the scale are consistent with each other. Items that are not internally consistent detract from the scale and are generally dropped during scale

TABLE 2.1. ESSENTIALS OF RATING SCALES IN DATA COLLECTION

Rating scales cannot be used alone to make a diagnosis; they are adjunctive tools used to complement a diagnostic evaluation.

Rating scales have several valuable roles in clinical practice including: diagnostic corroboration; establishing severity of a disorder or symptom; screening for a disorder or symptom; identifying treatment goals; and monitoring treatment response.

Rating scales' *utility* is highest when the scale is brief, easy to complete, and has a single total score, or several subscale scores, that can be easily derived and interpreted.

Rating scales must be *suitable*, i.e., they must be geared to the youth's developmental abilities. Therefore, scales developed with adults cannot be administered to youth without examining their functioning in this age group.

Rating scales for youth are best used with multiple informants in order to consider ecological, or contextual, aspects of a youth's disorder. Typical informants include: the youth, parents/guardians, teachers, coaches, other relevant adults, and sometimes peers.

The younger the child, the worse the agreement, or concordance, between the youth's own report and that of a relevant adult, demonstrating both developmental issues and personal perspective. Such discordance does not invalidate results.

Relevant adults show only poor to moderate agreement, or concordance, in their reports of a youth's behavior, demonstrating both contextual aspects of a youth's behavior and each individual's personal perspective. This does not invalidate any individual's report.

For self-report scales, reliability and validity are lower at younger ages and for youths with externalizing behaviors rather than internalizing symptoms.

construction. *Test-retest reliability*, or *stability*, assesses whether a scale is stable over time. If the construct measured has not changed, then repeated measurements should be similar. If stability has not been established, it is difficult to determine whether change measured over time is real or represents random error in the scale. Obviously, this could pose significant problems when monitoring treatment or measuring final treatment outcome. It should be noted that stability varies to some extent as a function of the construct being measured. Some constructs, such as impulsivity, are expected to be stable over time. Other constructs, such as anger, suicidality, and depression, are expected to wax and wane and may produce lower test-retest reliability coefficients. *Interrater reliability* represents the agreement, or *concordance*, between different informants. Such concordance may be between two different clinicians administering the same scale, for example, in determining diagnosis. However, for the scales presented here, *interrater reliability* will refer to scores between youths and relevant adults in their lives, or among these various adults.

Validity pertains to whether the scale accurately assesses what it was designed to assess. Lack of validity is referred to as "systematic error." Validity must be assessed against multiple criteria over time and in multiple applications. Therefore, newly developed scales may not have sufficient validity data, and there is some risk that a new scale does not really measure what it purports to measure. There are several types of validity.

Construct validity examines whether the scale taps a theoretic construct, such as aggression, anxiety, etc. *Factor validity* refers to whether a scale consists of meaningful subscales that measure somewhat different concepts related to the overall scale's construct. It is determined through a statistical procedure termed "factor analysis" and can be used to help support a scale's construct validity. For example, ADHD scales are expected to demonstrate separate inattentive and hyperactive-impulsive factors, consistent with the current DSM-IV diagnostic construct. *Content validity* assesses whether the scale's items represent the construct being measured. *Face validity* is a type of content validity that is determined by subjectively judging whether items measure the content area. That is, one looks at the items and, from clinical experience, determines that the items are indeed representative of the construct to be measured. *Criterion validity* is assessed in relation to other measures with established validity in measuring the same construct. There are two subtypes: *predictive validity* asks whether the scale correlates with an event that will occur in the future; *concurrent validity* refers to a scale's correlation with an event assessed at the same time the scale is administered. Concurrent validity includes *convergent validity*, or the extent of correlation with some other relevant variable, and *discriminant validity*, which compares scores for groups that do and do not have a particular problem or diagnosis. Finally, a scale's *sensitivity* and *specificity* are often evaluated to support validity. Sensitivity refers to a scale's ability to detect true cases, while specificity refers to the "false positives" a scale produces.

While the ideal scale would have established validities in all of these dimensions, this will not be the case in practice. Rather, the user must determine whether the validity data available support the intended application. For example, if a scale is to be used for screening, then good discriminant validity and sensitivity might be highly desirable. By contrast, if a scale is to be used to determine whether a youth could be discharged early from the hospital, then good predictive validity would be of particular importance.

Uniform guidelines do not apply across reliability and validity coefficients. The magnitude of reliability coefficients should generally be quite high, while validity estimates should be statistically significant but are often lower in magnitude. Among the various forms of reliability, there are differences in the expected range of coefficients. For example, adequate internal consistency reliability estimates are expected to be high, above 0.80. Short-term (a few weeks) test-retest reliability should also be above 0.80, but longer term (longer than 1 month) stability may be less conservative, that is, above 0.60. Interrater reliability coefficients should be above 0.80 for examiners concurrently scoring a youth's interview. However, as discussed above, agreement is often lower among adults who interact with the youth in different contexts, such as home versus school. Thus, interrater reliability estimates among lay adults in the 0.30 range are not uncommon and are not necessarily a prohibitive flaw. Validity correlations are typically lower than reliability estimates. High correlations above 0.90 would suggest that the new scale is redundant with the validating scale and that the new scale adds nothing new to the measurement of a particular construct. Adequate validity is indicated by statistically significant correlations, generally above 0.40, but sometimes even lower coefficients are adequate.

Obviously, interpreting psychometric data can be complicated. As this text seeks to present the essentials of using rating scales with youths suffering psychiatric disorders, psychometrics are presented qualitatively. This information should help the potential user to decide whether a particular scale might be useful for an intended application. If more quantitative information is needed, the interested reader is referred to the series of articles in the bibliography.

Presentation of the Scales

The scales are presented here in both text and tables. The text discusses the scales' applications, while the tables summarize their technical properties. In the tables, column 1 contains the acronym for the scale. Column 2 provides information on the appropriate reporter (e.g., self-report, parent report) and suitable age groups. Column 3 gives the publisher of the scale. Column 4 gives the number of items and number of scoring points. Column 5 provides the administration time. Columns 6 and 7 contain psychometric properties: reliabilities and validities, respectively.

All of these scales have adequate functioning for their intended purposes and are easy to complete, score, and interpret. They are suitable for youths and have high utility in practice. Most scales are commercially available, but some must be obtained through their authors or are in the public domain. Certainly, many other scales are available to tap the same constructs as the scales presented here, but we thought these scales were most relevant for general clinical practice.

BROADBAND RATING SCALES

Broadband scales assess a variety of problems, typically including both externalizing and internalizing problems. They have excellent utility for initial evaluations, as they cover a wide range of problems, can be completed by multiple informants in different settings, and help to focus further assessment. Broad coverage is particularly important in initial evaluation, as youths referred for specific concerns generally have other problems requiring assessment. Despite their utility, broadband scales suffer some limitations, such as a tendency to be lengthy. They may, therefore, be viewed as burdensome for respondents, particularly if multiple administrations are required, as in treatment monitoring, or if used with other measures. Finally, due to their breadth and the need to minimize respondent burden, they contain few items per subscale, that is, they lack depth in evaluating a specific problem. Thus, these scales are best used to identify problems needing further evaluation with interviews, observations, or narrow-band scales. The most popular broadband scales are shown in Table 2.2. They cover a range of problems in various settings, consider adaptive skills, have multiple reporter forms, and have computer scoring to integrate these forms and obviate cumbersome hand scoring that decreases utility.

The *Child Behavior Checklist* (CBCL) was originally developed in the 1960s and has been considered the "gold standard" among behavior rating scales. The CBCL is among a family of behavior rating scales, with multiple reporter forms and developmental variations. In addition to the CBCL, this system of scales includes: *Teacher Report Form* (TRF), *Youth Self-Report* (YSR), *Child Behavior Checklist 1¹/₂−5* (CBCL-1¹/₂−5), and *Caregiver-Teacher Report Form* (C-TRF) for preschoolers. The CBCL, TRF, and YSR include subscales with the following labels: Anxious/Depressed, Withdrawn/Depressed, Somatic Complaints, Social Problems, Thought Problems, Attention Problems, Rule-Breaking Behavior, and Aggressive Behavior. Composite scores for Internalizing, Externalizing, and Total Problems are also calculated. Scores can also be calculated for DSM-IV scales, which are labeled Attention Deficit Hyperactivity Problems, Oppositional Defiant Problems, Conduct Problems, Affective Problems, Anxiety Problems, and Somatic Problems. A series of items also assess youths' adaptive functioning. For the CBCL-1¹/₂−5 and C-TRF, scores are derived for subscales labeled: Emotionally Reactive, Anxious/Depressed, Somatic Complaints, Withdrawn Behavior, Sleep Problems, Attention Problems, and Aggressive Behavior. Composite scores for Internalizing, Externalizing, and Total Problems are also calculated. DSM-IV subscales are labeled Affective Problems, Anxiety Problems, Pervasive Developmental Problems, Attention Deficit Hyperactivity Problems, and Oppositional Defiant Problems. The CBCL-1¹/₂−5 also has a language screening scale due to the frequent overlap of language delays and behavior problems. These measures have recently been updated, with new normative data and several modifications to item content and subscale structure. Several problem behavior items in the CBCL system include blanks for parents to provide specific manifestations of a youth's problem. It is important to review parents' responses, as they may offer important clinical information or may reflect misunderstanding of the items. Additionally, several subscale labels are misleading. For example, the "Aggressive Behavior" subscale describes oppositional and defiant behaviors, with few items describing aggression. The "Thought Problems" subscale is loaded for inattention, and is not an index for thought disorder. Finally, the controversy regarding the use of DSM-IV with young children suggests caution in using these subscales for the CBCL-1¹/₂−5 and C-TRF. Overall, these scales have a wide range of applications across ethnic and language groups in clinical, community, and school settings. Their utility is immense.

TABLE 2.2. BROADBAND SCALES

Scale	Reporter and Age of Youth	Publisher and Cost	Items	Time	Reliability	Validity
CBCL/TRF	Parent or teacher 16–18 y/o	ASEBA $35 for manual	120 problem items	15–20 min	IC: moderate to excellent TR: fair to excellent over short term but poor to good over longer term; IR: fair to excellent between parents; poor to moderate between teachers; poor to low between parent and teacher	Adequate convergent and discriminant validity for parent and teacher forms
CBCL	Parent or teacher $1\frac{1}{2}$–5 y/o	ASEBA $35 for manual	102 problem items	15–20 min	IC: moderate to excellent TR: fair to excellent over short term but poor to good over longer term IR: fair to good between parents; poor to moderate between teachers; very poor to low between parent and teacher	Adequate convergent and discriminant validity for parent and teacher forms on behavior and language scales
C-TRF	$1\frac{1}{2}$–5 y/o		8 language items 310 vocabulary words			
YSR	Youth/Self 11–18 y/o	ASEBA $35 for manual	105 problem items	15–20 min	IC: fair to excellent TR: fair to excellent over short term but poor to fair over longer term IR: poor to fair between youth and parent; very poor to poor between youth and teacher	Adequate discriminant validity between referred and nonreferred youth

CBCL, Child Behavior Checklist; CBCL-1$\frac{1}{2}$–5/C-TRF, CBCL for ages 1–5 years old, C-TRF, Caregiver-Teacher Report Form; TRF, Teacher Report Form; YSR, Youth Self-report; IC, internal consistency reliability; TR, test-retest reliability; IR, interrater reliability.

See bibliography for information on obtaining the scales.

Narrow-Band Scales Assessing Externalizing Behaviors

Externalizing behaviors are publicly observable, and these youths are typically referred because of the problems they pose to parents and teachers (see Table 2.3). Youths generally underestimate their misbehaviors, and adults are considered the optimal informants. These scales are more likely than internalizing scales to demonstrate developmental relevance, as they were developed for elementary school children based on their behaviors at home and school. Less clear is their suitability for younger and older ages. Suitability for girls is also somewhat unclear, as these scales predominantly reflect behaviors displayed by boys.

RATING SCALES FOR ATTENTION DEFICIT HYPERACTIVITY DISORDER

Ongoing interest in ADHD has led to several scales being developed and/or updated to DSM-IV criteria. This basis in diagnostic criteria facilitates construct validity, and most scales include the expected subscales of Inattention and Hyperactivity/Impulsivity. For the most part, these scales are very similar. Choosing among them hinges on the intended application, assessment of comorbidity, other scales included in the assessment, and the need for adolescent self-report. Otherwise, there are subtle differences in these scales' characteristics, such as adequacy of the normative data and psychometric strengths and weaknesses, which may influence choice.

The *Conners Rating Scale–Revised* (CRS-R) is an updated version of this popular scale. It addresses prior deficits in factor structure, normative base, and empiric support. Consistent with earlier versions, the CRS-R covers core ADHD symptoms as well as a variety of comorbid problems such as ODD and CD. There are multiple indices to assess these constructs. The normative base, strong psychometrics, and multiple documented uses make the CRS-R excellent for the assessment of ADHD. Its discriminant validity and generally good sensitivity also make it effective in screening and group assignment. However, the lower sensitivity of the teacher version suggests the risk of missing cases at school. There are abbreviated versions that may facilitate monitoring in drug studies. Disadvantages relate to poorer functioning of the comorbidity indices than the ADHD indices. Thus, the CRS-R does not replace broadband scales for comprehensive assessment. Overall, the CRS-R has become the standard measure of ADHD and is a good choice for clinical practice.

The *Swanson, Nolan and Pelham-IV Questionnaire* (SNAP-IV) was the first of many scales to present DSM criteria in a rating scale format and has been updated with each DSM revision. It has been widely used in research. The shortened and most frequently used version of the SNAP-IV includes core DSM-IV–derived ADHD subscales along with summary questions in each domain. An extended version adds symptom criteria for comorbid DSM-IV disorders, making it more like the CRS-R. The SNAP-IV and scoring information are conveniently provided free at www.ADHD.net. Its free availability has made the SNAP-IV popular in clinical practice and an alternative to the CRS-R.

Normative and psychometric data for the SNAP-IV are very limited. However, the SNAP-IV's ADHD and ODD subscales resemble other DSM-IV–based ADHD scales, and their psychometric support may also support the SNAP-IV. The SNAP-IV is sensitive to treatment effects and is frequently used for monitoring treatment. Although the SNAP-IV is appealing, particularly due to its free online availability, the lack of adequate technical and normative information makes it more appropriate for research use.

TABLE 2.3. SCALES ASSESSING EXTERNALIZING BEHAVIORS

Scale	Reporter and Age of Youth	Publisher and Cost	Items	Time	Reliability	Validity
CRS-R	Parent, teacher and adolescent/self 3–17 y/o	Multi-health Systems, Inc. $46 for manual	80 items (parent); 59 items (teacher); 87 items (adolescent)	20–30 min for full versions; 10 min for brief versions	IC: moderate to excellent for all versions TR: very poor to moderate for parent version; low to good for teacher version; moderate to good for adolescent version IR: very poor to fair between parent and teacher and between adolescent and parent; very poor to low between adolescent and teacher	Adequate discriminant validity SENS/SPEC: 92%/94% (parent version); SENS/SPEC: 78%/91% (teacher version); SENS/SPEC: 81%/84% (adolescent version)
SNAP-IV	Parent or teacher 5–11 y/o	Available free at: www.ADHD.net	90 items for full version; 31 items for ADHD + ODD version	20–30 min for full version; 5–10 min for ADHD + ODD version	IC: good to excellent for teachers TR: not reported IR: poor between parent and teacher	No validity data reported
ECBI	Parent 2–16 y/o	Psychological Assessment Resources $40 for manual	36 items	5–10 min	IC: excellent TR: very good over short term but moderate over longer term IR: moderate between mothers and fathers	Adequate convergent and discriminant validity
SESBI-R	Teacher 2–16 y/o	Psychological Assessment Resources $40 for manual	38 items	5–10 min	IC: excellent TR: very good to excellent over short term IR: not reported	Adequate convergent and discriminant validity; some support for predictive validity
HSQ	Parent 4–11 y/o	Guilford Press $36 for manual	16 items	5–10 min	IC: good TR: fair to good over short term IR: poor to fair between mother and father	Adequate convergent and discriminant validity
SSQ	Teacher 4–11 y/o	Guilford Press $36 for manual	12 items	5–10 min	IC: good to excellent TR: moderate to good over short term IR: not reported	Adequate convergent and discriminant validity

ADHD, attention deficit hyperactivity disorder; ODD, oppositional defiant disorder; CRS-R, Conners, Rating Scales, Revised; SNAP-IV, Swanson, Nolan, and Pelham-IV questionnaire; ECBI, Eyberg Child Behavior Inventory; SESBI-R, Sutter-Eyberg Student Behavior Inventory, Revised; HSQ/SSQ, Home and School Situations Questionnaires; IC, internal consistency reliability; TR, test-retest reliability; IR, inter-rater reliability; SENS, sensitivity; SPEC, specificity.

See bibliography for information on obtaining the scales.

RATING SCALES FOR GENERAL DISRUPTIVE BEHAVIORS

Overall, there are few DSM-based scales specifically developed to assess ODD and CD. Further, such available scales are primarily research scales and, although there is great potential for clinical application, they have not been integrated into clinical practice. However, there are several scales that assess more general disruptive behaviors that are appropriate to clinical practice. These scales have considerable utility, particularly when used in conjunction with broadband and diagnosis-based scales.

The revised *Eyberg Child Behavior Inventory* (ECBI) and *Sutter-Eyberg Student Behavior Inventory Revised* (SESBI-R) are both commonly used scales that assess general behavior problems in the home and classroom setting, respectively. Though they are not identical in content, there is considerable overlap and the scales use a comparable format, allowing users to evaluate youths' behavior across settings. The scales are not DSM-based, though there is considerable overlap with ADHD, ODD, and CD constructs. These scales describe a behavior problem and ask respondents to indicate (a) whether the behavior is problematic for their child, and (b) to rate the severity or frequency of the problem. Composite scores are derived for the number of behavior problems and the severity or frequency of behavior problems. The use of these two scales allows for some assessment of the respondent's threshold for behavior problems. For example, a teacher may respond that a behavior is problematic but occurs relatively infrequently, suggesting a low threshold and perhaps unrealistic expectations. Normative and psychometric data are available, and the scales have been used extensively in clinical populations. Although normative data are available through early adolescence, the content of these scales makes them most appropriate for toddlers through school-aged children. They are not likely to be as useful for assessing the severe conduct problems of adolescents.

The *Home and School Situations Questionnaires* (HSQ, SSQ) are unique observer-rated scales for younger children. They focus on the environmental context in which deviant behaviors occur, rather than emphasizing the frequency of behavior problems. The scales include common household or classroom situations and, like the ECBI and SESBI-R, ask respondents to indicate whether the child's behavior is problematic in that setting. For situations rated as problematic, respondents then rate their severity. These data are used to prioritize targets for intervention, evaluate situational precipitants, and assess problematic times of the day that may relate to interventions. Modifications of the HSQ and SSQ are available, including versions specific to ADHD-related symptoms and a form relevant for adolescents.

The HSQ and SSQ are sensitive to treatment gains made with medication and behavioral interventions. The normative data are somewhat outdated. Thus, the scales are most useful for understanding an individual youth's daily functioning and monitoring treatment response rather than comparing a youth with peers. Further, because they do not focus on a specific diagnosis or construct, the scales are best used as adjuncts to diagnosis-based or construct-driven scales.

NARROW-BAND SCALES ASSESSING INTERNALIZING SYMPTOMS

Internalizing symptoms are best assessed by youth themselves as they provide information on their subjective experience (see Table 2.4). Most of these scales also have parallel parent reports and/or teacher reports that broaden the understanding of youths' difficulties by providing an observer's perception of the youth when depressed or anxious. Comparison of youths' and caregivers' reports suggests that adults often fail to appreciate the level and quality of the youth's distress.

TABLE 2.4. SCALES ASSESSING INTERNALIZING SYMPTOMS

Scale	Reporter and Age of Youth	Publisher and Cost	Items	Time	Reliability	Validity
BDI	Adolescent/self Adolescents	Psychological Corporation $40 for manual	21 items	<10 min for full version 5 min for brief version	IC: moderate to excellent TR: fair to good IR: not reported	Adequate concurrent, convergent, and discriminant validity SENS/SPEC: 82%/53% (with cutoff of 11) SENS/SPEC: 100%/93% (with cutoff of 16)
CDI	Child/self, also parent and teacher versions 7–18 y/o	Multi-Health Systems $37 for manual	27 items	<20 min for full version 5 min for brief version	IC: fair to good TR: poor to very good IR: low	Adequate convergent and concurrent validity; variable discriminant validity
CES-D	Youth/self, also a parent version Adolescents Parent	Public domain	20 items	<20 min for full versions 5 min for brief versions	IC: moderate (CES-D); good (CES-DC) TR: moderate (CES-D & CES-DC) poor (CES-D & CES-DC)	At least moderate to good concurrent, convergent, and discriminant validity for CES-D; moderate concurrent but poor discriminant validity for CES-DC
CES-DC	Children and adolescents	Public domain			IC: excellent TR: good	
Reynolds ADS	Youth/self 13–18 y/o	Assessment Resources, Inc. $62 for manual	30 items	<20 min	IR: not reported	Adequate to good concurrent and convergent validity for both RADS and RCDS
Reynolds CDS	Child/self, also a parent version for children	Assessment Resources, Inc. $34 for manual	30 items	<20 min <20 min	IC: good TR: good IR: not reported	
MRS	Clinician administered Adolescents	Public domain	11 items	15 min to complete and score, but considerable time to gather information	IC: good TR: not reported IR: not reported	Adequate concurrent, convergent, discriminant, and divergent validity per preliminary research

(Continued)

TABLE 2.4. (CONTINUED)

Scale	Reporter and Age of Youth	Publisher and Cost	Items	Time	Reliability	Validity
MASC	Youth/self, also a parent version; Children and adolescents	Multi-Health Systems $37 for manual	39 items	<25 min for full version <10 min for brief version	IC: fair to excellent TR: fair to excellent IR: poor	At least adequate convergent, discriminant, and divergent validity
SPAI-C	Youth/self 9–14 y/o	Multi-Health Systems $37 for manual	26 items	<30 min	IC: excellent TR: fair to good IR: not reported	At least adequate concurrent, convergent, and divergent validity SENS: 83% (with cutoff of 18) SENS/SPEC: 70%/80% (with cutoff of 20)
CPTS-RI	Clinician administered or youth/self	Available through author	20 items	20–45 min	IC: fair to good for children	Adequate convergent validity Adequate concurrent, convergent, discriminant, predictive validity
Reynolds SIQ	Youth/self 14–18 y/o	Psychological Assessment Resources $34 for manual	30 items	<30 min	IC: excellent TR: moderate IR: not reported	Adequate concurrent, convergent, discriminant, predictive validity
SIQ-Jr.	Youth/self 11–13 y/o	Psychological Assessment Resources $47.79 for manual	15 items	30 min	IC: excellent TR: not reported IR: not reported	Adequate concurrent, convergent, discriminant, predictive validity SENS/SPEC: 80%/86%
CASPI	Youth/self Children and adolescents	Available through author	36 items	20 min	IC: moderate to excellent TR: fair to moderate IR: not reported	Adequate convergent and discriminant validity SENS/SPEC: 80%/65% for suicide attempts SENS/SPEC: 70%/65% for any suicidality
BHS	Youth/self Adolescents	Psychological Corporation $38 for manual	20 items	<15 min	IC: good TR: not reported	Some support for convergent and discriminant validity but not yet well established
HSC	Youth/self Children and adolescents	Available through author	17 items	<15 min	IC: moderate to excellent TR: low IR: not reported	Adequate concurrent and convergent validity; some support for discriminant validity but not well established

BDI, Beck depression inventory; CDI, Children's Depression Inventory; CES-D, Center for Epidemiologic Studies-depression Scale; CES-DC, CES-D scale modified for children; Reynolds ADS, Reynolds Adolescent Depression Scale; Reynolds CDS, Reynolds Child Depression Scale; MRS, Mania Rating Scale; MASC, Multidimensional Anxiety Scale for Children; SPAI-C, Social Phobia Anxiety Inventory for Children; CPTS-RI, Children's Post Traumatic Stress-reaction Index; SIQ, Suicide Ideation Questionnaire, for high school students; SIQ-Jr, Suicide Ideation Questionnaire, for middle school students; CASPI, Child-Adolescent Suicidal Potential Index; BHS, Beck Hopelessness Scale; HSC, Hopelessness Scale for Children; IC, internal consistency reliability; TR, test-retest reliability; IR, interrater reliability; SENS, sensitivity; SPEC, specificity.

See bibliography for information on obtaining the scales.

Several aspects of internalizing symptoms affect the functioning of these scales. A youth's feelings of depression, anxiety, or suicidality fluctuate over time. As a result, longer-term test-retest reliability is difficult to establish. Nonetheless, to detect meaningful changes in symptoms over the course of treatment, a scale with good short-term stability is needed. Another difficulty relates to the overlap of internalizing symptomatology. This makes it difficult to differentiate depressive and anxiety-related symptoms. In other words, the presence of anxiety will result in elevated scores on most depression-rating scales, and vice versa. Also, the short-term experience of depressed mood and anxiety is common, making it difficult to discern normal fluctuations in mood from clinically meaningful symptomatology. Therefore, it is important to consider a scale's discriminant and divergent validity when used for the assessment of these conditions.

Rating Scales Assessing Mood Symptoms

Depressive disorders in youth were elucidated in the 1980s when most depression-rating scales were developed. Few of them continue to be widely used. Their shortcomings relate to laxity in the construct that they tap, so these scales may be better measures of distress than depression. Also, depressive symptoms are common in both clinic-referred and community samples, so discriminating depressed youths in any setting can be a daunting task.

The *Beck Depression Inventory* (BDI) is the most popular depression-rating scale for adolescents with high utility in diverse applications across ethnicity and language. It assesses the same components of depression with adolescents that it assesses with adults: cognitive, behavioral, affective, and somatic. The BDI functions somewhat better with community than clinical samples. The BDI appears to show good discriminant validity, differentiating outpatient-depressed teens from those with anxiety and CDs. This makes it a preferred scale for augmenting diagnostic assessment. Decreasing scores as youth recover from depression also make the BDI useful for monitoring treatment. Cutoff scores vary with gender, clinical status, and ethnicity. Disadvantages relate to the lack of a parent- or teacher-report form.

The *Children's Depression Inventory* (CDI) is a downward extension of the BDI to preadolescents, although it is often used with teens as well. It is the most studied and popular scale of juvenile depression and has great utility. Five subscales are most often found: Dysphoric Mood, Acting Out, Loss of Personal and Social Interest, Self-Deprecation, and Vegetative Symptoms. The Acting Out subscale demonstrates how children's misbehaviors are related to their depressive cognitions. For adolescents these two issues appear independent. The utility of the subscales is unclear, and total scores are usually used. The CDI shows good predictive validity for future functioning and sensitivity to change during therapy. However, discriminant validity and diagnostic sensitivity and specificity are poor, and the CDI may really measure distress rather than depression. Nevertheless, its ongoing multiple and diverse applications attest to its usefulness. The rich literature on the CDI ensures that the potential user can find appropriate studies to evaluate its applicability to their intended application.

The *Center for Epidemiological Studies-Depression Scale* (CES-D) is a popular scale as it is in the public domain, and therefore included here. It consists of items selected from other scales assessing depression in adults and has been widely used with adolescents. It has also been modified for children and adolescents [Center for Epidemiological Studies-Depression Scale modified for children (CES-DC)]. Unfortunately, the overall psychometric functioning of the CES-D is only moderate for adolescents and poor for children. Also, neither the CES-D nor the CES-DC adequately discriminates depressed youths from other clinical samples, although this is a difficult task for any depression scale. These scales show poor sensitivity and specificity.

Overall, the CES-D and the CES-DC are appealing in their ready availability in the public domain, brevity, and format, along with some adequate psychometric properties for adolescents. However, the CES-DC does not appear suitable for children. The CES-D may be most useful in community samples as a first stage for screening or for monitoring treatment of individual youths, but not for comparing the progress of different youths. In any application, both the CES-D and CES-DC probably detect general psychopathology rather than depression.

The *Reynolds Adolescent Depression Scale* (**RADS**) and the *Reynolds Child Depression Scale* (**RCDS**) are two related scales based on DSM-III criteria for depression, thus facilitating construct validity and their discrimination of depression from distress. These scales function very well with diverse samples of ethnically heterogeneous community and clinical samples, although their main focus has been in the schools. They offer the opportunity to assess children and adolescents with similar but developmentally suitable scales, making them useful for longitudinal applications. They have found many applications assessing violence, affective disturbances, suicidality, and impairment.

One caveat is needed with the RADS and RCDS. Contemporary research and advancement in diagnostic criteria have made these scales somewhat outdated. Potential users should be aware that the RADS and RCDS construct of depression based on DSM-III is somewhat discordant with the DSM-IV construct or diagnostic criteria. Nonetheless, the DSM-IV construct of depression is sufficiently similar to the DSM-III construct so that this is not a prohibitive flaw in prioritizing the selection of a scale for assessing depression. Also, as the RADS and RCDS are the only depression-rating scales that have clear diagnostic constructs, it is important that clinicians have the option of such a scale. Finally, due to the paucity of well-established rating scales for depression, these scales appropriately continue to receive wide use.

The *Mania Rating Scale* (**MRS**) is a clinician-administered scale that assesses manic symptomatology in adults. There is preliminary evidence of its functioning with youth diagnosed with bipolar disorder including assessment of its factor structure. The MRS is completed by the clinician after interviewing a youth, his or her parents, and possibly staff or other caregivers who regularly interact with the youth. Thus, considerable time is expended in gathering information needed to rate this brief scale. It has shown some ability to discriminate bipolar disorder from ADHD and some divergent validity in relation to ADHD and depression. The MRS has also shown sensitivity to treatment with mood stabilizers. However, the MRS has not yet been adequately examined to establish its suitability with children or adolescents or its utility for clinical applications. Nonetheless, it is increasingly used with youths diagnosed with bipolar disorder and there is an increasing body of work regarding its functioning with youths.

Rating Scales Assessing Anxiety Symptoms

Anxiety was among the first juvenile symptoms evaluated with rating scales. Older, but still widely used, scales had questionable suitability and focused on trait versus state anxiety, a distinction that has not shown clinical relevance. Additionally, even transient anxiety in youths may produce elevated scores. Several newer anxiety-rating scales have overcome these difficulties. In particular, they have good stability and discriminant and divergent validity to aid in differentiating anxiety from other internalizing symptoms.

The *Multidimensional Anxiety Scale for Children* (**MASC**) assesses a spectrum of anxiety symptoms rather than a single anxiety construct. It was developed with youths from heterogeneous clinical and community settings. It has four major subscales, three of which can be subdivided: Physical Symptoms (Tense/Restless and Somatic/Autonomic), Social Anxiety (Humiliation/Rejection and Public Performance Fears), Harm Avoidance (Perfectionism and Anxious Coping), and Separation Anxiety. Two factors match the DSM-IV diagnoses of Social Phobia and Separation Anxiety Disorder, while the total score matches Generalized Anxiety Disorder. This is the first scale to validate the hypothesized division of anxiety into physical symptoms and approach-avoidance behaviors. Particular strengths include an inconsistency index that identifies invalid profiles due to random responding and an anxiety disorders index that discriminates anxious youths with 88% accuracy. There is also evidence of divergence from depression and from other anxiety disorders. The scale appears sensitive to treatment. Overall, the MASC has become the most popular, and perhaps the preferred, anxiety-rating scale.

The *Social Phobia and Anxiety Inventory for Children* (SPAI-C) differs from the other anxiety-rating scales in that it measures a specific construct of social anxiety over three subscales: Assertiveness, Traditional Social Encounters, and Public Performance. Its moderate validities support the SPAI-C's measurement of a construct that differs from general anxiety. This is one of few scales to discriminate among anxiety disorders. The SPAI-C classifies 67% of youths with social phobia and 74% with other anxiety disorders. Its sensitivity to treatment needs clarification, as it has detected benefits of medication but not psychotherapy. The SPAI-C has many uses with school and clinical samples. It is the scale most often used for socially anxious youth, although other scales have recently been developed.

The *Children's PTSD-Reaction Index* (CPTS-RI) is the most widely used measure of posttraumatic stress disorder (PTSD) symptoms for youths. It is a clinician-administered scale that can also be used as a self-report for youths over 8 years old. The items were based on DSM-III-R–defined PTSD with three subscales: Reexperiencing/Numbing, Fear/Anxiety, and Concentration/Sleep. This structure partially overlaps with the three DSM-IV factors of Reexperiencing, Arousal, and Avoidance. It functions well in relation to various types of trauma including bone marrow transplantation, sexual abuse, natural disasters, and war victimization across cultures. The CPTS-RI is a widely used measure of PTSD symptoms for children and adolescents. It is a clinician-administered scale that can be used as a self-report scale with youths over 8 years old. The items were based on an adult measure of PTSD derived from DSM-III. However, it deviates from DSM-III. The CPTS-RI items ask about a decrease in the enjoyment of activities, whereas DSM-III asks about a decrease in the amount of activities, for example, decrease in the enjoyment of sleep compared with decrease in the amount of sleep. Factor analysis of the CPTS-RI has revealed three factors, Reexperiencing/Numbing, Fear/Anxiety, and Concentration/Sleep, similar to the three DSM-IV factors of Reexperiencing, Arousal, and Avoidance. Sensitivity and specificity for a diagnosis of PTSD are moderate to good. It has also shown sensitivity to psychotherapy. The CPTS-RI is one of the best studied and most used scales for evaluating traumatized youth. However, the CPTS-RI does not measure all of the DSM-IV–defined PTSD symptoms and deviates somewhat from the DSM in its approach to symptoms. Finally, the overall utility is diminished by the costs associated with clinician administration, although a self-report format may obviate this disadvantage for older youths.

Rating Scales Assessing Suicidality and Hopelessness

The construct of suicidality ranges from ideation to completion. It is unclear whether youths with suicidal ideation, attempts, and completed suicides comprise distinct, overlapping, or identical samples. Furthermore, base rates for completed suicide are low.

Therefore, it is difficult to attain strong predictive validity with suicide scales. Given the potential consequences of failing to identify high-risk youths, the main goal of a screening scale is high sensitivity. This often results in scales that overidentify at-risk youths. Interestingly, despite increasing social awareness and concerns over youths' suicidality, few scales are available to assess this problem. More popular has been the use of scales assessing hopelessness, which demonstrate high correlation with suicidality and are often used in place of, or in addition to, suicide-rating scales.

The *Reynolds Suicide Scales* include the *Suicide Ideation Questionnaire* (SIQ) for high school and the *SIQ-Jr* for middle school students. Both scales measure the intensity and frequency of suicidal ideation. They form the screening stage in a 2-stage evaluation program. The second stage uses the *Suicidal Potential Interview* (SPI) to evaluate ideation endorsed on the SIQ/SIQ-Jr. The SPI begins with four questions regarding current emotional state, stressors, negative life events, and positive life aspects. The remaining questions pertain directly to suicidal thoughts, intent, plans, preparatory actions, and suicidal history. The sequential use of the SIQ/SIQ-Jr and the SPI comprises a model suicide prevention curriculum. One downside is length of the screening step and the need for a clinician to administer the SPI. Also, the SPI is not commercially available but must be obtained from its author. The scales function well in elucidating the relationship of suicidality to hopelessness, depression, and loss.

The *Child-Adolescent Suicidal Potential Index* (CASPI) is a newer scale that assesses risk for suicide. It covers multiple domains identified in past studies with the Child Suicide Potential Scales (CSPS), a comprehensive clinician interview that is more relevant to specialty clinics and research than to general office practice. However, the CASPI can be quickly completed in the office. The CASPI has three major subscales: Anxious-Impulsive Depression, Suicidal Ideation or Acts, and Family Distress. The Suicidal Ideation or Acts subscale best discriminates suicidal youths. It provides cutoff scores for both attempts and any suicidality. Possible concerns relate to the surprising lack of age and gender effects for the second subscale. Also, the "yes/no" scoring facilitates comprehension by children but may diminish sensitivity to treatment effects. The CASPI is new and requires further applications to establish its strengths and weaknesses. However, given the dearth of relevant scales, its use should be considered.

The *Beck Hopelessness Scale* (BHS) was developed for adults but has been widely used with adolescents. Hopelessness is correlated with depression but more powerfully predicts suicidal ideation and eventual suicide. Like suicidality, hopelessness measures a state, rather than trait, construct. The proposed subscales of the BHS have not been consistently reported with adolescents: Feelings about the Future, Loss of Motivation, and Future Expectations. The BHS discriminates suicidal from nonsuicidal adolescents and predicts serious suicide attempts independent of depression. However, its 2-point scoring and lack of stability data may obfuscate the detection of treatment effects in adolescents. Examination with the intended sample is recommended prior to routine use.

The *Hopelessness Scale for Children* (HSC) is a downward modification of the BHS, developed with inpatient children but widely used with adolescents. Hopelessness in children relates to a negative attributional style fostered through aversive development and correlates with depression and suicidality, but not with anxiety. The HSC functions better with children than with teens. It has been used with diverse samples and offers rich comparative data across psychiatric and medical applications to guide the potential user in determining whether the HSC is relevant to their intended application. High scores on the HSC along with high scores on scales measuring depression or distress should alert a clinician to serious risk for self-harm.

RATING SCALES ASSESSING FUNCTIONAL IMPAIRMENT

The term "functional impairment" refers to specific deficits in role performance across various domains of functioning, often developing in conjunction with a psychiatric disorder. The domains considered in functional assessment generally include cognitive level, verbal abilities, academic achievement, social interactions, capacity for self-care, and use of leisure time.

Functional impairment is often confused with severity of a disorder. However, severity of illness is a *characteristic of a disorder* that indicates the extent to which the disorder is manifested or its seriousness. Severity of illness may affect an individual's functioning and influence the types of interventions used. However, it does not explicitly identify the domains of life in which the individual struggles, areas that may be preserved, nor how the individual has adapted to the illness. By contrast, functional impairment is a *characteristic of the individual* that indicates in a more global way how the individual functions across life's roles.

Interest in measuring functional impairment has developed due to its relevance in determining "caseness." That is, symptomatology by itself does not define a psychiatric disorder. There must also be psychosocial dysfunction. This is why DSM-IV incorporates "Axis V," a measure of functional status. Functional impairment is also important to families, health care administrators, and policy makers who are interested in how well clinical interventions improve the quality of an individual's life. Furthermore, functional recovery often lags behind syndromal resolution. Thus, a measure of functional impairment helps to elucidate whether an individual is returning to premorbid levels of functioning. These scales will be of interest mostly to clinicians working in community clinics or with multidisciplinary health care professionals (see Table 2.5).

Scales assessing functional impairment vary with the population assessed and the purpose of measurement. For service utilization, a scale may be needed that quantifies specific impairments that determine the level of services the youth could receive, that is, outpatient services or more costly inpatient services. In clinical practice, a scale may be needed to determine youths' strengths and weaknesses in structuring interventions. Both global rating scales and multidimensional impairment scales have been developed for such measurements. All of these scales should be used as adjuncts to diagnosis-based or symptom-based rating scales.

Unidimional or Global Scales

Unidimensional, or global, scales synthesize a youth's functioning over many domains to describe overall impairment. A single score allows for comparison of functional impairment between groups of patients with different diagnoses as well as for ease of measuring functional change over time. However, global scales do not disentangle functioning from symptomatology and do not consider which domains should be targeted for intervention. Nevertheless, they are popular because of their ease of use and the intuitive appeal of a single score.

The *Children's Global Assessment Scale* (CGAS) is a clinician-rated scale that rates the youth's functioning based on data obtained during clinical assessment. Of course, the downside is that such data are generally geared toward symptomatology, not functioning. A nonclinician's CGAS that can be administered by lay persons has also been developed for epidemiologic research and possibly for other settings where clinician rating is not feasible.

The CGAS's stability makes it appropriate for monitoring interventions, and the good concordance between raters allows multiple raters to be used in different settings. Its validity, especially its discriminant validity, makes the CGAS appropriate for differentiating clinical from nonclinical subjects, psychiatric outpatients from inpatients, and for differentiating children at risk. Scores below 61 predict service utilization and thus may be considered a good clinical cutoff. Thus, the CGAS is appropriate for establishing "caseness," screening, and monitoring treatment.

TABLE 2.5. SCALES ASSESSING FUNCTIONAL IMPAIRMENT

Scale	Reporter and Age of Youth	Publisher and Cost	Items	Time	Reliability	Validity
CGAS	Clinician 4–16 y/o	Public domain	1 item	5 min	IC: NA TR: very good over short term and longer term IR: very good to excellent	Adequate convergent and discriminant validity; some support for predictive validity
CIS	Lay interview 10–17 y/o Lay interview with parent about child 7–9 y/o	Public domain	13 items	5 min	IC: very good for parent; moderate for youth TR: very good for parent; moderate for youth over short term IR: not reported	Adequate convergent and discriminant validity
VABS	Clinician administered to parent of youth Birth–18 y/o	American Guidance Service $155.99 for manual	297 items	20–60 min	IC: moderate to excellent; excellent for autism scales TR: moderate to excellent over short term IR: good to excellent overall	At least adequate convergent and discriminant validity
CAFAS	Clinician rating or parent interview 5–16 y/o	Functional Assessment Systems $19 for manual	164 items	<30 min	IC: moderate TR: good to excellent IR: moderate to excellent	Adequate convergent, discriminant, and predictive validity

CGAS, Children's Global Assessment Scale; CIS, Columbia Impairment Scale; VABS, Vineland Adaptive Behavior Scales; CAFAS, Child and Adolescent Functional Assessment Scale; IC, internal consistency reliability; TR, test-retest reliability; IR, interrater reliability.

See bibliography for information on obtaining the scales.

Further, information on its sensitivity and specificity would be helpful especially to further determine its screening abilities. The CGAS can easily be incorporated into office practice. However, caution is needed in using the CGAS with developmentally disabled youths, as it does not consider their limitations and may artificially classify them as in need of services.

The *Columbia Impairment Scale* (CIS) is a "respondent-based" global impairment scale that can be administered by a lay interviewer, definitely an advantage in an office practice. Respondent-based means that the interviewer does not make a clinical judgment but relies instead on patient responses to items. There are separate parent-report and adolescent-report versions that cover a youth's functioning in interpersonal relations, schoolwork or job, use of leisure time, and psychopathology.

The CIS has good stability but its sensitivity to change has not been established, making its utility for treatment monitoring unclear. However, both the parent and child versions of the CIS discriminate clinical samples of youths, making it useful for detecting differences between different groups of youths. Also, the CIS appears to perform better than standard checklists in detecting youth in need of mental health treatment, making it a good screening tool. Overall, the CIS has good utility for applications requiring a brief lay measure requiring little training and allowing comparison of parents' and youth's perceptions of a youth's functioning.

Multidimensional Scales

Multidimensional scales contain multiple subscales that describe different aspects of youths' functioning that may be impaired by mental illness. Each subscale, or domain, may only minimally overlap with the other subscales, depending on the specific instrument. Thus, low internal consistency reliability is typically found between these subscales and is not considered a flaw. The development of these scales underscores many issues relevant to understanding the effects of mental illness on youths' lives. For example, assessing *impairments* might inform clinicians about how mental illness leads to social disability. On the other hand, measuring *adjustment* to illness might elucidate areas that are more resilient and how to prevent handicap.

The *Vineland Adaptive Behavior Scales* (VABS) *Survey Form* comprises the prototypical multidimensional measure of youths' functioning. These scales have been extensively used with developmentally disabled youths. The VABS is completed as a semi-structured interview with caregivers. The interview follows a standardized administration though specialized training is not required. There is also a Classroom Edition for teachers. The VABS Survey Form addresses developmental skills in four domains: Daily Living Skills; Communication; Socialization; and for ages birth to 5 years old, Motor Skills. Each domain is broken down into smaller subscales. For example, in the communication domain, scores are derived for expressive, receptive, and written communication. Daily living skills are broken down into Personal, Domestic, and Community subscales. There is also an optional maladaptive behavior domain for ages 5 years and older only. Rather than administering all items, estimated starting points are provided by age, and basal and ceiling rules are used to ensure that a youth's abilities are adequately represented. The VABS has nationally representative and ethnically diverse normative data for youth from birth to 18 years old, as well as supplementary data for special clinical populations, such as autistic youths.

The VABS has been examined over many years with adequate psychometric properties and validity data, making it appropriate for most clinical applications. Parents' and teachers' agreement is better for the VABS than for other scales. The broad age-range is a strength, as it ensures adequate coverage for developmentally delayed youths. One of its most common applications is the assessment of functioning in conjunction with intelligence tests to establish "caseness" for youths in need of services or disability coverage. The VABS has longevity and is the standard measure of impairment for developmentally challenged youths.

The *Child and Adolescent Functional Assessment Scale* (CAFAS) is a clinician-administered interview that assesses impairment secondary to emotional, behavioral, or substance abuse problems. It consists of five subscales: Role Performance, Behavior Toward Self and Others, Thinking, Moods/Emotions, and Substance Abuse. The caregiver subscales include: Basic Needs and Family/Social Support. Each of the youths' five subscales contains specific behavioral descriptors to help determine severity level. These descriptors can then be used in treatment planning and monitored to provide evidence-based treatment and develop a dialogue with families about a youth's progress in different contexts. Although the scoring itself is brief, considerable clinical data must be gathered prior to scoring.

The suboptimal internal consistency among the subscales reflects their measuring different areas of functioning, the goal of such scales. More important is the evidence of adequate interrater reliability and stability over 1 week. The CAFAS' validity is evident in its ability to discriminate different levels of clinical severity. The CAFAS has also predicted service utilization, juvenile recidivism, legal involvement, and poor school attendance. It has shown sensitivity to treatment effects and serves as an efficient screening tool. The author provides training for potential users, and there is a website to update users on new information (www.cafas.com). The CAFAS is used by 30 states to determine eligibility for state-funded programs or for measuring programmatic outcomes.

Conclusions

The scales presented here do not substitute for diagnostic assessment and good clinical judgment. They do provide an idea of how the clinician can individualize an assessment battery to particular youths and clinical need. They offer the opportunity to better understand youths' difficulties, to quantify those difficulties in a manner that can be followed during treatment, and in the process to increase accountability in clinical practice.

Case Vignettes

Case vignette #1: Adolescent with internalizing symptoms

EJ is a 15-year-old girl who had separation anxiety in elementary school and continues to be somewhat timid and perfectionistic, though she has generally done well. However, in her freshman year of high school, EJ refused to attend school regularly. Her grades dropped in part due to missing school but also due to decreased concentration. She complained about several physical symptoms, which showed no organic etiology. She expressed lots of worry about her family and potential disasters. She was irritable and withdrawn from usual activities.

When interviewed, EJ endorsed a depressed and irritable mood but no suicidality. She endorsed considerable cognitive symptoms, such as initial insomnia due to "thinking too much" and "too many thoughts in my head." She jumped around a lot in describing her symptoms and seemed "pressured." However, she also expressed lots of self-doubt.

EJ met criteria for major depression but the other symptoms were perplexing. To understand her internalizing symptoms, several self-report scales were administered. The

BDI showed a high score, probably indicating her depression and distress. Additionally, due to her seeming "pressured," there was a concern about mania, and the MRS was administered. The score was within normal limits. Due to her earlier separation anxiety, lifelong timidity, and perfectionism, the clinician then decided to focus on an anxiety disorder. EJ completed the MASC. She showed severely elevated scores on the subscales of Physical Symptoms (Tense/Restless and Somatic/Autonomic) and Harm Avoidance (Perfectionism and Anxious Coping), but lower scores on Separation Anxiety and Social Anxiety (Public Performance Fears and Humiliation/Rejection). Also, the total score of the MASC was high, consistent with generalized anxiety disorder. Further discussion with EJ revealed that her anxiety had long preceded the depression. Her physician started selective serotonin reuptake inhibitors (SSRI) medication at low dose so as not to exacerbate her anxiety. Also, to facilitate her getting back to school quickly he started a 2-month trial of low dose clonazepam. She also started psychotherapy. BDI and MASC scores were followed every other week while in treatment. Over the next 6 months, her depression and anxiety symptoms resolved and ratings on the BDI and MASC normalized.

Case vignette #2: Prepubertal child with externalizing behaviors

JT was a 9-year-old boy who had struggled academically and socially but maintained adequate grades and social skills at a private school, largely through intensive parental involvement. Then in the fourth grade, due to his parents' separation, he moved to a public school and started to fall behind academically and to develop social difficulties. The teacher spoke with his mother who noted oppositional and defiant behaviors at home. The teacher and mother decided to ask the pediatrician about ADHD and possibly medication. After an initial evaluation, the pediatrician asked the teacher to complete the TRF and the mother to complete the CBCL. Both scales noted difficulties in attention/concentration as well as hyperactivity. However, the teacher's TRF also noted an elevated Internalizing Scale, and the mother's CBCL indicated an elevated Aggression Subscale that indicates opposition and defiance. JT had a mixed profile with both externalizing and internalizing problems. To better sort this out, the pediatrician had the teacher and mother complete the CRS-R, which corroborated his initial diagnosis of ADHD. As JT seemed so unhappy, he also completed the CDI. Results suggested that JT was depressed. Further history with JT confirmed the diagnosis of dysthymic disorder.

The pediatrician initially treated the ADHD symptoms with a stimulant medication and monitored JT's ADHD symptoms with monthly ratings on the abbreviated CRS-R. He did better but seemed to still struggle throughout the day. The pediatrician then had the mother complete the HSQ and the teacher complete the SSQ. These scales indicated that JT had problems in transitioning from one setting or one activity to another. Therefore, the pediatrician had the teacher and parents develop a behavior plan for helping JT through daily transitions.

However, over the next month, even as his academic and social behaviors improved, JT's mood still seemed low. He was clearly distraught about his parents' separation. The pediatrician knew that antidepressant medications are not so useful for childhood depression. Therefore, he referred JT for counseling. The counselor completed the CAFAS due to concerns about the family's overall needs. Results indicated that the mother needed help, as she was depressed. Therefore, the mother was enrolled in therapy and was started on an antidepressant. Over the next 8 months, the counselor monitored JT's depressive symptoms with monthly CDIs. His distress gradually improved, he was promoted to the fifth grade, and he completed summer camp.

BIBLIOGRAPHY

Collett BR, Ohan JL, Myers KM. Ten-year review of rating scales. V: scales assessing attention-deficit hyperactivity disorder. *J Am Acad Child Adolesc Psychiatry* 2003a;42:1015–1037.

Collett BR, Ohan JL, Myers KM. Ten-year review of rating scales. VI: scales assessing externalizing behaviors. *J Am Acad Child Adolesc Psychiatry* 2003b;42:1143–1170.

Kazdin AE. *Research design in clinical psychology*, 3rd ed. Boston, MA: Allyn and Bacon, 1998:245–302.

Myers K, Winters NC. Ten-year review of rating scales. I: Overview of scale functioning, psychometric properties, and selection. *J Am Acad Child Adolesc Psychiatry* 2002a;41:114–122.

Myers K, Winters NC. Ten-year review of rating scales. II: Scales for internalizing disorders. *J Am Acad Child Adolesc Psychiatry* 2002b;41:634–659.

Ohan JL, Myers K, Collett BR. Ten-year review of rating scales. IV: Scales assessing trauma and its effects. *J Am Acad Child Adolesc Psychiatry* 2002;41:1401–1422.

Winters NC, Myers K, Proud L. Ten-year review of rating scales. III: Scales for suicidality, cognitive style, and self-esteem. *J Am Acad Child Adolesc Psychiatry* 2002;41:1150–1181.

Winters NC, Collett BR, Myers K. Ten-year review of rating scales. VII: Scales assessing functional impairment. *J Am Acad Child Adolesc Psychiatry (in press)*.

SUGGESTED READINGS

American Psychiatric Association. *Handbook of psychiatric measures*. Washington, DC: American Psychiatric Press, 2000.
(For clinicians interested in detailed knowledge about rating scales. This text also includes a CD-ROM so that the scales can be downloaded and printed out.)

American Academy of Child and Adolescent Psychiatry. *Practice parameters of the American academy of child and adolescent psychiatry.*
(For clinicians seeking guidelines for the evaluation and treatment of psychiatric disorders in youth.

Multiple practice parameters are now available. They are periodically summarized in a supplement to the Journal of the American Academy of Child and Adolescent Psychiatry, also available at www.aacap.org.)

Sajatovic M, Ramirez L. *Rating scales in mental health*, 2nd ed. Los Angeles, CA: Lexi Comp, 2003.
(Reviews over 100 scales; ideal for clinicians as well as administrators seeking to incorporate more evidenced-based practice into their work.)

OBTAINING THE SCALES *(in order of presentation in text)*

Child Behavior Checklist (CBCL)/ Teacher Report Form (TRF)/Youth Self Report (YSR)

Achenbach TM, Rescorla LA (2000), *Manual for the ASEBA school-age forms & profiles*. University of Vermont, Research Center for Children, Youth, and Families, Burlington, VT. Available from: Achenbach System of Empirically Based Assessment (ASEBA), Room 6436, 1 South Prospect Street, Burlington, VT 05401-3456, 1-802-656-8313 or 1-802-656-2608; www.aseba.org.

Child Behavior Checklist 1¹/₂–5 years old (CBCL 1¹/₂–5) / Caregiver-Teacher Report Form (C-TRF)

Achenbach TM, Rescorla LA (2001), *Manual for the ASEBA preschool forms & profiles*. University of Vermont, Research Center for Children, Youth, and Families, Burlington, VT. Available from Achenbach System of Empirically Based Assessment (ASEBA), Room 6436, 1 South Prospect Street, Burlington, VT 05401-3456, 1-802-656-8313 or 1-802-656-2608; www.aseba.org.

Conners Rating Scales-Revised (CRS-R)

Conners C(1997), *Conners' rating scales-revised technical manual*. Multi-Health Systems, 908 Niagara Falls Blvd., North Tonawanda, NY 14120-2060; 1-800-456-3003; www.mhs.com.

Swanson, Nolan, and Pelham-IV Questionnaire (SNAP-IV)

Swanson J, Schuck S, Mann M, et al. (2001b), Categorical and dimensional definitions and evaluations of symptoms of ADHD: the SNAP and SWAN ratings scales. Available at http://www.adhd.net. Accessed February 16, 2005.

Eyberg Child Behavior Inventory (ECBI) and Sutter-Eyberg Student Behavior Inventory Revised (SESBI-R)

Eyberg SM, Pincus D (1999), *Eyeberg child behavior inventory and Sutter-Eyberg student behavior inventory-revised, professional manual*. Psychological Assessment Resources, 16204 N. Florida Avenue, Lutz, FL 33549, 1-813-968-3003; 1-800-331-8378; www.parinc.com.

Home Situations Questionnaire (HSQ) and School Situations Questionnaire (SSQ)

Barkley RA (1997), *Defiant children: a clinician's manual for assessment and parent training*, 2nd ed. Guilford Press, 72 Spring St., New York 10012; 1-800-365-7006; 1-212-431-9800; www.info@guilford.com.

The Beck Depression Inventory (BDI)

Beck A, Steer RA (1993), *Beck depression inventory (BDI) manual*, 2nd ed. Psychological Corporation, 555 Academic Court, San Antonio, TX 78204-2498; 1-800-211-8378; www.psychcorp.com.

Children's Depression Inventory (CDI)

Kovacs M (1992), *Children's depression inventory manual*. Multi-Health Systems, 908 Niagara Falls Blvd., North Tonawanda, NY 14120-2060; 1-800-456-3003; www.mhs.com.

Center for Epidemiologic Studies-Depression Scale (CES-D)

Radloff LS (1977), The CES-D Scale: a self-report depression scale for research in the general population. *Applied Psychol Meas* 1:385–401. Currently available from: National Institutes of Health, Epidemiology Branch, 5600 Fishers Lane, Rockville MD 20857.

Also available in: Radloff LS, Locke BZ (2000), Center for epidemiologic studies depression scale (CES-D). In: American Psychiatric Association, eds. *Handbook of psychiatric measures*. American Psychiatric Association, Washington, DC, Chapter 24, Mood Disorders Measures, 523–526.

The Reynolds Depression Scales

Reynolds WM (1987), *Reynolds adolescent depression scale (RADS) and Reynolds child depression scale (RCDS)*. Psychological Assessment Resources, 16204 N. Florida Avenue, Lutz, FL 33549, 1-813-968-3003; www.parinc.com.

Young Mania Rating Scale (Y-MRS)

Young RC, Biggs JT, Ziegler VE, et al. (1978), A rating scale for mania: Reliability, validity and sensitivity. *Br J Psychiatry* 133:429–435.

Also available in: Young RC, Biggs JT, Ziegler VE, et al. (2000), Young mania rating scale (YMRS). In: American Psychiatric Association, eds. *Handbook of psychiatric measures*. American Psychiatric Association, Washington, DC, Chapter 24, Mood Disorders Measures, 540–542.

Manual for the Multidimensional Anxiety Scale for Children (MASC)

March JS (1997), *Manual for the multidimensional anxiety scale for children (MASC)*. Multi-Health Systems, 908 Niagara Falls Blvd., North Tonawanda, NY 14120-2060; 1-800-456-3003; www.mhs.com.

Social Phobia and Anxiety Inventory for Children (SPAI-C)

Beidel DC, Turner SM, Morris TL (1988), *Social phobia and anxiety inventory for children (SPAIC-C)*. Multi-Health Systems, 908 Niagara Falls Blvd, North Tonawanda, NY 14120-2060; 1-800-456-3003; www.mhs.com.

The Child Post Traumatic Stress-Reaction Index (CPTS-RI)

Pynoos RS (2002), *The child post traumatic stress-reaction index (CPTS-RI)*. Available from: Robert Pynoos, MD, Trauma Psychiatry Service, UCLA, 300 UCLA Medical Plaza, Los Angeles, CA 90024-6968; rpynoos@npih.medsch.ucla.edu.

The Reynolds Suicide Scales

Reynolds CR (1987), *Suicidal ideation questionnaire (SIQ): professional manual*. Psychological Assessment Resources, 16204 N. Florida Avenue, Lutz, FL 33549, 1-813-968-3003; www.parinc.com.

Child and Adolescent Suicide Potential Index (CASPI)

Pfeffer CR (2002), *Child and adolescent suicide potential index (CASPI)*. Available from: Cynthia R Pfeffer, MD, Cornell University, Department of Psychiatry, 21 Bloomingdate Rd, White Plains, NY 10605-1596; cpfeffer@med.cornell.edu.

The Beck Hopelessness Scale (BHS)

Beck A (1993), *Beck hopelessness scale (BHS) manual*. Psychological Corporation, 555 Academic Court, San Antonio, TX 78204-2498; 1-800-211-8378; www.psychcorp.com.

The Hopelessness Scale for Children

Kazdin AE (2003), *The hopelessness scale for children (HSC)*. Available from the author: Alan Kazdin, PhD, Yale University, 1-203-432-9993; Alan.Kazdin@yale.edu.

The Children's Global Assessment Scale (CGAS)

Bird HR (1999), The assessment of functional impairment. In: Shaffer D, Lucas CP, Richters JE, eds. *Diagnostic assessment in child and adolescent psychopathology*. New York: Guilford Press, 209–229.

Also available from the author: David ShafferMD, Department of Child Psychiatry, College of Physicians and Surgeons, Columbia University, 1051 Riverside Dr., New York, NY 10032.

Also in: Shaffer D, Gould MS, Bird H, et al. (2000), Children's global assessment scale (CGAS). In: American Psychiatric Association, eds. *Handbook of psychiatric measures*. American Psychiatric Association, Washington, DC, Chapter 19, Child and Adolescent Measures of Functional Status, 363–365.

The Columbia Impairment Scale (CIS)

Bird HR (1999), The assessment of functional impairment. In: Shaffer D, Lucas CP, Richters JE, eds. *Diagnostic assessment in child and adolescent psychopathology*. New York: Guilford Press, 209–229.

Also available from the author: Hector R, Bird MD, Division of Child Psychiatry, NY State Psychiatric Institute, Unit 78, 1051 Riverside Dr., New York, NY 10032; Tel: (212) 543-5191; Fax: (212) 543-5730.

Also available in: Bird HR (2000), Columbia impairment scale (CIS). In: American Psychiatric Association, eds. *Handbook of psychiatric measures.* American Psychiatric Association, Washington, DC, Chapter 19, Child and Adolescent Measures of Functional Status, 367–369.

Vineland Adaptive Behavior Scales: Interview Edition Survey Form Manual

Sparrow SS, Balla DA, Cicchetti DV (1984), *Interview edition survey form manual: Vineland adaptive behavior scales.* American Guidance Service, Circle Pines, MN, AGS Publishing, 4201 Woodland Road, Circle Pines, MN 55014-1796; Tel: 1-800-328-2560; Fax: (651) 287-7220 or 1-800-471-8457; customerservice@agsnet.com.

The Child and Adolescent Functional Assessment Scale (CAFAS)

Hodges K (1994), *The child and adolescent functional assessment scale (CAFAS), self training manual.* Eastern Michigan University, Department of Psychology, Ypsilanti, MI. To obtain: Kay Hodges PhD, Functional Assessment Systems, LLC, 2140 Old Earhart Rd, Ann Arbor, MI 48105; Tel: (734) 769-9725; Fax: (734) 769-1434; Hodges@provide.net; www.cafas.com.

Also available in: Hodges K (2000), Child and adolescent functional assessment scale (CAFAS). In: American Psychiatric Association, eds. *Handbook of psychiatric measures.* American Psychiatric Association, Washington, DC, Chapter 19, Child and Adolescent Measures of Functional Status, 365–367.

CHAPTER 3

Psychological Assessment

NORMAN H. REED

Introduction

The benefits of using psychological assessments in psychiatric and primary care settings are substantial. Information collected from different settings using multiple methods provides a better clinical picture and can lead to improved diagnosis and treatment planning. The opposite is also true. In a review of the literature by Perry in 1992, reliance on a single method of assessment (e.g., semistructured interview) by a single clinician yielded a 70% error rate in personality diagnoses when compared to a complex assessment process.

However, in the current health care climate, managed health care organizations are hesitant to allow physicians to refer patients for in-depth or comprehensive assessments, preferring simple, single method ratings with quick turnaround and a superficial survey of symptoms. As a result, clinical planning decisions often rely on unstructured interviews and informal observations obtained over a short period of time, and subsequent treatment plans may not address the complexity of a patient's needs. While an interview with the patient and family is a good place to start information collection, children, adolescents, and their parents can be poor historians or biased informants. For example, the patient's agenda when presenting at an evaluation may be to obtain medication, prove there are no problems, or affix blame on certain individuals or circumstances. A further source of error can be the context of the interview, often leading to denial or exaggeration of presenting problems. For example, a youth may believe that the outcome of treatment will be that he/she is required to take medication for the rest of his/her life and therefore admits to no symptoms during the interview.

Effective treatment requires that errors in assessment and diagnosis be minimized. Appropriate use of psychological assessment can minimize diagnostic errors and provide a sound basis for subsequent treatment planning.

When Assessment Is Useful

Psychological assessment improves the accuracy and reliability of diagnosis and treatment planning. Despite the added cost and time required for the use of psychological assessments, many patients ultimately benefit from fewer false starts at treatment and avoidance of inappropriate interventions. Not every patient requires psychological assessment. Psychological consultations are indicated when patients present with an unclear diagnosis or with complex, multidimensional problems. Other patients who can benefit from psychological assessments are those who have been unresponsive to past treatments, dissatisfied with previous mental health treatment, difficult to engage in treatment, or suspected of secondary gains or symptoms. Finally, as noted in Table 3.1, psychological assessment is useful when liability risk appears high and when patients seek certain medications or medical treatments that are of questionable benefit.

Testing Versus Assessment

It is important to distinguish between psychological testing and psychological assessment. A *psychological test* is a systematic procedure for measuring a relatively narrow dimension of behavior. Systematic procedure means that the tests are designed to be consistently administered, thereby minimizing measurement error related to situational variables, clinician error, and clinician–patient interaction. Psychological tests also allow

---

TABLE 3.1. COMMON INDICATIONS FOR PSYCHOLOGICAL ASSESSMENT

- Difficult to engage patients/families
- Histories are biased or unreliable
- Suspicions of secondary gain
- Presence of complex and/or multiple presenting problems
- Poor responsiveness to multiple treatment interventions
- Questions about risk of harm to self or others
- Being faced with litigious family/youth situations

for incorporation of developmental and normative descriptions. For example, the score on an Attention Deficit Hyperactivity Disorder (ADHD) or Depression-rating scale can be compared to a large group of individual scores previously collected and studied and judged to be high, average, or low for the age group represented by the patient. Some tests provide critical "cutoff" scores suggesting the significant presence of the construct that the test measures.

A correctly developed psychological test relies on empirically quantified information, standardized administration, and construct validity. However, many tests use only one type of evaluation, such as self-reports, observer ratings, or performance tasks, which can yield single method bias and may only measure a single diagnostic construct. Again, using the simple ADHD or Depression symptom checklist as an example, raters assign a level of disorder or quantity score to each symptom or behavior about themselves or someone else. In the case of patients self-reporting, they may have little self-awareness, be seeking certain treatments, exhibit intense denial or resistance, or have exaggerated symptoms in the narrow situational context of a single test. Clinicians may have known their patients for only a short time, view them in limited settings, such as in physical education or academic classes or at youth group outings, or have a biased preconceived view that influences their observations. In addition, these simple tests often do not measure sufficient domains of behaviors to differentiate between various diagnostic subtleties. For example, when inattention is rated high on an ADHD rating scale, this may also represent the attention problems that afflict depressed or anxious children.

Psychological assessment uses a number of scores obtained through multiple methods and tests and combines the data in the context of historic and referral information, interview data, and behavior observations in order to generate a cohesive and comprehensive understanding of the patient. Psychological assessment examines multiple test scores from a battery of tests in the context of current situational circumstances, developmental history, and family social system factors. In Case Vignette #1, the high score obtained on a self-report ADHD scale would be compared to the low scores obtained from teachers, the high anxiety scores on a performance test, the history of average school performance, the recent episode of sexual abuse by a peer at school, and information that a parent has recently dropped out of treatment for methamphetamine abuse. The experienced psychologist can take multiple sources of information and develop an accurate description of the patient's diagnosis as well as a more precise and relevant treatment plan.

While the formal psychological assessment process can provide a more reliable and accurate clinical picture than reliance on a single clinician using a single method (i.e., an interview), this process cannot be completed by a minimally trained clinician. Psychological assessment requires an extensive knowledge of psychopathology, personality, psychological measurement, research methods, and assessment methods to integrate information with complex history, situational context, and developmental information.

The Standards for Educational and Psychological Testing suggest that publishers of psychological tests use competency-based qualification guidelines in determining who can purchase and administer various tests. This is to ensure ethical test use and appropriate interpretation of test results. Publishers assign each test one of several qualification levels. Reputable suppliers request credentials when selling these tests. Psychological Assessment Resources, Inc. uses the following qualification guidelines:

- Qualification level A indicates no special qualifications are required.
- Qualification level B indicates a degree from an accredited 4-year college in psychology or related field plus satisfactory completion of coursework in testing.
- Qualification C indicates all qualifications for Level B plus an advanced professional degree that provides appropriate training in the administration and interpretation of

psychological tests or a license from an agency that requires training and experience in ethical and competent use of psychological tests.

- Qualification level S requires a degree or license to practice in a health care profession or occupation including the following: clinical psychology, medicine, neurology, neuropsychology, nursing, occupational therapy, and other allied health care professions, physicians' assistants, psychiatry, school psychology, social work, speech-language pathology, plus appropriate training and experience in the ethical administration, scoring, and interpretation of clinical behavior assessment instruments.

Common Tests Used with Children and Adolescents

There are numerous psychological tests used to assess children and adolescents. These tests differ based on content and method of measurement. The various types illustrated here and most likely utilized in a good assessment include the following: achievement, behavioral problems, adaptive behavior, intelligence, personality self-report, personality projective, neuropsychological, and parenting/family.

The purpose of *achievement testing* is to measure an individual's development, strengths, and weaknesses in various areas of learning such as written expression, reading, spelling, math, nonverbal reasoning, language skills, or expressive and receptive vocabulary. Often, a child has behavioral problems in school or with peers due to learning and processing problems. These tests help to identify learning disabilities in academic content areas that require special focus.

The purpose of *behavioral problem ratings* is to get a concrete description of functioning across various living environments or settings, such as school, home, day care, and restaurants. Scales with a broad sampling of behavioral items are more useful than narrow samples. Scales that use ratings from various individuals in the patient's life (such as teacher, parent, friend, sibling, or self) are far more useful than single rater forms. Some tests group responses into different scales, such as aggression, level of isolation, externalizing behavior, or internalizing behavior. These are most useful to determine what behaviors are most excessive, in which environments they are most excessive, and whether the behavior is excessive for age.

Adaptive behavior techniques usually consist of semistructured interview formats. Adaptive behavior skills are important for personal responsibility, self-care, daily living, social functioning, and independent living. This is an important measurement in assessing for developmental disabilities. In developmentally disabled youth with normal intelligence quotients, the use of an adaptive behavior instrument is required to determine eligibility for disability services through most county and state funding agencies.

Intelligence testing measures performance on a number of verbal and nonverbal tasks. These tasks represent certain abilities, including the ability to learn or understand from experience, the ability to retain knowledge, reasoning ability, the ability to respond to new situations, and the ability to direct behavior. School settings use intelligence tests to help determine placement, handicapping conditions, or appropriate modalities of treatment. For example, a highly verbal reasoning type of therapy is inappropriate for a child with low verbal skills.

Personality tests measure the way in which a person may typically respond emotionally, cognitively, and behaviorally in various situations. These tests often measure manifest symptoms as well as coping mechanisms, defenses, affect, perception of reality, thinking processes, ego functioning, conflicts, drives, motivators, and level of distress. Personality tests are broken into two methods of measurement: self-report scales and projective techniques. Self-reports usually require a true or false response to a number of statements or a selection from a short continuum ranging from "no, never" to "all the time." Projective tests involve the presentation of ambiguous stimuli in order to measure how personality influences the way in which the individuals perceive, organize, and interpret their environment and experiences. Personality tests are often used to establish differential diagnosis, treatment plans, and risk assessment.

Neuropsychological testing is concerned with the measurement of brain-behavior relations. This type of assessment examines areas of learning, information processing, planning, sensory-motor functioning, perceptions, memory, executive functioning, attention, and personality changes. Neuropsychological testing is most useful when clinicians suspect that damage to the brain is interfering with a youth's performance and adaptive functioning.

Parent/Family types of tests are used to describe parent–child relationships, family functioning, stressful areas of parent–child interactions, strength of the child-rearing alliance between parents, and parenting skills. These tests identify context issues affecting a youth's symptom presentation.

Examples of the actual tests most commonly used by psychologists for the assessment of child and adolescent disorders are presented in Table 3.2 by type of test, appropriate age ranges, and where the test can be purchased.

When to Refer

Psychological assessment can be used for a number of purposes. Referrals can be made for issues pertaining to description of current functioning, confirmation or refutation of clinical impressions, differential diagnosis, identification of treatment needs and appropriate treatment interventions, predictions of outcome, monitoring treatment over time, and risk management.

When making referrals for psychological assessment, it is important to be specific about the goal of the assessment. Often, specific tests are requested without reference to the goal of the assessment or how the information will be used. A preferable method of referral makes clear the questions being asked by the referring clinician, family, patient, or agency so that the psychologist picks the appropriate methods given the situational and personal characteristics of the child. Some typical questions to pose to the testing psychologist include: "Is the child suffering from depression or is there some other difficulty present?" "What seems to be the meaning of the child's poor attention or restlessness?" "What is behind the youth's aggression?" "Is there some way to effectively treat his/her aggression?" "Does the child exhibit any suicidal or homicidal risk?" Other typical questions are summarized in Table 3.3.

Once the referral is made, the psychologist will select the battery of tests most useful to answer the referral questions. The psychologist will develop a battery that uses multiple sources or samples of information gathered with multiple methods. A common battery for children or youths will include historic information, baseline observations gathered over multiple sites (i.e., home and school) with multiple raters (i.e., parents, teachers, or self), interview data, self-report data, projective testing, and intelligence/achievement measures. When selecting a battery, patient characteristics such as age, ethnicity, ability to read, language disabilities, and physical disabilities are taken into consideration. Issues such as prior testing history, time constraints, and who will have access to the results (i.e., estranged parents, juvenile court, insurance companies, etc.) are also taken into consideration.

TABLE 3.2. COMMONLY USED TESTS FOR THE ASSESSMENT OF CHILDREN AND YOUTH

Test Category	Test Name	Test Age Range	Supplier
Intelligence	Stanford-Binet	Ages 2 to 23 yr	a
	Wechsler Preschool and Primary Scale of Intelligence III	Ages 2:6 to 7:3 yr	b
	WISC IV	Ages 6 to 16:11 yr	b
	WASI	Ages 6 to 89 yr	b
	K-ABC-II	Ages 2:5 to 12:5 yr	c
	Test of Nonverbal Intelligence	Ages 6 to 85 yr	c
Achievement	KTEA	Ages 4:6 to 90 yr	d
	WIAT	Ages 4 to 85 yr	b
	Wide Range Achievement Test	Ages 5 to 85 yr	b,c
Adaptive	AAMR	Ages 3 to 21 yr	c
	Adaptive Behavior Assessment System-II	Ages 0 to 89 yr	b
	Vineland Adaptive Behavior Scales-II	Ages 0 to 18:11 yr	d
Behavior problems	BASC-2	Ages 2:6 to 18:11 yr	d
	Achenbach System of Empirically Based Assessment	Ages 1:5 to 59 yr	e
Personality— self-report	Jesness Inventory Revised	Ages 8 yr and older	f
	MMPI	Ages 14 yr and older	g
	Personality Inventory for Youth	Ages 9 to 19 yr	b,c
	Millon Adolescent Clinical Inventory	Ages 13 to 19 yr	g
	Trauma Symptom Checklist for Children	Ages 8 to 16 yr	b,c
Projective	Rorschach	Ages 5 yr and older	b,c,g
	Thematic Apperception Test	Ages 4 yr and older	b,c,g
Neuropsychological tests	NEPSY	Ages 3 to 12 yr	b,c
	WRAML 2	Ages 5 to 90 yr	b,c
Memory	Rey-Osterrieth Complex Figure Test	Ages 5 to 94 yr	c
	Wisconsin Card Sorting Test	Ages 6:5 to 89 yr	c
Parenting/family	Family Assessment Measure	Ages 10 yr to adult	c
	Parenting Stress Index	Parents–child, 0 to 12 yr	b,c
	Parenting Satisfaction Scale	Parents of elementary child	b

WISC, Wechsler Intelligence Scale for Children; WASI, Wechsler Abbreviated Scale of Intelligence; K-ABC-II, Kaufman Assessment Battery for Children, second edition; KTEA, Kaufman Test of Educational Achievement; WIAT, Wechsler Individual Achievement Test II; AAMR, Adaptive Behavior Scale; BASC-2, Behavior Assessment System for Children, second edition; MMPI, Minnesota Multiphasic Personality Inventory; NEPSY, A Developmental Neuropsychological Assessment; WRAML 2, Wide Range Assessment of Memory and Learning, second edition.

Suppliers

(a) Riverside Publishing Company, www.riverpub.com
(b) PsychCorp, www.harcourtassessment.com
(c) Psychological Assessment Resources, www.parinc.com
(d) AGS Publishing, www.agsnet.com
(e) ASEBA Research Center, www.ASEBA.org
(f) Multi Health Systems, www.mhs.com
(g) Pearson Assessments, www.pearsonassessments.com

Psychological Reports

Results from a psychological assessment are often written out in the form of a report rather than only being reported as specific test scores. These reports, along with the actual testing data, are considered confidential, and the psychologist is ethically bound to maintain the confidentiality of their patients. Confidentiality rules vary according to the individual state and should be similar to those followed for any medical record document.

Reports can vary greatly depending on the psychologist's training and the referral question, but primary components of a good report share basic components as shown in Table 3.4. Psychological assessment reports usually include the presenting problem, relevant background

TABLE 3.3. EXAMPLES OF REFERRAL QUESTIONS FOR PSYCHOLOGICAL ASSESSMENT

- Does this child qualify for a handicapping condition and special education services?
- Does this child qualify for MRDD services?
- Does this child's attention problem suggest ADHD, juvenile mania, or an anxiety disorder?
- Does this child's impulsivity and attention problems relate to a brain injury?
- Are this child's behavior problems related to trauma?
- Is this child a dangerous sex offender?
- Should this child be placed in 24-h care for the safety of others?
- Does this child's complaints of hearing voices in the absence of other psychotic symptoms represent the development of a thought disorder?
- Is this child's aggression and irritability related to depression or conduct problems?
- Is this child a homicidal or suicidal risk?

MRDD, mental retardation/developmental disorders; ADHD, attention deficit hyperactivity disorder.

information, interview information with the youth and parents, testing results, a formulation or summary of data collected, and recommendations or answers to the referral questions. The psychologist will go over these results and conclusions with the youth (if age appropriate) and his or her parents. Turnaround time of the report depends on many factors, including the availability of the patient, difficulty in testing the patient, difficulty of the referral questions, and workload of the clinician. However, a 1- to 2-week turnaround for more extensive assessment protocols is a guideline to utilize. Forensic assessments are often more time consuming and require more data gathering, making for a longer turnaround time.

Conclusions

Psychological assessment provides a valuable adjunct to optimize the evaluation and treatment planning of youths with mental health and developmental problems. A variety of clinical problems can be addressed ranging from the broad evaluation of symptoms and behaviors, to in-depth assessment of a specific symptom, to elucidation of broad constructs such as intelligence and personality. Psychological assessment offers such evaluation in a comprehensive yet efficient testing battery. While psychological assessment is often thought to increase the cost of mental health evaluation and treatment, it may instead ensure that the most appropriate treatment is implemented in the most timely manner. Clinicians seeking to integrate psychological assessment into their evaluation and treatment will profit from collaborating with a few psychologists whose work they can get to know well. In that manner, referring clinicians can best hone their referral questions and the psychologists can best hone their feedback so that the referral process ensures the best clinical service for young patients.

TABLE 3.4. ESSENTIAL COMPONENTS OF A CHILD AND ADOLESCENT PSYCHOLOGICAL ASSESSMENT REPORT

- Specific referral question
- List of specific data gathering techniques
- Relevant background history
- Interview with significant adults in child's or adolescent's life (parents, teachers, other family)
- Interview with child or adolescent
- Behavioral rating scales collected from multiple environments and multiple observers
- Testing—varied depending on question to address but usually covers multiple domains
- Summary of data or formulation of results
- Diagnostic impression if requested
- Recommendations or conclusions addressing specific referral questions

Case Vignettes

Case vignette #1

A pediatrician was presented with a 9-year-old girl and ADHD behavior rating scales completed by school staff and parents. Ratings yielded noteworthy scores for the inattentiveness, hyperactivity, and other ADHD behavior scales. Both parents and a teacher had completed the rating instrument, and all had high scores consistent with the presence of ADHD. However, in gathering background information, the pediatrician noted that the biologic mother had a great aunt with a history of depression and possible bipolar disorder, the child had no history of overactivity or poor attention in the classroom or home prior to this last 6 months, and the child was recently discovered to be playing doctor with a neighborhood boy 1 year her junior. Rather than immediately prescribing a stimulant, the pediatrician determined that the diagnostic picture was unclear and, therefore, referred the youth to a child psychologist with the goal of obtaining a differential diagnosis and treatment suggestions.

In examining the referral, the psychologist noted the primary symptoms could be observed in a child suffering from bipolar disorder, posttraumatic stress disorder, ADHD, or even a general anxiety disorder caused by recent family upheaval. Thus, any selected tests needed to sort out these various symptoms. The battery chosen included the Child Behavior Checklist and Teacher's Report forms, which are behavioral ratings covering various diagnostic and psychopathology constructs and have extensive developmental data to help sort out significant behavioral problems for different age levels. In addition, there are a number of research articles suggesting the use of the Child Behavior Checklist for the differential diagnosis of ADHD and juvenile mania. The psychologist also chose to use the Trauma Symptom Checklist for Children; Personality Inventory for Youth, which is filled out by the child; a more extensive Developmental History Questionnaire; a Home Situation Questionnaire Revised; and a Rorschach test and the Wechsler Intelligence Scale for Children-III. The latter was utilized because it has been noted that children with intellectual delays sometimes have difficulty focusing in a classroom setting or in the home. Upon presenting the standardized testing to the young girl, the psychologist noted she had difficulty concentrating, was restless, and answered impulsively. In addition, she was aggressive and boisterous with her siblings and mother during the family interview, and she complained of difficulty falling asleep. The intelligence testing yielded scores in the average range for her age and suggested, despite her impulsive style, that she was able to express her intelligence adequately. Behavioral ratings compared to other girls of her age yielded high scores on the aggression, inattention, and depression scales by parents and teachers. This is a pattern often seen with children who may be exhibiting early symptoms of juvenile mania. The girl's responses on the Personality Inventory for Youth yielded significantly high scores on the Psychological Discomfort scale, particularly on the Depression and Sleep Disturbance subscales, and the Impulsivity/Distractibility scale, particularly the Brashness and Distractibility/Overactivity subscales. The Trauma Symptom Checklist for Children indicated no significant problems in any of the areas such as sexual concerns, dissociation, defensive avoidance, or anxiety, but did have elevations on the Depression subtest. In addition, the girl's responding was considered to be consistent and did not exhibit a pattern of malingering or deceptiveness. Finally, the Rorschach test indicated severe problems with mood and a tendency toward depression or hypomania, aggression, and disorganized thinking in emotionally charged situations. There was an indication of a pattern similar to those found suffering from juvenile mania or bipolar disorder. There was also indication, given her age, that she may have been having some difficulty with processing information in emotionally charged, ambivalent situations. Altogether, these different testing results suggest the child suffers from a juvenile bipolar disorder. Based on this diagnosis, the treatment approach would be much different from that based on the originally suggested diagnosis of ADHD.

In the field of child and youth mental health, use of behavioral ratings to measure treatment effectiveness has become increasingly more prevalent. The American Academy of Child and Adolescent Psychiatry has, in their standards of practice, recommended the integration of behavioral ratings from multiple settings with interview and observational data if ADHD is suspected; it also recommends using a series of behavioral rating measures to evaluate the success of medication treatment over time. Use of depression or anxiety-rating scales is also encouraged for use with children or youths to measure treatment effectiveness with medication. Referrals for behavioral ratings aimed at measuring the effect of a treatment protocol are also common. Thus, data are gathered using standard single construct behavior rating scales to obtain baseline information about symptoms before medication and psychosocial treatment are started and at various points along the way to help determine whether the treatment is working. In such monitoring applications, it is not necessary to be concerned with developmental norms or with multiple diagnostic constructs as the diagnosis is already made and monitoring is only measured against an individual's own baseline. In such cases, psychological testing can help reduce potential legal liability for health care professionals by providing a "baseline" reference point or outside opinion should a patient claim a provider was negligent, committed malpractice, or damaged the patient with the treatment provided. In this vignette, however, the pediatrician was being asked to make a diagnosis based upon limited behavioral ratings and could easily have gone down the wrong treatment path.

Case vignette #2

In this example, a 13-year-old girl who was being treated for depressive symptoms was not responding well to standard treatment. She was subsequently referred for psychological assessment to aid with diagnosis and treatment planning. At the time of the referral, she was residing in a psychiatric state hospital and exhibiting symptoms of withdrawal, lethargy, sleep dysregulation, complaints of anxiety in school, and difficulty in concentrating. She had periodic aggressive outbursts where she hurt younger children. These symptoms were exhibited in the context of a divorced family where her father had maintained limited contact and her mother had abandoned all contact. She had been exposed to neglect and parental substance abuse. She had been in a foster home placement, in the psychiatric state hospital, and had a history of prior psychiatric hospitalizations. The psychologist chose a testing battery including intelligence testing with the Wechsler Intelligence Scale for Children (WISC-III); the Child Behavior Checklist, completed by hospital staff, as her parents were unavailable; the Youth Self-Report, which is a version of the Child Behavior Checklist completed by the patient; the Personality Inventory for Youth; and the Rorschach test. The presenting problem suggests the presence of depression, anxiety, and possibly ADHD. In getting the results, it was noted that the teenager tended to respond slowly to the standardized testing. Her responses to the Similarities subtest on the WISC-III, which measures verbal abstract reasoning, suggests some very loose associations or overly concrete associations. She obtained a score in the low average range of intelligence both in the Verbal and Performance portions of the intelligence testing. The Child Behavior Checklist completed by both swing and day staff indicated high scores on the Thought Problem scale, Depression scale, Attention Deficit scale, and Anxiety scales. Her own report indicated problems with depression and anxiety. In particular, she reported symptoms suggestive of being fearful, somewhat hypervigilant, and lacking in self-worth. The Personality Inventory for Youth indicated high scores on the clinical scales of Reality Distortion (Feelings of Alienation, Hallucinations, and Delusions subscales), psychological discomfort (Depression subscale), social withdrawal (Isolation subscale), and social skill deficit (limited peer status).

Finally, the Rorschach test indicated problems with reality testing and logical reasoning. Overall, these findings suggested a pattern significantly similar to those who suffer from an incipient psychosis. The depression was not as evident on this particular assessment. Based on these findings, the treatment plan was adjusted to focus more on addressing poor reality testing, social interactions, and emotional controls that are associated with the presence of a psychotic disorder. She was prescribed an antipsychotic medication and showed rapid improvement over a short period of time. Soon after medication initiation, she was released from the hospital to community treatment. As this case vignette demonstrates, a battery of psychological tests can help to organize and differentiate complicated and overlapping symptoms and place them in proper context when data are gathered using multiple methods.

BIBLIOGRAPHY

AACAP. Practice parameters for the assessment and treatment of children, adolescents, and adults with attention-deficit/hyperactivity disorder. *J Am Acad Child Adolesc Psychiatry* 1997;36(10 Suppl): 85S–121S.

Franzer MD, Berg RA. *Screening children for brain impairment*, 2nd ed. New York: Springer, 1998.

Groth-Marnat G. *Handbook of psychological assessment*, 4th ed. New York: John Wiley and Sons, 2003.

Meyer GJ, Finn SE, Eyde LD, et al. *Benefits and costs of psychological assessment in healthcare delivery:* *report of the Board of Professional Affairs Psychological Assessment Work Group, part I.* Washington, DC: American Psychological Association, 1998.

Perry JC. Problems and considerations in the valid assessment of personality disorders. *Am J Psychiatry* 1992;149:1645–1653.

Reynolds CR, Kamphaus RW. *Handbook of psychological and educational assessment of children*, 2nd ed., Vols. 1 & 2. New York: Guilford Publications, 2003.

SUGGESTED READINGS

Gabel S, Oster G, Butnik S. *Understanding psychological testing in children: a guide for health professionals*. New York: Plenum Publishing, 1986. *(A review of psychological testing in children.)*

Hebben N, Milberg W. *Essentials of neuropsychological assessment*. Chichester: John Wiley and Sons, 2002. *(A comprehensive guide to basic tests and practical issues related to neuropsychological assessment.)*

Olin JT, Keatinge C. *Rapid psychological assessment*. New York: John Wiley and Sons, 1998. *(A practical and concise assessment book that contains essential information on a variety of tests used in the clinical assessment of patients of all ages.)*

Psychiatric Syndromes

CHAPTER 4

Attention Deficit Hyperactivity Disorder

DOROTHY E. STUBBE

Introduction

Attention deficit hyperactivity disorder (ADHD) is the most commonly diagnosed psychiatric disorder of childhood and is characterized by deficits in attention, concentration, activity level, and impulse control. ADHD is often associated with significant comorbidity with other psychiatric disorders, both externalizing [such as oppositional defiant disorder (ODD) and conduct disorder (CD)] and internalizing (such as major depression and anxiety disorders), as well as bipolar disorder. The impact of ADHD on the child, his or her family, schools, and society is enormous, with billions of dollars spent annually for school services, mental health services, and increased use of the juvenile justice system. This disorder is a major public health problem. ADHD children frequently experience peer rejection and engage in a broad array of impulsive and disruptive behaviors, with subsequent negative consequences on self-esteem and adaptive coping. In contrast with historic notions, children do not typically "outgrow" ADHD. Morbidity and disability often persist into adult life. This chapter will review current understanding of ADHD including its phenomenology, etiology, course, diagnostic considerations, controversies surrounding the disorder, and treatment.

HISTORIC NOTES

The conceptualization and diagnostic terminology related to ADHD have changed dramatically over the years. Historically, three views of the disorder have dominated: (a) behavioral (e.g., hyperactivity); (b) etiologic [e.g., minimal brain dysfunction (MBD)]; and (c) cognitive (e.g., attention deficit disorder). The fluctuations in conceptualization over time have led to changes in diagnostic criteria, research designs, epidemiologic prevalence rates, and treatment interventions.

The first "modern" description of ADHD was proposed in 1902 by Still, in which he described a group of children who were hyperactive, unable to concentrate, and had learning and conduct difficulties described as "morbid defects of moral control." He posited both organic and environmental causes for the disorder.

A shift to a more purely organic brain disorder conceptualization of the syndrome occurred around the time of World War I. The change was partly a result of the observation that children who suffered and survived the sequelae of encephalitis associated with the influenza epidemic sometimes developed a severe behavior disorder with overactivity and impulsivity. In 1947, Strauss and Lehtinen described a group of mentally retarded children with hyperactivity, impulsivity, and perseveration, which they conceptualized as minimal brain damage syndrome. In 1962, Clements and Peters proposed the term MBD for nonretarded individuals with high levels of hyperactivity and impulsivity.

The disorder was renamed and reconceptualized in 1968 with the second edition of the *Diagnostic and Statistical Manual of Mental Disorders* (DSM-II) and the corresponding *International Classification of Diseases* (ICD-9) as hyperkinetic syndrome of childhood. This disorder remains in the ICD-10 (used in the United Kingdom and Europe and for billing coding in the United States) and includes children with pervasive overactivity and inattention (IA) but excludes children with co-occurring conduct difficulties. The DSM criteria used in the United States include children with co-occurring conduct difficulties, thus consisting of a larger population of children. The lack of unified international diagnostic criteria has added confusion regarding the applicability of study results across countries.

A conceptual shift occurred in the late-1970s, in which the disorder was coined attention deficit disorder, and the core deficiency of the disorder was postulated as a failure to regulate attention, arousal, and inhibitory control. Subsequent revisions of the DSM have alternately included or excluded the overactivity and restlessness as key to ADHD. The present conceptualization in the fourth edition of the DSM (DSM-IV) published in 1994 consists of three subtypes: predominant symptoms of inattention (ADHD-IA), predominant symptoms of hyperactivity with impulsivity (ADHD-HI), or the combination of the two (ADHD-Combined).

CURRENT CONTROVERSIES

ADHD is the most common and the most intensively studied childhood psychiatric disorder, with over 1,000 articles published annually on the topic. Despite the scientific data on the etiology, prevalence, and effective treatments for the disorder, ADHD has been particularly steeped in controversy in the lay public, the media, and even among medical and mental health professionals. Some have questioned the existence of the disorder entirely, arguing that the symptoms may represent the far end of the normal continuum of activity level. The issue of conceptualization of ADHD as comprising the extreme and dysfunctional end of a normal continuum of activity level and attentiveness (dimensional conceptualization) versus a qualitatively different behavioral syndrome (categoric conceptualization) remains unclear. Some researchers have suggested that the functional brain scanning technique of single photon emission computed tomography (SPECT) may be used to diagnose ADHD and its subtypes, thus guiding more specific interventions. Imaging studies suggest lower than normal blood flow in a variety of brain regions, especially the prefrontal cortex. The ability to subtype ADHD for treatment purposes using this technology, however, remains an area of debate.

However, the most controversial area regarding ADHD surrounds the use of medication for the disorder. There is concern that stimulant drugs may be overprescribed or used as a method of controlling children's behavior rather than as an effective treatment of a serious long-term disorder. Public mistrust has been fueled by the burgeoning number of stimulant prescriptions written in the United States. Indeed, the number of prescriptions has doubled every 5 years. The rise in the number of stimulant prescriptions can be attributed to an increase in the population of patients treated, as well as an increasing acceptance of medication treatment as effective for ADHD symptoms. Medications are increasingly being used with younger children (preschool children), adolescents, adults, and for the inattentive type of ADHD. A recent study by Olfson et al. concerning national trends in the treatment of ADHD suggests that outpatient treatment for ADHD increased almost fourfold between 1987 and 1997. Among children who received treatment for ADHD, there was a significant decrease in the number of treatment visits but an increase in the number of stimulant prescriptions. Up to three fourths of children with a diagnosis of ADHD are currently prescribed medication. However, only a fraction of the children and adolescents in need of psychiatric services obtain them. This means that there are many children with ADHD who are not diagnosed and not in treatment, many of whom are not treated with stimulants, but also inevitably children without ADHD who do receive treatment. There is considerable regional variability in the rates of diagnosis of ADHD and medication treatment of children and adolescents in the United States. The functional disability of the disorder, the risk for poor long-term outcome, and the enormous comorbidity with multiple other psychiatric disorders (conduct difficulties, substance abuse, mood disorders, anxiety, and learning problems) underscore the need for continued intensive research regarding safe and effective interventions with this group of children.

Clinical Features

As shown in Table 4.1, the core symptoms or criteria needed to make a diagnosis of ADHD cover cognitive and/or motor symptoms grouped as inattention, hyperactivity, and impulsivity, or the combination of both sets of symptoms. A variety of other psychiatric disorders may present with difficulties with sustained attention (such as anxiety, depression, or psychotic disorders), high levels of activity (such as bipolar disorder), or both. Thus, the clinician must differentiate the core symptoms of ADHD from the secondary effects of the other psychiatric disorders. Because there is a high degree of comorbidity of ADHD with other psychiatric conditions (especially with ODD and CD, but also with internalizing mood and anxiety disorders), the clinician must complete a thorough assessment to clarify the diagnosis and disabling symptoms. The onset of ADHD impairment must be in early childhood, at least before age 7, even if it was not diagnosed until later in life. There must be functional impairment in a variety of life settings (home, school, work, etc.). ADHD should not be diagnosed if it presents only concomitantly with a pervasive developmental disorder or psychotic disorder.

Epidemiology

ADHD is relatively common, affecting an estimated 2% to 12% of school-aged children, depending on definition and study. As is true for most developmental and psychiatric disorders of childhood onset, there is no definitive diagnostic test for ADHD. This

TABLE 4.1. *DIAGNOSTIC AND STATISTICAL MANUAL OF MENTAL DISORDERS*, **FOURTH EDITION, TEXT REVISION DIAGNOSTIC CRITERIA FOR ATTENTION DEFICIT HYPERACTIVITY DISORDER**

Inattention	• Often fails to give close attention to details or makes careless mistakes in schoolwork, work, or other activities
	• Often has difficulty sustaining attention in tasks or play activities
	• Often does not seem to listen when spoken to directly
	• Often does not follow through on instructions and fails to finish schoolwork, chores, or duties in the workplace (not due to oppositional behavior or failure to understand instructions)
	• Often has difficulty organizing tasks and activities
	• Often avoids, dislikes, or is reluctant to engage in tasks that require sustained mental effort (such as schoolwork or homework)
	• Often loses things necessary for tasks or activities (e.g., toys, school assignments, pencils, books, or tools)
	• Is often easily distracted by extraneous stimuli
	• Is often forgetful in daily activities
Hyperactivity/ impulsivity	• Often fidgets with hands or feet or squirms in seat
	• Often leaves seat in classroom or in other situations in which remaining seated is expected
	• Often runs about or climbs excessively in situations in which it is inappropriate (in adolescents or adults, may be limited to subjective feelings of restlessness)
	• Often has difficulty playing or engaging in leisure activities quietly
	• Is often "on the go" or often acts as if "driven by a motor"
	• Often talks excessively
	• Often blurts out answers before questions have been completed
	• Often has difficulty awaiting turn
	• Often interrupts or intrudes on others (e.g., butts into conversations or games)
Other features	• Some hyperactive-impulsive or inattentive symptoms that caused impairment were present before age 7 yr
	• Some impairment from the symptoms is present in two or more settings [e.g., at school (or work) and at home]
	• There must be clear evidence of clinically significant impairment in social, academic, or occupational functioning
	• The symptoms do not occur exclusively during the course of a pervasive developmental disorder, schizophrenia, or other psychotic disorder and are not better accounted for by another mental disorder (e.g., mood disorder, anxiety disorder, dissociative disorder, or a personality disorder)

Note: The DSM-IV-TR denotes the following about the three subtypes of ADHD where symptoms are maladaptive and inconsistent with developmental level and persist for at least 6 mo:

Attention deficit hyperactivity disorder (combined type): six or more symptoms from the inattention list plus six or more symptoms from the hyperactivity/impulsivity list

Attention deficit hyperactivity disorder (predominantly inattentive type): six or more symptoms from the inattention list

Attention deficit hyperactivity disorder (predominantly hyperactive-impulsive type): six or more symptoms from the hyperactivity/impulsivity list

From American Psychiatric Association. *Diagnostic and statistical manual of mental disorders*, 4th ed, Text rev. Washington, DC: American Psychiatric Association, 2000, with permission.

makes epidemiologic reliability and validity more difficult. The classroom teacher is a particularly valuable source of information in diagnosing ADHD, along with parents and the child. Epidemiologic estimates of the prevalence of ADHD have increased substantially with the DSM-IV classification of ADHD into three categories: inattentive type, hyperactive/impulsive type, or combined type. This diagnostic nomenclature has led to an increase in prevalence, a broadening of the disorder to include more girls, preschoolers, and adults, and has impacted the educational services and treatment modalities utilized. It has also led to greater discrepancies with rates of ADHD found in Europe, where behavioral aspects of the disorder are de-emphasized.

In community samples of children, boys are diagnosed with ADHD-Combined in a frequency of 3:1 as compared with girls. Clinic samples tend to be higher, approaching a 9:1 male-to-female ratio, most likely due to the higher proportion of disruptive behaviors in boys with ADHD-Combined, which may promote referral for treatment. Indeed, ADHD is diagnosed in as many as half of children referred for mental health services. ADHD-IA is not associated with an increase in disruptive behaviors and is more nearly equal in prevalence between boys and girls.

Psychosocial correlates with ADHD include low income/poverty, urban residence, family dysfunction, and parents with psychiatric disorders. These psychosocial risk factors suggest that there may be multiple pathways leading to the clinical constellation of ADHD in vulnerable children. This information is important for public health prevention efforts and may guide early intervention efforts.

Clinical Course

Although many of the symptoms of ADHD may remit, it has become clear that ADHD is frequently a chronic disorder, which leads to a negative impact on functioning throughout the life cycle. Studies following children with ADHD into adolescence have fairly consistently shown that ADHD children, as compared with controls, exhibit impaired academic functioning, perform more poorly on cognitive tasks, and are characterized by lower self-esteem and poor social functioning. About three fourths of these children continue to show symptoms of ADHD into adolescence, and pervasive conduct problems are common.

Follow-up studies into adulthood show that 40% to 50% of individuals diagnosed with ADHD continue to suffer from clinically significant symptoms of ADHD. Furthermore, up to 33% of ADHD individuals versus 1% to 9% of controls drop out of high school. ADHD children obtain less education overall (by 2–3 years), and fewer complete a graduate degree. Likewise, the ADHD cohort demonstrates significantly lower occupation rankings at the age of 25. Children with ADHD are also at increased risk for developing antisocial personality disorder and substance use disorders in adulthood.

Etiology and Pathogenesis

GENETIC FACTORS

Although the exact etiology of ADHD remains unknown, data from family genetic, twin, adoption, and segregation analysis strongly suggest a genetic etiology. Heritability coefficients are very high ($\mu = 0.8$).

ADHD is thought to be a complex genetic disorder that does not follow classic Mendelian inheritance patterns, but is believed to result from the combined effects of several genes and interactions with the environment. Preliminary molecular genetic studies have implicated candidate genes associated with the dopamine system, including the dopamine D2 and D4 receptors and the dopamine transporter. There is also preliminary evidence that genes involved in norepinephrine modulation are affected in some patients. Given the importance of these catecholamines for the modulation of attentional circuits, it is not surprising that alterations in these systems would result in impaired attention regulation. However, there is a great deal of study left to be done on the role of genes and the gene-environment interaction in the etiology of ADHD.

NEURODEVELOPMENTAL FACTORS

Prefrontal, parietal, and temporal association cortices, and their projections to the striatum, make distinct contributions to the core ability to focus attention. In particular, the prefrontal cortex uses working memory to guide overt responses (movement) as well as covert responses (attention), allowing us to inhibit inappropriate behaviors and to attenuate the processing of irrelevant stimuli. The neurotransmitters of dopamine and norepinephrine are both intricately involved in modulating prefrontal cortical functioning. There is evidence that moderate amounts of these neurotransmitters are essential to prefrontal cortical functioning, but that high levels (as are found in extreme stress) may actually impair optimal functioning.

Barkley has postulated that the primary deficit in the disorder of ADHD-combined is one of behavioral disinhibition. Behavioral disinhibition is conceptualized as fundamental to problems with working memory, self-regulation of affect, motivation and arousal, the capacity for reasoning and reflection, and goal-directed behavior. Brown has argued that the common etiologic deficit in all types of ADHD is one of impaired executive functioning. Developmental difficulties with activation, focus, sustaining effort, modulating emotions, utilizing working memory, and regulating behaviors are all subsumed under the rubric of executive functioning impairment.

Early neurodevelopmental problems such as obstetric complications, prematurity, other genetic abnormalities (such as fragile X disorder and others), and exposure *in utero* to alcohol, cocaine, or other toxins may predispose to ADHD. It is postulated that fetal insults, particularly during the second trimester during the height of neural development, may cause subtle functional abnormalities to the frontal cortex and other brain structures, resulting in the disorder. Early findings are also provocative regarding the neuronal-environmental interactions as related to brain functioning. Specifically, the efficiency of brain functioning may be molded in the perinatal period via neuronal pruning, which is enhanced by appropriate levels of stimulation and nurturance. Severe psychosocial adversity in infancy thus may predispose to less efficient neuronal tracks and potentially to subtle neurodevelopmental disorders such as ADHD.

NEUROIMAGING FINDINGS

Imaging studies of ADHD have focused on the prefrontal cortex, basal ganglia, and cerebellum. Although results have been mixed, there is evidence of structural and functional differences in the brains of children and adults with ADHD. Volumetric measures have detected smaller right-sided prefrontal regions overall in boys with ADHD. These reductions correlated with performance on tasks that require response inhibition. Girls with ADHD have been found to have smaller left and total caudate volumes. A consistent finding has been reduced volume of the posterior–inferior cerebellar vermis, a region that exhibits a high degree of dopamine receptor reactivity.

Functional neuroimaging with positron emission tomography (PET) has demonstrated decreased frontal cerebral metabolism in adults with ADHD. Decreased blood flow has been reported in ADHD subjects in the striatum and prefrontal cortex. Although functional magnetic resonance imaging has not been conclusive, early results also indicate subtle deficits in frontal lobe activity. Preliminary results of PET imaging examining the neuropharmacology of ADHD support the notion that catecholamine dysregulation is central to the pathophysiology of the disorder and not just to its treatment.

Assessment

ADHD is a clinical diagnosis. There is no definitive diagnostic test for ADHD, but rather the diagnosis is established by clinical judgment based on a comprehensive assessment that involves multiple domains, informants, methods, and settings. The essentials of assessment for ADHD are summarized in Table 4.2.

A complete history, screening physical, and neurologic exam are necessary to provide accurate assessment of ADHD in children and adolescents. A careful assessment of the child's prenatal and developmental history, current symptoms, psychosocial functioning, and family psychiatric history are important when making a diagnosis. Whenever possible, the history should be gathered from multiple sources, including the parents or primary caretakers, teachers, the pediatrician, and the child. These reporters will likely not fully agree in their observations or assessment of the child. Even parents living in the same home with the child may demonstrate only moderate concordance in reporting their child's behaviors. The younger the child, the poorer will be his or her concordance with the reports of his or her parents or other adults. Low concordance does not necessarily negate the diagnosis of ADHD. Rather, it reflects the ecologic aspects of ADHD (and other psychiatric disorders) as well as the contextual factors that affect the child's behavior across settings and individuals. The diagnosis of ADHD cannot be made by only observing the child in the physician's office. The structured setting, individualized attention, and novelty may mask the ADHD.

Many parents will note difficult temperament and poor impulse control from an early age. Often, early gross motor development with more delayed fine motor and language development are described. The psychiatric history should focus on presenting symptoms, the longitudinal timeline of symptom development, and associated features and/or confounding factors (e.g., mood disorders, developmental problems, recent stress or traumas, or substance abuse). Often a rating scale of symptoms (e.g., the Conners' scales) is useful in quantifying the symptoms and their severity.

A physical examination, including height, weight, and vital signs, is indicated. If there is suspicion of neurologic, toxic, or endocrine abnormalities, these should be

TABLE 4.2. ESSENTIALS IN THE ASSESSMENT OF ATTENTION DEFICIT HYPERACTIVITY DISORDER

1. Multiple historic informants (parents, teachers, child) should be included in the evaluation process. Discrepancies among these reporters should be expected and do not negate the diagnosis.
2. Hyperactivity does not need to be present during the mental status exam to make the diagnosis of ADHD.
3. There are no specific laboratory tests, neuroimaging procedures, rating scales, neurologic or attentional assessments, or psychological tests that have been established to be individually diagnostic for ADHD. Although the computerized continuous performance test (CPT) may be a helpful adjunct in diagnosis, it is not a conclusive test for the disorder.
4. Concomitant learning disabilities or cognitive deficits should be ruled out as a cause of the inattention or increased motor activity, although they may be comorbid with ADHD.
5. Possible comorbid disorders should be evaluated.
6. There are no specific physical features associated with making the diagnosis of ADHD.
7. ADHD is a clinical diagnosis based on careful history taking and clinical examination.
8. ADHD is not a diagnosis of exclusion, although many other psychiatric disorders and psychosocial factors need to be ruled out, or excluded, in making the diagnosis of ADHD.
9. Baseline and follow-up rating scales are helpful in monitoring the effectiveness of treatment interventions and medication regimens. Such scales cannot establish a diagnosis of ADHD.

ADHD, attention deficit hyperactivity disorder.

followed up with the appropriate diagnostic tests. For example, lead toxicity should be considered for children living in poor neighborhoods or old houses. Environmental stress should also be assessed, as a highly distressed child may present as inattentive and overactive. Assessment of comorbidity is crucial. Reportedly, 40% to 60% of ADHD children are diagnosed with at least one other psychiatric disorder. Comorbidity may affect the level and type of pathology encountered, the response to treatment, and long-term outcome. ADHD associated with childhood comorbidity suggests a more serious clinical course and worse prognosis. Thus, both the ADHD and the comorbid condition must be the focus of treatment.

Psychoeducational testing to assess intellectual ability, academic achievement, and possible learning disabilities is a crucial component of a thorough assessment. At times, more complete neuropsychological testing to assess executive functioning and more subtle deficits of the disorder may be indicated. The Continuous Performance Test (CPT) is a computerized test that assesses attentional abilities and impulsivity of response style. Although not specifically diagnostic, it may help in the complete diagnostic assessment. Preliminary studies have shown that CPTs may be helpful in distinguishing ADHD from mania. Children with ADHD usually show improved CPT scores after treatment with stimulant medications. Children with mania do not show improved CPT scores after stimulant treatment. Children with ADHD frequently have learning problems, but these must be well delineated to ensure appropriate educational services. For example, learning problems may exacerbate a child's inattention and hyperactivity as he or she may not understand the school work and avoids it. On the other hand, the ADHD may prevent a child from attending long enough to retain material that he or she is capable of learning. Reports from the teacher regarding behavior, learning, and attendance should be obtained as well as grades and test scores.

Comorbidity and Differential Diagnosis

Individuals with ADHD are at increased risk of suffering from other psychiatric disorders. The most common comorbidities are summarized in Table 4.3.

It is important to diagnose comorbid disorders since the ADHD child with a comorbid condition may have a different clinical presentation, life course, and response to treatment. The most common comorbidities with ADHD are disruptive behavior disorders, learning disorders, mood disorders (bipolar disorder and major depressive disorder), and anxiety disorders.

It is estimated that 50% of children with ADHD meet criteria for either ODD or CD. In general, ADHD comorbid with conduct difficulties suggests an increase in impairment and risk. In one study, ADHD boys without delinquency were no different from controls on neuropsychological measures, whereas the ADHD delinquents were impaired in the

TABLE 4.3. COMMON COMORBID DISORDERS ASSOCIATED WITH ATTENTION DEFICIT HYPERACTIVITY DISORDER

Disorder	Estimated % Associated with ADHD
Oppositional defiant disorder or conduct disorder	50%
Learning disabilities	40% (20%–60%)
Anxiety disorder	30% (25%–33%)
Major depression	30% (3%–75%)
Bipolar disorder	10%–20% of clinical samples

ADHD, attention deficit hyperactivity disorder.

areas of verbal skill, visual motor integration, and visuospatial skills. Additionally, children with ADHD and CD have a much stronger family history of antisocial behavior in relatives. There is evidence that positive response to stimulant medications in comorbid children may also lead to a decrease in antisocial behaviors in addition to inattentiveness and hyperactivity.

Learning disabilities are common in children suffering from ADHD—an estimated 20% to 60% suffer from reading, spelling, or arithmetic disorders. Both ADHD and reading disorder have strong genetic components but seem to be inherited independently. Children with learning disabilities alone do not respond to stimulant medications, but children with comorbid ADHD and reading disability show increased reading achievement when inattentiveness is successfully controlled with medication.

The prevalence of comorbid bipolar disorder is an area of considerable controversy. Because hyperactivity and mania have similar symptoms of overactivity and impulsivity, parceling out their unique symptom profiles is sometimes quite difficult. However, there is an increasing body of research (especially from groups in St. Louis and Massachusetts General Hospital) suggesting that prepubertal mania is more common than originally estimated, and that it may frequently be comorbid with ADHD. Children with comorbid mania and ADHD demonstrate more grandiosity, elated or irritable mood, racing thoughts, and hypersexuality than children suffering from ADHD alone. These children tend to respond better to mood stabilizing medications with or without stimulant medications than to stimulant medications alone. Major depressive disorder comorbid with ADHD is also of unclear prevalence in prepubertal children. Estimates have ranged from 3% to 75%, and clinically referred children demonstrate higher rates of depression than do ADHD children in community samples. Depressive symptoms generally have an onset after the ADHD symptoms. When major depressive disorder is clearly diagnosed, its course is independent of ADHD symptoms (unlike the demoralization that frequently occurs in children with ADHD alone).

About 25% to 33% of children with ADHD will meet criteria for an anxiety disorder, compared with 5% to 15% of the general population. Children with ADHD and comorbid anxiety report anxiety symptoms more frequently than do their parents, suggesting that parents may be unaware of their children's internalizing symptoms. Children with comorbid ADHD and anxiety tend to report a greater occurrence of social difficulties. Additionally, there is a correlation with pregnancy problems and developmental delays, and these children have generally experienced more stressful life events than children with ADHD alone. Genetic studies suggest that anxiety and ADHD are inherited independently of each other.

ADHD must be differentiated from age-appropriate overactivity and other disorders. The differential diagnosis for ADHD is extensive, as summarized in Table 4.4.

Many medications or other substances may cause overactivity or activation. Asthma medications, prednisone, allergy medications, lead intoxication, and substance abuse, to name a few, should be ruled out. Additionally, other medical disorders, such as hearing or vision impairment, seizure disorder, genetic abnormalities, thyroid disorders, and poor nutrition may present with ADHD symptoms. Traumatized children who have experienced severe psychosocial adversity may be anxious and inattentive. Other anxiety disorders may also interfere with the child's ability to attend and/or sit quietly. Children with mild pervasive developmental disorders frequently present with high levels of distractibility and overactivity, which may present as ADHD. Mood disorders (especially bipolar disorder) are frequently very difficult to differentiate from severe ADHD and may be comorbid as well. Children with conduct problems may have comorbid ADHD, or the oppositionality and defiance may be mistaken for ADHD if attention and the actual motor components are not clearly assessed.

TABLE 4.4. ESSENTIAL DIFFERENTIAL DIAGNOSIS FOR ATTENTION DEFICIT HYPERACTIVITY DISORDER

Psychiatric disorders
Oppositional defiant disorder
Conduct disorder
Mood disorders (depression and bipolar disorder)
Anxiety disorders
Tic disorders
Substance use disorders
Pervasive developmental disorder
Learning disorders
Posttraumatic stress disorder
Mental retardation or borderline intellectual functioning

Psychosocial conditions
Abuse and/or neglect
Poor nutrition
Neighborhood violence
Chaotic family situation
Being bullied at school

Medical disorders
Partial deafness or poor eyesight
Seizure disorder
Fetal alcohol syndrome/effects
Genetic abnormalities (such as fragile X)
Sedating or activating medications
Thyroid abnormality
Heavy metal poisoning

Treatment

ADHD is a complex disorder affecting every area of functioning and thereby requires a comprehensive treatment program. The essentials of an effective treatment plan are summarized in Table 4.5 and include: psychosocial interventions, medication treatment, and ensuring an appropriate educational plan.

The Multimodal Treatment Study of ADHD (MTA) was a large (n = 579) study sponsored by the National Institute of Mental Health (NIMH) investigating the effects of various treatment modalities on children with ADHD-combined type over a 14-month time period. The aim of the study was to compare the effectiveness of medication treatment combined with intensive and broad-based psychosocial treatment with medication management or psychosocial treatment alone, and to compare these treatment programs with regular community care. In the MTA study, the psychosocial treatments provided included an 8-week, all-day summer treatment program that utilized contingency management and included social skills training. Additionally, parent training and teacher consultation on classroom behavior management were included. The medication used was methylphenidate, adjusted on a monthly basis with monthly teacher feedback and family interview. Children in the community care arm of the study also frequently received medication, but overall they received lower dosages than the children in the study.

The study found that for the core symptoms of ADHD, combined treatment was not superior to medication management alone and medication management was also superior to behavioral treatment alone and treatment in the community. However, for non-ADHD areas of functioning, the combined treatment was superior to the other groups in

TABLE 4.5. ESSENTIALS OF TREATMENT FOR ATTENTION DEFICIT HYPERACTIVITY DISORDER

1. Treatment should include more than just medication management. Parental guidance and counseling and psychoeducation are cornerstones of treatment.
2. Unsuccessful treatment of ADHD often occurs when comorbid diagnoses are not identified and addressed.
3. Collaboration with a child's school is usually critical to ensure academic progress.
4. Medication holidays over the summer or during weekends do not decrease the effectiveness of stimulants.
5. Medication holidays should be individualized to the child's unique situation and utilized only if the child's social functioning and safety will not be severely compromised.
6. Treatment with stimulants does not increase the likelihood of substance use disorders and may actually lower the risk.
7. In general, failure of an initial stimulant trial should be followed with one or two subsequent stimulant trials before treating with a different class of psychotropic medication.

ADHD, attention deficit hyperactivity disorder.

the treatment of oppositional and aggressive symptoms, internalizing symptoms, teacher-rated social skills, parent–child relations, and reading achievement.

PSYCHOSOCIAL TREATMENTS

Psychosocial treatments may include psychoeducation, parent training in behavioral management skills, classroom interventions, contingency management, social skills training, cognitive behavior therapy, and individual psychotherapy of the child. Of these, parent training, classroom interventions, contingency management, and social skills training have demonstrated efficacy. Psychoeducation, which includes intensive support and education of the family, is essential in developing an ongoing therapeutic alliance between the therapist, the child, and his or her family to ensure collaboration in the complex task of helping the child achieve optimal functioning.

School is where ADHD symptoms may be most disabling, as the demands to sit quietly, pay attention, and work cooperatively are inherent in the school setting. School interventions include ensuring that learning needs are appropriately assessed and addressed. Additionally, contact with teachers regarding the diagnosis and effectiveness of treatment is required. It is crucial that the teacher understands the disorder, and that he or she provides a classroom environment that optimizes the child's learning. Preferential seating (seating within the class to optimize paying attention and minimize distractions), a behavioral management plan that highlights positive reinforcement for desired work habits and behavior, social skills groups, and other interventions may help the child gain school success. More intensive interventions (a small self-contained classroom, special educational services, or a more intensive therapeutic educational plan) may be required for children who are more impaired by the disorder and/or comorbidities.

MEDICATION TREATMENT

As highlighted in the MTA study, medication treatment may be highly effective in addressing the core symptoms of ADHD. There is a large body of literature documenting the efficacy of stimulants on core features of ADHD (motoric overactivity, impulsivity, and inattentiveness) as well as their substantial effects on cognition, social function, and aggression. The stimulant medications are the best studied medications in child and adolescent psychiatry and have demonstrated safety and efficacy in over 200 controlled studies. Despite concerns of many families about the abuse potential of the medication, and the risk of precipitating addiction, treatment with stimulant medications has not been demonstrated to increase illicit substance use. In fact, there is evidence that children and adolescents in treatment are at decreased risk for substance abuse, legal difficulties, and other sequelae of poor impulse control. Finally, concerns that stimulant medication might be responsible for the smaller brain structures found in ADHD children do not appear supported.

At times, medication "holidays" may be indicated, for example, when the child does not take ADHD medication during nonschool periods of time. Although this practice may be helpful for children in whom appetite and sleep are disturbed with the medication, many children may require the medication even when not in school to maintain appropriate social behavior, to be able to enjoy and benefit from group activities, and to decrease highly impulsive behavior that may pose a safety issue.

PSYCHOTROPICS AS SINGLE AGENTS IN THE TREATMENT OF ATTENTION DEFICIT HYPERACTIVITY DISORDER

There are several treatment options for ADHD tailored to patient need, an algorithm for which is presented in Table 4.6. In general, the stimulant medications are considered first line in the treatment of the core symptoms of ADHD. Atomoxetine is an antidepressant that has recently been marketed as a long-acting, noncontrolled medication monotherapy for ADHD, and some clinicians are beginning to use this medication first line, although the body of data on efficacy and effectiveness remains small. Common side effects of the stimulant medications are appetite suppression, sleep disturbances, and some changes in pulse and blood pressure. Stimulants may precipitate or exacerbate tics. At times, stimulant medications may cause more serious side effects, such as dsyphoria, irritability, or even hallucinations. These symptoms may be more common in very young children. Clonidine (Catapres) or guanfacine (Tenex) may be considered first-line treatment of patients with ADHD and tics. However, stimulants have been used successfully in some patients with tic disorders if the dosages are started and increased slowly.

TABLE 4.6. MEDICATION ALGORITHM FOR TREATING ATTENTION DEFICIT HYPERACTIVITY DISORDER

Considered first line
Methylphenidate: Ritalin[a], Ritalin SR[a], Concerta[a], Metadate[a], Focalin[a]
Dextroamphetamine: Dexedrine[a], Dextrostat[a]
Amphetamine salts (Adderall[a])

Second line
Atomoxetine (Straterra[a])
Bupropion (Wellbutrin)
Venlafaxine (Effexor)
TCAs: nortriptyline, desipramine, imipramine
Guanfacine (Tenex)
Clonidine (Catapres)

Considered when most other medications are ineffective
MAOIs: phenelzine, tranylcypromine, selegine
Pemoline (Cylert[a])
Atypical antipsychotics: risperidone, olanzapine, Quetiapine, ziprasidone
Typical antipsychotics: haloperidol[a], thioridazine[a], Thorazine[a]

TCAs, tricyclic antidepressants; MAOIs, monoamine oxidase inhibitors.
[a]Food and Drug Administration (FDA) approved for treatment of ADHD.

Second-line medications for the treatment of ADHD include antidepressants in the tricyclic [tricyclic antidepressant (TCA)] class, bupropion, venlafaxine, and the α-adrenergic agonists clonidine and guanfacine. Tricyclic medications are well studied and have demonstrated efficacy for ADHD in children for whom stimulant medications are ineffective or have marked side effects. However, several reports of sudden death in children taking desipramine and the need for careful drug blood level and cardiac conduction monitoring have decreased the use of the tricyclic medications. Additionally, there is a high risk of fatality in overdose. Mixing with other medications may lead to dangerously high serum levels. However, TCAs may be the first-line medications in patients with marked anxiety or severe tics. The antidepressants in the selective serotonergic reuptake inhibitors (SSRIs) class have demonstrated little effectiveness in treating core symptoms of ADHD.

The α-adrenergic agonists clonidine and guanfacine have preliminary data to suggest enhanced cognitive functioning in the prefrontal cortex. These medications may be particularly indicated in the treatment of ADHD and tic disorders, as they are also effective medications for mild tics. However, several reports of death in children who had received clonidine and other medications, without known causality, suggest that caution is advised in prescribing these medications. In addition to monotherapy, clonidine and guanfacine are sometimes used in combined therapy with stimulants. Clonidine may be used at night for sleeplessness, as it tends to be sedating. Additionally, the α-agonists tend to help with the "rebound" hyperactivity in the afternoon when the stimulant medication wears off or may be used concomitantly to target hyperactivity and overarousal. There were concerns that the combination of methylphenidate and clonidine may have contributed to sudden death in several children, but review of the cases has not supported this claim.

The antipsychotic medications may be helpful in treating the agitation and aggression of children and adolescents with ADHD but are used only third line and usually in low dose in combination with other ADHD medications. They are also sometimes used for ADHD children with comorbid tics that are not responsive to the α-agonists. The monoamine oxidase inhibitors (MAOIs) are antidepressants with preliminary studies suggesting effectiveness for ADHD symptoms. Currently, dietetic restrictions (no tyramine-containing foods) and drug–drug interactions limit the use of MAOIs in juveniles. However, the development of reversible and transdermal preparations may lead to MAOIs with a more favorable safety profile. Practical aspects of using these medications with youths are summarized in Table 4.7.

General principles of pharmacotherapy should be followed in the medication treatment of children, adolescents, and adults with ADHD. These include beginning with one medication and slowly titrating medication dosages up as needed until optimal effectiveness is achieved with minimal side effects. At times, changing dosage timing may help decrease such side effects as appetite suppression or sleep disturbance. Routine monitoring of vital signs (blood pressure and pulse), height, and weight are indicated. If stimulant medications successfully treat ADHD, but comorbid symptoms (such as depression) persist, addition of an antidepressant medication may be indicated. Several studies have described safety and efficacy of combined SSRI and stimulant pharmacotherapy. Alternatively, the use of an antidepressant medication with secondary ADHD effects (such as bupropion or venlafaxine) may be considered. However, both the SSRIs and venlafaxine have been recently implicated in increased suicidal behavior for adolescents. Pemoline has been associated with hepatitis and should be used only when other medications have been tried and only with close blood monitoring of liver function every 2 weeks.

TABLE 4.7. MEDICATIONS FOR ATTENTION DEFICIT HYPERACTIVITY DISORDER

Medication Class	Preparations Available	Recommended Schedule/Dosage	Duration of Effect	Mechanism of Action	Common Adverse Effects/Comments
STIMULANTS					
METHYLPHENIDATE					
Short-acting					Common side effects: decreased appetite, insomnia, rebound hyperactivity, benign increase in HR and BP. May unmask or induce tics.
Focalin	2.5, 5, 10 mg tabs	Initial: 2.5 mg bid Max: 20 mg/d	3–5 h	Dopamine presynaptic release and reuptake	Less common side effects: "hyperfocus" phenomenon, depression, psychosis
Ritalin and generics					• Safety/effectiveness not studied in patients <6 yr
Methylin	5, 10, 20 mg tabs	Initial: 5 mg bid with/after breakfast and lunch Max: 60 mg/d May require tid in some pts	3–5 h		• Monitor vital signs, growth, and weight • Give with/after food • Longer-acting preparations—less rebound, more coverage through day, but may have greater problematic effects on evening appetite and sleep
Intermediate-acting					
Metadate ER	10, 20 mg tabs	Initial: 10 mg q am	6–8 h		• Capsule formulations may be opened and sprinkled on food
Methylin ER	10, 20 mg tabs	Initial: 10 mg q am			• Tablets should be swallowed whole
Ritalin SR	20 mg tabs	Initial: 20 mg q am			
Generics		Max: 60 mg/d May require bid dosage in some pts			
Long-acting					
Metadate CD Ritalin LA	20 mg caps 20, 30, 40 mg caps	Initial: 1 20 mg cap q am Max 60 mg/d	8 h		
Concerta	18, 27, 36, 54 mg tabs	Initial: 18 mg tab q Max: 54 mg/day	12 h		
AMPHETAMINES					Common side effects: decreased appetite, insomnia, rebound hyperactivity, benign increase in HR and BP. May unmask or induce tics.
Short-acting					Less common side effects: "hyperfocus" phenomenon, depression, psychosis
Adderall generics	5, 7.5, 10, 12.5, 15, 20, 30 mg tabs	3–5 yr: 2.5 mg qd-bid ≥6 yr: 5 mg qd-bid Max: 40 mg/d	4–6 h	Dopamine presynaptic release and reuptake	

Drug	Preparations	Duration	Dosage	Mechanism	Comments
Dexedrine generics	5 mg tabs	4–6 h	3–5 yr: 2.5 mg bid-tid ≥6 yr: 5 mg bid-tid Max: 40 mg/d		• Safety/effectiveness not studied in patients <6 yr • Monitor vital signs, growth, and weight • Give with/after food
Dextrostat	5, 10 mg tabs 5, 10 mg tabs	4–6 h	3–5 yr: 2.5 mg bid-tid ≥6 yr: 5 mg bid-tid Max: 40 mg/d		• Longer-acting preparations—less rebound, more coverage through day, but may have greater problematic effects on evening appetite and sleep • Capsule formulations may be opened and sprinkled on food Tablets should be swallowed whole If one preparation does not work, another stimulant may be effective
Intermediate-acting					
Dexedrine spansule	5, 10, 15 mg caps	6–8 h	≥6 yr: 5–10 mg qd-bid Max: 40 mg/d		
Long-acting					
Adderall XR	5, 10, 15, 20, 25, 30 mg caps	10–12 h	≥6 yr: 10 mg qd Max: 30 mg/d		
Pemoline (Cylert)	18.75, 37.5, 75 mg tabs 37.5 mg chewable	24 h	Initial: 18.75 qd Max: 112.5 mg		Potential for serious hepatotoxicity • Q 2 wk LFTs
ANTIDEPRESSANTS					
Atomoxetine (Strattera)	10, 18, 25, 40, 60 mg caps	Lasts into evening or longer	Initial: 0.5 mg/kg q am or div bid Increase ≥3 d to 1.2 mg/kg q am or div bid Max: 1.4 mg/kg/d or 100 mg/d	Selective norepinephrine reuptake inhibitor	Indicated for patients who have not responded to, or have unacceptable side effects from, stimulants; or those who have tic disorder or object to controlled substances • Safety/effectiveness not studied in patients <6 yr • May decrease appetite, cause sleep disturbance • Monitor vital signs, growth, and weight • May take days/weeks to note effectiveness
Aminoketone					
Bupropion (Wellbutrin SR, Zyban)	75, 100 mg tabs 100, 150 mg tabs	12 h or more	Initial: 75 mg qd Max: 6 mg/kg/d in div bid dosages	Mixed dopaminergic and norepinephrine reuptake blockade	Lowers seizure threshold. May cause irritability, insomnia, tic exacerbation • Contraindicated in bulimics • Also used to treat depression, smoking cessation • No FDA approval for children

(Continued)

TABLE 4.7. CONTINUED

Medication Class	Preparations Available	Recommended Schedule/Dosage	Duration of Effect	Mechanism of Action	Common Adverse Effects/Comments
TRICYCLICS					Cardiovascular effects (generally dose-dependent) • Increased diastolic BP and ECG conduction parameters • Overdoses can be fatal • Reports of sudden death on desipramine of unclear etiology
Tertiary amines Imipramine Imipramine pamoate (Tofranil)	10, 25, 50, 75, 100, 125, 150 mg tabs	Initial: 10–25 mg qhs Max: 5 mg/kg/d in q d or bid divided dosages			
Secondary amines Desipramine (Norpramin)	10, 25, 50, 75, 100, 150 tabs	Initial: 25 mg qhs Max: 3 mg/kg/d in qd or bid dosages	Up to 24 h coverage	Norepinephrine > dopamine presynaptic reuptake blockade	Treatment requires serum level and ECG monitoring Risk of seizures May be first line in patients with comorbid depression, anxiety, or tic disorders
Nortriptyline (Pamelor)	10, 25, 50, 75 mg caps	Initial: 10–25 mg qhs Max: 3 mg/kg/d in qd or bid dosages	Up to 24 h coverage	Anticholinergic, antihistamine, α-1 postsynaptic effects	Side effects similar to SSRIs • Irritability • Insomnia
Venlafaxine (Effexor)	25, 37.5, 50, 75, 100 mg tabs	Initial: 75 mg/d in divided bid or tid dosage (qd for XR preparations)	Up to 24 h coverage	Serotonergic-noradrenergic reuptake inhibitor	• GI symptoms • Headache • Potential withdrawal symptoms
(Effexor XR)	37.5, 75, 150 mg caps	Max: 3 mg/kg/d	Up to 24 h coverage	mechanism of action. Weak dopamine reuptake inhibitor	• BP changes

NORADRENERGIC MODULATORS

α-2 AGONISTS

Clonidine (Catapres)	0.1, 0.2, 0.3 mg tabs	Initial: .05 mg qhs Max: 0.5 mg/d in bid, tid, qid div doses	About 4 h	α-2 noradrenergic agonist, which decreases overall adrenergic tone	Cardiovascular side effects • Hypotension • Possible rebound hypertension—must taper to D/C • ? ECG monitoring needed • Reports of death in children who received clonidine and other medications (all with confounding factors)
Guanfacine (Tenex)	1.0, 2.0 mg tabs	Initial: 0.5 mg qhs Max: 5 mg/d in qd, bid, or tid divided doses	About 6–8 h	Guanfacine is more selective α-2a agonist	May be used for sleep disturbances with/without use of stimulants Effectiveness for hyperactivity and impulsivity, hyperarousal, tic disorders • Delayed action for up to 5 wk • Not effective for primary inattention and distractibility Side effects: • Sedation (frequent) • Depression • Dry mouth • Confusion at high doses

BP, blood pressure; HR, heart rate; FDA, Food and Drug Administration; ECG, electrocardiogram; SSRIs, selective serotonergic reuptake inhibitor; GI, gastrointestinal.

Case Vignette

Case vignette #1

Will is a 7-year-old boy who is very impulsive. Most of the time he talks out of turn and interrupts conversations of those around him. He is very inattentive in his first-grade classroom and rarely completes assignments without one-to-one supervision. Will frequently gets sent to the principal's office for oppositional and disruptive behavior. He has difficulty playing games with peers because he rarely can wait for his turn and becomes overly upset when he loses. Will has a normal physical exam and no history of significant medical illnesses. He is not taking any medications at this time except a multivitamin with fluoride. His eyesight and hearing are also normal. He has a first cousin who was diagnosed with ADHD without hyperactivity and dyslexia. Family history is negative for any other psychiatric problems. School testing revealed a normal IQ without any specific learning disabilities.

Will was diagnosed with ADHD-HI and started on a trial of methylphenidate (Ritalin). Weighing 20 kilograms, he had a good response to a dose of 10 mg before school and 5 mg at noon. School behavior problems were greatly reduced on this regimen. His mother, however, noted a problem with intense hyperactivity and emotional instability in the evenings. This affective lability was not present on the weekends when Will did not receive methylphenidate. "Ritalin rebound" was diagnosed, and a trial of Adderall was instituted. Will's psychiatrist reasoned that Adderall, with its longer half-life, might not cause the stimulant-rebound phenomenon experienced with Ritalin. On a dose of 5 mg with breakfast and 2.5 mg at lunch, the problem with evening hyperactivity resolved. Will maintained his improved behavior and academic performance at school. Two weeks later, however, Will developed loud vocal tics which could be heard in the adjacent classrooms. His parents immediately took him back to his psychiatrist. In William's case his psychiatrist discontinued the Adderall and started guanfacine. William's tics decreased in frequency and severity after a 2-month treatment course, but his residual ADHD symptoms were still quite troubling to him and his classmates. The guanfacine also caused a significant amount of sedation. Will was subsequently taken off the guanfacine and given a trial of olanzapine. Within 2 months his tics had resolved, but the olanzapine did not help with Will's hyperactivity and inattention. He was glad when the olanzapine was discontinued because of the lethargy he experienced while treated with this medication. William's psychiatrist suggested a trial of long-acting methylphenidate to treat his continuing ADHD symptoms. Because of his parents' fears of a reexacerbation of tics, they elected not to restart any stimulants. His schoolwork problems were addressed with the assignment of a one-to-one instructional aide and behavioral modification protocols. He was also enrolled in a social skills group led by the school counselor. By the end of the school year, he was completing more of his assignments and getting along better with his peers. (Sometimes clinicians forget improved school performance can be achieved without medication.) It is interesting to note that Will still receives olanzapine periodically for tics. Fortunately, a course of 3 to 5 days results in the cessation of a tic episode.

BIBLIOGRAPHY

AACAP. Practice parameter for the use of stimulant medications in the treatment of children, adolescents and adults. *J Am Acad Child Adolesc Psychiatry* 2002;41(Suppl. 2):26S–49S.

Arnsten AFT, Castellanos FX. Neurobiology of attention regulation and its disorders. In: Martin A, Scahill L, Charney DS, Leckman JF, eds. *Pediatric psychopharmacology: principles and practice.* New York: Oxford University Press, 2003:99–109.

Barkley RA. *Attention deficit hyperactivity disorder: a handbook for diagnosis and treatment*, 2nd ed. New York: Guilford Press, 1998.

Biederman J. Resolved: mania is mistaken for ADHD in prepubertal children, affirmative. *J Am Acad Child Adolesc Psychiatry* 1998;37:1091–1093.

Brown TE. *Attention-deficit disorders and comorbidities in children, adolescents and adults.* Washington, DC: American Psychiatric Press, 2000.

Byrne JM, DeWolfe NA, Bawden HN. Assessment of attention-deficit hyperactivity disorder in preschoolers. *Child Neuropsychol* 1998;4:49–66.

Castellanos FX, Swanson J. Biological underpinnings of ADHD. In: Sandberg S, ed. *Hyperactivity and attention disorders of childhood: Cambridge monographs in child and adolescent psychiatry.* Cambridge: Cambridge University Press, 2002.

Clements SD, Peters JE. Minimal brain dysfunction in the school-age child. *Arch Gen Psychiatry* 1962;6:185–197.

Conners CK. *Conners ADHD DSM-IV scales for parents and teachers: technical manual.* North Tonowanda, New York: Multi Health Systems, 1997.

Dulcan M, Benson RS. Practice parameters for the assessment and treatment of children, adolescents and adults with attention-deficit/hyperactivity disorder. *J Am Acad Child Adolesc Psychiatry* 1997;36(Suppl. 10):85S–121S.

DuPaul GJ, McGoey KE, Eckert TL, et al. Preschool children with attention deficit/hyperactivity disorder: impairment in behavioral, social, and school functioning. *J Am Acad Child Adolesc Psychiatry* 2001;40:508–515.

Faraone SV, Biederman J. The neurobiology of attention deficit hyperactivity disorder. In: Charney DS, Nestler EJ, Bunney BS, eds. *Neurobiology of mental illness.* New York: Oxford University Press, 1999:788–801.

Jensen PS, Kettle L, Roper MT, et al. Are stimulants overprescribed: treatment of ADHD in four US communities. *J Am Acad Child Adolesc Psychiatry* 1999;38:797–804.

Jensen PS. ADHD comorbidity and treatment outcomes in the MTA. *J Am Acad Child Adolesc Psychiatry* 2001;40:134–136.

Mannuzza S, Klein RG, Bessler A, et al. Adult psychiatric status of hyperactive boys grown up. *Am J Psychiatry* 1998;155:493–498.

MTA Cooperative Group. A 14-month randomized clinical trial of treatment strategies for attention deficit/hyperactivity disorder. *Arch Gen Psychiatry* 1999;56:1073–1086.

MTA Cooperative Group. Moderators and mediators of treatment response for children with attention-deficit/hyperactivity disorder. *Arch Gen Psychiatry* 1999;56:1088–1096.

National Institutes of Health. National Institutes of Health Consensus Development Conference statement: diagnosis and treatment of attention deficit hyperactivity disorder (ADHD). *J Am Acad Child Adolesc Psychiatry* 2000;39:182–193.

Olfson M, Gameroff MJ, Marcus SC, et al. National trends in the treatment of attention deficit hyperactivity disorder. *Am J Psychiatry* 2003;160:1071–1077.

Pelham WE, Wheeler T, Chronis A. Empirically supported psychosocial treatments for Attention Deficit Hyperactivity Disorder. *J Consult Clin Psychol* 1998;27:190–205.

Still GF. The Coulston lectures on some abnormal physical conditions in children. *Lancet* 1902;1:1008–1012.

Strauss AA, Lehtinen LE. *Psychopathology and education in the brain injured child.* New York: Grune & Statton, 1947.

Stubbe DE. Attention-deficit/hyperactivity disorder. *Child and adolescent psychiatric clinics of North America 9.* Philadelphia, PA: WB Saunders, 2000.

Szatmari P. The epidemiology of attention-deficit hyperactivity disorders. In: Weiss G, ed. *Attention-deficit hyperactivity disorder.* Philadelphia, PA: WB Saunders, 1992:361–371.

Taylor E. Development of clinical services for attention-deficit/hyperactivity disorder. *Arch Gen Psychiatry* 1999;56:1097–1099.

Weiss G, Hechtman LT. *Hyperactive children grown up: ADHD in children, adolescents, and adults*, 2nd ed. New York: Guilford Press, 1993.

Zito JM, Safer DJ, dosReis S, et al. Trends in the prescribing of psychotropic medications to preschoolers. *JAMA* 2000;283:1025–1030.

SUGGESTED READINGS

Newsletters/online resources for parents and public

Attention! The Magazine of Children and Adults with Attention Deficit Disorders, 449 N.W. 70th Avenue, Suite 208, Plantation, FL 33317

Challenge: The First National Newsletter on Attention Deficit (Hyperactivity) Disorder. P.O. Box 2001, West Newbury, MA 01985

Children and Adults with Attention-Deficit/Hyperactivity Disorder (CHADD). http://www.chadd.org

National Attention Deficit Disorder Association (ADDA). http://www.add.org

Readings for parents, patients, and teachers

Barkley RA PhD. *Taking charge of ADHD: the complete, authoritative guide for parents.* New York: Guilford Press, 1995.

(A comprehensive reference volume on all aspects of ADHD for parents and teachers.)

Braswell L, Bloomquist M, Pederson S. *A guide to understanding and helping children with attention deficit hyperactivity disorder in school settings.* Minneapolis, MN: University of Minnesota, Department of Professional Development and Conference Services, Continuing Education and Extension, 315 Pillsbury Drive S.E., 55455, 1991;612:625–3504.

Clark L. *The time-out solution: a parent's guide for handling everyday behavior problems.* Chicago, IL: Contemporary Books, 1989.

(Lots of detail on using time-out, but also other punishments and positive ways of increasing appropriate behavior. Includes examples, checklists, and tear-out reminder sheets.)

Fowler MC. *Maybe you know my kid: a parent's guide to identifying, understanding and helping your child with attention deficit hyperactive disorder.* New York: Carol Publishing Group, 1990.

Garber SW, Garber MD, Spizman RF. *Is your child hyperactive? Inattentive? Impulsive? Distractible? Helping the ADD/Hyperactive child.* New York: Villard Books, 1995.

(A practical program for changing behavior with or without medication.)

Hallowell EM, Ratey JJ. *Driven to distraction: recognizing and coping with attention deficit disorder from childhood through adulthood.* New York: Pantheon Books, 1994.

(Written by two psychiatrists who have ADHD themselves. Especially strong on the diagnosis and treatment of ADHD in adults.)

Hallowell EM, Ratey JJ. *Answers to distraction.* New York: Pantheon Books, 1994.

(The sequel to Driven to Distraction: Recognizing and Coping with Attention Deficit Disorder from Childhood through Adulthood.)

Ingersoll B. *Your hyperactive child: a parent's guide to coping with attention deficit disorder.* New York: Doubleday, 1988.

(A comprehensive book with many examples. Includes brief guidelines for teachers and an appendix with behavioral management programs for classroom use.)

Ingersoll B, Goldstein S. *Attention deficit disorder and learning disabilities: realities, myths and controversial treatments.* New York: Doubleday Main Street Books, 1993.

(A review by two psychologists focusing on causes and treatment. Good coverage of common myths and unfounded claims.)

Kelly K, Ramundo P. *You mean I'm not lazy, stupid or crazy?* New York: NY Fireside Books, 1996.

(A book targeted for youths with ADHD.)

Nadeau K. *Survival guide for college students with ADD or LD.* New York: Magination Press, 1994.

(A handy practical guide for the ADHD college student.)

For clinicians

The ADHD Report. New York: Guilford Press, 72 Spring St., 10012.

CHAPTER 5

Oppositional Defiant Disorder and Conduct Disorder

FRANCHESKA PEREPLETCHIKOVA
ALAN E. KAZDIN

Introduction

Oppositional defiant disorder (ODD) and conduct disorder (CD) encompass a range of dysfunctional behaviors that emerge over the course of childhood. Both ODD and CD include hostile and defiant behavior toward authority, such as disobedience, temper tantrums, argumentativeness, and refusal to comply with requests. However, individuals with ODD do not exhibit the more severe and persistent behavior patterns of CD, such as aggression toward others, destruction of property, theft, and deceit. Although this chapter covers both ODD and CD, greater attention is accorded the latter disorder. Much more is known about the onset, clinical course, and long-term outcomes of CD. Also, CD has more deleterious consequences for the individual, the family, and society at large.

Disruptive behaviors encompass a variety of acts that reflect social rule violations and actions against others. Many of these behaviors such as argumentativeness, temper tantrums, resentfulness, lying, fighting, and bullying others are relatively common among children over the course of normal development. The diagnoses ODD and CD are reserved for instances in which disruptive behaviors lead to impairment in everyday functioning, as reflected in unmanageability at home and at school or disorderly acts that affect others.

Contemporary diagnosis, as reflected in the 1994 *Diagnostic and Statistical Manual of Mental Disorders*, Fourth Edition (DSM-IV), has recognized an increased number of disorders among children and adolescents. Antisocial, disruptive, obstreperous, oppositional, unmanageable, and delinquent child behaviors have been acknowledged throughout history even though their identification as part of psychiatric diagnosis is quite recent. The behaviors have been attributed to possession by the devil, criminality, and, only quite recently, mental illness. Extreme measures often have been allowed. For example, early in the history of the United States (in Massachusetts), there was a law that such children could be killed if their parents approved. The fact that conduct problems represent dysfunction that warrants intervention has not been questioned. The challenge and advances within the past 25 years have been to delineate the disorders of conduct and to identify ways to treat or prevent them.

Clinical Features

ODD and CD are closely related, as evidenced by the work of Rowe et al. Several somewhat different models of the nature of this relationship have been proposed. Because all features of ODD are evident in CD, ODD is usually viewed as a precursor to CD. CD is also seen as a more severe form of ODD. Furthermore, ODD is sometimes viewed as a subtype of CD. Finally, because these disorders are similar in etiology, the distinction between CD and ODD itself has been questioned. In short, the precise nature of the relationship between these disorders is still a matter of debate and empirical attention.

DIAGNOSTIC CRITERIA FOR OPPOSITIONAL DEFIANT DISORDER

DSM-IV delineates ODD as a recurrent pattern of negativistic, hostile, and defiant behavior. Table 5.1 lists the main symptoms. A diagnosis of ODD is provided if the individual shows at least four symptoms within the past 6 months. To meet the criteria, the behavior must occur more frequently than is typically observed in individuals of compatible age and developmental level and must be associated with impaired functioning.

TABLE 5.1. MAJOR DIAGNOSTIC SYMPTOMS OF OPPOSITIONAL DEFIANT DISORDER

1. Often loses temper.
2. Often argues with adults.
3. Often actively defies or refuses to comply with adult's requests or rules.
4. Often deliberately annoys people.
5. Often blames others for his or her mistakes or misbehavior.
6. Is often touchy or easily annoyed by others.
7. If often angry or resentful.
8. Is often spiteful or vindictive.

From American Psychiatric Association. *Diagnostic and statistical manual of mental disorders*, 4th ed, Text rev. Washington, DC: American Psychiatric Association, 2000, with permission.

DIAGNOSTIC CRITERIA FOR CONDUCT DISORDER

Current diagnosis using the DSM-IV delineates CD as the violation of basic rights of others and age-appropriate societal norms as the essential features. Table 5.2 lists the main symptoms. A diagnosis of CD is provided if the individual shows at least three symptoms occurring within the past 12 months, with at least one of the symptoms evident in the last 6 months. To meet the criteria, the behaviors must be repetitive and persistent and be associated with impaired functioning.

Many ways of subtyping have been proposed. Historically, the greatest evidence has accumulated for aggressive and nonaggressive subtypes. These are characterized by youths who engage primarily in fighting as opposed to stealing. Some youths are of a mixed type, show symptoms of both, and have a particularly untoward prognosis. In current research, another way of delineating subtypes has focused on age of onset. Two types are distinguished that vary in the nature of conduct problems, developmental course and prognosis, and gender ratio.

Childhood-onset CD is characterized by aggressive behavior. Symptoms usually emerge early in childhood. Individuals with this subtype are usually boys, are aggressive, have disturbed peer relationships, have more persistent CD, and are more likely to develop adult antisocial personality disorder than are those with adolescent-onset CD. These individuals usually had ODD during early childhood and have symptoms that meet the full criteria for CD before puberty.

Adolescent-onset CD is defined by the absence of CD symptoms prior to age 10. Individuals with this type usually have more normative peer relationships and are less likely to display aggressive behaviors, have persistent CD, and develop antisocial personality disorder than those with childhood-onset type. Moreover, the adolescent-onset type is more evenly distributed among boys and girls. Symptoms are more likely to reflect vandalism and illegal behaviors than aggressive acts.

There has been support for the subtypes but a great deal more work is needed to identify whether there are key characteristics that can be identified to refine this grouping further. Also, age of onset in childhood versus adolescence is not very sensitive to large differences seen clinically. For example, among prepubertal children (all considered child-onset types), onset, symptom pattern and severity, family history, and long-term course can vary widely.

TABLE 5.2. MAJOR DIAGNOSTIC SYMPTOMS OF CONDUCT DISORDER

1. Bullying or threatening others.
2. Fighting.
3. Using a weapon that can cause serious physical harm to others.
4. Being physically cruel to people.
5. Being physically cruel to animals.
6. Stealing while confronting a victim (e.g., mugging, purse snatching, extortion, armed robbery).
7. Forcing someone into sexual activity.
8. Fire setting.
9. Destroying property of others.
10. Breaking into someone else's house, building, or car.
11. Frequent lying or "conning" others.
12. Stealing without confronting a victim.
13. Staying out late at night despite parental prohibitions.
14. Running away from home.
15. Being truant from school.

From American Psychiatric Association. *Diagnostic and statistical manual of mental disorders*, 4th ed, Text rev. Washington, DC: American Psychiatric Association, 2000, with permission.

LIMITATIONS IN CONTEMPORARY DIAGNOSIS OF OPPOSITIONAL DEFIANT DISORDER AND CONDUCT DISORDER

There are several limitations to the DSM-IV diagnostic criteria of ODD and CD. First, the criteria for diagnosis of ODD and CD are somewhat arbitrary. For example, there is no firm empiric basis for selecting the minimal number of symptoms or a time period as part of the criteria. Variation in the number of symptoms or time period on either side of the cutoff points does not appear to be clinically or prognostically meaningful. Furthermore, diagnosis of ODD relies on the subjective estimation of whether the behavior occurs more frequently than is typically observed in normal development. Such decisions are arbitrary because no specific criterion is present or is based on evidence that would consider sex, cultural, and ethnic differences. Second, the diagnostic criteria do not include a core set of symptoms. This allows for a vast heterogeneity of symptom patterns within the diagnosis. Indeed, the requirement of at least 3 of 15 criteria yields an astonishing 32,647 ways in which the CD diagnosis may be met. Third, features of ODD and CD are observable in other disorders, which raise concerns about the meaningfulness of the current categorical delineation of disruptive behavior problems. Fourth, diagnosis of CD seems to be age-biased. The diagnostic symptoms are the same or applied in the same way across ages. However, some behaviors, such as stealing, running away, and fire setting, may be less evident in younger ages. There is a need for a more flexible system with symptoms varying depending on age. Finally, DSM-IV criteria do not account for sex differences. Diagnostic symptoms of CD focus on aggressive and violent actions that are more likely in boys. Girls, on the other hand, are more likely to engage in less obvious acts, such as stealing or lying. Such bias may account for the higher prevalence of CD among boys.

Differential Diagnoses and Comorbid Disorders

OPPOSITIONAL DEFIANT DISORDER

ODD is comorbid with attention deficit hyperactivity disorder (ADHD), anxiety disorders, and depressive disorders, as detailed by Angold and Costello. The comorbid condition of ODD and ADHD is associated with greater family conflict, teen management difficulties, rebelliousness, antisocial acts, and earlier substance abuse. Furthermore, symptoms of ODD are sometimes evident in individuals with mental retardation. A diagnosis of ODD is given only if the oppositional behavior is markedly greater than is commonly observed among individuals of comparable age, gender, and severity of cognitive problems.

Features of ODD can be evident in other disorders, such as mood disorder, psychotic disorders, and disorders of language comprehension. Differential diagnosis is based on the associated behavioral patterns and accompanying symptoms. Both ODD and CD include hostile and defiant behavior toward authority, such as disobedience, argumentativeness, temper tantrums, and refusal to comply with requests. However, individuals with ODD do not exhibit more severe and persistent behavior patterns such as aggression toward others and destruction of property. When a behavior pattern meets both diagnoses, the diagnosis of CD takes precedence. Oppositional behavior is a common feature of mood and psychotic disorders and should not be diagnosed separately if symptoms occur exclusively during the course of these disorders. ODD should also be distinguished from a failure to follow directions that results from impaired language comprehension, such as in hearing loss and mixed receptive-expressive language disorder.

CONDUCT DISORDER

CD has a high rate of comorbidity over the course of childhood and adolescence, especially with ADHD, depressive disorders, anxiety disorders, and substance use disorders, as described by Angold and Costello. The combination of ADHD and CD is especially common, with estimates from 45% to 70% of children with one of these disorders also meeting criteria for the other. Children with both diagnoses show high levels of conduct problems, peer rejection, school problems, and conflictual interactions with parents. Comorbid anxiety disorder has been linked to lower levels of aggression and violence (at least in younger children) but higher rates of shyness and social withdrawal. Comorbid among adolescents, depression is strongly associated with suicide, especially when coupled with substance use disorders.

Features of CD are also evident in other disorders, including adjustment disorders, mania, child or adolescent antisocial behavior, and antisocial personality disorder. Differential diagnoses can be discerned from the onset and course of each disorder, associated behavioral patterns, and accompanying symptoms. A manic episode can occur in children and adolescents with conduct problems. The episodic course and accompanying core symptoms of mood elevation distinguish a manic episode from CD. Adjustment disorders with disturbance of conduct are differentiated from CD by an associated psychosocial stressor preceding the conduct problems. Isolated behavior problems that do not meet criteria for CD or adjustment disorder can be coded as child or adolescent antisocial behavior. Antisocial personality disorder is diagnosed when the individual is at least 18 years old, meets criteria for CD before the age of 15 years, and continues antisocial behavior. For individuals over age 18, a diagnosis of CD is given only if the criteria for antisocial personality disorder are not met.

Epidemiology

The prevalence of a disorder refers to the percentage of cases in the population at a given point in time. Among school-aged community samples, the prevalence of ODD and CD combined is approximately 2% to 16%. This estimate is conservative in representing the scope of the problem because research suggests that meeting the diagnostic criteria cutoff is not meaningful in relation to the course of ODD and CD. Children who approach, but do not quite meet, the diagnostic criteria are also likely to have significant impairment in their everyday lives and poor long-term prognoses, especially in the case of CD.

ODD is more prevalent in boys than in girls, especially before puberty. Such differences can be explained by more consistent parental expectations and reinforcement of girls and more unresponsive and rejective parenting of boys. Parents also tend to tolerate more excessive behaviors from boys. Furthermore, girls may have more difficulty in expressing anger and are more inclined to refrain from behaviors that would negatively affect relationships such as oppositionality, which evokes frustration and annoyance.

Boys also show approximately 3 to 4 times higher rates of CD than girls. The sex differences may also be explained by the above factors and by differences in predispositions toward responding in aggressive ways and the base rates in the different symptoms that comprise CD. Age variations reveal interesting patterns in prevalence rates. Rates of CD tend to be higher for adolescents (approximately 7% for youths ages 12–16) than for children (approximately 4% for children ages 4–11 years). Childhood onset and adolescent onset CD are often considered to represent distinguishable patterns in light of the symptom patterns, sex distribution, and long-term course, as highlighted later.

The prevalence does not convey the scope of the problem from a clinical or social perspective. Symptoms of CD represent clinically important criteria for referring one third to one half of youth for inpatient and outpatient treatment. Moreover, CD has been identified as the most costly mental health problem, at least in the United States. This is due in large part to the findings that children referred for treatment are likely to become involved in several service systems (e.g., mental health, juvenile justice, special education), and this may continue throughout childhood and well into adulthood.

Clinical Course

Typically, ODD becomes evident before age 8. In a significant proportion of cases, ODD is a developmental precursor of CD. Little is known, however, about the outcomes of children with ODD who do not develop antisocial and aggressive symptoms. As discussed previously, CD can emerge in childhood or in adolescence. Adolescent onset is more common and is more equally distributed among boys and girls. Childhood onset is considered to be a more severe form of CD as it usually leads to more severe outcomes. Longitudinal studies show that CD in childhood predicts aggressive and antisocial behavior up to 30 years later. Among CD youths identified in childhood, slightly less than 50% continue their CD into adulthood. If all comorbid diagnoses are considered, apart from CD, slightly over 80% are likely to show a psychiatric disorder as adults. Psychiatric disorder in adulthood is only one of many untoward prognostic features. As highlighted in Table 5.3, individuals with a history of CD evince a broad range of negative outcomes.

Etiology and Pathogenesis

RISK FACTORS

There is no single defining set of symptoms that constitute ODD or CD. Children who meet the diagnosis for either of these disorders may not share any symptoms in light of the heterogeneity of the current diagnostic criteria. Consequently, on *a priori* grounds it is unlikely

TABLE 5.3. LONG-TERM PROGNOSIS OF YOUTHS IDENTIFIED AS CONDUCT DISORDERED: MAJOR CHARACTERISTICS LIKELY TO BE EVIDENT IN ADULTHOOD

Major Characteristics	Prognosis
Psychiatric status	Greater psychiatric impairment including antisocial personality, alcohol and drug abuse, and isolated symptoms (e.g., anxiety, somatic complaints); also, greater history of psychiatric hospitalization.
Criminal behavior	Higher rates of driving while intoxicated, criminal behavior, arrest records, conviction, and period of time spent in jail.
Occupation adjustment	Less likely to be employed; shorter history of employment, lower status jobs, more frequent change of jobs, lower wages, and depend more frequently on financial assistance (welfare). Served less frequently and performed less well in the armed services.
Educational attainment	Higher rates of dropping out of school; lower attainment among those who remain in school.
Marital status	Higher rates of divorce, remarriage, and separation.
Social participation	Less contact with relatives, friends, and neighbors; little participation in organizations such as church.
Physical health	Higher mortality rate; higher rate of hospitalization for physical problems.

Note: These characteristics are based on comparisons of clinically referred children identified for conduct disorder relative to control clinical referrals or normal controls or from comparisons of delinquent and nondelinquent youths (see Pepper and Rubin, 1991; Peters, McMahon, and Quinsey, 1992).

that there would be a simple etiology. The diagnosis may require finer distinctions in terms of subgroups, time of onset, and clinical course before advances will be made. A great deal is known about the onset of CD, which has been studied much more thoroughly than ODD.

Rather than etiology, research focuses on multiple risk factors that contribute to the onset. This shift is in recognition that there are multiple factors that contribute to CD and multiple paths. *Risk factors* refer to characteristics, events, or processes that increase the likelihood (risk) for the onset of a problem or dysfunction. Risk factors, as antecedents to the dysfunction, may provide clues as to the development and progression of CD, possible mechanisms and processes through which the dysfunctions come about, and foci for possible intervention. Several factors that predispose children and adolescents to behavior problems are highlighted in Table 5.4.

PROTECTIVE FACTORS

Even under very adverse conditions with multiple risk factors present, many individuals will not experience adverse outcomes. Protective factors refer to characteristics, events, or

TABLE 5.4. FACTORS THAT PLACE YOUTHS AT RISK FOR THE ONSET OF OPPOSITIONAL DEFIANT DISORDER AND CONDUCT DISORDER

Child factors

Child Temperament: a more difficult child temperament (on a dimension of "easy to difficult"), as characterized by more negative mood, lower levels of approach toward new stimuli, and less adaptability to change.

Neuropsychological Deficits and Difficulties: deficits in diverse functions related to language (e.g., verbal learning, verbal fluency, verbal IQ), memory, motor coordination, integration of auditory and visual cues, and "executive" functions of the brain (e.g., abstract reasoning, concept formation, planning, control of attention).

Subclinical Levels of Conduct Disorder: early signs (e.g., elementary school) of mild ("subclinical") levels of unmanageability and aggression, especially with early age of onset; multiple types of antisocial behaviors, and multiple situations in which they are evident (e.g., at home, school, the community).

Academic and Intellectual Performance: academic deficiencies and lower levels of intellectual functioning.

Parent and family factors

Prenatal and Perinatal Complications: pregnancy and birth-related complications including maternal infection, prematurity and low birth weight, impaired respiration at birth, and minor birth injury.

Psychopathology and Criminal Behavior in the Family: criminal behavior, antisocial personality disorder, and alcoholism of a parent.

Poor Parental Practices: coercive parent-child communications, inconsistent disciplining, harsh or corporal punishment, and permissive or overcontrolling parenting.

Monitoring of the Child: poor supervision, lack of monitoring of whereabouts, and few rules about where youths can go and when they can return.

Quality of the Family Relationships: less parental acceptance of their children, less warmth, affection, and emotional support, and less attachment.

Marital Discord: unhappy marital relationships, interpersonal conflict, and aggression of the parents.

Family Size: larger family size (i.e., more children in the family).

Sibling with Antisocial Behavior: presence of a sibling, especially an older brother, with antisocial behavior.

Socioeconomic Disadvantage: poverty, overcrowding, unemployment, receipt of social assistance ("welfare"), and poor housing.

School-related factors

Characteristics of the Setting: attending schools where there is little emphasis on academic work, little teacher time spent on lessons, infrequent teacher use of praise and appreciation for school work, little emphasis on individual responsibility of the students, poor working conditions for pupils (e.g., furniture in poor repair), unavailability of the teacher to deal with children's problems, and low teacher expectations.

Note: The list of risk factors highlights major influences. Identified factors are generally stronger predictors of conduct disorder than oppositional defiant disorder. The number of factors and the relations of specific factors to risk are more complex than the summary statements noted here (see Burke, Loeber, and Birmaher, 2002; Hendren, 1999; Kazdin, 1995; Stoff, Breiling, and Maser, 1997).

processes that decrease the impact of a risk factor and the likelihood of an adverse outcome. Protective factors are identified by studying individuals known to be at risk (who show several risk factors) and by delineating subgroups of those who do, versus those who do not, later develop CD. Among a high-risk sample, children are less likely to develop CD if they are first-born, are perceived by their mothers as affectionate, show high self-esteem and locus of control, and have alternative caretakers in the family (in addition to the parents) and a supportive same-sex model who played an important role in their development. Other factors that reduce or attenuate risk include above-average intelligence, competence in various skill areas, getting along with peers, and having friends.

The mechanisms through which risk and protective factors may exert their influence is not known. As an exception, parenting practices (e.g., harsh punishment, attending to aggressive child behavior) have been well studied. These practices directly contribute to aggressive and antisocial behavior. Moreover, altering these practices reduces aggressive and antisocial child behavior, as evidenced by Reid et al.

Antisocial behavior runs in families. Twin and adoption studies indicate a genetic influence on antisocial behavior and deviance in general. Advances in molecular genetics will no doubt lead to breakthroughs that move closer to understanding mechanisms of action and subgroups of youths. For example, Caspi found that children who are maltreated are especially likely to develop antisocial behavior if they have a gene encoding a specific neurotransmitter-metabolizing enzyme. Further research relating genotype of vulnerability to subsequent risk factors will add considerably to the identification of subgroups and pathways involved in CD.

Assessment

ODD and CD are usually evaluated using multiple assessment modalities. These modalities have been described in detail separately by Kazdin and Sommers-Flanagan. Each modality may be more or less relevant for the purposes of a particular assessment and may yield information not attainable by other forms of assessment. For example, raters can have limited knowledge about a child's conduct problems. Conclusions about symptoms, severity of dysfunction, and changes over time will vary for different measures. Furthermore, youths with behavior problems tend to exhibit symptoms in some settings but not others. Therefore, utilizing multimethod, multirater, and multisetting assessment approaches would provide a better picture of each psychopathology. Table 5.5 presents the essentials of assessment.

TABLE 5.5. ESSENTIALS OF ASSESSMENT OF OPPOSITIONAL DEFIANT DISORDER AND CONDUCT DISORDER

1. Multimethod, multirater, and multisetting assessment approaches should be utilized in the evaluation of ODD and CD.
2. There are no specific assessment instruments that have been established to be individually diagnostic for ODD and CD.
3. There are no core symptoms associated with making the diagnosis of ODD and CD.
4. When a behavior pattern meets both diagnoses, the diagnosis of CD takes precedence.
5. Parental practices, parent-child interactions, parental psychopathology, and child's peer relationships should be assessed for treatment planning and delivery.
6. Educational assessment should be performed if school or learning problems are suspected.
7. Functional analysis of the behavior patterns, including baseline and follow-up ratings, should be performed to evaluate the effectiveness of treatment.

ODD, oppositional defiant disorder; CD, conduct disorder.

SELF-REPORT MEASURES

Self-report measures are used in the assessment of childhood psychopathologies because they can elicit information not apparent to parents, not obtainable from institutional records, or not evident through direct observations. Children over 10 years old and adolescents readily report their disruptive behavior and can provide a valid account of their conduct. However, younger children rarely identify themselves as having a problem. The ability of children to report their psychological maladjustment is not as clear as that of adolescents or adults, at least in relation to conventional self-report measures. Although, for these reasons, self-report inventories are not usually used as primary measures among young children, they are still regarded as a valuable source of important information.

Several self-report measures are currently available to assess disruptive behavior problems. Selected examples of the measures that have been studied extensively include the *Children's Action Tendency Scale* by Deluty, the *Adolescent Antisocial Self-Report Behavior Checklist* by Kulik, Stein, and Sarbin, and the *Self-Report Delinquency Scale* by Elliott, Dunford, and Huizinga. The *Children's Action Tendency Scale*, intended for ages 6 to 15 years, is a 30-item questionnaire that asks a child to select what he or she would do in an interpersonal situation. The format is forced–choice, and responses fall along three dimensions: aggressiveness, assertiveness, and submissiveness. The *Adolescent Antisocial Self-Report Behavior Checklist* measures a broad range of behaviors from mild misconduct to serious antisocial acts. It consists of 52 items rated on a 5-point scale (from never to very often). Items load on four factors: delinquency, drug use, parental defiance, and assaultiveness. The *Self-Report Delinquency Scale* is intended for ages 11 to 21. This instrument asks about the occurrences of delinquent acts at home, at school, and in the community over the last year. The measure consists of 47 items rated on a 4-point scale (from $1 =$ once to $4 =$ four or more times). The items encompass theft, property damage, illegal services (e.g., peddling drugs), public disorder, status offenses (e.g., running away), and index offenses (e.g., assaults).

REPORTS OF SIGNIFICANT OTHERS

Reports of significant others (e.g., parents, relatives, teachers) are most frequently used as a measure of childhood psychopathology. Parents are in a unique position to provide accounts of a child's functioning and changes over time. Their reports correlate significantly with clinical judgments. Furthermore, such inventories are easy to administer and can cover a wide range of symptoms. However, reports of significant others have their own limitations. Parents sometimes are unaware of covert acts such as stealing and substance abuse. Also, parental evaluations can be influenced by parental stress and psychopathology.

The *Eyberg Child Behavior Inventory* is a frequently used and well-studied measure for oppositional and conduct problems completed by significant others. This measure is intended for ages 2 to 17. This 36-item inventory is designed to assess a frequency of a wide range of behavior problems that occur at home. A parent is asked to endorse whether each item is a problem (yes, no) and specify the frequency of occurrences on a 7-point scale (from never to always). The scores reflect the number of items endorsed as a problem and the intensity of problems.

Scales that can be applied to conduct problems, but also across the full spectrum of symptoms, are commonly used. The most widely used measure is the *Child Behavior Checklist* by Achenbach. The measure has multiple versions completed by different raters (parent, teacher, adolescent/child) and provides scores to evaluate externalizing and internalizing behaviors. The utility of this measure derives from widespread use and standardization among clinic and nonclinic samples. Also, broad and specific scales are available to assess aggression, delinquency, and ADHD to provide fine-grained analyses of individual symptom domains.

DIRECT OBSERVATION

Observations directly sample behaviors and do not have to rely on recollections or general impressions. Also, observations can provide actual frequencies of particular behaviors. However, they have several drawbacks and limitations. Covert acts and infrequently occurring behaviors are not readily observable directly. Also, the act of observation, if evident to the child or parent, can influence performance. Furthermore, direct observations may require extensive training to ensure accuracy and reliability, which makes them quite costly and time consuming.

An example of a relatively elaborate direct observational measure is the *Family Interaction Coding System* by Reid. This system is designed for ages 3 to 12. It records parent-child behaviors in the home. The occurrences and nonoccurences of 29 different behaviors are coded by observers within small intervals of 1 hour each day for a period of several days. Individual behaviors are usually summarized with a total aversive behavior score.

INSTITUTIONAL AND SOCIETAL RECORDS

Institutional records are frequently used to measure antisocial behavior because they represent a significant indicator of the impact of the problem on society, can reveal important social trends, facilitate decisions about allocation of resources and services, and can be utilized to evaluate interventions designed to reduce dysfunctional behavior problems. However, official records can greatly underestimate the occurrence of antisocial behavior because most delinquent acts are not observed or recorded. Examples of institutional and societal records include school attendance, grades, graduation, suspensions, expulsions, contacts with police, arrest records, and convictions.

Treatment

Many different treatments have been applied, including pharmacotherapy; psychotherapy; home, school, and community-based programs; residential and hospital treatment; and assorted social services. Relatively few treatments have been carefully evaluated in controlled studies and been shown to reduce ODD and CD problems and to improve functioning of the child in everyday life. Table 5.6 presents treatment essentials of ODD and CD, and key points are elaborated below.

PHARMACOLOGIC TREATMENT

Pharmacotherapy is rarely reported or studied for ODD. Medications for CD have been used primarily to alleviate aggression, reduce reactivity preceding aggressive behaviors, and moderate levels of emotional arousal as reported by multiple investigators including Burke et al.; Gerardin et al.; Green; Waslick et al.; and Werry and Aman. Medication-based interventions are predicated on research findings that disruptive behavior problems are at least partially attributable to disturbances in neurobiologic mechanisms. Because few randomized controlled trials have been performed to establish the effectiveness of medications, ODD and CD have no standard pharmacologic treatment. Medications that have been variably useful in treating disruptive behavior problems include stimulants,

TABLE 5.6. ESSENTIALS OF TREATMENT OF OPPOSITIONAL DEFIANT DISORDER AND CONDUCT DISORDER

1. Pharmacologic treatment alone is not sufficient in the management of the majority of CD cases.
2. Evidence-based psychosocial treatments should be utilized.
3. Treatment planning should consider child's age, severity and range of problems, family needs, and commitment.
4. Comorbid diagnoses should be identified and treated.
5. Parental guidance is critical in the management of ODD and CD.
6. Parental psychopathology and stress should be considered.
7. All areas and setting in which a child exhibits behavior problems should be identified and addressed.

CD, conduct disorder; ODD, oppositional defiant disorder.

adrenolytic drugs, mood stabilizers, and neuroleptics. Table 5.7 highlights major therapeutic classes of medications and their clinical and side effects.

Psychostimulants, such as amphetamine and methylphenidate, are thought to exert their primary neuropharmacologic effects by facilitating the release of neurotransmitters that positively correlate with levels of aggression. They appear to have a dose-dependent effect. Low doses stimulate aggressive behaviors, while moderate-to-high doses suppress aggressive behaviors. Stimulants have been demonstrated to reduce aggressive behaviors primarily in children with ADHD. There is some recent evidence, however, supporting their usefulness in reducing aggressive behaviors in children with ODD and CD, with and without ADHD. Stimulants are relatively safe in the application to childhood disorders and are recommended as a good initial choice for the aggressive child with underlying ADHD.

Mood stabilizers, such as lithium and anticonvulsants, reduce aggressive behaviors and are recommended for impulsivity, explosive temper, and mood lability. Adrenolytic drugs such as clonidine and propranolol are also useful in the treatment of behavior problems as

TABLE 5.7. PHARMACOLOGIC AGENTS USED IN TREATMENT OF OPPOSITIONAL DEFIANT DISORDER AND CONDUCT DISORDER

Therapeutic Class	Medication	Clinical Effect	Negative Side Effects
Psychostimulants	Methylphenidate Amphetamine	Dose-dependent effect; Diminish aggression; decrease motor activity level; reduce disinhibited behavior	Potentially addictive; loss of appetite; insomnia; tachycardia; nervousness; abdominal pain; and weight loss
Mood stabilizers	Lithium Anticonvulsants: Carbamazepine Valproic acid	Reduce aggression; decrease behavioral dyscontrol and manic excitement	Fine tremor; polydipsia; polyuria; nausea; malaise; sedation; weight gain; anorexia; hair loss; gastrointestinal upset
Antipsychotics	Chlorpromazine Thioridazine Haloperidol Clozapine Risperidone Droperidol	Reduce level of CNS activation	Tardive dyskinesia sedation; weight gain; anxiety; rigidity; hyperthermia; fluctuating vital signs
Adrenergic agents	Clonidine Guanfacine Propranolol Pindolol Nadolol Metoprolol	Reduce anger and aggression; decrease agitation and rage; increase frustration tolerance	Sedation; worsening or induction of depressive symptoms; fatigue; headache; insomnia; dizziness

CNS, central nervous system.

they help to mute aggression, reduce agitation and rage, and increase frustration tolerance, possibly by reducing adrenergic output.

Neuroleptics, or antipsychotic medications, such as chlorpromazine, haloperidol, and the newer atypical neuroleptics, such as risperidone and olanzapine, have reduced aggressive and violent behavior, hyperactivity, and social unresponsiveness. However, because of possible chronic tardive dyskinesia and other adverse side effects, it is recommended to utilize them primarily in severely aggressive CD. There may be a larger role for the atypical neuroleptics as their side effect profile is more benign than the traditional neuroleptics.

PSYCHOTHERAPIES

Over 550 therapies are in use for children and adolescents. A very small portion has been subjected to empiric tests. Interestingly, a few treatments have been well studied in relation to ODD and CD and qualify as evidence-based treatments in light of replications in controlled clinical trials.

Parent-management training refers to a treatment in which parents are trained to interact with the child in ways that promote prosocial behavior. The treatment focuses on the use of antecedents (e.g., prompts, setting events), reinforcement (e.g., praise, tokens), development of prosocial behavior, and other techniques to develop adaptive child behavior. Extensive research has shown that many parent–child interaction patterns in the home unwittingly foster and escalate child oppositional and aggressive behavior. Parent training teaches skills to the parent, develops interactions between parents and the child that promote positive parent and child behavior, and, in the process, decreases disruptive behavior.

Cognitive problem-solving skills training is based on research showing that youths with aggressive and antisocial behavior often show distortions in various cognitive processes (e.g., how individuals perceive, code, interpret, and experience the world, as reflected in beliefs, attributions, and expectations). A variety of cognitive processes pertain to interactions with others, including the ability to generate solutions to interpersonal problems and consequences of action (e.g., what would happen after a particular behavior). Problem-solving skills therapy develops skills in approaching interpersonal situations and teaches ways to identify prosocial or adaptive solutions and alternative consequences of actions. Children practice the approach in treatment sessions and in other settings (home, school) outside of treatment.

Multisystemic therapy focuses on the child behavior within the context of various systems (e.g., the family, peer group, schools) that may contribute to the child's problem behavior or could be used to help alter that behavior. A focus on the family as a system is designed to build better communication, to reduce negative interactions, and to improve the ability of the parents to function. Factors that can affect these interactions and the child's problems, such as stress that the parent experiences, marital conflict, and association of the child with a deviant peer group, are also a focus of treatment. Many different techniques are applied to address these areas. Parent-management training and problem-solving skills training often are incorporated into treatment. Several studies, especially with adjudicated adolescents, have attested to the efficacy and durability of the effects of multisystemic therapy.

The three treatments noted here are well studied. Others such as *anger-management training* and *functional family therapy* also have evidence on their behalf. Although there are now evidence-based treatments for ODD and CD, they are not widely available. In most clinical settings, general relationship therapy, play therapy, or psychodynamically oriented psychotherapy are more likely to be practiced.

Prevention

Early intervention programs with the family have been effective in reducing disruptive behaviors. These programs have been described by several investigators including McCord and Tremblay as well as Mrazek and Haggerty. High-risk families are identified, usually by such factors as low socioeconomic status, low educational attainment, and high-stress living conditions. Intervention programs sometimes begin before the child is born to provide counseling related to maternal care, to provide support in the home to reduce stress, and to prepare the parents for child-rearing demands. After the infant is born, the program may continue for a few years to help support parents, to develop the cognitive skills of the child, and to enroll the child in a preschool program. In adolescence, children who had received such programs show lower arrest rates, higher levels of educational attainment, and less substance use and abuse than other youths who did not receive early intervention.

During early and middle childhood, prevention programs are often conducted in the schools because there are opportunities to provide programs to youths in larger numbers, in the context of peers, and on a regular basis for extended periods. Programs often focus on developing positive skills and success experiences at home and at school. The reason for this focus is that bonding to deviant peers and poor family connections are risk factors for delinquency and substance abuse. Developing such success experiences in the schools with elementary school children has increased bonding to families and decreased rates of defiant and antisocial behavior and substance abuse. To date, the evidence shows that preventive interventions can have significant impact on aggressive and antisocial behavior.

Conclusions

ODD and, to a much greater extent, CD in children and adolescents are significant clinical problems because of its prevalence and referral rates for services. CD is a large and costly social problem because it continues over the course of development and brings the child in contact with multiple special education, social, mental health, and juvenile justice services. The costs, monetary and social, extend to others. The symptoms often lead to the disturbance or victimization of others in the form of oppositional or aggressive acts and, as the child enters into adulthood, abuse and domestic violence. Efforts to understand the underpinnings and paths leading to ODD and CD continue to advance. The heterogeneity of these disorders and the multiple risk factors involved introduce challenges.

Treatment has advanced considerably in the past 20 years. A few medications look promising for key symptoms of CD. The strongest evidence is for stimulants and mood stabilizers. As yet, there is no established medication with support in multiple, randomized, controlled trials. Three psychotherapies were mentioned. Each has multiple replications in controlled trials and has been shown to reduce symptoms of ODD or CD and to improve prosocial functioning. Prevention was mentioned in passing because advances have been made here as well. Now that promising interventions are available, a key challenge is disseminating them to mental health professionals so they can be implemented as standard care.

For many individuals, severe antisocial behavior and associated dysfunction in multiple spheres represents a lifelong pattern. Because these disruptive disorders are often passed from parents to children, efforts to understand and intervene are critically important. Many questions remain about ODD and CD and their course. Even so, much of the available knowledge can have an impact on the problem.

Case Vignette

Case vignette #1

A family and their son David, a teenager with CD, present to a clinic service (Yale Child Conduct Clinic) that is an outpatient service for children (ages 2–13) who are referred for oppositional, aggressive, and antisocial behavior. We can only offer highlights of the child and family here.

"I cannot take it anymore. It is so frustrating that sometimes I feel like running away from my own home," said David's mother during a clinical interview. David is a 13-year-old biracial boy, who was referred to the outpatient clinic for physical and verbal aggression, noncompliance, destruction of property, running away, and disruptive behavior in school. His mother reports that he lies frequently and refuses to do homework and chores. David responds to requests with anger and, when frustrated, punches holes in doors. He was also recently charged with carrying a dangerous weapon, assault, and a risk of injury to a minor when he shot a girl with a BB gun. He is currently on probation due to these charges. Furthermore, he was involved in thefts outside of the home with confrontation of another person.

According to his mother, David has difficulty getting along with his siblings. He is particularly aggressive with his sister, who is 2 years younger. His mother indicated that David does not tolerate anything from his sister and takes every comment the wrong way. He also has problematic relationships with peers. At school, he argues and fights with children and has been suspended several times for behavior problems. He is not liked by his peers, which makes him angry, resentful, and aggressive. His mother states that children at school "pick on him and start with him," and he tends to react and fight back. In extracurricular activities, such as basketball, he loses his temper and is sometimes asked to leave the field. His mother also noted that none of David's friends or acquaintances are positive role models and that he spends too much time fooling around, getting into trouble, or just hanging out with delinquent peers.

David also shows academic difficulties. His intelligence is in the borderline range (full-scale IQ score of 77 on the Wechsler Intelligence Scale for Children-Revised). He is now two grades behind in school and also stayed back in the first and fifth grades. He was in special education in several grades and tested out for sixth grade, in which he is currently placed. His teachers report that he is very disruptive in class, disrespects instructors, lacks motivation and attention, and is physically aggressive.

During assessment, David's mother indicated that she does not closely monitor his academic performance, rarely supervises his activities, and is not spending enough time with him after school or on weekends. Furthermore, she noted using physical, harsh verbal, and prolonged punishment, such as verbal threats, frequent corporal punishment, criticizing in front of others, and taking away privileges for more than 1 week. She also indicated that her disciplining is inconsistent as she would often retract the punishment or would ignore David's negative behavior one day and punish it the next day.

Several characteristics of David's family are noteworthy. He resides with his biological mother and three siblings in a high-crime neighborhood. David is the oldest child in the family and has two younger sisters and a baby brother. All children have different fathers. David's parents were never married; however, he has weekly contact with his biological father. His mother is currently separated from her last husband. She works part-time as a unit clerk in a hospital and receives public assistance. Her highest educational level is junior high school. As a child, David's mother was also in trouble with the law, ran away on several occasions, was a member of a gang, got into fights on a regular basis, and was arrested as a teenager. She also reported having a drug and alcohol problem as a teenager but never sought treatment. However, she was in therapy for mental health problems as a child.

DISCUSSION OF VIGNETTE

Case vignette #1 illustrates key symptoms of CD and also many of the contextual issues involved related to the child, parents, family, and living conditions. With both ODD and CD, research has advanced considerably by focusing on child symptom patterns, disorders, and related features within the child (e.g., comorbidity). What is often most striking about CD, in particular, is the fact that it is deeply embedded in contexts that extend well beyond features of the child's presenting symptoms. The risk factors for onset of CD illustrate many of the characteristics of families that continue to be present long after onset of the disorder. This makes delivery of treatment a special challenge. Advances in evidence-based treatments are remarkable. At the same time, delivering these treatments often requires attention to a host of parent and family dysfunctions that clinical trials of treatment rarely discuss.

Acknowledgment

Completion of this chapter was facilitated by support from the William T. Grant Foundation (98-1872-98) and National Institute of Mental Health (MH59029).

BIBLIOGRAPHY

Achenbach TM. *Manual for the child behavior checklist/4–18 and 1991 profile*. Burlington, VT: University of Vermont, Department of Psychiatry, 1992.

American Psychiatric Association. *Diagnostic and statistical manual of mental disorders*, 4th ed. Washington, DC: American Psychiatric Association, 1994.

Angold A, Costello EJ. Toward establishing an empirical basis for the diagnosis of oppositional defiant disorder. *J Am Acad Child Adolesc Psychiatry* 1996;35:1205–1212.

Angold A, Costello EJ. The epidemiology of disorders of conduct: nosological issues and comorbidity. In: Hill J, Maughan B, eds. *Conduct disorder in childhood and adolescence*. Cambridge: Cambridge University Press, 2001.

Burke JD, Loeber R, Birmaher B. Oppositional defiant disorder and conduct disorder: a review of the past 10 years, part II. *J Am Acad Child Adolesc Psychiatry* 2002;41:1275–1293.

Caspi A, McMClay J, Moffitt TE, et al. Role of genotype in the cycle of violence in maltreated children. *Science* 2002;297:851–854.

Deluty RH. Children's Action Tendency Scale: a self-report measure of aggressiveness, assertiveness, and submissiveness in children. *J Consult Clin Psychol* 1979;47:1061–1071.

Elliott DS, Dunford FW, Huizinga D. The identification and prediction of carrier offenders utilizing self-reported and official data. In: Burchard JD, Burchard SN, eds. *Preventing delinquent behavior*. Newbury Park, CA: Sage Publications Inc, 1987.

Eyberg SM, Robinson EA. Conduct problem behavior: standardization of a behavioral rating scale with adolescents. *J Clin Child Psychol* 1983;12:347–354.

Gerardin P, Cohen D, Mazet P, et al. Drug treatment of conduct disorder in young people. *Eur Neuropsychopharmacol* 2002;12:361–370.

Green WH. *Child and adolescent clinical psychopharmacology*, 2nd ed. Baltimore, MD: Williams & Wilkins, 1995.

Hendren RL. Disruptive behavior disorders in childhood and adolescents. In: Oldham JM, Riba RM, eds. *Review of psychiatry*. Washington, DC: American Psychiatric Press, 1999.

Kazdin AE. *Conduct disorder in childhood and adolescence*, 2nd ed. Thousand Oaks, CA: Sage Publications Inc, 1995.

Kazdin AE. *Psychotherapy for children and adolescents: directions for research and practice*. New York: Oxford University Press, 2000.

Kulik JA, Stein KB, Sarbin TR. Dimensions and patterns of adolescent antisocial behavior. *J Consul Clin Psychol* 1968;32:375–382.

McCord J, Tremblay RE. *Preventing antisocial behavior*. New York: Guilford Press, 1992.

Mrazek PJ, Haggerty RJ. *Reducing risks for mental disorders: frontiers of preventive intervention research*. Washington, DC: National Academy Press, 1994.

Pepper DJ, Rubin KH. *The development and treatment of childhood aggression*. Hillsdale, NJ: Lawrence Erlbaum Associates, 1991.

Peters RD, McMahon RJ, Quinsey VL. *Aggression and violence throughout the life span*. Newbury Park, CA: Sage Publications Inc, 1992.

Reid JB. A social learning approach to family intervention. *Observation in home settings*. Eugene, OR: Castalia Press, 1978.

Reid JB, Patterson GR, Synder J. *Antisocial behavior in children and adolescents: a developmental analysis and model for intervention*. Washington, DC: American Psychological Association, 2002.

Rowe R, Maughan B, Pickles A, et al. The relationship between DSM-IV oppositional defiant disorder and conduct disorder: finding from the Great Smoky Mountains Study. *J Child Psychol Psychiatry* 2002;43:365–373.

Sommers-Flanagan J, Sommers-Flanagan R. Assessment and diagnosis of conduct disorder. *J Counsel Dev* 1998;76:189–197.

Stoff DM, Breiling J, Maser JD. *Handbook of antisocial behavior*. New York: John Wiley and Sons, 1997.

Waslick B, Werry JS, Greenhill LL. Pharmacotherapy and toxicology of oppositional defiant disorder and conduct disorder. In: Quay HC, Hogan AE, eds. *Handbook of disruptive behavior disorders*. New York: Plenum Publishing, 1999.

Werry JS, Aman MG. *A practitioner's guide to psychoactive drugs for children and adolescents*, 2nd ed. New York: Plenum Publishing, 1998.

CHAPTER 6

Substance Use Disorders

KEITH CHENG

Introduction

The use of drugs and alcohol is arguably one of the rites of passage for American youths. Unfortunately, the use of these substances can lead to misuse and addiction. In fact, substance use disorders (SUDs) are among the most prevalent psychiatric disorders in young people. For clinicians treating the medical and mental health needs of children and adolescents, a constant vigil for the development of SUDs is part of any ongoing caregiving relationship. Not only do SUDs themselves cause major morbidity and dysfunction for youths, they are often associated with serious comorbid disorders. Overall, SUDs cause much distress for youths, their families, and society.

Definitions

SUD comprises one of two major categories included in the *Diagnostic and Statistical Manual of Mental Disorders*, Fourth Edition, Text Revision (DSM-IV-TR) nomenclature of psychiatric disorders termed "Substance-related Disorders." These disorders include the use of both legal and illicit substances. There are over 100 specific substance-related disorders that are further subcategorized into: Substance-induced Disorders and SUDs. Substance-induced disorders are comprised of intoxication and withdrawal states as well as substance-induced delirium and dementia. SUDs are comprised of substance abuse and substance dependence. These latter two disorders are the focus of this chapter as they comprise the major areas of psychopathology for youths with substance-related disorders. The DSM-IV-TR specifically outlines diagnostic criteria for abuse, dependence, intoxication, and withdrawal states for nicotine, alcohol, cannabis, inhalants, amphetamines, cocaine, opioids, hallucinogens, phencyclidine (PCP), and other substances such as caffeine and sedative-hypnotics. Drug use alone does not meet criteria for an SUD. There must be a maladaptive pattern of substance use leading to clinically significant impairment or distress. The criteria for substance abuse and substance dependence are outlined in Table 6.1.

Substance abuse is diagnosed when one or more of the four diagnostic criterion items listed in Table 6.1 are present during a 12-month period. Substance dependence is diagnosed when at least three or more of the seven diagnostic criterion items listed in Table 6.1 are present during a 12-month period. The criteria for substance dependence are more extensive and severe than the criteria for substance abuse in that they include the findings of tolerance, withdrawal, or a pattern of compulsive use.

Clinical Presentations

Compared to adults, adolescents with SUDs present with a greater number of drugs used at any time. While substance-dependent youths frequently present with symptoms of tolerance, they present less often with symptoms of withdrawal or other symptoms of dependence noted

TABLE 6.1. *DIAGNOSTIC AND STATISTICAL MANUAL OF PSYCHIATRIC DISORDERS,* FOURTH EDITION, TEXT REVISION CRITERIA FOR SUBSTANCE ABUSE AND SUBSTANCE DEPENDENCE

DSM-IV-TR Substance Abuse Criteria	DSM-IV-TR Substance Dependence Criteria
Recurrent substance use resulting in failure to fulfill major role obligations	Tolerance
Recurrent substance use in situations which are physically hazardous	Withdrawal
Recurrent substance-related legal problems	Substance taken in larger amounts and for a longer period than was intended
Continued substance use despite having persistent or recurrent social problems secondary to use	Persistent desire or unsuccessful efforts to cut down or control substance use
Symptoms do no meet criteria for substance dependence	Great deal of time spent in activities necessary to obtain the substance
	Important social, occupational, or recreational activities given up because of substance use
	Substance use continued despite knowledge that medical or psychological problems are secondary to use

DSM-IV-TR, *Diagnostic and Statistical Manual of Mental Disorders,* Fourth Edition, Text Revision.

From American Psychiatric Association. *Diagnostic and statistical manual of mental disorders,* 4th ed, Text rev. Washington, DC: American Psychiatric Association, 2000, with permission.

in Table 6.1. In adults, severe dysfunction in the workplace is common in SUDs. In youths, the equivalent dysfunction is poor school performance. As with adults, increases in deviant and risk-taking behaviors are common. However, minors using tobacco and alcohol are demonstrating more risk-taking behaviors than substance-using adults. By definition, minors are breaking the law when smoking cigarettes or drinking alcohol. Minors must resort to stealing or purchasing and possessing these items illegally. These factors along with the increasing cognitive impairments and poor judgment lead to criminal behaviors in later stages of substance abuse and dependence. Thus, SUD youths often have comorbid conduct disorders.

TOBACCO

The active addictive ingredient in tobacco products is nicotine. Nicotine is extremely addictive. It acts as both a sedative and stimulant to the central nervous system (CNS). Nicotine is readily absorbed through smoke in the lungs and directly through the oral mucosa when tobacco is chewed. Entry into the CNS takes only seconds. One episode of administration of nicotine usually lasts about 30 minutes. Stimulation of the CNS by nicotine is followed directly by a period of depression and fatigue as the nicotine level decreases, which leads to more nicotine-seeking behavior. Psychiatric symptoms of increased anger, hostility, aggression, and loss of social cooperation result within 24 hours of nicotine cessation in chronic smokers.

ALCOHOL

The clinical presentation of youths using alcohol varies widely. Initial signs of alcohol use or abuse are minimal, so parents and clinicians may not recognize that the youth is drinking. The effects of alcohol on the body and behavior follow a general pattern based on blood levels. In blood alcohol levels of less than 0.1%, individuals feel mildly euphoric, they become disinhibited, and may be more self-confident or daring. Attention span is shortened and social judgment is impaired. Physically, individuals may appear flushed. At blood alcohol levels of 0.1% to 0.25%, individuals become sedated, body movements are uncoordinated, individuals have trouble remembering things, and vision becomes blurry. In blood levels between 0.2% and 0.4%, overt confusion is evident, slurred speech is severe, gait is staggering, and incoherence is the primary finding. When blood levels approach 0.5%, individuals are generally in a stupor or coma. They lose muscle function and any motor response to physical stimuli. Individuals at this level of intoxication cannot stand or walk and lapse into and out of consciousness, large muscle group reflexes are depressed, pupillary reflexes cease, bradycardia develops, and temperature regulation and respiratory drive begin to fail.

The chronic use of alcohol by youths may result in many negative sequelae. Adolescent drinkers score worse than nondrinkers on vocabulary, general information, and memory tests. Neuropsychological deficits may develop in early to middle adolescents (ages 15 and 16) with extensive alcohol use. Adolescent drinkers perform worse in school and are more likely to fall behind. They have an increased risk of social problems, depression, suicidal thoughts and violence, and completed suicide associated with intoxication. Alcohol affects the sleep cycle, resulting in impaired learning and memory as well as the disrupted release of growth hormone necessary for maturation.

MARIJUANA

Marijuana is usually smoked in cigarettes (joints), cigars (blunts), or in a pipe (bong). Marijuana may also be ingested when mixed in food or beverages. The primary active psychoactive substance in marijuana is δ-9-tetrahydrocannabinal (THC). THC is rapidly absorbed into the lungs when marijuana is smoked and passes into the CNS. In the brain, THC binds to specific cannabinoid receptors. This receptor binding leads to the pleasurable effects of THC including mild euphoria and a sense of well-being. Other short-term effects include increased heart rate, memory loss, distorted perceptions, loss of coordination, impaired problem solving, and learning impairment. Long-term physical effects in adults include cardiovascular disease and increased risk for cancer. The Drug Abuse Warning Network (DAWN) is a national public health surveillance system sponsored by the Substance Abuse and Mental Health Services Administration (SAMHSA) that monitors trends in drug-related emergency department visits and deaths. Data from DAWN have indicated that a user's risk of heart attack quadruples in the first hour of smoking marijuana. It is also notable that smoke from marijuana is estimated to have 50% to 75% more carcinogens than tobacco smoke. Psychiatric and psychosocial sequelae of chronic heavy use of marijuana include depression, anxiety, personality disturbances, and poor school and work performance. Students who smoke marijuana are less likely to graduate from high school when compared to their nonsmoking peers. College students who smoked marijuana daily for a 30-day period were found to have impaired memory and learning skills. Youths who are dependent find it difficult to stop marijuana because of intense withdrawal symptoms of anxiety, irritability, and insomnia.

INHALANTS

Despite being the most common drug of abuse in preadolescents, inhalants are frequently overlooked by parents or clinicians that suspect their child or patient of abusing drugs. Inhalants can be classified in three main categories: solvents, gases, and nitrites. Solvents often abused include paint thinner, dry-cleaning fluid, gasoline, glue, felt-tip marker fluid, and correction fluids. Gases used for abuse may include butane, solvents used in spray paints, propane, hair spray, ether, and nitrous oxide. Nitrites known for abuse are room deodorizers, amyl nitrites, and butyl nitrites. Nearly all abused inhalants produce short-term effects like anesthetics. Most inhalants have effects that last a few minutes. Initially, users feel stimulated. Successive inhalations result in feelings of disinhibition and loss of control. Solvents and aerosol sprays also decrease the heart and respiratory rates and impair judgment. Amyl and butyl nitrites can cause rapid pulse, headaches, and involuntary passing of urine and feces. With extensive use, unconsciousness may occur. Chronic use can result in irreversible hearing loss (spray paint, glue, and correction fluids), peripheral neuropathies (gasoline, nitrous oxide, model glue), CNS damage (toluene, spray paint, glue, and dewaxers), and bone marrow suppression (gasoline, benzene). Reversible liver and kidney damage occurs with chlorinated hydrocarbons found in correction and dry-cleaning fluids. Abuse of amyl nitrites has been associated with the development of Kaposi sarcoma.

AMPHETAMINES

Amphetamines, in general, and methamphetamines, specifically, have an especially high potential for abuse and dependence. Amphetamines are usually taken orally or intranasally ("snorted"). Amphetamine users may also smoke or inject themselves with this drug. When used in this fashion there is usually an immediate euphoria or "rush." This intense experience is usually highly pleasurable and lasts for a few minutes. Oral and intranasal users feel euphoric with administration but not with the same sudden intensity experienced when smoking or injecting. Amphetamines cause increased heart rate and blood pressure. They also cause insomnia and anorexia. In high doses they can cause cardiovascular collapse, confusion, tremors, seizures, severe anxiety, paranoia, aggressiveness, and frank psychosis. Occasionally, hyperthermia and convulsions cause death.

Methylphenidate is the most commonly prescribed stimulant for the treatment of attention deficit hyperactivity disorder (ADHD). During the 1990s, there were increasing reports of its abuse. When used to get "high," methylphenidate pills are usually crushed and then snorted intranasally. In the low doses used for the treatment of ADHD, the typical euphoria or "high" is not experienced. Typically, abusers self-administer amounts that are several times higher than the therapeutic doses used to treat ADHD.

COCAINE

Cocaine may be the most addictive drug of abuse. After one trial of cocaine, most individuals cannot prevent or control the extent of future use. Common routes of administration are snorting, injecting, and smoking. "Crack" is the street name for cocaine that is processed from cocaine hydrochloride to freebase for smoking. "Freebasing" cocaine is a method of using chemicals such as ether to convert the powder into a solid substance that can be smoked. Smoking "crack" allows very high doses to reach the brain rapidly and brings on an intense and immediate euphoria. Physical effects of cocaine use include tachycardia, hypertension, constricted peripheral blood vessels, dilated pupils, and increased temperature. The duration of cocaine effects varies with dose and route of administration. Usually, the faster the absorption, the shorter is the duration of action. The euphoria from snorting lasts around 15 to 30 minutes compared to 5 to 10 minutes for smoking. When dependent cocaine users stop using cocaine, they experience a profound depression. Suicide is not uncommon during these depressive states if the user is unable to restart cocaine use.

OPIOIDS

Opioids such as heroin and morphine are highly addictive. The short-term pleasurable effects of opiates start immediately when administered by injection. The surge of euphoria accompanied by flushing of the skin usually lasts for a few hours. Following the initial euphoria, users become drowsy and mental functioning is diminished as CNS depression occurs. Physical signs of opiate use may include respiratory depression, miosis (mydriasis occurs in severe respiratory depression), dry mucous membranes, hypotension, and bradycardia. If used regularly, withdrawal states result from cessation of the drug. Typical withdrawal symptoms include craving, restlessness, muscle and bone pain, insomnia, diarrhea, vomiting, cold flashes, and piloerections. Heavy users may experience withdrawal symptoms within hours of their last drug administration. Chronic users may develop cardiac infections, collapse of veins, abscesses, cellulitis, pneumonia, liver disease, and human immunodeficiency virus (HIV) infections or acquired immunodeficiency syndrome (AIDS).

HALLUCINOGENS: LYSERGIC ACID DIETHYLAMIDE

Lysergic acid diethylamide (LSD) is one of the most commonly used drugs in the hallucinogen category. The effects of LSD are unpredictable and vary from user to user. Symptoms can be dose related. Physical signs of LSD use include dilated pupils, elevated temperature, mild tachycardia and hypertension, sweating, loss of appetite, insomnia, dry mouth, and tremor. In addition to delusions and hallucinogens, LSD is associated with synesthesias (for example, tasting colors) and distorted sense of time. The effects of the drug usually occur 30 to 90 minutes after administration. These "good" or "bad" trips may last up to 12 hours. Some users may experience extreme dysphoria, terrifying thoughts and feelings, and fears of going crazy. Reports of fatal accidents during LSD intoxicated states are not uncommon. LSD is not considered an addicting drug, as it does not produce compulsive drug-seeking behavior like that seen with opioid, cocaine, amphetamine, nicotine, and alcohol use. Tolerance, however, does occur in LSD users. Chronic users need to take more LSD to achieve the same state of intoxication experienced during early LSD use.

PHENCYCLIDINE

Phencyclidine (PCP) was originally developed in the 1950s as an anesthetic. Its use as an anesthetic was discontinued in 1965 because of side effects now commonly seen in emergency rooms (ERs). The most troublesome side effects presenting to the ER include agitation, delusions, and irrational thinking. At low doses, PCP use results in mild tachypnea and moderate tachycardia and hypertension. Generalized numbness, lack of muscle control, flushing, and sweating are also commonly associated symptoms of PCP use. At high doses PCP can cause hypotension, bradycardia, and respiratory depression. Nausea, vomiting, blurred vision, drooling, and loss of balance often result from high-dose PCP use. Occasionally, seizures, coma, and death occur in PCP intoxication. The most common routes of recreational PCP administration are smoking, snorting, and ingestion. For smoking, PCP is sometimes applied to leafy materials such as mint, parsley, or marijuana. PCP is considered addicting. PCP use frequently leads to psychological dependence, craving, and compulsive drug-seeking behavior. PCP can also cause symptoms that are similar to what is seen in schizophrenia. Delusions, hallucinations, catatonia, and disorganized thinking are common psychiatric symptoms seen with PCP use. Memory loss, speech and language dysfunction, depression, and weight loss result from long-term use. These symptoms may persist up to a year after PCP cessation.

3,4-METHYLENEDIOXYMETHAMPHETAMINE (ECSTASY)

3,4-methylenedioxymethamphetamine (MDMA) or "ecstasy" is well known for its use at "raves." A rave is a dance party that lasts all night featuring electronically synthesized music and drug use. Popular with American youths at "raves" or other club scenes, MDMA has both stimulant effects similar to methamphetamine and hallucinogenic effects similar to LSD. It is usually taken in pill form, but sometimes it is taken through injection or suppository. MDMA is associated with tachycardia and hypertension. Other physical symptoms include muscle tension, involuntary teeth clenching, nausea, blurred vision, dizziness, chills, and sweating. In high doses, MDMA can cause malignant hyperthermia that can lead to cardiovascular collapse, rhabdomyolysis, and renal failure. Psychiatric symptoms with MDMA are similar to those found with methamphetamine and cocaine including confusion, depression, sleep dysregulation, severe anxiety, and paranoia.

STEROIDS

Anabolic steroids were first developed in the 1930s to facilitate growth of skeletal muscles in laboratory animals. Since then, athletes have used them to improve their performance in athletic competitions. First used by body builders, steroid use has become so widespread that nearly every level of sports competition has documented cases of steroid use. Anabolic steroids can cause many psychiatric symptoms including euphoria, increased energy, sexual arousal, mood swings, distractibility, forgetfulness, and confusion. In high doses, steroid abusers report increased irritability and aggressiveness. Some users link their steroid use with episodes of physical fighting, destruction of property, and even armed robbery. Steroid use can lead to dependence. Steroid users often continue their use even in the face of negative social relations, irritability, and nervousness. Withdrawal symptoms include mood swings, fatigue, anorexia, loss of libido, and insomnia. The most dangerous withdrawal symptom is depression because it sometimes leads to suicide attempts.

Epidemiology

In 2003, SUDs were the second most commonly diagnosed psychiatric disorders in youths evaluated in community settings, as noted in Table 6.2. Second only to the disruptive behavior disorders category, it is estimated that over 5 million youths, by age 16, have met the diagnostic criteria for an SUD.

Costello et al. estimate the cumulative prevalence of SUDs in American youths by age 16 to be 12.2%. Recent and past research show that boys outnumber girls in rates of substance use. By age 16, 14% of boys and 10% of girls will have experienced an episode of SUD. Researchers at Johns Hopkins University postulate that this gender difference is due to boys having greater opportunities for using substances. When given equal access to drugs and alcohol, the gender rates are more equal.

Since 1975 the National Institute on Drug Abuse (NIDA) has been sponsoring the "Monitoring the Future" (MTF) survey to study the extent of drug and alcohol abuse in the United States. Currently, the MTF collects incidence and prevalence data on substance use by 8th, 10th, and 12th graders across ethnicity and gender. The substances investigated include tobacco, alcohol, marijuana, inhalants, amphetamines, cocaine, opioids, LSD, PCP, MDMA or "ecstasy," and steroids. The MTF data reveal important trends in youths' substance use over the past 25 years, including the persistence of ethnic and gender differences, the decreased use of some substances, the increased use of others, and the "niche" use of selected drugs.

For the 2002 survey, more than 43,000 students in 394 schools nationwide were interviewed about lifetime, past year, past month, and daily use of drugs. Substance-use trends for these grades demonstrate the lowest prevalence in 8th grade increasing through 10th grade and the highest in 12th grade, with the exception of inhalants, which are inversely related to grade level. During 2000 to 2002, the most commonly used substances were tobacco, alcohol, and marijuana as summarized in Table 6.3.

TABLE 6.2. PREDICTED CUMULATIVE PREVALENCE OF PSYCHIATRIC DISORDERS BY AGE 16

DSM-IV Disorders in Youths	Prevalence (%)
Disruptive behavior disorders	24.4
ADHD	4.1
Oppositional defiant disorder	11.3
Conduct disorder	9.0
Substance use disorders	12.2
Anxiety disorders	9.9
Depressive disorders	9.5

DSM-IV, *Diagnostic and Statistical Manual of Mental Disorders*, Fourth Edition; ADHD, attention deficit hyperactivity disorder.

From Costello EJ, Mustillo S, Erkanli A, et al. Prevalence and development of psychiatric disorders in childhood and adolescence. *Arch Gen Psychiatry* 2003;60:837–844, with permission.

TABLE 6.3. MONITORING THE FUTURE SURVEY: 2002 DRUG USE TRENDS

Drug	8th Graders (%)	10th Graders (%)	12th Graders (%)
Tobacco cigarettes last 30 d	10.7	17.7	26.7
Tobacco cigarettes daily	2.1	4.4	9.1
Alcohol last 30 d	19.6	35.4	48.6
Alcohol daily	0.7	1.8	3.5
Marijuana last 30 d	8.3	17.8	21.5
Marijuana daily	1.2	3.9	6.0
Inhalants last 30 d	3.8	2.4	1.5
Amphetamines last 30 d	2.8	5.2	5.5
Cocaine last 30 d	1.1	1.6	2.3
Opioids (heroin) last 30 d	0.5	0.5	0.5
Hallucinogens (LSD) last 30 d	0.7	0.7	0.7
MDMA (ecstasy) last 30 d	1.4	1.8	2.4
Steroids last 30 d	0.8	1.0	1.45

LSD, lysergic acid diethylamide; MDMA, 3,4-methylenedioxymethamphetamine.

From Johnson LD, O'Malley PM, Bachman JG, et al. *Monitoring the future national results on adolescent drug use: overview of key findings*, 2003. Bethesda, MD: NIDA, NIH Publication No. 03-5374, 2004, with permission.

TOBACCO

The MTF study shows that *on a daily basis*, tobacco is the substance most commonly used by youths with 10% of high-school seniors smoking at least a half pack of cigarettes a day. On average, 26.7% of high-school seniors report smoking tobacco in the past 30 days. Although cigarette use has declined slightly during the 2001 to 2002 MTF measurement period, these percentages are still greater than at any time since the 1970s. Overall, it is estimated that 4.1 million (18%) American youths between the ages of 12 and 17 use cigarettes.

Ethnic differences are important in tobacco use. Daily smoking declined among all ethnic groups between 1976 and 1990, then leveled off before beginning to increase modestly between 1996 and 2000. Native Americans were most likely to smoke and African-Americans the least likely. Within ethnic groups, Native American 12th grade girls smoke more than Native American 12th grade boys. While female and male white American 12th graders smoke at the same rate, African American, Mexican American, and Asian American 12th grade women smoke less than their respective male peers.

ALCOHOL

Based on use *during the past 30 days*, alcohol is the most commonly used substance by American youths according to the MTF study. The average age of a first drink is 12 years old, and nearly 20% of 12- to 20-year olds are considered binge drinkers. Approximately 49% of high-school seniors report using alcohol in the last 30 days, and 3.5% admit using alcohol on a daily basis. Between 2001 and 2002, 8th and 10th graders have reported decreased use of alcohol.

Ethnicity is also an important risk factor for alcohol use. Native Americans were most likely to report heavy drinking (five or more drinks in a row within the past 2 weeks), while Asian American and African American 12th graders reported the lowest prevalence of heavy drinking. Within each ethnic group there were no gender differences. However, overall, girls, regardless of ethnic background, were less likely than boys to report heavy alcohol use, and the prevalence for both girls and boys over the 25-year period ending in 2000 generally decreased.

MARIJUANA

While tobacco and alcohol are legal substances for adults but not for minors, marijuana use is illegal at all ages. Marijuana is the illicit drug most commonly used by adolescents according to the MTF study. In 2001, over 12 million youths 12 years of age and older used marijuana at least once in the last 30 days. Daily marijuana use is actually greater than daily alcohol use in high-school seniors, with 6% reporting daily marijuana use and 21% reporting marijuana use in the last 30 days.

Among ethnic groups, Native Americans were most likely and Asian Americans least likely to have used marijuana within the past month. Overall, 12th-grade boys in all ethnic groups are somewhat more likely than girls to have used marijuana within the past 30 days. Overall, prevalence rates for both girls and boys declined between 1976 and 1990, held steady until 1995, and then increased between 1996 and 2000.

INHALANTS

Inhalants, the third most commonly abused legal substance, are notable for their greater rate of use in 8th graders compared to 12th graders. Current studies indicate that over 12.8 million Americans have abused inhalants at least once in their lives. The MTF study found that approximately 20% of 8th graders abused inhalants at a high point of use in the 1990s. During the past several years, inhalant use declined. In 2002, use among 8th and 10th graders was at its lowest since inclusion in the 1991 MTF survey. Among 8th graders, lifetime use decreased from 17% in 2001 to 15% in 2002. Rates of use among 12th graders are the lowest in 20 years.

AMPHETAMINES

Amphetamines are the second most commonly abused illicit substance. About 5% of high-school students illicitly use stimulants on a monthly basis, and 10% report using amphetamines in the past 12 months. From 2001 to 2002, 8th graders reported decreased illicit use of amphetamines during the past year and over their lifetimes. Nonmedical use of methylphenidate (Ritalin) was stable, with past year rates at 2.8% for 8th graders, 4.8% for 10th graders, and 4.0% for 12th graders in 2002.

COCAINE

Cocaine (powder) use remained statistically unchanged across all grades from 2001 to 2002. This comes after declines in cocaine use among 10th graders from 2000 to 2001 and among 12th graders between 1999 and 2000. Past year use of powder cocaine was reported by 1.8% of 8th graders, 3.4% of 10th graders, and 4.4% of 12th graders. Past year use of cocaine in any form was reported by 2.3% of 8th graders, 4.0% of 10th graders, and 5.0% of 12th graders. Crack use, however, showed a significant increase in past year use among 10th graders in 2002, returning to its 2000 level following a decline in 2001.

HALLUCINOGENS

In 2001 almost 1.4 million youths aged 12 to 17 used hallucinogens at least once in their lifetimes. Hallucinogen use over the lifetime, past year, and past month decreased among 12th graders and also decreased over the past year among 10th graders. LSD, in particular, showed major declines. For example, from 2001 to 2002, past year use declined from 2.2% to 1.5% among 8th graders, 4.1% to 2.6% among 10th graders, and 6.6% to 3.5% among

12th graders. These are the lowest rates of LSD use in the history of the MTF survey for each grade.

African Americans are less likely than whites, Asians, or Hispanics to have used any hallucinogen in their lifetimes. Perhaps this relates to African Americans and Hispanics being more likely to perceive great risk in trying LSD once or twice.

3,4-METHYLENEDIOXYMETHAMPHETAMINE (ECSTASY)

Rates of MDMA (ecstasy) use decreased significantly among 10th graders, with past year use down from 6.2% in 2001 to 4.9% in 2002 and past month use down from 2.6% to 1.8%. Use by 8th and 12th graders also declined. However, in metropolitan areas, MDMA use has been increasing. Usually limited to urban "club scenes" in Boston and New York, MDMA appears to be spreading to the "inner-city" youth populations.

STEROIDS

Use of anabolic and androgenic steroids remained stable from 2001 to 2002 in each grade and category. In 2002, 0.8% of 8th graders, 1.3% of 10th graders, and 1.4% of 12th graders reported using steroids in the past 30 days. By 12th grade, 4% of youths have used steroids at least once.

Clinical Course

In contrast to adults, polysubstance use by adolescents seems to be the rule rather than the exception; therefore, adolescents often present with multiple SUD diagnoses. Typically, substance use in youths starts as midadolescent experimentation with cigarettes and alcohol. For most youths, the use of substances stops there. For others there is a progression into marijuana use. Marijuana is considered a "gateway" drug to other substances, usually illicit drugs. The 1970s studies by Kandel et al. have described the gateway effect, with the risk of using illicit drugs being relatively low prior to marijuana use. As substance abuse progresses into later stages, individuals use hallucinogens, cocaine, and opiates. It is important to note that this general sequence of substance use does not necessarily lead to the later stages of abuse and dependence. Individuals have the highest risk for continuous lifelong problems with substances if they started using them before the age of 15 years. Robins and McEvoy report that the earlier the onset of substance use and the more rapid the progression through the stages of use, the more likely a youth is to sustain an SUD. The risk for using any substance usually peaks in the late teens and early twenties. With the exceptions of cocaine and prescription drugs, most drug use tends to decrease after individuals reach 25 years of age.

Risk Factors, Etiology, and Pathologenesis

The causes of SUDs are unknown. There is, however, strong evidence for a genetic component. Genetic research has consistently shown high rates of alcoholism in first-degree relatives of alcoholic individuals. Some studies have shown 25% of fathers or brothers of an alcoholic individual will also have alcoholism. The concordance rate for alcoholism is higher in identical twins than fraternal twins. Furthermore, children of parents with SUDs, who are adopted at birth to non–drug-using families, have a higher rate of developing an SUD than does the general population. The risk factors for the development of SUDs are many and varied, as summarized in Table 6.4.

TABLE 6.4. ESSENTIAL RISK FACTORS FOR SUBSTANCE USE DISORDER

- Chaotic home environment
- Parental substance abuse
- Parental mental illness
- Ineffective parenting
- Lack of parental involvement
- Failing school performance
- Poor social coping skills
- Association with conduct-disordered peers
- Perceived parental/peer/community approval of drug use

NIDA has identified family factors as most crucial in promoting drug abuse by youths, and much of the research over the past decade has focused on family function. Children of parents with SUDs and/or mental illness are at high risk for abusing or becoming dependent on drugs and alcohol. Poor parental attachment, nurturing, and monitoring, particularly with children who have other mental disorders, also increase risk for developing a SUD.

Recent research has delineated the structural and functional effects of substance use in the CNS. For example, chronic inhalant abuse has long been linked to widespread brain damage and cognitive abnormalities that can range from mild impairment to severe dementia. Rosenberg et al. at the University of Colorado compared magnetic resonance imaging (MRI) scans of chronic inhalant abusers with the scans of chronic cocaine abusers. The MRI scans of the inhalant users showed more abnormalities in the basal ganglia, cerebellum, pons, and thalamus. Swan has noted in *NIDA Notes* that new MRI technology that measures blood flow in the brain corroborates earlier studies using positron emission tomography (PET). These studies show evidence of brain abnormalities caused by methamphetamine abuse. Perfusion magnetic resonance imaging (pMRI) measures blood flow in key brain regions by producing images based on hundreds of electronic cross sections showing brain structure and blood flow. In methamphetamine abusers, these scans reveal increased blood flow in sections of the parietal regions (the left temporoparietal white matter and right posterior parietal area). Scans also show decreased blood flow in the frontal, other parietal, and basal ganglia regions (specifically, the left and right putamen and insular areas and the right lateral parietal area). Increased blood flow in parietal regions suggests that glial cells, designed to protect or repair nerve cells in harm's way, are responding to drug-induced injury. Neuroimaging researchers point out that these changes in brain function provide additional evidence that methamphetamine and other drugs of abuse are substantially toxic to the brain.

Assessment

The components for a comprehensive SUD assessment include a careful history from multiple informants including the youth and relevant adults, a mental status examination (MSE), physical examination, substance-use rating scales, and drug testing. The salient points for gathering an SUD history are summarized in Table 6.5.

Because of time constraints, clinicians may concentrate on eliciting basic information such as which drugs are being used, how much, and for how long. For treatment planning, asking about family functioning, peer relationships, and academic performance is also critical. Children and adolescents must be interviewed separately from parents to provide them more freedom to disclose drug use without a disapproving environment. They should also be interviewed with their parents to observe family interactions and to collect data about family functioning.

TABLE 6.5. ESSENTIALS OF SUBSTANCE USE DISORDER ASSESSMENT

- Because substance-using youths commonly keep their substance-using behaviors covert, there is a need to gather information from multiple sources, including parents, siblings, teachers, caseworkers, and peers if available.
- Polysubstance use by adolescents is the rule rather than the exception; therefore, adolescents often present with multiple SUD diagnoses. Determine how many psychoactive substances are being used and how available they are to the youth.
- Many adolescents use drugs and alcohol, but to make the diagnosis of an SUD look for the hallmarks of associated psychosocial dysfunction, decreased academic performance, and timing of onset of these problems.
- Determine whether there is substance use or abuse occurring by other members in the home or whether there is a lack of rules against substance use by juvenile members of the family.
- Take a thorough social history to determine who are the youth's peers and associates and whether they use substances or are involved in conduct-disordered behaviors.
- Determine where the youth uses substances. Does he or she use alone or tend to be with groups of certain people and settings?
- Be sure to assess for other psychiatric disorders as there is a high level of comorbidity, and many symptoms of SUD can mimic psychiatric symptoms.
- Substance abuse rating instruments can be helpful in screening for SUDs and for monitoring treatment response. "Lie scales" can be especially helpful in identifying youths that deny their substance use.
- The use of urine drug screens can be helpful in identifying SUDs in youths that are skilled in hiding their drug use from adults. However, a single negative drug screen does not rule out drug use, abuse, or dependence; and a single positive drug screen does not establish an SUD.

SUD, substance use disorder.

Rating scales, while not mandatory to make the diagnosis of SUD, can be helpful when the history is conflicted or unclear or to establish a baseline for future assessment of treatment. However, in special populations like antisocial youths, these instruments may have limited value. Most screening instruments have been developed for adults. One of the most commonly used instruments in adults and older adolescents is the CAGE Questionnaire. "CAGE" is a mnemonic for attempts to *cut* back on drinking, being *annoyed* at criticisms about drinking, feeling *guilty* about drinking, and using alcohol as an *eye* opener. This instrument is normed for individuals over 16 years old. There are also instruments developed specifically for youths 12 to 18 years old including, the Substance-Abuse Subtle Screening Inventory (SASSI), Personal Experience Screening Questionnaire (PESQ), and Adolescent Diagnostic Interview (ADI). The SASSI and PESQ are self-report questionnaires that do not require any special training for administration or interpretation. They require 10 to 15 minutes for completion. Developed by Glenn Miller in the 1980s, the SASSI is intended for clinical populations in both inpatient and outpatient settings. It consists of 78 items that are interpreted with eight subscales. The SASSI is notable for having validity and lie scales, particularly relevant to this population. The National Institute on Alcohol Abuse and Alcoholism notes that the SASSI's resistance to efforts at faking may well be its most important attribute. It is especially effective in identifying individuals with early stages of chemical dependency who are either in denial or deliberately trying to conceal their chemical dependency. The PESQ target group is the general adolescent population. It is especially useful in schools, juvenile detention centers, medical clinics, and other settings where routine screening rather than an in-depth interview evaluation is the goal. This instrument contains 40 items that are scored using three subscales that examine drug use history, problem severity, and psychosocial factors. The ADI is a clinician-administered interview and, therefore, requires training for administration. Clinical social workers and nurses can be trained to administer the ADI. The ADI consists of 213 interview questions and takes about 45 minutes to complete depending on how many substances the youth endorses using. In addition, eight psychiatric status screens alert the interviewer to the presence of other difficulties often associated with substance abuse: depression, mania, eating disorders, delusional thinking, hallucinations, attention deficit disorders, anxiety disorders, and conduct disorders. Primary care clinicians and other busy clinicians may find this instrument valuable in documenting the need for referral to substance-abuse specialists but would likely want another professional to administer the ADI due to its length. The psychiatric screening questions also alert clinicians to the need for further evaluation or treatment of comorbid psychiatric illness.

The physical examination of youths with SUDs usually does not yield as many findings as the examination of adult substance abusers because medical complications require chronic substance use that adolescents have not had sufficient time to develop. Furthermore, during states of intoxication, the common clinical presentations outlined above may not be consistently present. The physical examination may be more helpful with regard to associated high-risk complications such as sexually transmitted infections, including HIV infections, and pregnancy.

The use of serum and urine toxicology can be helpful in detecting substances in youths who are skilled at hiding their drug use. While a positive drug screen cannot be used by itself to make the diagnosis of an SUD, its presence can be used to confront denial by the youth and guardians and result in a more candid history. Adolescents can be adept at escaping drug testing by offering many excuses for their drug-related behaviors. Also, they may contaminate urine samples, use increased hydration, or even use diuretics to invalidate laboratory drug screening. They are often knowledgeable about time frames for drug clearance (see Table 6.6) and thus escape detection by manipulating the time at which they provide a sample for testing. Clinicians can also use drug testing for ongoing assessment. Furthermore, the possibility of detection by random drug screens may foster motivation for sobriety in some recovering youths and provide parents a tool for managing this problem.

Differential Diagnosis

The first issue in differential diagnosis is distinguishing nonpathologic substance use from a frank SUD. One or more episodes of intoxication is not sufficient for diagnosing an SUD. The presence of impaired psychosocial functioning does distinguish nonpathologic from pathologic use.

Perhaps the most difficult differential diagnostic question is whether a youth has a primary depressive or anxiety disorder (including posttraumatic stress disorder) and is using substances to "self-medicate" versus having a primary drug problem with another psychiatric disorder developing secondary to the substance use. In particular, observation for signs of depression or anxiety after a period of sobriety can help clarify this diagnostic issue.

TABLE 6.6. URINE DRUG SCREEN DETECTION PARAMETERS

Drug	Detection Period
Alcohol	6–10 h
Marijuana and hashish	1 d–5 wk
Amphetamines	1–2 d
Cocaine	1–4 d
Codeine, morphine, heroin, opium	1–2 d
LSD	8 h
Phencyclidine	2–8 d
Oral anabolic steroids	Up to 3 wk
Injected anabolic steroids	Up to 3 mo

LSD, lysergic acid diethylamide.

Another important issue involves the frequent history of head trauma in youths with SUDs. These youths may present with cognitive psychopathology, and it can be unclear whether these deficits are due to preexisting head trauma or the SUD. Careful history with special attention to a timeline of symptom evolution and symptom assessment may help to establish whether these cognitive symptoms are due to the earlier head injury or the SUD. Of course, sustained sobriety is the best way to sort this out. Psychosis may also develop in youths with histories of hallucinogen abuse. Waiting for the psychotic symptoms to resolve after a period of sobriety usually resolves this diagnostic question.

In the end, these issues of primacy of diagnosis might not be resolved as youths with SUDs may have various comorbid conditions. In a meta-analysis of general population comorbidity data, Costello et al. reported that there was a high level of comorbidity of SUDs with disruptive behavior disorders, an intermediate level of comorbidity with depressive disorders, and a low level of comorbidity with anxiety disorders. An SUD was associated with a twofold increase in the likelihood of a comorbid anxiety disorder and a six- to eight-fold increase in disruptive behavior disorders. A review of the literature reveals a range of comorbidities with SUDs: 30% to 50% for ADHD, 25% to 80% for conduct disorder, and 20% to 30% for mood disorders.

Treatment

According to the 2000 National Household Survey on Drug Abuse (NHSDA), of an estimated 1.1 million youths 12 to 17 years old, 4.9% needed treatment for an illicit SUD. Of this group, only 0.1 million youths, 10.2% of the 12- to 17-year-olds, who needed treatment received treatment. Thus, an estimated 1.0 million youths did not receive needed treatment.

The development of evidence-based treatments for youths with SUDs lags far behind the development of adult interventions. Since the early 1990s, however, a plethora of youth-treatment strategies has been developed that focuses on multimodal family-based and community-based interventions with special attention to youths' development and family function, as summarized in Table 6.7.

The SUD risk factors identified during the evaluation should guide multimodal treatment planning. Treatment modalities may include psychosocial interventions, individual psychotherapies, group therapies including 12-step approaches, family therapy, community-based interventions, and pharmacotherapies.

PSYCHOSOCIAL INTERVENTIONS

The most important psychosocial intervention is parental and family psychoeducation. In addition to basic knowledge about the substances and treatment modalities, parents need

---

TABLE 6.7. ESSENTIALS OF SUBSTANCE USE DISORDER TREATMENT

- Current research emphasizes family and multimodal approaches to treatment.
- Family involvement is critical to a comprehensive treatment plan. Family functional weakness can help determine treatment interventions. For example, lack of parental involvement in the child's life, lack of family rules, and untreated parental SUDs can all be focal points for treatment interventions.
- Clinicians and families who are discouraged about the substance-using youth need to be reminded that drug abuse is a preventable behavior and drug addiction is a treatable disorder.
- While abstinence is the obvious long-term goal, the treatment team must help the family remain patient and supportive despite the chronic and relapsing nature of SUDs.

SUDs, substance use disorders.

to be educated about the relapsing nature of SUDs. Parents are frequently frustrated with their child's multiple relapses and cease to participate in treatment. This can be prevented with education about the nature of recovery. Continuous parental support for their child to be drug free is critical for successful treatment. Psychosocial approaches like those used in multisystemic therapy (MST) concentrate on removing drug-using youths from environments that trigger substance use. Another goal of psychosocial interventions is to reduce and, if possible, eliminate associations with peer groups that are involved in substance abuse. Removal of drug-using peer groups may be the most important intervention. This process can occur in a clinician's office as follows. The first step would include eliciting a list of persons and places a youth should avoid to remain sober. The second step would be to have the youth share this list with his or her parents. The third step would be to obtain a commitment from the youth to his or her parents that he or she would agree to avoid these "triggers" to substance use. The fourth step would include the parents in developing a list of principles and activities to which they would commit to help their child stay sober. While the content of this process is quite straightforward, the core component is helping the substance-using youth and his or her parents develop concrete ways of working together.

PSYCHOTHERAPEUTIC INTERVENTIONS

To date, there are no controlled studies showing the efficacy of individual psychotherapies such as psychodynamic, cognitive-behavioral, or interpersonal psychotherapies in the treatment of SUDs. Cognitive therapy for depression has been well established. Cognitive approaches may also be successful through the identification and modification of thinking errors associated with substance abuse. For example, Bukstein and Van Hasselt have described the use of a cognitive-behavioral approach to relapse prevention. Self-control is developed through the identification of environmental and thinking triggers to substance use and relapse, as well as the creation of strategies for dealing with these triggers. Case reports suggest that psychodynamic and interpersonal therapies may also have a role in treating youths with SUDs. Youths with comorbid depression or anxiety are most likely to benefit from psychodynamic and interpersonal psychotherapies, but only after they have achieved sobriety. Since antisocial adults do not respond well to these psychotherapies, the use of psychodynamic and interpersonal approaches should probably be avoided in substance-abusing youths with conduct-disordered behaviors.

GROUP THERAPIES AND 12-STEP APPROACHES

Group therapy for youths with SUDs has been a staple of treatment at all levels of intervention from outpatient to inpatient programs. Twelve-step programs used with adolescents are based on Alcoholics Anonymous and Narcotics Anonymous programs used with adults. Adolescent group therapies are present in most urban settings. Youths attending these groups are thought to benefit from peer confrontation of denial and peer support for continued sobriety. Grouping high-risk youths for prevention, however, may harm more than help. Dishion et al. found that with group interventions youths at high risk for conduct disorders and SUDs exhibited worse behavior than youths given nongroup interventions. The 11- to 14-year-old youths appeared to negatively influence each other through a type of "peer deviancy training." Dishion hypothesized that negative peer influences are most dangerous in younger adolescents who are at the initial phases of drug use. Treatment planning should consider these developmental issues when including group therapy in a treatment plan.

FAMILY THERAPY

Family therapy is critical in the treatment of youths with SUDs, as many risk factors are family related. Common goals of family treatment include psychoeducation of parents and family members about SUDs, improving family communication, decreasing family denial and resistance to treatment, assisting the family to initiate and maintain efforts to get the adolescent into appropriate treatment and stay sober, assist the family in establishing structure with consistent limit setting, and careful monitoring of the adolescent's activities. Examples of specific family interventions include behavioral skills training, supportive interventions, and structural family therapy. Behavioral skills training is one of the most basic forms of family intervention. In this educational intervention, parents are coached on limit setting and effective communication with their children. Supportive approaches provide encouragement to parents to maintain efforts to keep resistant youth in treatment and cope with the consequences to the family of the youth's SUD. Structural family therapy focuses on helping the family understand the interdependence of SUDs with all the relationships in the family system. With this understanding, maladaptive interactions, destructive control dynamics, scapegoating, poor boundaries, and individual maladaptive roles in the family are identified, changed, and eliminated.

COMMUNITY-BASED INTERVENTIONS

During the 1990s, community-based treatments for youths with SUDs emerged. NIDA has sponsored several community-based prevention programs that indicate potential benefits in preventing SUDs. For example, Spoth et al. have shown that family skills training designed for general populations delay the onset of alcohol use in early adolescence. They estimated that their prevention programs provide substantial financial savings to society by preventing teenagers from starting to drink at an early age, which yields higher rates of adult alcoholism. MST is another example of a community-based treatment. Created by Henggler et al., MST was originally developed to treat conduct disorders using family-oriented, comprehensive, flexible, and individualized interventions that focus on the specific weaknesses of a youth and his or her family. Studies released in the 1990s have shown reductions in substance use and deviant behaviors without expensive hospitalizations or residential care. Follow-up studies indicate sustained benefits of MST several years after cessation of treatment. These benefits include increases in school attendance and decreases in juvenile detention. Thus, MST is an evidence-based treatment that appears to be more effective than residential and hospital interventions that have not shown long-term positive outcomes but are much more costly for families and society.

PHARMACOTHERAPIES

In adult SUD treatment, pharmacologic interventions are aimed at treating intoxicated states and withdrawal conditions, preventing continued use, and providing narcotic maintenance. Common adult interventions include the use of naltrexone and disulfiram for alcoholism, benzodiazepines for withdrawal states, and methadone for heroin addiction.

There is a paucity of controlled research studies, however, regarding pharmacologic treatment of SUDs in youths. Because of this, caution should be exercised when extrapolating from adult to youth samples. Factors that may prompt more aggressive and immediate pharmacologic treatment are situations in which psychiatric symptoms clearly predate substance abuse and past pharmacologic treatments have been effective in treating these symptoms. If a clinician uses psychotropic medications to treat a youth's SUD, it is critical that the consent process includes the risks involved in using psychotropic medications concurrently during substance use. Furthermore, because of the lack of research data or Food and Drug Administration (FDA) approval for using psychotropic medications for SUDs, these facts should be communicated to parents or guardians in the consent process.

The use of psychotropic medications in youths with SUDs usually targets comorbid psychiatric illness rather then prevention of ongoing use of drugs of abuse or dependence. There are a few case studies describing the use of psychotropic agents with substance-abusing youth. Kaminer described the use of desipramine in the treatment of cocaine-dependent youths, and Myers et al. described the use of disufiram in alcohol-dependent youths. They both concluded that because of the lack of convincing evidence, these medications should be reserved for youths that are severely dependent and resistant to other forms of treatment. Several studies show that pharmacologic treatment of mood disorders may reduce alcohol consumption in the adult. The American Academy of Child and Adolescent Psychiatry Practice Parameter for SUDs recommends that, before treating depression in substance-abusing youths, the youth be observed for several weeks off of any substances to determine whether depressive symptoms persist. If symptoms do persist after several weeks of complete sobriety, clinicians should then consider psychopharmacologic intervention. It should be noted that Riggs and Bukstein have recently reported that depression does not remit as readily for adolescents as for adults after abstinence. Therefore, nonmedical substance-abuse treatments alone are often not adequate treatment for youths with comorbid depression and substance use.

ADHD is another common comorbid disorder that presents special concerns for pharmacologic interventions. The use of stimulants in substance-abusing youths seems contraindicated. However, recent studies by Wilens et al. show that ADHD youths who are not treated with stimulants appear to have a greater risk of developing substance abuse than either normal controls or ADHD youths who are treated with stimulants. Ironically, for those worried about stimulant treatment causing an SUD, the treatment of ADHD may actually prevent substance use. Fortunately, there are also nonschedule II medications that provide effective treatments for ADHD. Atomoxetine was FDA approved in 2002 and is considered a first-line medication for ADHD in youths with a comorbid SUD. Prior to the development of atomoxetine, bupropion was the preferred pharmacotherapy for ADHD in SUD youth. As noted in the MTF study, the abuse of stimulant medications by youths is becoming more prevalent. In these cases, α-2a agonists, such as guanfacine and clonidine, or tricyclic antidepressants, such as imipramine and desipramine, should also be considered before using stimulants.

LEVELS OF CARE

Depending on the stage of abuse or severity of symptoms, treatment settings can range from the most restrictive level, that is, inpatient residential or hospital programs, to the least restrictive, that is, traditional outpatient settings. Intermediate levels of care include day treatment programs. Using the least restrictive treatment setting is preferred for a variety of reasons. The cost of outpatient treatment is much less than inpatient programs. But more importantly, outpatient programs do not disrupt school attendance and allow for daily family interaction. In general, inpatient programs are reserved for youths that have failed outpatient treatment settings, are unable to stop their drug use in less restrictive settings, and are using potentially fatal types or amounts of drugs. Hospital settings are necessary when there are medical complications from drug use. Residential settings are indicated when the youth with SUD needs a locked or secure setting or 24-hour supervision that cannot be provided at home. Day treatment programs are useful when youths need daily monitoring and psychotherapeutic interventions but do not need 24-hour supervision.

CONSENT ISSUES

In comparison to adults, youths with SUDs are almost always forced into treatment by their parents, guardians, or the courts. This poses special problems. While parents may consent to treatment on behalf of their child, this does not ensure active participation by the youth. A less common problem arises when a youth himself or herself wants to consent for treatment. Youths under the age of 18 years (ages vary from state to state) may enroll in treatment without parental consent or support. A minor can also be court-ordered into treatment against parental wishes. In these two latter scenarios, lack of family and parental involvement poses an impediment to successful treatment. As family support is critical to successful treatment, options that do not include parental consent should be avoided when possible.

Prevention

Current prevention programs are based on research that has identified factors that protect against substance use, as summarized in Table 6.8.

These programs emphasize the strengthening or development of these protective factors. The most prominent factors include strong family attachments; clear family rules; active parental involvement in the lives of their children; success in school performance; strong family affiliations with prosocial institutions such as family, school, and religious organizations; and the adherence to conventional norms about drug use. NIDA has categorized research-based drug abuse prevention programs into three types: universal programs, selective programs, and indicated programs.

Universal programs are intended to reach the general population, such as all students in a school. *Selective programs* target groups at risk or subsets of the general population, such as children of drug users or poor school achievers. *Indicated programs* are designed for people who are already experimenting with drugs or who exhibit other risk behaviors. The bulk of these prevention programs use psychoeducation for substance-using youths and their families. For youths, emphasis is put on the development of drug resistance skills. Other skill-building education focuses on self-management and general life and social skills. Family interventions focus on the development of good communication skills, promotion of parent-child bonding, and improved family functioning. Early research has shown promise. It remains to be seen whether these prevention strategies have more lasting effects than the current follow-up studies that have been of short duration.

TABLE 6.8. PROTECTIVE FACTORS AGAINST SUBSTANCE USE DISORDERS

- Strong family attachments
- Clear parental rules about behavior within the family and in the community
- Active parental involvement in the lives of their children
- Active parent monitoring of behavior
- Academic success
- Internalization of societal norms against drug use

Case Vignettes

Case vignette #1

Joe is a very independent 14-year-old who had developed a life separate from his parents. He is a straight-A student who is now spending more of his time with friends than at home with his family. His alcohol dependence came to his parents' attention when they found him unconscious in the bathroom. After being evaluated in the local hospital emergency room, Joe's parents were informed that he had passed out from alcohol poisoning. As Joe had been very responsible until this episode, his parents accepted his explanation that he had not realized how much he had drunk for the first time at a party. He promised never to drink again. His parents were less worried when there were not any signs of drinking after a 2-month period, and they decided to go on a trip and leave Joe at home with his older sister. When they returned, they checked the liquor cabinet and found many of the bottles almost empty. Joe blamed his sister and his sister blamed him. Alcohol was eliminated from the home. A month later, Joe's parents received a call from the parents of one of Joe's friends. They reported Joe was passed out in their home and they were missing some alcohol. When Joe returned home they found a plastic bag filled with vodka in the inside pocket of his jacket. Joe was angry and told his parents they did not have to worry about him. "I'm old enough to take care of myself," he emphasized. "You can't do anything for me." For the next week he avoided talking to his parents and stayed away from home during the day and returned only to sleep, usually after midnight. The parents consulted with their primary care physician.

Joe's doctor outlined the three possible interventions: inpatient, intensive day treatment, and traditional outpatient. Given the fact that Joe had at least two known episodes of unconsciousness from alcohol intoxication and now was stealing alcohol from outside the home, it was likely that he was alcohol dependent. As Joe did not appear to be able to stop his impulses to drink in an unsupervised environment, his doctor thought he needed residential or inpatient treatment. The doctor decided to use the strategy of offering the least restrictive setting, that is, outpatient treatment, only if Joe would agree to be enrolled in a residential program if he relapsed. This would provide some modicum of assent to treatment from Joe. An intervention meeting was held in the doctor's office. Joe agreed to the outpatient plan with the promise to cooperate with an inpatient program if he relapsed. Two weeks later, after he was again found unconscious at the home of a friend, he went without resistance to a residential program.

Case vignette #2

Amy is a 17-year-old who came on her own to a neighborhood mental health clinic. She was depressed and admitted to drinking heavily for the past several months. Her parents are immigrants from Eastern Europe and do not speak English. Amy preferred that they not be involved in her treatment. Actually, she was quite angry with them because they did not spend enough time with her or her siblings. She had developed her own social life and spent all of her free time with her friends. She also complained that her father drank too much. When offered disulfiram, she agreed to a trial. At her insistence, she provided her own consent. She was initially sober for the first several months of treatment. However, after 6 months of treatment, she began missing appointments and admitted that she would stop taking the disulfiram before going to parties and getting drunk. She subsequently dropped out of treatment and did not answer any phone calls or letters from the clinic.

In retrospect, the treatment team determined that Amy's treatment was unsuccessful because of the failure to engage Amy's family in treatment planning. Amy presented as a mature 17-year-old holding a full-time job after dropping out of school. She was getting on with her life despite living in a home where she felt little parental interest or nurturing. There was a subtle but palpable tendency for the treatment staff to exclude the family as a bad influence on Amy. In a case review, the team noted that even in adult cases, treatment success is much greater when the family is involved. They had colluded with Amy and her family's desire to not make family interventions a major part of the treatment plan.

Case vignette #3

James is a 10-year-old boy from a religious upper middle-class family. His parents have brought James to his pediatrician because they are worried about recent behavioral changes. James was noted to look more distant and bored at home. Often, he was confused and disoriented. Usually an "A" student, James began bringing home failing grades. His parents wondered if he had a viral infection. After obtaining a negative physical examination and unremarkable screening laboratory tests for heavy metal poisoning, anemia, endocrine pathology, and electrolyte abnormalities, the pediatrician directed the family to look for sources of drug use. The parents were indignant but complied. No drugs or alcohol paraphernalia could be located. Concurrent urine drug testing was negative. What did the pediatrician ask the parents to check for next?

The parents were directed to look in the home for signs of missing cleaning agents or gasoline. To their chagrin, the gasoline container for the lawn mower was almost empty. When confronted, James admitted he had been "huffing" gasoline for several months. Some new peers were enrolled in his class at school. They encouraged him to sniff gasoline with them. James wanted to fit in and soon his social huffing turned into a chronic habit.

BIBLIOGRAPHY

Bukstein OG, Van Hasselt VB. Alcohol and drug abuse. In: Bellack AS, Hersen M, eds. *Handbook of behavior therapy in the psychiatric setting.* New York: Plenum Press,1993:453–475.

Brown SA, Tapert SF, Granholm E, et al. Neurocognitive functioning of adolescents: effects of protracted alcohol use. *Alcohol Clin Exp Res* 2000;24:164–171.

Chambers R, Taylor JR, Potenza MN. Developmental neurocircuitry of motivation in adolescence: a critical period of addiction vulnerability. *Am J Psychiatry* 2003;160:1041–1052.

Chang L, Ernst T, Speck O, et al. Perfusion MRI and computerized test abnormalities in abstinent methamphetamine users. *Psychiatry Res Neuroimaging* 2002;114:65–79.

Costello EJ, Mustillo S, Erkanli A, et al. Prevalence and development of psychiatric disorders in childhood and adolescence. *Arch Gen Psychiatry* 2003;60:837–844.

Dishion TJ, Poulin F, Burraston B. Peer group dynamics associated with iatrogenic effects in group interventions with high-risk young adolescents. In: Nangle DW, Erdley CA, eds. *New directions for child and adolescent development: friendship and psychological adjustment.* San Francisco, CA: Jossey-Bass, 2001;79–92.

Deas D, Riggs P, Langenbucher J, et al. Adolescents are not adults: developmental considerations in alcohol users. *Alcohol Clin Exp Res* 2000;24:232–237.

Henggeler SW, Borduin CM, Melton GB. Effects of multisystemic therapy on drug use and abuse in serious juvenile offenders: a progress report from two outcome studies. *Fam Dynam Addict Q* 1991;1:40–51.

Johnson LD, O'Malley PM, Bachman JG. University of Michigan, Institute for Social Research. *Monitoring the future national results on adolescent drug use: overview of key findings*. Bethesda, MD: NIDA, NIH, Publication No. 03-5374,2003.

Kaminer Y, Jellinek S. Contingency management reinforcement procedures for adolescent substance abuse. *J Am Acad Child Adolesc Psychiatry* 2000;39:1324–1326.

Kandel D. Stages in adolescent involvement in drug use. *Science* 1975;190:912–914.

Kandel DB, Johnson JG, Bird HR, et al. Psychiatric comorbidity among adolescents with substance use disorders: findings from the MECA study. *J Am Acad Child Adolesc Psychiatry* 1999;38:693–699.

Martin CS, Arria AM, Mezzich AC, et al. Patterns of polydrug use in adolescent alcohol abusers. *Am J Drug Alcohol Abuse* 1993;19:511–522.

Miller GA. The Substance Abuse Subtle Screening Inventory (SASSI): manual, 2nd ed. Springfield, IN: The SASSI Institute, 1999.

Myers WC, Donahue JE, Goldstein MR. Disulfiram for alcohol use disorders in adolescents. *J Am Acad Child Adolesc Psychiatry* 1994;33:484–489.

Riggs PD, Baker S, Mikulich SK, et al. Depression in substance dependent delinquents. *Am Acad Child Adolesc Psychiatry* 1995;34:764–771.

Robins LN, McEvoy L. Conduct problems as predictors of substance abuse. In: Robins LN, Rutter M, eds. *Straight and devious pathways from childhood to adulthood*. Cambridge: Cambridge University Press, 1990:182–204.

Rosenberg NL, Grigsby J, Dreisbach J, et al. Neuropsychologic impairment and MRI abnormalities associated with chronic solvent abuse. *J Clin Toxicol* 2002;40:21–34.

Rowe CL, Liddle HA. Substance abuse. *J Marital Fam Ther* 2003;29:97–120.

Shrier LA, Harris SK, Kurland M, et al. Substance use problems and associated psychiatric symptoms among adolescents in primary care. *Pediatrics* 2003;111:e699–e705.

Sloboda Z, David SL. *Preventing drug use among children and adolescents: a research based guide*. Bethesda, MD: NIDA, NIH, Publication No. 04-4212A, 2003.

Spoth R, Reyes ML, Redmond C, et al. Assessing a public health approach to delay onset and progression of adolescent substance use: latent transition and log-linear analyses of longitudinal family preventive intervention outcomes. *J Consult Clin Psychol* 1999;67(5):619–630.

Swan S. Exploring the Role of Child Abuse in Later Drug Abuse. *NIDA Notes*. 2003;18(2).

Van Etten ML, Neumark YD, Anthony JC. Male-female differences in the earliest stages of drug involvement. *Addiction* 1999;94:1413–1419.

Wilens TE. Does stimulant therapy of attention-deficit/hyperactivity disorder beget later substance abuse? A meta-analytic review of the literature. *Pediatrics* 2003;111:179–185.

Williams JS. Grouping high-risk youths for prevention may harm more than help. *NIDA Notes* 2003;17:1–6.

SUGGESTED READINGS

Lowinson J, Ruiz P, Millman R, Langrad J, eds. *Substance abuse: a comprehensive textbook*. Baltimore, MD: Lippincott Williams & Wilkins, 1997. *(This textbook has detailed information for the clinician.)*

Schaefer D, Espeland P, eds. *Choices and consequences: what to do when a teenager uses drugs/alcohol: a step-by-step system that really works*. New York: New American Library Trade, 1998. *(A book for bewildered parents with practical advice for handling drug-abusing teens.)*

Tartar R, Vanyukov, M, eds. *Etiology of substance-use disorders in children and adolescents: emerging findings from the center for education and drug abuse research*. Binghamton, NY: Haworth Press, 2002.

(For clinicians interested in a review of research findings.)

The Work Group on Quality Issues, American Academy of Child and Adolescent Psychiatry. *Practice parameters for the assessment and treatment of children and adolescents with substance use disorders*. Washington, DC: American Academy of Child and Adolescent Psychiatry, 1997.

Todd T, Selekman M. *Family therapy approaches in adolescents with alcoholism*. Boston: Allyn & Bacon, 1991. *(Family interventions for clinicians working with families.)*

CHAPTER 7

Anxiety Disorders

BEVERLY JEAN BRYANT
KEITH CHENG

Introduction

As a group, anxiety disorders are the most common, but least diagnosed, category of psychiatric disorders affecting American youths. Anxiety was first noted as a disorder in adults in 1871 when DaCosta described "Irritable Heart Syndrome" in a Civil War veteran. The syndrome was characterized by chest pain, palpitations, and dizziness and came to be known as "Soldier's Heart." Freud described childhood anxiety symptoms in the famous case of "Little Hans," a preschooler who developed a phobic response to horses. In 1941, Johnson coined the term "School Phobia" to describe a child's reluctance to attend school due to anxiety about separation from his mother. These early observations of childhood anxiety have been elaborated upon over the past 50 years to distinguish the dual roles of anxiety in both normal development and psychopathology, as first eloquently described in the work of Anna Freud. In normal development, anxiety has an ethological role alerting the child to danger in his environment and activating responses that ensure self-preservation. This role of normal anxiety applies to psychological development as well as physical development. For example, Daniel Stern noted the anxious dilemma that the toddler faces in separating from his mother to individuate into his or her own competent person. While the child may want to be his or her own person, separation and individuation risk loss of, or loss of the love of, his or her mother. This certainly creates an anxious situation, one that must be resolved for healthy development.

As child and adolescent psychiatrists have learned more about early development over the past two decades, investigators like Charles Zeanah have reported how anxiety in either the infant or the parent may lead to disordered relationships and clinically impaired anxiety for the child that may persist into later life. Research over the past 2 decades has also shown that the roots of anxiety may be constitutional. Some toddlers show a temperament that is extremely inhibited, or very shy, that predisposes to anxiety, perhaps regardless of environmental contributions. Thus, anxiety provides investigators and clinicians with much to contemplate regarding the roles of "nature and nurture" in the development of childhood psychopathology.

During normal development, anxiety has an adaptive function serving to alert an individual to potential danger, and for children there are different dangers at each developmental stage. Anxiety is not defined as a symptom if it is a normal feature of development. For example, a certain degree of anxiety is expected when young children are separated from their primary caregivers. Anxiety becomes pathologic when it interferes with normal development by preventing youth from mastering major developmental tasks such as academics, social integration, and self-perception.

The multiple types of anxiety disorders and the many domains of functioning that they impede underscore how important anxiety is to childhood development. This chapter focuses on the presentation, evaluation, and treatment of separation anxiety disorder (SAD), generalized anxiety disorder (GAD), specific phobias, social phobia (which is also called Social Anxiety Disorder), and panic disorder. Posttraumatic stress disorder (PTSD) and obsessive–compulsive disorder (OCD) are discussed in separate chapters due to their unique features and treatment implications.

Clinical Features

Fear is defined as a response to actual threat. Most children experience various fears throughout their childhood, and some of these fears are specific to developmental stage. In contrast to fear, anxiety is defined as an anticipatory response to *perceived* threat, either internal or external. Both fear and anxiety are characterized by distressing "fight or flight" reactions and a plethora of other physiologic responses that may affect multiple systems including cardiac, pulmonary, gastrointestinal, and neurologic. Anxiety is often further characterized by cognitive symptoms such as feelings of losing control or losing one's mind, unwelcome or intrusive thoughts, inattention, insomnia, and even perceptual disturbances such as depersonalization or vague visual images. Similar to adults, anxious youths often interpret their symptoms as indicative of underlying physical illness, resulting in overutilization of medical services and frustration for health care providers. Young people's burden surpasses that of anxious adults as anxiety interferes with normal development and impedes the acquisition of skills needed to successfully prepare for independence in adulthood. Typically, these youths are cautious in approaching new situations, cannot easily integrate socially, and avoid participating in physical activities in which they could get hurt, such as gym class or sports, or in social situations in which they could be embarrassed. Their peers may perceive them as different, exclude them, or even taunt them.

The *Diagnostic and Statistical Manual of Psychiatric Disorders*, Fourth Edition, Text Revision (DSM-IV-TR) requires that the same criteria be used to diagnose anxiety disorders in childhood and adolescence as in adulthood. In each of these anxiety disorders, some of the aforementioned nonspecific physical and cognitive symptoms may occur. In addition, each anxiety disorder has its own distinguishing features that occur in both adults and youths, but developmental factors may obscure their easy identification in youths. Thus, the clinician is challenged to look for specific anxiety symptoms within a developmental framework. The diagnostic features of the various anxiety disorders are summarized in Tables 7.1 and 7.2 and reviewed below.

TABLE 7.1. CARDINAL SYMPTOMS OF ANXIETY DISORDERS

Separation anxiety disorder	Developmentally inappropriate and excessive anxiety concerning separation from home or loved ones, characterized by three or more of the following: • Worries about loss or harm befalling loved ones • Fear of separation or anticipated separation • Refusal to go to school because of fear of separation (not simple school refusal) • Reluctance to be alone or to go to sleep without an attachment figure present • Nightmares involving themes of separation • Somatic complaints such as stomachaches, nausea, vomiting, and headaches when separated from (or anticipating separation from) major attachment figures
Generalized anxiety disorder	Excessive worry that is difficult to control associated with at least one of the following six symptoms: • Restlessness or the feeling of being on edge • Fatigue • Difficulty concentrating or mind going blank • Irritability • Muscle tension • Sleep disturbance
Specific phobia	Excessive and unreasonable fear of a specific object or situation; exposure to the phobic stimulus provokes an immediate anxiety response which may take the form of a panic attack (see Table 7.2). There are several specific subtypes of fears including: • Animals • Natural environment (heights, storms, water) • Blood, injection, injury • Situational (airplanes, elevators, enclosed places)
Social phobia	A marked and persistent fear of one or more social or performance situations in which the person is exposed to unfamiliar people or to possible scrutiny by others. Children fear that they will act in a way that will be humiliating or embarrassing. Other criteria include: • There must be evidence of the capacity for age-appropriate relationships • Exposure to the feared social situation almost invariably provokes anxiety manifested by crying, tantrums, "freezing," or shrinking from social situations with unfamiliar people • The anxiety must occur in peer settings • Recognizing that the fear is excessive or unreasonable, a criteria for adults, may not be present in children • Avoidance or distress of the feared situations interferes significantly with the child's normal routine or functioning • Duration is at least 6 mo
Panic disorder	Recurrent unexpected panic attacks followed by a month or more of: • Persistent worry about having additional panic attacks • Fear of losing control • A significant change in behavior related to the panic attacks Agoraphobia is characterized by: • Fear of being in places or situations from which escape might be difficult or embarrassing, such as being in a crowded or public place • Exposure to such stimuli are avoided or endured with great distress

From American Psychiatric Association. *Diagnostic and statistical manual of mental disorders*, 4th ed, Text rev. Washington, DC: 2000, with permission.

TABLE 7.2. CRITERIA FOR PANIC ATTACK

Criteria for panic attack	A discrete period of intense fear or discomfort in which four or more of the following symptoms develop abruptly and reach a peak within 10 min:
	• Palpitations
	• Sweating
	• Trembling
	• Shortness of breath
	• Feeling of choking
	• Chest pain
	• Abdominal distress
	• Dizziness
	• Feelings of unreality or being detached from oneself
	• Fear of losing control or going crazy
	• Fear of dying
	• Numbness or tingling sensations
	• Chills or hot flushes
	For children, panic attacks may be expressed by crying, temper tantrums, "freezing up," or clinging behaviors.

From American Psychiatric Association. *Diagnostic and statistical manual of mental disorders*, 4th ed, Text rev. Washington, DC: 2000, with permission.

SEPARATION ANXIETY DISORDER

The DSM-IV-TR separates disorders that are usually first diagnosed in infancy, childhood, or adolescence from disorders that more commonly begin during adulthood. The only anxiety disorder specifically described as beginning in childhood and not categorized with the other anxiety disorders is SAD. SAD is characterized by developmentally inappropriate anxiety when faced with separation, or anticipated separation, from home or loved ones. The anxiety is alleviated by reunion with the loved one, a major factor distinguishing SAD from other anxiety disorders. Children with SAD often worry that they or loved ones (including pets) will be killed, lost, or kidnapped. They are afraid to go to sleep by themselves and often sleep with their parents long after such behavior should have ceased. If parents refuse to let them sleep in their bed, these children may sleep on the floor outside the parents' bedroom, or parents may need to sit with them until they fall asleep. They may also have unusual experiences, such as seeing monsters or feeling that they are being watched. Sleep may be further impaired by nightmares about catastrophic events that destroy the family, such as fire or earthquakes. Children with SAD are fearful of being alone in a room. They may want their parent in eyesight at all times, even following the parent into the bathroom.

Somatic complaints such as stomachaches, headaches, dizziness, nausea, and vomiting are common in children with SAD, sometimes prompting referral to gastroenterologists or neurologists. These somatic complaints are especially common in the morning on school days, as these children claim that they are too ill to attend school; but once they are allowed to stay home, they function well. School refusal, or school phobia, can be an especially debilitating manifestation of SAD, particularly when the parent, who is often depressed or anxious, is complicit with the child's fear of leaving the parent and home. Once at school, these children may frequently ask to call home or claim physical symptoms to get sent home from school. Weekends may be symptom free, but these children play close to home. When faced with separation, they can become aggressive. Severe prolonged tantrums are common. Such aggression and affective dyscontrol is confusing to adults because SAD children do not readily recognize or verbalize the precipitant to their dyscontrol, that is, the feared separation. The symptoms of SAD must have onset before age 18, persist at least 4 weeks, and cause significant impairment in functioning.

GENERALIZED ANXIETY DISORDER

Children with GAD are characterized by worry, worry, worry. They worry about school, family, friends, athletic performance, the safety of their loved ones, the possibility of earthquakes or nuclear war, and what other people think of them. The attacks on the World Trade Center on September 11, 2001 caused many people to worry about further terrorist attacks. However, children with GAD are more likely to feel paralyzed by these fears. They also express many somatic concerns. Complaints about headaches, stomachaches, tiredness, and muscle pains are most common, leading to many doctor visits. Cognitive symptoms such as decreased concentration and irritability are also common. This excessive worry interferes with usual daily functioning in children and adolescents, taking the form of difficulty completing assignments, "freezing up" on an examination, avoidance of school activities, or reluctance to participate in sports or other activities in which they think they might not do well or could get hurt. Younger children with GAD will repeatedly ask their parents questions about perceived threats, dangers, or unanticipated difficulties they may face, and they are not easily reassured. They do not feel confident to cope with all the dangers they think could occur. Their "antennae" are constantly up, looking for dangers, potential threats, and the unexpected. They do not like surprises. Their affect is often tense and they are commonly "wide-eyed" or vigilantly scanning their environment.

Parents are frequently frustrated by the oppositional behaviors and tantrums of their anxious children. In these cases, anxious defiance is interpreted as being naughty, disrespectful, or willful rather then being scared or worried or experiencing surges of uncontrollable anxiety. Some of the most oppositional and stubborn children suffer unrecognized anxiety. In adults, GAD symptoms often affect work performance or marital relationships. Similarly, in school-aged children with untreated GAD, social and academic derailment occurs. They may become so troubled that they limit participation with their peers. While most school-aged children enjoy Halloween and Fourth of July holiday activities, children with GAD may find "trick-or-treating" or fireworks worrisome and overstimulating and stay close to home. They also constantly seek reassurance from their parents. Peers find such avoidance odd and shun them, further restricting these children's lives. Recent research has shown that children with GAD do not do as well as their peers in school, in part due to their reluctance to speak up and ask for help from their teachers and in part due to being too distracted by their worries.

As these children enter adolescence, the symptoms of GAD continue to limit their participation in usual teen activities. Rather than being interested in driving the family car, they may insist on being driven by their parents. They limit their peer relationships to a select few, if they have any close friends at all. They may decline to go on family vacations or out to dinner because they are feeling ill or worried about getting sick or hurt. Adolescents with GAD are prone to brooding, which tends to distance them from their family and friends. Dropping out of school is a risk, due to complaints of feeling ill or unsafe in the school environment or not being able to keep up with peers socially. By adolescence, the common sequelae to GAD found in adults may occur, that is, the development of depression or substance use.

PHOBIC DISORDERS

Phobic disorders are heterogeneous, consisting of specific phobias, which involve a single feared object or situation, and social phobia, also called social anxiety disorder, a more serious and impairing condition. Phobic disorders need to be differentiated from the normal episodes of fear often seen in childhood. The difference between having a phobic disorder or an age-appropriate episode of fearfulness is based on developmental considerations, the length and intensity of fearful affect, and the severity of accompanying impairment of everyday functioning. Toddlers are at times terrified of being separated from their parents, kindergarten-aged children are frequently frightened of dark places or of "monsters" under the bed, school-age children are scared of using public bathrooms, and teenagers are often afraid of undressing for gym class or giving a speech in class. These examples of age-appropriate fearfulness or anxiety are usually transient in nature, do not prevent engagement in the usual activities of childhood, and are not of sufficient severity to cause developmental derailment.

Specific phobias

With specific phobias, fear and avoidance occur in response to exposure to a specific object or situation. Common phobias involve animals, storms, bridges, costumed characters, and vomiting. The essential feature of a phobic response is the development of an intense and immediate anxiety. Indeed, children may appear panicked with physiologic arousal when they are frightened by the object or situation. For example, children with a fear of dogs frequently insist on staying in the house if the neighbors own dogs. At the sight of a dog, large or small, phobic children become agitated and frightened. They may become obsessed with possibly meeting their feared object and think of how they can avoid the neighborhood dogs, and they may escalate to agitation when hearing a dog bark or viewing a dog on television. Phobias frequently interfere with social relationships as children may refuse to visit the home of a best friend for fear of meeting the family pet. However, when contact with the feared object is not experienced as a threat, these youths function normally.

Social phobia or social anxiety disorder

While not as common in children as in adults, social phobia, or social anxiety disorder, can be debilitating. Social phobia is described by the DSM-IV-TR as an anxiety disorder with a marked and persistent fear of one or more social situations; that is, there is fear of being placed in social situations. Avoidance of these situations is prominent as intense anxiety is experienced when placed in these social settings. Children suffering from social phobia dislike situations in which others scrutinize them. They withdraw from group activities and stay on the periphery. Often, they cling to familiar adults. Many socially phobic children also have symptoms of separation anxiety. However, the anxiety of social phobia is not predicated on separation from a loved one, and these youth are overly "shy" in public even with a parent present, although not "shy" at home. At school, they are terrified of having to read in front of the classroom or write on the blackboard. They do not answer questions in class and sometimes remain mute if a teacher calls on them. Classmates may jeer them because they refuse to dress for gym class and avoid going to dances or parties. With the aforementioned problems, social phobia can lead to school refusal with subsequent school failure and even truancy charges. The simple task of eating may become aversive for children with social phobia, especially eating in front of others. Some may even appear paranoid as they avoid talking to adults or are reluctant to answer the phone. In response to all these worries, socially phobic youth frequently avoid all meaningful social relationships. As teenagers, these youth forgo developing peer groups or romantic attachments and frequently become loners. In contrast to adolescents and adults, children with social phobia may not realize their concerns are excessive or unreasonable, thus impeding treatment.

PANIC ATTACKS AND PANIC DISORDER

Panic attacks are discrete episodes of intense anxiety that begin without warning and generally peak within 10 minutes. They are characterized by autonomic arousal such as chest pain, palpitations, numbness and tingling, diaphoresis, chills, hot flashes, nausea and vomiting, trembling, and dizziness. Cognitive symptoms also occur including feelings of being unreal or detached from oneself and fears of dying or going crazy. For children who cannot easily describe their feelings, panic attacks often manifest as unprovoked tantrums. The child is described as "being crazy" or "manipulative and controlling." Throwing chairs and destroying objects can be part of these tantrums. Because these episodes of irrational and agitated behaviors are not recognized as symptoms of a panic attack, affected children are thought to have a behavior problem rather than be suffering from an anxiety disorder. This may lead to harsh discipline when more supportive interventions are indicated.

Panic attacks are a cardinal symptom of panic disorder as defined by the DSM-IV-TR and are summarized in Table 7.2. According to the DSM-IV-TR, in order to meet criteria for panic disorder, panic attacks must occur at least four times per week, followed by at least 1 month of apprehension about additional attacks, concern over the consequences of another attack, or a significant change in behavior related to the attack. In contrast to adults, children with panic disorder are more likely to become irritable and have tantrums without warning rather than being worried about when their next panic attack will occur or the consequences of losing control. While panic attacks can occur with many psychiatric syndromes such as mood disorders, PTSD, and substance use disorders, they are generally more frequent and intense when occurring as part of panic disorder.

Some children with panic disorder become withdrawn rather than more disruptive. Those who normally enjoy going to the mall become concerned about "freaking out" in public, especially in front of peers. Consequently, they make many excuses about why they cannot go out. Parents complain that they cannot get their child out of the house, sometimes not even to the yard. This may lead to panic disorder with agoraphobia.

The essential feature of agoraphobia is fear of being in a situation where escape would be impossible or embarrassing in the event of a panic attack, such as a shopping center or football game. Avoidance of public places ensues. Agoraphobia does not always accompany panic disorder and can occur independently, although the circumstances of onset are then more difficult to establish. Often, children with agoraphobia can play in the house without problems, but if they are expected to go outside, they become distressed, withdrawn, or refuse to leave their houses. Most commonly, they make multiple excuses to avoid leaving their homes. Obviously, impairment in most domains of life ensues.

Epidemiology

As a group, anxiety disorders affect 20% of youth up to age 18 years. Clinically, anxiety disorders are diagnosed equally in men and women, but in epidemiologic samples they are more frequently found in women. SAD has an estimated prevalence ranging from 2.0% to 5.4%, with a higher prevalence in younger children, most commonly becoming evident around the age of 11 years old.

In the DSM-III-R, overanxious disorder (OAD) was classified under "Disorders Usually First Diagnosed in Infancy, Childhood, or Adolescence." Subsequently, however, the DSM-IV required the same criteria be used to diagnose anxiety disorders across the developmental spectrum. As OAD was a disorder limited to childhood, but with considerable overlap with GAD, it was dropped from the DSM-IV and the subsequent revision. Youths with features of OAD or GAD have been subsumed under the diagnosis of GAD. Therefore, earlier prevalence studies of GAD in children also include OAD. These estimated prevalence ranges from 3% to 6%, with higher rates in older children and adolescents. In younger children, the disorder is equally represented in boys and girls. However, as children mature, girls are increasingly represented.

Specific phobias affect 2.4% to 3.3% of children, and there seems to be a higher prevalence in girls than boys. The common specific phobias of childhood include fear of the dark, fear of specific animals, fear of going to school, fear of the doctor or dentist, and fear of dying. Phobias wane with age.

Recent research with adults has found social phobia, or social anxiety disorder, to be much more prevalent than previously estimated, affecting 3% to 13% of adults over their lifetimes, thus making it one of the most common psychiatric illnesses. Many of these cases appear to have an onset in childhood and adolescence. In epidemiologic studies over the past 2 decades, social phobia has been estimated to affect 1% of children and adolescents at any point in time. Considering that the lifetime prevalence may be as high as 13% in adults, a point prevalence of 1% may underestimate the lifetime prevalence of social phobia during childhood and adolescence. Future studies may find higher rates of social phobia as more becomes known about this disorder in early life.

Clinical Course

SEPARATION ANXIETY DISORDER

SAD may begin quite early in life with increasing identification as the child starts school, although it may start during later school years or after a stressful life event such as the death of a loved one or pet. More often, the onset is not associated with any identifiable event. However, there may be environmental factors that facilitate the development of SAD, most often a depressed mother, marital strife, or family loss. A small number of youths with SAD will develop agoraphobia. Younger children often recover from SAD completely with little residual impairment. Older age of onset, higher intelligence, other comorbid psychiatric disorders, greater severity, and prolonged SAD symptoms (over 1 year) portend poorer prognosis with a chronic course characterized by periodic exacerbations and more persistent symptoms. These children overutilize medical services and, if left untreated, often experience derailed personal, social, and academic development. SAD is not diagnosed in adulthood, but it may evolve into other anxiety disorders, in particular, panic disorder and agoraphobia. Major depressive disorder is an even more likely outcome.

GENERALIZED ANXIETY DISORDER

The mean age of onset of GAD in childhood is 8 years old. The onset of GAD, however, can occur at any age in later childhood, adolescence, or adulthood. The presentation may be abrupt or gradual and the course may vary with time. Although little is currently known about the progression of GAD, there is some evidence that GAD presents in a consistent way over the lifespan, and it may not be necessary to require fewer somatic complaints in children than adults in order to meet diagnostic criteria. Prognosis is influenced by the coexistence of other disorders such as major depression but is usually associated with gradual improvement. Although GAD may affect multiple domains of functioning, most youths persevere and have many successes.

PHOBIC DISORDERS

Many types of specific phobias have a childhood onset. In particular, natural environmental-type phobias (i.e., heights and animals) as well as blood, injection, and injury phobias generally have their onset in childhood. Most specific phobias remit during the course of development.

Social phobia has a bimodal age of onset with a peak in childhood and another in young adulthood. The course of social phobia is not so well delineated. Some cases appear to become chronic into adulthood, but others may remit with maturity.

PANIC ATTACKS AND PANIC DISORDER

Like social phobia, little is known about the long-term clinical course of individuals with childhood-onset panic attacks or panic disorder. Some children may experience a panic attack without recurrence. However, for most youth the course appears to be chronic and tends to fluctuate in severity. If agoraphobia develops, it usually does so within the first year of panic symptoms. Agoraphobia can be one of the most debilitating sequelae of panic disorder. Resolution of panic attacks does not always resolve symptoms of agoraphobia. Unfortunately, there is little information about the progression of agoraphobia into young adulthood. Panic attacks are either uncommon in youth or, alternatively, not often recognized, thus leading to inadequate examination in clinical or epidemiologic studies and inadequate information regarding their sequelae and course.

Etiology and Risk Factors

Many theories have been postulated to explain the origins of anxiety disorders. In Freud's case of "Little Hans," psychoanalysts postulate that Hans's fear of horses resulted from his Oedipal complex or displaced fear of his father onto the horse. Behaviorists focus on the role of learning theory and classic and operant conditioning in the development of phobic responses. Pairing of an anxiety-provoking experience with the sight of a horse being injured or falling down would condition a phobic response to horses. A geneticist would be more interested in identifying phobias or other anxiety disorders in Hans's relatives. Developmental psychologists might be interested as to whether Hans showed behavioral inhibition in his earlier years of life. During the past 2 decades, emphasis has been on understanding the genetic, environmental, neurobiologic, and temperamental factors associated with the development of anxiety disorders, that is, a biopsychosocial integration. Many investigators postulate that children are born with biologically or constitutionally predetermined temperaments, some of which are a liability for the development of anxiety disorders. These vulnerabilities are then variably affected by environmental factors to form clinically significant anxiety symptoms. The environmental factors may be diverse including neurobiologic insults, exposure to trauma, a depressed mother who is not attuned to her child's needs, or, for the most vulnerable youth, simple uncertainties such as peer teasing or parental discord.

Since the 1970s, temperament has assumed increasing importance in the conceptualization of anxiety disorders, especially social phobia. Chess et al. described the dimension of approach/withdrawal in young children in terms of response to unfamiliar situations, people, and objects. The response can be inhibited (shy, cautious, and withdrawn) or uninhibited (bold and curious). Children with "inhibited temperaments" are at risk for the development of social phobia. A study by Schwartz et al. has shown links between extreme behavioral inhibition in toddlers and later social anxiety in adolescents and adults. Inhibited girls appear more likely than boys to develop social anxiety during adolescence. Prospective studies have shown an increased risk of multiple anxiety disorders in middle childhood for children who were classified as behaviorally inhibited as preschoolers. By school age, children with persistent behavioral inhibition begin to manifest anxiety disorders. The stress of school entry is a common environmental trigger.

There is a large body of evidence to support a familial component to anxiety disorders, which is now being investigated in relation to temperament. Anxiety disorders are more common in children of parents with anxiety disorders. As mentioned earlier, familial factors, both genetic and environmental, contribute to SAD. There is a higher rate of panic disorder in the mothers of children with SAD and higher rates of SAD in first-degree biologic relatives than in the general population. Children who have recently suffered from a serious illness, disruptive change in the school or home environment, or death or illness of a loved one are also at increased risk.

To understand the relative contributions of genetic and environmental risk factors for anxiety disorders, Kendler et al. studied identical twins, raised together and apart. If a disorder is genetically determined, the rate of concordance in identical twins should be close to 100%. If a disorder has no genetic contribution, the rate of concordance in identical twins raised apart should be no different from that of unrelated individuals. Kendler et al. found that the same genetic risk factors contribute to the risk for both GAD and major depression and that common or familial environment played no role in GAD. In contrast, environmental factors accounted for twice the liability of genetic factors in the development of social phobia. It also appears that anxiety disorders and depressive disorders aggregate in families. The patterns of genetic contribution vary somewhat according to the specific diagnoses and will be reviewed in the discussion of specific disorders.

Biologic and genetic factors are also important in other ways as gleaned from studies with adults. There is a distinction between the anatomic circuitry in the brain that processes the reaction to a specific threat and that which responds to the context in which the threat occurs. Inherited differences in the construction of these circuits may place certain individuals at risk for either social anxiety or phobic anxiety. This is supported by the higher occurrence of social phobia in first-degree biologic relatives of afflicted individuals and also by animal studies, which have demonstrated that phobic behavior can be bred into dogs. In fact, specific phobias aggregate within families, particularly with regard to fears of blood and injury.

The hypothalamic-pituitary-adrenal (HPA) axis and various neurotransmitters such as γ-aminobutyric acid (GABA), norepinephrine (NE), serotonin (S), neuropeptide-Y (NPY), and cholecystokinin (CCK) have been implicated in the neurochemical processes associated with anxiety. For example, when under stress, the body produces endorphins. When stress ends, the body produces CCK to counteract the endorphins. Exogenous administration of CCK can cause panic symptoms. This is currently being used as a tool to study the neurobiologic mechanisms involved in panic disorders.

The use of regional cerebral blood flow studies such as positron emission topography (PET), computerized electroencephalograms (EEGs), functional magnetic resonance imaging (fMRI), and volumetric computerized axial tomography (CAT) scans have contributed to theories about the neurobiologic basis of anxiety disorders in adults. Functional brain imaging studies in adult panic disorder patients at the National Institute of Mental Health have implicated both the anterior and posterior cingulate in the regulation of anxiety. PET scan studies by Neumeister et al. have shown serotonin receptor site dysregulation in the cingulated areas and the raphe in the midbrain. On the basis of new neuroimaging studies, it is hypothesized that anticipatory anxiety and phobic anticipatory anxiety are associated with the cingulated portion of the limbic system, phobic avoidance is associated with the prefrontal cortex, and panic is associated with the brainstem. Similar studies have not yet been conducted with youths, although these adult studies are likely relevant. Like many psychiatric and medical illnesses that have an onset early in life, the etiologies of pediatric anxiety disorders are probably multifactorial and complex. Future research will elucidate how genetic, biologic, and environmental factors interact to produce anxiety symptoms in youths.

Assessment

The initial evaluation of anxiety disorders includes screening for physical and psychiatric disorders that might be comorbid with or mistaken for anxiety disorders as outlined in Table 7.3. A wide variety of medical illnesses may masquerade as an anxiety disorder. For example, asthma produces dyspnea that is similar to the shortness of breath experienced during intense episodes of anxiety. Hyperthyroidism is associated with nervousness and agitation. Cardiac arrhythmias can produce chest tightness and palpitations similar to that experienced during panic attacks. If potential medical causes of anxietylike symptoms are not identified, subsequent treatment will be ineffective, and iatrogenic complications may follow. The medical history often reveals multiple visits to the emergency room, the primary care physician, or even to medical specialists for unexplained physical symptoms. Protracted recovery times from minor illnesses are common. The presence of medication that could produce anxiety symptoms should also be investigated, such as phenylpropanolamine, theophylline, β-blockers, and anticholinergics.

Anxious children are typically reticent to talk about their worries. Therefore, in addition to obtaining clinical information individually from an anxious child, it is important to gather information from parents and other sources. Such information may include data from schoolteachers, counselors, principals, primary care clinicians, and mental health therapists as indicated in Chapter 1. Since teachers interact with children on a daily basis in a social context, they are in the best position to observe socially phobic behaviors in addition to excessive worries about failure and school avoidance. School history often reveals patterns of chronic absences, disparity between potential and actual achievement, or social problems such as being bullied or isolated. The therapists of children who have been in mental health treatment can provide valuable information about the severity and quality of anxiety symptoms, family dynamics, and past treatment. Parents and teachers often focus more on the behavior than the emotions associated with the presentation of anxiety disorders in children. Thus, parents are better reporters of the behavioral concomitants of anxiety disorders, while children are better reporters of their internal, or subjective, experiences.

After establishing rapport with the anxious child, it is appropriate to ask about "worries." If anxious children feel comfortable with their therapist, they may spill out descriptions of worries about death, dying, storms, illnesses, and so on, which sometimes surprises parents who are unaware of their children's inner lives. It is helpful to ask the

TABLE 7.3. ESSENTIALS OF ASSESSMENT OF ANXIETY DISORDER IN CHILDREN AND ADOLESCENTS

1. Rule out physical causes such as hyperthyroidism, side effects to medications (allergy/asthma medications; hypoglycemic agents; etc.), substance abuse, or other medical conditions.
2. Children are often reticent to talk about their worries, so it is important to obtain data from other sources including parents, teachers, coaches, therapists, and primary care physicians.
3. Younger children may better communicate their anxieties through drawings, play with family figures, or other play techniques.
4. Determine the trigger(s) for the anxiety. Does the anxiety occur in response to a specific stimulus? Does it occur "out of the blue?" Does it occur in anticipation of something (e.g., going to school, taking an examination, visit with a family member, etc.)?
5. Understand environmental and familial factors that may affect the youth's anxiety. What is the family history of anxiety? How does the parent react to the anxiety? Are there family conflicts contributing to the anxiety?
6. Screen for comorbid psychiatric disorders: mood disorders, psychosis, eating disorders, and disruptive behavior disorders.
7. Consider the use of symptom rating scales to better categorize, understand, and monitor the child's anxieties.

children about specific worries such as the death of a pet or fear of tornadoes. Parents will then remember associated material, such as examples of the child hiding in the closet during a thunderstorm. Concerns about family health and safety are important to elicit, as these children are typically worried about those around them.

The developmental history can identify predisposing temperament such as an inhibited or cautious style. Special consideration should be focused on stranger and separation responses, flexibility in new situations, response to change, the rhythm of physiologic processes, the presence of fears, and behavioral inhibition. All these factors that suggest an overtly cautious or inhibited child should raise concerns about underlying anxiety.

In looking for the presence of DSM-IV-TR diagnostic criteria, evaluators should also determine the impact of anxiety symptoms on the daily life of the child. Normal children have anxiety from time to time, but children with anxiety disorders have more intense symptoms, symptoms of long duration, or symptoms that impair functions. This level of symptomatology interferes not only with activities of daily living such as going to social activities, sleeping alone, using the bathroom, or eating at a restaurant, but also limits children from health-promoting activities such as visits to the dentist or doctor, immunizations, or other medical procedures. Anxiety symptoms that cause considerable distress need treatment before they cause developmental derailment. Missing an excessive number of school days and being too anxious to concentrate in class can cause academic delays and isolation from peers.

Several techniques are used to gather data from anxious children. Younger children often best describe their fears through play or drawings. Evaluators should provide this age group with appropriate toys that can be used to tell a story, for example, family puppets, dolls, or animals. A play city or dollhouse provides a good setting for stories of worry to unfold. Drawings with simple implements such as crayons, markers, or pencils provide a projective device for eliciting children's inner themes of anxiety, such as characters being chased by monsters or harm befalling helpless figures. Asking children to be storytellers is also a fruitful and easy way for them to describe their worries. For those children who do not want to talk, the creation of a storybook or cartoon strip can be a creative substitution. Older children are often willing to author an autobiography. While frightening themes of aggression, violence, and being injured may be elicited with these techniques, clinicians need to remember that the presence of these findings by themselves is not diagnostic of an anxiety disorder.

On mental status examination, anxious children show many characteristic signs and symptoms. They may avoid eye contact and if asked about poor social grace, they generally respond that it makes them feel "funny" or uncomfortable. They may also appear inhibited in the interview room and approach toys tentatively, awaiting direction from an adult. They may prefer to sit near their parents, hide behind them, or want the parents to speak for them. Anxious children draw pictures of monsters or scary scenarios from their internal worries like being chased by "bad guys." Those with obsessive or compulsive traits may also request an eraser to correct their pictures over and over until they are "perfect." When asked for their three wishes, they often say, "I wish Mommy would live forever" or "I wish no one would ever die or get sick." Children with school refusal often say that they wish they never had to go to school or that they could be with their parents all day long. Any assessment of anxiety should test the ability of the child to separate from adult caretakers. Interestingly, parents may have a greater problem separating than do their children. Such a scenario is valuable to understanding the dyadic aspect of children's anxiety and for treatment planning. When they are asked to separate from their parents, anxious children even may have a tantrum. Some may have a panic attack in a physician's office if they anticipate some anxiety-provoking event such as receiving an immunization. Cold and clammy tremulous handshakes are a common finding in children with anxiety disorders. Visual inspection reveals damaged fingernails and cuticles from nail biting, skin excoriations or rashes from excessive nervous rubbing, or, in severe cases, hair missing from the scalp secondary to anxiety-driven hair pulling. Anxious children appear tense and uncomfortable, are often hyperalert, sit on the edge of their chairs, or are restless. Some are filled with worries about their health with multiple nonspecific aches and pains. Since the World Trade Center disaster of 2001, it has not been unusual for anxious children to worry about world events like war and the possibility of terrorist attacks in the United States. The presentation of anxious adolescents varies from being subdued and unwilling to participate to being overly verbal or overinclusive in their responses. Their thought content focuses on themes such as losing control or fears about getting in trouble. Many also have specific concerns about their health. Socially immature teens are often less cooperative than school-age children because of their developmental tendency to oppose adults.

Rating scales can provide an additional source of clinical information regarding children's response to treatment. Commonly used rating scales include the Multidimensional Anxiety Scale for Children (MASC), the Screen for Child Anxiety-Related Emotional Disorders (SCARED), the Social Phobia and Anxiety Inventory for Children (SPAI-C), and the Fear Survey Schedule for Children-R (FSSC-R). For details, see Chapter 2. These rating scales provide an overall assessment of anxiety as well as help clinicians to identify specific anxiety problem areas. For example, the MASC assesses physical harm avoidance and social aspects of anxiety, the SCARED measures DSM-IV subtypes of anxiety disorders, and the SPAI-C specifically assesses social phobia. Clinicians can then create more appropriate treatment plans. Rating scales are especially helpful to track the effectiveness of psychotherapy, medications, and other interventions. Essentials of assessment are summarized in Table 7.3.

Differential Diagnosis and Comorbidity

The differential diagnosis of anxiety disorders in children should include screening for physical conditions that may mimic anxiety disorders as well as psychiatric disorders that may be comorbid with or misdiagnosed as anxiety disorders.

Differentiation of clinical subtypes of anxiety disorders can be difficult. At least one third of children with an anxiety disorder meet criteria for two or more anxiety disorders, and children with anxiety disorders often suffer from other psychiatric disorders as well. The two most common disorders that need to be differentiated from anxiety disorders are attention deficit hyperactivity disorder (ADHD) and major depression.

ADHD and anxiety disorders are difficult to differentiate because they share several key manifestations. Anxious children tend to show inattention, similar to the inattention criteria of ADHD, but are less likely to manifest the hyperactive and impulsive behaviors. The history and endorsement of severe and intense worries are probably the strongest discriminators of an anxiety disorder from ADHD. Anxious children may also be differentiated by their hypervigilant affect. While anxiety disorders must be discriminated from ADHD, these two disorders may also be comorbid. Between 15% and 24% of children with anxiety disorders also meet criteria for ADHD. Conversely, 25% of children with ADHD are found to also have an anxiety disorder. The comorbidity is important to identify because it complicates treatment. For example, an anxiety disorder can impede the response of ADHD to usual treatments, particularly stimulant treatment. Also, stimulant medication may exacerbate anxiety. Thus, children with both ADHD and an anxiety disorder frequently present as disruptive children who have failed stimulant medication trials.

Children with depressive disorders also share many of the same symptoms found in children with anxiety disorders including sleep dysregulation, irritability, social withdrawal, poor concentration, negativity about themselves and the future, and finicky eating. The sleep problem of anxious children is usually early insomnia. Depressed children may also have problems with staying asleep, terminal insomnia, and sometimes hypersomnia.

The irritability of anxiety disorders is usually associated with the situations or objects that trigger worry or fear, while the irritability in depressive disorders is more autonomous and pervasive. The social withdrawal of anxious children is tied into their fears of being exposed or teased, while depressed children are anhedonic, disinterested in social interaction, or feel no one likes them. The rate of anxiety disorders comorbid with major depression in children ranges from 28% to 69%. Children with comorbid anxiety and depression are older at evaluation and have more severe symptoms of anxiety than those with anxiety disorders alone.

Psychotic disorders need to be ruled out. This is most commonly encountered in youths suffering panic attacks. These children's complaints that they feel like they are losing their mind, losing control, or having perceptual alterations may be mistaken for psychosis. However, anxious children have intact reality testing; they are able to tell the difference between make-believe and real life. With early school-aged children and preschoolers, however, it is harder to discern the presence of intact reality testing as they are less able to verbally describe their inner experiences. Moreover, they are likely to act out their anxiety through disruptive behaviors.

Some oppositional children have underlying anxiety disorders. It can be confusing for adults to realize that a child who refuses to bathe or do chores outside is reacting to underlying anxiety. Tantrums result when the child encounters an anxiety-provoking trigger or feels overwhelmed by pressures when placed in unsafe situations. While anxious children often feel remorseful for their defiance or behavioral aggression, children with oppositional defiant disorder (ODD) have no guilt and externalize blame onto others. It is not uncommon for a child with severe anxiety to be labeled as ODD. This unfortunately leads to ineffective treatment and more disruptive behavior patterns.

Refusing to go to school, alternately called school refusal or school phobia, deserves special attention. School refusal can be secondary to all of the anxiety disorders discussed in this chapter, as well as secondary to other disorders and problems. For example, a child may be labeled as "school phobic" to account for school refusal behaviors, but may actually refuse to attend school due to a panic disorder and agoraphobia. More commonly, a child refuses school due to SAD. In this case, the child may have no problem attending school as long as the parent remains at school the whole day. School phobia is not to be confused with truancy in which the youth simply skips school, often to pursue antisocial activity, without any underlying anxiety, depression, or concerns about being harmed at school.

Treatment

Early intervention is needed to prevent developmental derailments. However, by the time most children come to psychiatric attention, they already are experiencing major difficulties. The importance of early intervention programs is accentuated by Mattison's research that suggests children who suffer from severe anxiety are more likely to become anxious adults. Furthermore, early intervention programs can decrease the development of anxiety disorders in youths.

Effective assessment and treatment of anxiety disorders in children and adolescents require a multimodal approach, taking into account developmental as well as cultural factors. Behavioral, cognitive, psychodynamic, and family therapies have been used effectively. While there is preliminary evidence of pharmacologic efficacy for the treatment of some anxiety disorders, they should never be used as the sole intervention. Child and adolescent psychiatrists and collaborating clinicians usually integrate several approaches in treating youths with anxiety disorders, as summarized in Table 7.4.

TABLE 7.4. TREATMENT ESSENTIALS FOR ANXIETY DISORDERS IN CHILDREN AND ADOLESCENTS

1. Treatment interventions must be multimodal. Intervention strategies should include school staff, family members, primary care clinicians, and therapists.
2. Educate the primary caregivers about the nature of anxiety, how it can affect family relationships (how the child's anxiety symptoms "control" the family), how family members can inadvertently perpetuate the symptoms through their own anxiety, and how to support the child in overcoming the anxiety. Assist family members in setting appropriate limits for the child (i.e., insisting that the child go to school and helping the child to succeed in doing so).
3. Parents of children with separation anxiety disorder need to develop a "shared-vision" with the treatment team on the antecedents to separation symptoms and the types of effective interventions.
4. Anxious youths and their parents should be warned to minimize or eliminate intake of caffeine, a known cause of anxiety.
5. Cognitive behavioral therapy should comprise the first-line treatment; the use of standardized manualized treatments is preferred due to their evidence base for efficacy.
6. Pharmacotherapy should be reserved for treatment-resistance cases or to augment psychotherapeutic interventions so as to maximize effectiveness in the most timely manner.

BEHAVIORAL THERAPY

Behavioral therapy is focused on modifying the child's current behavior and the response of those who care for him within the context of the school, the family, and other important settings. Two of the most well-known and best-studied forms of therapy are cognitive behavioral therapy (CBT) and exposure and response prevention (ERP). Eye movement desensitization reprocessing (EMDR) is being used increasingly with children, although systematic studies are still needed.

CBT uses a behavioral approach combined with a focus on identifying automatic "thinking errors" that perpetuate the anxiety. "Thinking errors," or negative cognitive processes, refer to a wide range of internal thought constructs that organize how children perceive, code, and experience their world and then fuel their emotions. In CBT treatments, youths are taught to identify "thinking errors" such as black and white thinking (only dishes washed in a dishwasher are free of germs), overgeneralization (all dogs are going to bite me), and catastrophic thinking (I just know this plane is going to crash) and then to realistically evaluate these negative cognitions in light of objective evidence. Youths are taught to restructure their thinking and develop a plan to cope with anxiety arousal by stressful situations. A key component of CBT is the completion of "homework" assignments. Practicing coping skills helps reinforce changes in pathologic cognitions. A number of studies have shown that parents rate their children as improved after completion of CBT. They notice a decrease in generalized anxiety and depression and an increase in coping and social skills. Treatment gains also tend to be maintained at 3-year follow-up. However, in at least one study comparing "attention" placebo-control treatment to CBT, both groups made significant improvement. This may indicate that the therapeutic relationship alone was the effective agent in helping children to overcome their anxiety. Alternatively, an attitude of "readiness to change" may be present when children come to treatment, and that attitude may propel them forward, regardless of the specific therapy.

ERP focuses on identifying a hierarchy of fearful stimuli, teaching the child relaxation techniques, and desensitizing the child to fearful stimuli via graded exposure. This approach is especially successful for treatment of specific phobias, social phobia, and agoraphobia. For example, children with fears of animals would be exposed to a small "nonthreatening" dog or picture of a dog. This causes anxiety and distress, but no catastrophic event follows, and children use their previously learned relaxation skills to decrease their discomfort. Subsequently, a decrease of anxiety symptoms occurs. After mastery of the milder anxiety aroused by a small animal, larger or more frightening animals may be used as the fear-provoking stimuli. The ERP process is repeated until treatment goals are obtained, that is, until the child can contain his anxious response and tolerate the anxiety-provoking stimulus.

The Coping Cat program was developed by Kendall et al. and is specifically indicated for children with SAD, GAD, and social phobia. There is a companion program called the Childhood Anxiety Treatment, or C.A.T. Project which is available for teens. The "Coping Cat" program is a manual-based psychotherapy program that incorporates the principles of CBT, ERP, and psychoeducational work with parents. The program consists of 16 to 18 individual sessions with several parent sessions. Individual sessions are focused on helping children to recognize the psychological and physiologic signs of anxious arousal, identify the cognitive processes associated with these signs, and develop specific plans to counter maladaptive patterns of behavior. Negative self-talk ("Kids will think I'm a loser") can be managed with replacement cognitions ("Lots of kids make mistakes from time to time and they still have friends"). Anxious children may be taught to recognize physical signs of anxiety such as hyperventilation and to use relaxation techniques such as deep breathing exercises and guided imagery. Children are given homework assignments and also allowed to practice coping skills while being exposed to anxiety-provoking situations. Parents are involved in a supportive role as consultants (not as coclients). The first part of the program is devoted to the development of the F.E.A.R. (Feeling frightened, Expecting bad things to happen, Attitudes and actions that will help, Results and rewards) plan, which is outlined in Table 7.5. The second half is devoted to exposure and practice of coping skills. Randomized clinical trials to examine the efficacy of the "Coping Cat" have been promising. One trial indicated that 64% of children who received the treatment no longer met diagnostic criteria for their primary diagnosis versus 5% of wait-list controls. Furthermore, these gains were maintained 1 year later. A second study found that 50% of cases no longer met criteria for the primary diagnosis after treatment. These programs are summarized in Table 7.5.

Barrett and Short developed the F.R.I.E.N.D.S. (Feeling worried, Relax and feel good, Inner thoughts, Explore plans, Nice work, Don't forget to practice, Stay Calm) program for adolescents based on similar concepts to the "Coping Cat" program. The components of this program are summarized in Table 7.6. In this program, the parents are also taught coping skills and learn how to support the child in identification of negative thoughts and implementation of adaptive responses. Parents are encouraged to model good coping skills and to form support networks with other parents. Group strategies have also been found to be effective. Randomized clinical trials have compared the efficacy of individual CBT (Coping Cat and F.R.I.E.N.D.S.) versus individual CBT plus family involvement. After treatment, 56% of the children with individual treatment alone no longer met criteria for the primary anxiety disorder versus 71% of the children who had individual treatment plus family involvement versus 25% of wait-list controls. Thus, family involvement augments the benefits of individual therapy.

TABLE 7.5. THE FEAR PLAN

F = Feeling frightened? The child learns how to recognize the symptoms of anxiety and practices relaxation techniques.

E = Expecting bad things to happen? The child learns to recognize negative self-talk and is trained to challenge thinking errors.

A = Attitudes and actions that will help. The child learns how to use positive self-talk and problem solving skills.

R = Results and rewards. Adaptive behavior is rewarded and the child is taught to expect partial results and not perfection. Children are encouraged to rate themselves and to give self-rewards.

TABLE 7.6. THE F.R.I.E.N.D.S. PROGRAM

F = Feeling worried? Children are taught to recognize the symptoms of anxiety.
R = Relax and feel good. Relaxation skills are taught and practiced.
I = Inner thoughts. Children identify negative self-talk.
E = Explore plans. Problem-solving skills are taught and practiced.
N = Nice work so reward yourself. Children learn to evaluate their performance and reward themselves for partial success (not necessarily perfection).
D = Don't forget to practice. Children are encouraged to role-play and practice the skills they have learned.
S = Stay calm. Children are reminded that they can stay calm because they now know how to cope with their worries.

Another therapy that focuses on ERP principles is EMDR. EMDR is a specific technique for desensitizing patients to fearful stimuli that has generated much controversy. Rothbaum studied EMDR compared to prolonged image exposure in rape victims and found that EMDR was preferred by both patients and therapists due to its shorter duration of treatment and the relatively decreased amount of induced emotional distress. There have been at least seven published, randomized, controlled studies, which support EMDR's superiority to wait-list, routine care, and active treatment controls in the treatment of PTSD. One of these studies included children. Allen argues that EMDR can be viewed as a variant of exposure therapy that incorporates elements of cognitive behavior therapy, relaxation therapy, and self-regulation. More studies are needed in this area, particularly with children.

FAMILY THERAPY

The goal of family therapy is to evaluate the family system in terms of areas of competence and dysfunction and to help the family change maladaptive patterns. As noted earlier, many children with anxiety disorders have parents who are also afflicted with anxiety. Dysfunctional family patterns can result, which serve to unwittingly perpetuate these disorders. Enmeshment and parental control can be important factors. For example, children with separation anxiety disorder may have parents who aggravate anxiety responses by not allowing their children to make any decisions on their own or engage in any activities without direct parental supervision. This intrusive parenting style driven by parental anxiety prevents the development of autonomous functioning. The child becomes anxious about being able to cope without the parent. Hence, family interventions should focus on decreasing the level of enmeshment between the child and parents, increasing appropriate boundaries, and developing autonomous functioning by the child. Parent training can also be an effective part of family intervention as demonstrated by the efficacy of the F.R.I.E.N.D.S. program described above.

PHARMACOTHERAPY

In contrast to ADHD, there is a dearth of research supporting the use of psychotropic medications for the treatment anxiety disorders occurring in youths except for OCD. Thus, the Food and Drug Administration (FDA) has not approved any psychotropic medication for the treatment of childhood anxiety disorders except for OCD. Despite this lack of data, several pharmacologic agents are routinely used in clinical practice to treat severe child and adolescent anxiety disorders. Of these, the selective serotonin reuptake inhibitors (SSRIs) have been the best studied and show the most promise. Other potentially helpful medications include benzodiazepines, anticonvulsants, β-blockers, α-2a agonists, and antipsychotics.

TABLE 7.7. PSYCHOTROPIC MEDICATIONS FOR TREATING ANXIETY DISORDERS

1st line: *SSRIs*—remember that SSRIs can induce anxiety or even panic symptoms in vulnerable individuals, so "start low and go slow." Sometimes, benzodiazepines are started concurrently with an SSRI and later tapered once the SSRI confers therapeutic benefits.

2nd line: *Benzodiazepines*—such as alprazolam, lorazepam, and clonazepam can be useful in the short-term treatment of anxiety, e.g., to reintegrate the child into school. Oxazepam is a good alternative for youth who are oversedated by the aforementioned agents. These agents need to be tapered slowly to avoid anxiety associated with withdrawal.

3rd line: α-2a *Agonists*—guanfacine and clonidine may be more useful for symptoms of hyperautonomic arousal such as palpitations and tachypnea.

Tricyclic antidepressants—with appropriate monitoring, can be used in youths without any cardiac problems.

Others: *Buspirone*—shown to be effective in a handful of case reports. Usually considered more effective in mild anxiety. Few associated side effects. No risk for the development of abuse or dependence.

Anticonvulsant agents—case reports mostly in adults support the use of anticonvulsants such as valproate, gabapentin, topiramate, and oxcarbazepine. Consider using when other agents have been ineffective.

Antipsychotic agents—may be useful when all other medications have not been successful or in children with borderline reality testing.

SSRIs, selective serotonin reuptake inhibitors.

An algorithm for psychotropic medications commonly used to treat anxiety disorders is summarized in Table 7.7.

Pediatric psychopharmacologists suggest that SSRIs and atypical antidepressants such as venlafaxine be used as first-line medications for the treatment of anxiety disorders. The SSRIs are generally well tolerated, do not require routine serum monitoring, and have an advantageous side effect profile. Several double-blinded placebo-controlled studies have shown efficacy of these antidepressants in the treatment of anxiety disorders in youths. For example, fluvoxamine (Luvox) is efficacious in treating phobias, GADs, and SAD in children. Paroxetine (Paxil) has been efficacious for social phobia and venlafaxine (Effexor) for GAD. Nevertheless, the 2004 FDA advisory against the use of all SSRIs with children and adolescents challenges clinicians to consider other nonpharmacologic interventions first. (See Chapters 22 and 24.) The most problematic complication of the SSRIs with children, especially those with anxiety disorders, is an "activation phase" that often occurs sometime during the first several weeks of treatment. Suicidal ideation and aggression may occur in a small percentage of youths. This "activation" may be minimized by starting with low doses of SSRIs, doses lower than what is used for depression. During this phase, children may be physically active, talkative, may feel jittery, and have trouble falling asleep. As these adverse reactions typically occur before the therapeutic effects develop, many parents discontinue the medication prematurely. Anticipating this response and obtaining full consent is essential to encouraging compliance. If such a reaction develops, lowering the dose may suffice. Fluoxetine (Prozac) is approved for the treatment of depression in children, while sertraline (Zoloft) and fluvoxamine (Luvox) are approved for treatment of OCD. No medications are approved for treatment of SAD, GAD, panic disorder, or phobic disorder. While the SSRIs have shown promise in various investigations, further study to determine their safety, efficacy, and range of responses is clearly needed.

Because of concerns of prolonged QT syndrome and sudden cardiac arrest noted in several children prescribed desipramine in the 1980s to 1990s, tricyclic antidepressants (TCAs) are considered second-line agents for the treatment of anxiety disorders. There are only a few double-blind placebo-controlled studies of imipramine in the treatment of school phobia and SAD, and results have been equivocal. One investigation by Gittelman-Klein and Klein supports the use of imipramine to treat SAD with or without school refusal. Another investigation by Bernstein et al. supports combining imipramine and CBT for anxious and depressed teens. Three negative studies were hindered by small sample size or inadequate imipramine dosage. Thus, it appears that imipramine and other TCAs may have a limited role in treating juvenile anxiety disorders but should only be considered when SSRIs are not effective. If TCAs are prescribed, serum monitoring is recommended. Baseline and intermittent follow-up electrocardiograms (ECGs) with dosage changes are also often obtained, even in the presence of normal serum levels.

Buspirone (Buspar) and combination psychotropic regimens are considered third-line agents. Although there has been little evidence to support its use in youths, buspirone, a nonbenzodiazepine anxiolytic, may be useful when other treatments fail. Buspirone has been shown to be effective in adults and is appealing because it does not pose the risk for abuse and dependence. Despite the lack of double-blinded controlled studies, several open-label and case studies suggest potential efficacy.

To date, there are no double-blind placebo-controlled studies of adequate statistical power that support the use of benzodiazepines in youths. Despite this of lack efficacy data, the benzodiazepines are considered a second-line treatment for anxiety disorders in children and adolescents. Their use is complicated because of the possibility of physiologic dependence, sedation, and decreased mental acuity. Furthermore, the benzodiazepines are often behaviorally disinhibiting with children and adolescents. It is prudent to give a test dose and to determine whether disinhibition, or a paradoxical reaction, results before prescribing a routine regimen. The use of benzodiazepines should usually be limited to 2 to 3 weeks to minimize the development of dependence. These agents are often used in the short term to alleviate acute symptoms of anxiety while awaiting the therapeutic effects of other agents, such as SSRIs, for example, to facilitate reentry into school. Lorazepam, clonazepam, and alprazolam are benzodiazepines used with pediatric populations. There is now a time-release preparation of alprazolam, which offers convenient once daily dosing.

Some anticonvulsants may have a role in the treatment of anxiety disorders because of their effects on GABA. β-blockers and α-2 adrenergic agonists have also been used to reduce arousal associated with anxiety. These agents are most commonly used in the treatment of explosive rage in children and adolescents, particularly associated with PTSD.

Antipsychotic agents have not been routinely recommended for the treatment of anxiety disorders in children and adolescents unless comorbid psychosis is present. In adults, trifluoperazine (Stelazine) has an FDA indication for the time-limited treatment of GAD, but because of risks of tardive dyskinesia and extrapyramidal (EPS), traditional antipsychotics are avoided at all ages. Because atypical antipsychotics have a lower occurrence of motor and cognitive side effects, they are sometimes used when other pharmacologic interventions have failed or when anxiety causes poor reality testing. They have most often been used for PTSD and OCD, but panic disorder and SAD can also demonstrate irrational anxiety that could require treatment with an antipsychotic medication.

Conclusion

The assessment, diagnosis, and treatment of childhood and adolescent anxiety disorders are complex in part due to the high degree of comorbidity with other anxiety disorders as well as with other psychiatric disorders and the developmental context in which anxiety disorders begin. Anxiety disorders affect a large portion of children and adolescents, causing them tremendous suffering in multiple domains of functioning. The risks are often too great to delay treatment, even in the absence of clear evidence-based treatment guidelines. Currently, cognitive behavioral treatments are the best supported interventions and should comprise the first line of treatment. Pharmacotherapy can augment psychosocial treatments as individualized to each youth's circumstances and response to psychotherapeutic interventions.

In Case vignette #2 (below), Alexandra's case illustrates how anxiety can develop a life of its own, becoming a "monster" which plagues children, adolescents, and their families. As more is learned about the biologic, psychological, cultural, and social factors that contribute to anxiety, improved treatment strategies can be developed. This underscores the need for further research.

Case Vignettes

Case vignette #1

Mark is an 8-year-old boy who was referred by his pediatrician due to problems in school. Teachers noted that he could not concentrate in class, took a long time in completing assignments, and was often forgetful and easily distracted. He was prescribed stimulant medication for the presumptive diagnosis of ADHD, but his mother reported that his symptoms actually seemed worse and she stopped the medication. His mother noted that he would follow her from room to room in the house, refusing to let her out of his sight. He explained that when he was at school, he was afraid that his mother had been killed in a car accident. He cried every morning before going to school and often missed the school bus, forcing his mother to drive him to school. Once there, he would become irritable and angry and, within an hour of being dropped off, he would go to the office complaining that he was going to throw up. On several occasions, he actually vomited, prompting school officials to call his mother to take him home. His symptoms lessened on the weekends, but by Sunday night, complaints about headaches and stomach upset began again. A thorough physical workup and referral to a pediatric gastroenterologist failed to resolve the problem. Although Mark was a very bright student, he was at risk for failing the third grade, and his mother was in danger of losing her job.

After a psychiatric evaluation, Mark was diagnosed with SAD. It turns out that his mother had similar problems when she was a child and had been depressed for several years. He was prescribed low dose sertraline, titrated up to a dose of 25 mg over a 2-week period. The school was advised to allow him to leave class if he was physically ill, but only to go to the counselor's office until he recovered and could return to class. Mark's symptoms were explained as his body's response to anxiety and that his worries, stomachaches, and headaches should gradually improve with treatment. The teachers were educated about sertraline's potential activation effects as well as expected therapeutic response. At 4-week follow-up, Mark and his family were markedly relieved. Indeed, he had become almost "hyperactive" for a while consistent with "activation," but these symptoms were resolving and the family noted marked improvement in his anxiety as well as his mood. He also began attending school without argument or requests to return home. He was still having difficulty falling asleep, but that was also improving as his parents were using a behavioral system to encourage him to sleep in his own bed at night.

Case vignette #2

Alexandra is a 10-year-old girl. She was a straight-A student in the gifted studies program when she became paralyzed by the fear of vomiting. She had always had a high degree of anxiety, but it had not interfered with her functioning until after her parents divorced. At that point, she began avoiding school or leaving school due to a variety of somatic complaints. Her grades dropped. At the peak of her anxiety, she reported that she saw and heard "monsters" that came to her at night. She complained of shortness of breath, rapid heart rate, and cried uncontrollably in a panic. Alexandra's story underscores many of the pathognomonic characteristics of anxiety disorders in children. In addition to school refusal, Alexandra developed a phobic response to vomiting.

Alexandra was experiencing such severe panic attacks that it was impossible to take her to school. She was prescribed alprazolam 0.125 mg 3 times a day, titrated up to a dose of 0.25 mg 3 times a day over the next 3 days. She was somewhat sleepy, but panic symptoms resolved and she was able to return to school. After resumption of school attendance, a low dose of sertraline was prescribed, titrated up to a dose of 37.5 mg over 4-weeks (sertraline was increased by 12.5 mg every 2 weeks). She also enrolled in weekly cognitive behavioral psychotherapy to address both her overt anxiety symptoms and her catastrophic negative thinking and worry related to her parents' recent divorce.

Eventually, Alexandra was able to sleep through the night, she began going to school regularly, and she started to tolerate and redirect her grief over her parents' divorce. Over the ensuing 4 months, she tapered off of alprazolam, maintained the sertraline, and continued in psychotherapy. Symptoms returned after several episodes of family crises, but Alexandra was able to get back on track with "tune ups" of therapy and pharmacotherapy.

BIBLIOGRAPHY

Allen JG, Lewis L. A conceptual framework for treating traumatic memories and its application to EMDR. *Bull Menninger Clin* 1996;60:238–263.

Barrett PM, Shortt A. Parental involvement in the treatment of anxious children. In: Kazdin AE, Weisz JR, eds. *Evidence-based psychotherapies for children and adolescents*. New York: Guilford Press, 2003.

Beidel DC, Alfano C, Yeganek R, et al. Pharmacological and psychosocial treatments for childhood social phobia. *Child Adolesc Psychopharmacol News* 2002;7:4–7.

Beidel DC, Turner SM, Hamlin K, et al. The Social Phobia and Anxiety Inventory for Children (SPAI-C): external and discriminative validity. *Behav Ther* 2000;31:75–87.

Berney T, Kolvin I, Bhate SR. School phobia: a therapeutic trial with clomipramine and short-term outcome. *Br J Psychiatry* 1981;138:110–118.

Bernstein GA, Borchardt CM, Perwien AR. Imipramine plus cognitive-behavioral therapy in the treatment of school refusal. *J Am Acad Child Adolesc Psychiatry* 2000;39:276–283.

Bernstein GA, Garfinkle BD, Borchardt CM. Comparative studies of pharmacotherapy for school refusal. *J Am Acad Child Adolesc Psychiatry* 1990;29:773–781.

Bernstein GA, Shaw K. Practice parameters for the assessment and treatment of anxiety disorders. *J Am Acad Child Adolesc Psychiatry* 1993;32:1089–1098.

Birmaher B, Khetarpal S, Brent D, et al. The Screen for Child Anxiety Related Emotional Disorders (SCARED): scale construction and psychometric characteristics. *J Am Acad Child Adolesc Psychiatry* 1997;36:545–553.

Busatto GF, Buchpiguel CA, Zamignani DR, et al. Regional cerebral blood flow abnormalities in early onset obsessive compulsive disorder: an exploratory SPECT study. *J Am Acad Child Adolesc Psychiatry* 2001;40:347–354.

Chemtob CM, Tolin DF, Van der Kolk BA. Eye movement desensitization and reprocessing. In: Foa EB, Keane TM, Friedman MJ, eds. *Effective treatments for PTSD: practice guidelines from the international society for traumatic stress studies*. New York: Guilford Press, 2000:139–155, 333–335.

Chess S, Thomas A, Birch HG. Implications of a longitudinal study of child development for child psychiatry. *Am J Psychiatry* 1960;117:431–441.

FDA Public Health Advisory (2004), Food and Drug Administration Website. At: http://www.fda.gov/cder/drug/antidepressants/AntidepressantsPHA.htm. Accessed April 1, 2004.

Gittelman-Klein R, Klein DF. Controlled imipramine treatment of school phobia. *Arch Gen Psychiatry* 1971;25:204–207.

Gittelman-Klein R, Klein DF. School phobia: diagnostic considerations in the light of imipramine effects. *J Nerv Ment Dis* 1973;156:199–215.

Hahn ME, Hewitt JK, Henderson ND, et al. *Developmental behavioral genetics: neural, biometrical, and evolutionary approaches.* New York: Oxford University Press, 1990.

Kendall PC, Aschenbrand SG, Hudson JL. Child focused treatment of anxiety. In: Kazdin AE, Weisz JR, eds. *Evidence-based psychotherapies for children and adolescents,* New York: Guilford Press, 2003:81–100.

Kendler KS, Neale MC, Kessler RC, et al. Major depression and generalized anxiety disorder: same gene, (partly) different environments? *Arch Gen Psychiatry* 1992;49:716–722.

Livingston R. Anxiety disorders. In: Lewis M, ed. *Child and adolescent psychiatry: a comprehensive textbook.* Baltimore, MD: Williams & Wilkins, 2000:674–684.

March JS, Parker JD, Sullivan K, et al. The Multidimensional Anxiety Scale for Children (MASC): factor structure, reliability, and validity. *J Am Acad Child Adolesc Psychiatry* 1997;36:554–565.

Masi G, Mucci TC, Toni M, et al. Paroxetine in children and adolescent outpatients with panic disorder. *J Child Adolesc Psychopharmacol* 2001;11: 151–157.

Mattison RE. Suicide and other consequences of childhood and adolescent anxiety disorders. *J Clin Psychiatry* 1988;suppl 49:9–11

Neumeister A, Bain E, Nugent AC, et al. Reduced serotonin type 1A receptor binding in panic disorder. *J Neurosci* 2004;21:589–591.

Ollendick TH. Reliability and validity of the Revised Fear Survey Schedule for Children (FSSC-R). *Behav Res Ther* 1983;21:685–692.

Rothbaum BO. A controlled study of eye movement desensitization and reprocessing in the treatment of posttraumatic stress disordered sexual assault victims. *Bull Menninger Clin* 1997;61: 317–334.

Sallee R, Greenwald J. Neurobiology. In: March JS, ed. *Anxiety disorders in children and adolescents.* New York: Guilford Press, 1995:3–34.

Schwartz CE, Snidman N, Kagan J. Adolescent social anxiety as an outcome of inhibited temperament in childhood. *J Am Acad Child Adolesc Psychiatry* 1999;38:1008–1015.

Silverman W, Ginsburg G. Specific phobia and generalized anxiety disorders. In: March JS, ed. *Anxiety disorders in children and adolescents.* New York: Guilford Press, 1995:151–180.

Stern DN. *The interpersonal world of the infant: a view from psychoanalysis and developmental psychology.* New York: Basic Books, 2000.

Westenberg PM, Siebelink BM, Warmenhoven NJ, et al. Separation anxiety and overanxious disorders: relations to age and level of psychological maturity. *J Am Acad Child Adolesc Psychiatry* 1999;38: 1000–1006.

Zeanah CH, Boris NW, Larrieu JA. Infant development and developmental risk: a review of the past 10 years. *J Am Acad Child Adolesc Psychiatry* 1997;36:165–178.

SUGGESTED READINGS

DuPont Spencer E, DuPont R, DuPont C. *The anxiety cure for kids: a guide for parents.* Hoboken, NJ: John Wiley and Sons, 2003.
(A text for parents, but good for teachers, coaches, therapists, and nurses too, that helps them understand how to help anxious children with many practical tips.)

Kendall PC. *Cognitive-behavioral therapy for anxious children: therapist manual,* 2nd ed. Philadelphia: Temple University, 2000.

(Therapists interested in using the Coping Cat Workbook should use this manual which contains general strategies used in the treatment of anxiety in youth.)

Ollendick TH, March J, eds. *Phobic and anxiety disorders in children and adolescents: a clinician's guide to effective psychosocial and pharmacological interventions.* New York: Oxford University Press, 2003.
(A comprehensive textbook on youth anxiety disorders for clinicians.)

CHAPTER 8

Obsessive–Compulsive Disorder

JAMIE L. SNYDER

Introduction

Symptoms of obsessive–compulsive disorder (OCD) are described as far back as 1467, though in the frame of reference of that time people with OCD symptoms were considered to be possessed by the devil. Religious texts in the 1600s described "scrupulosity," excessive devotion, and extremes of religious doubting. Pioneers in psychiatry began studying the phenomena as early as 1838. Freud noted obsessions and compulsions early in his professional career (1953), and Anna Freud proposed that ego deficits and conflicting drives led to obsessional neuroses. For many years it was thought that environmental factors and, especially, family problems, played a major role in the development of OCD, leading to blaming and guilt during psychoanalytic treatment, which was the predominant treatment for many years. However, the ineffectiveness of psychoanalytic treatment for OCD has led to newer conceptualizations and treatments for this serious and tenacious disorder, which frequently has its onset during childhood.

Since the 1980s there has been an explosion of research in OCD related to the discovery that serotonin-specific reuptake inhibitors (SSRIs), for example, fluoxetine (Prozac), paroxetine (Paxil), fluvoxamine (Luvox), sertraline (Zoloft), and citalopram (Celexa), can help many patients with OCD. The development of techniques like magnetic resonance imaging (MRI) to better examine brain structure as well as positron emission tomography (PET) and single photon emission computed tomography (SPECT) scanning to study brain metabolism and function have played important roles as well. Studies regarding the prevalence of OCD have found that it is neither as rare as was once thought, nor as prevalent as initial studies reported. Evidence has been found for genetic transmission and possibly an infective etiology. Thus, work over the past two decades has considerably increased our understanding and treatment of children and adolescents with OCD.

Clinical Features

DEFINITION

In the *Diagnostic and Statistical Manual of Mental Disorders,* Fourth Edition, Text Revision (DSM-IV-TR), OCD is defined as one of the anxiety disorders. Individuals with OCD experience their symptoms as anxiety-provoking and distressing in ways that are similar to the other anxiety disorders, but with precipitators that we define as obsessions and attempts to alleviate the anxiety that we call compulsions. Obsessions are defined as recurrent and persistent ideas, thoughts, impulses, or images that are experienced as intrusive and inappropriate and cause marked anxiety or distress. They are more than simply excessive worries about real-life problems; the person recognizes that they are the product of his or her own mind and tries to ignore or suppress them. Compulsions are defined as repetitive behaviors or mental acts that the person feels driven to perform and are aimed at preventing distress or some dreaded event. They are not realistically connected with what they are designed to prevent or are clearly excessive. Repetitive stereotypic behaviors often observed in youths with mental retardation or pervasive developmental disorders (MR/PDD) differ from compulsions as they are not as complex as compulsions, are not aimed at neutralizing an obsession, and are usually more nonfunctional (rocking or head banging).

OCD requires either obsessions or compulsions accompanied by marked distress, consuming more than 1 hour per day, or interfering with functioning. At some point the individual has recognized his or her symptoms as excessive or unreasonable, though the DSM-IV-TR notes that this criteria does not apply to children. Symptoms should not be due to a substance or a general medical condition. If another diagnosis is present, the content of the obsessions should be different from the symptoms typical of the comorbid disorder, for example, more than eating obsessions in an eating disorder or more than hair pulling in trichotillomania.

The presentation of OCD can vary widely. For those children who are secretive about their difficulties, the presenting parental concerns may be temper tantrums, decreased school performance, food restrictions, or dermatitis rather than OCD. Temper tantrums in children with OCD tend to occur when their compulsions are prevented or interrupted. Decreased school performance occurs for a variety of reasons: (a) children sometimes redo their work until some impossible level of perfection is reached, (b) they will often refuse to turn in their work if it is not perfect; (c) classes may be missed while performing bathroom rituals at school; or (d) performing other rituals like repeatedly going in and out doors or up and down stairs even to the point of missing classes altogether. Food refusals or restrictions may be based on obsessive fears about contamination, fears of becoming fat, ordering rituals about food placement on the plate, or foods not touching one another.

Dermatitis can result from washing compulsions. Sometimes cleaning compulsions can present as a toilet stopped up from repeated wiping after defecation or with high volume use of soap, water, towels, or excessive clothing changes.

Systematic studies have shown heterogeneity in the onset and course of children's illness, as well as age at onset, comorbid diagnoses, and accompanying neurologic symptoms such as tics or choreiform movements. The typical presentation includes both obsessions and compulsions, often multiple; however, having only obsessions may be more common. This presentation can include all the symptoms of obsessions without the compulsions; thus, these children present with the internal distress and anxiety characteristics of obsessions but without the repetitive habits characteristic of compulsions. If children have insight, that is, an understanding that their thoughts are unusual or irrational and/or that there is something wrong with them, and can report their distress, this diagnosis is no more difficult to make. However, if children lack insight, that is do not feel there is anything wrong with them or perhaps feel that others are unreasonable, or are unable to describe their inner distress (for example, due to a language disorder or pervasive developmental disorder), the diagnosis can be difficult. Over time, the objects and content of obsessions and compulsions may change. Most patients in one long-term study endorsed all of the common symptoms at some point during their course of illness.

In an adolescent study, the most common categories of obsessions were contamination fears, fears regarding safety of themselves or loved ones, exactness or symmetry, and religious scrupulousness. Less common were concerns regarding bodily functions, lucky numbers, and sexual or aggressive preoccupations (in adults, aggressive and sexual preoccupations are more common). Obsessional slowness is a potentially disabling presentation in which a child moves dramatically slowly. Careful assessment may reveal preoccupation with multiple mental rituals that interfere with normal activities.

The most common compulsions in an adolescent study, in descending order of frequency, were cleaning rituals, repeating actions (doing and undoing), and checking rituals. Less common were rituals to protect themselves/others from illness or injury (i.e., avoiding "contaminated" objects), ordering maneuvers, and counting behaviors. Although some compulsions are tied to a specific worry/obsession, many consist of repeating an action until it "feels right." For example, these youths may go in and out through a door or up and down stairs until they "get it right." The sense of closure or completion that the child seeks may require symmetry, such as repeating an action with both left and right hands or repeating actions an odd or even number of times. Compulsive rereading or rewriting can interfere with school performance. Mental rituals may consist of silent praying, repetition, counting, or having to think about or look at something in a particular way until it feels "right." Children with OCD are less able than adults to specify what their rituals are intended to avert beyond a vague idea of something bad happening.

Compared to the general clinical population, children with OCD may be more selectively impaired. On the surface, they may appear to function well. School and social performance may be preserved until the symptoms become quite severe. This is partly due to awareness that their thoughts/symptoms are odd or unusual, so they can be quite embarrassed and secretive about the severity of their impairment. They often engage their families in assisting them in their rituals, such as cleaning or checking for them, or "covering" for them, such as making excuses if they miss school. Some patients can accept that something is done "right" if the parent does it for them. The child may become angry with the parents for trying to seek assistance for the problems. The parents want to believe that the symptoms are "just a phase." Often by the time they come to clinical attention, the whole family revolves around the child and his or her symptoms, often not realizing how much time or money they spend supporting the child's symptoms, for example, by doing many loads of laundry, using numerous bars of soap, and paying increased water bills for a child with contamination fears. Frequently, the initial manifesting symptoms can be perceived as adaptive, such as thinking that cleanliness is good, perfect homework is a good thing, and organizing is a positive behavior. The child does not always share the disturbing thoughts with parents, so well-meaning clinicians sometimes reassure parents that all is well/"normal" without asking all the right questions. Parents often prefer to accept reassurances rather than accept that there is something wrong with their child.

Epidemiology

As with any disorder presenting in childhood, the context of what is "normal for age" must be understood. Mild or transient obsessions and compulsions are common in the general population. A survey mailed to parents of children less than 6 years old found that urges to make things "just right" and preoccupations with symmetry and rules are very common in this group. A recent study of nonclinical samples found that 60% of fourth graders reported preoccupations with guilt about lying, as well as engaging in checking behaviors, while 50% reported contamination and germ fears.

The difficulty in assessing the prevalence of OCD comes in distinguishing the *disorder* from *symptoms* that occur as common experiences and as developmental phenomena. Screening tools used in various population studies throughout the years have varying levels of sensitivity and appear to differ greatly from clinical assessment tools, making it difficult to compare prevalence rates across studies.

The first prevalence reports for childhood OCD ranged from 0.2% to 1.2%. A rigorous study of a general adolescent population in 1988 reported a weighted point prevalence of 1%, with a lifetime prevalence of 1.9%. Many investigators have used the term *subclinical* OCD to describe subjects reporting substantial symptoms without the severity needed to meet the full OCD criteria. Depending on the definition used, prevalence estimates of subclinical OCD in adolescence range from 4% to 19%.

Boys and girls appear to be equally affected, though male patients may have an earlier age of onset. In a 1991 study, 35% of adult men reported that they had onset of their symptoms between the ages of 5 and 15 years, compared with 20% of women. In another study, boys were more likely to have early onset and a family member with OCD or Tourette disorder, while girls were more likely to have adolescent onset. There do not appear to be any differences in prevalence based on race/ethnicity or geography.

Clinical Course

The onset of OCD may occur quite early; there are case reports of children as young as 5 years and the modal age of onset in one study was 7 years old, while the mean age of onset was 10.2 years. This may imply the existence of an early onset as well as an adolescent-onset group.

Symptoms may exist an average of 5 to 8 years before patients reach clinical attention. This may be due to secretiveness, as most patients recognize their symptoms as unusual and so hide them, or lack of awareness about the disorder and treatment availability. Parental perception of the severity of the child's symptoms plays a major role in determining when the child is brought to treatment. Often, parents have spent years learning to accommodate the child's symptoms, erroneously believing that the child is just "going through a phase," or that by aiding the child in his or her compulsions that they are helping relieve the child's anxiety. They will sometimes minimize the severity of the symptoms and the amount of time the family and/or child spends coping with the symptoms. If the parents have any symptoms themselves, their recognition of the abnormality of their child's symptoms will frequently be impaired. Teachers, pediatricians, and primary-care physicians are frequently the people responsible for initiating an assessment.

OCD in children and adolescents appears to be a chronic condition with a waxing and waning course. In a large systematic follow-up study of pediatric OCD, 54 patients at National Institutes of Mental Health (NIMH) were evaluated 2 to 7 years after treatment. At follow-up, 43% still met diagnostic criteria for OCD, with only 6% reportedly symptom free.

Outcome studies in children and adolescents have not revealed any factors promoting recovery or persistence of OCD. Patient age, sex, and socioeconomic status have failed to predict response to treatment in two different studies or to predict relapse with desipramine substitution. Children who acknowledge the senselessness of their obsessions and are distressed by their rituals, that is, they have insight, may be more motivated to participate in treatment, though insight is not a prerequisite for treatment effectiveness. Situations complicated by oppositional behavior and/or family chaos may make treatment more challenging as illustrated by one finding that high "expressed emotion" may exacerbate OCD, while a calm, supportive family may improve the outcome.

Etiology and Pathogenesis

Genetic studies show evidence for a genetic component in OCD. Concordance rates are elevated in monozygotic compared to dizygotic twins, and higher rates for OCD are seen among first-degree relatives of clinical patients with OCD. An additional finding was that earlier age of onset was associated with greater "familiality," that is, a greater likelihood of OCD among relatives.

Elevated rates of OCD among patients with Tourette disorder and elevated occurrence of tics and a family history of tics among OCD patients suggest that the two disorders may have a similar genetic origin.

A number of structural and functional neuroimaging studies have examined patients with OCD compared to never-ill controls, both adults and adolescents. While studies are not conclusive yet, several computed tomography (CT) studies in the 1980s and structural MRI studies of the 1990s suggested abnormalities in the frontal cortex and the caudate nuclei of patients with OCD. Functional studies using PET in the 1980s and early 1990s reported increased activity in the orbital gyri and the caudate nuclei, which reversed with medication treatment. A functional MRI study in 1996 pointed to elevated activity in the frontal cortex, the caudate and lenticular nuclei, and the amygdala. Finally, functional magnetic resonance spectroscopy studies in 2000 found elevated glutamate levels in the caudate nuclei of 11 treatment-naïve pediatric subjects. After treatment with paroxetine, levels were equivalent to those in normal controls.

Pediatric autoimmune neuropsychiatric disorders associated with streptococcal infections (PANDAS) may be an important mechanism in the development of OCD in 10% to 20% of OCD patients. Typically, symptoms arise, or exacerbate, acutely after a streptococcal infection, often accompanied by the development of tics. This phenomenon may be related to obsessive–compulsive symptoms seen in Syndenham chorea. Similar to rheumatic carditis, there is some evidence that antineuronal antibodies formed against group A β-hemolytic streptococcal cell wall antigens cross-react with caudate neural tissue. Reviewing numerous studies that have been done in the last decade looking at PANDAS, the findings are equivocal, and it appears that immunologically curbing treatment such as plasmapheresis or immunoglobulin are only worth considering for acute infection-related onset or severe exacerbation of symptoms.

Assessment

Evaluation of any child or adolescent must consist of gathering information from as many relevant sources as appropriate. This always includes the child and his primary caregiver, as well as other sources who might be able to assist in the development of a complete picture of the child and his difficulties. These other sources could include a teacher, a noncustodial parent, extended family members, a day-care provider, a former foster family, and previous treatment providers. A thorough assessment is the only way to distinguish normal developmental variations, subclinical symptoms, differential diagnoses, and comorbidities, as well as examine any psychological problems that might be supporting the symptoms or otherwise complicating the clinical picture. A comprehensive evaluation of the child's development, social and academic functioning, and medical and family histories is essential, including a careful assessment of current and past obsessive–compulsive symptoms and any comorbid conditions. A family assessment is an important part of the evaluation, not only for the information they can provide about the patient, but to assess their understanding of their child, their responses to the child's behaviors, and their ability to participate in their child's treatment (potential parental psychopathology). Family history of OCD, tic disorders, or anxiety disorders should be assessed since these are often familial and can impact the child's treatment.

As previously discussed, some repetitive, perfectionistic, or ritualistic behaviors are common in children at various stages of development. Thus, in an assessment, it is important not only to identify specific symptoms but also assess their context, frequency and the severity of associated distress, and dysfunction. It is also important to note the child's efforts to resist the obsessions and compulsions and his or her success in these efforts. Determining the child's ability to resist gives some idea of the child's insight and motivation for therapy.

Over time, a child's OCD may manifest in many different ways, and the clinician should inquire about all the various categories of obsessions and compulsions. Some typical obsessions and compulsions are summarized in Table 8.1.

If the family presents for evaluation using the terms *obsessions* or *compulsions*, it is important to ask them to describe the behavior as such terms can vary greatly from family to family. Once the potential diagnosis of OCD is suspected, instruments such as the Children's Yale-Brown Obsessive Compulsive Scale (CY-BOCS) can be used to rate and record symptom severity. The CY-BOCS was developed as a clinician-administered interview and as such it can require considerable time to complete. However, some clinicians forego the formal interview format, instead using it to summarize areas to be assessed. There is also a brief self-report screening version that patients can fill out to give clinicians some guidelines for further intervention. The Children's Version of the Leyton Obsessional Inventory (CV-LOI) is also useful to assess children older than 10 years old. A

TABLE 8.1. TYPES OF OBSESSIONS AND COMPULSIONS

Types of Obsessions/Fears	Types of Compulsions/Behavior
Aggressive	Cleaning/washing
Contamination	Checking
Sexual	Repeating rituals
Hoarding/saving	Counting
Religious/scrupulosity	Ordering/arranging
Need for symmetry	Hoarding/collecting
Somatic	Miscellaneous
Miscellaneous	

major advantage of the CV-LOI is that it has population norms and includes obsessive–compulsive personality traits.

Given the close association between tic disorders and OCD, specific assessment of any history of motor or vocal tics should be conducted. More complex tics, such as tapping and touching patterns, may be difficult to distinguish from compulsive behavior as both may be preceded by premonitory physical sensations, urges, and mental perceptions that persist until the action is completed. In general, if there is no history of simple tics, then complex tics can be ruled out, thereby increasing the likelihood that such behaviors represent a compulsion. When tics are present, one should inquire whether they are accompanied by specific fears or a vague discomfort that something bad might happen if the behaviors are not completed, which also would increase the likelihood that the behavior is a compulsion. Clinicians should also inquire about compulsive habits such as nail-biting, hair pulling, or skin picking. Generally tics, perseverative or stereotyped behaviors, and habits are not as complex as compulsions, are not aimed at neutralizing an obsession, and are usually more nonfunctional (rocking or head banging).

There are no pathognomonic laboratory findings in OCD. Any laboratory evaluations should be based on the findings of the comprehensive evaluation. Baseline electrocardiogram (ECG), child behavior check (CBC), electrolytes, liver function, and blood, urea, nitrogen (BUN)/Creatinine levels may be necessary before beginning medications. If tics, chorea, or psychotic symptoms are present, measurements of serum copper for Wilson disease should be considered. CT or MRI is only necessary if focal neurologic findings are found. An electroencephalogram (EEG) is only indicated if a seizure disorder is suspected.

A child with acute onset of tics and/or OCD symptoms needs careful consideration of medical illnesses during the preceding months. A throat culture and an antistreptolysin O or antistreptococcal DNAase B titer may be worth considering.

Psychological tests such as the Wechsler Intelligence Scales for Children, third edition (WISC-3) can be helpful to assess any concerns with intellectual function, severity of internal stressors, and characteristic defense mechanisms used by the child. Behavior-rating scales such as the Achenbach Child Behavior Checklist could be useful in screening for comorbid conditions or evaluating behavioral problems. The essential aspects of assessing a child for OCD are summarized in Table 8.2.

TABLE 8.2. ESSENTIALS OF ASSESSMENT OF OBSESSIVE–COMPULSIVE DISORDER

1. Since some repetitive, perfectionistic, or ritualistic behaviors are common in children at various stages of development, identify symptoms, their frequency, severity, and context within a developmental framework.
2. A comprehensive evaluation should include the child's development, social and academic functioning, and medical history along with a careful assessment of current and past OCD symptoms and comorbid conditions.
3. Family history of OCD, tic disorders, or anxiety disorders should be assessed as these disorders are often familial, can impact the child's treatment, and may guide treatment decisions.
4. As a child's OCD may manifest in many different ways, the clinician should inquire about the major categories of obsessions and compulsions as summarized in Table 8.1.
5. In order to determine severity, assess symptom context, frequency, and associated distress/dysfunction, as well as the child's efforts to resist the obsessions and compulsions and his or her success in these efforts.
6. Instruments such as the Children's Yale-Brown Obsessive Compulsive Scale can be used to rate and record symptom severity and can be helpful to summarize the areas to be assessed.
7. Given the association between tic disorders and OCD, assessment for motor or vocal tics should be conducted.
8. Any laboratory or other evaluations should be based on the findings of the clinical evaluation.

OCD, obsessive–compulsive disorder.

Differential Diagnosis and Comorbidity

There are many disorders that either coexist with OCD or have obsessions or compulsions as part of their manifestation, as summarized in Table 8.3.

Some authors argue that to organize a whole group of heterogeneous disorders and comorbid features under the term OCD based on the presence of a single symptom seems arbitrary. There is also some evidence for various "types" of OCD, such as tic related versus non-tic related. Care must be taken not to equate *subclinical* obsessions and compulsions with OCD, especially in adolescents who may be demonstrating signs and symptoms of obsessive–compulsive personality disorder (OCPD).

OBSESSIVE–COMPULSIVE PERSONALITY DISORDER

Characteristics of OCPD are listed in Table 8.4.

OCPD is, as the name suggests, a personality disorder that is coded on Axis II of the DSM-IV nomenclature. As a personality disorder, symptoms of OCPD represent a stable characteristic pattern of daily functioning, as opposed to the waxing and waning symptoms of OCD, which appear to represent an illness superimposed on an individual's personality. These two disorders do not appear to represent a simple continuum of obsessive–compulsive symptomatology, and some investigators have bemoaned the similar terminology. Patients with OCPD do not usually experience their obsessional and compulsive behaviors as ego-dystonic; that is, the symptoms do not provoke anxiety in them, and ordinarily the symptoms do not result in significant functional impairment except perhaps in social or intimate relationships. OCPD does tend to exacerbate with a person's level of stress, but persists at some level all the time. Most patients with OCD do not exhibit OCPD, but it does appear to be more common among patients with OCD and their relatives than in the general population, especially among those with hoarding symptoms. This may reflect a spectrum of conditions with vertical transmission.

TIC DISORDERS

At least 50% of children and adolescents with Tourette disorder develop obsessive–compulsive symptoms or disorder by adulthood. Conversely, a personal or family history

TABLE 8.3. DIFFERENTIAL DIAGNOSIS FOR OBSESSIVE–COMPULSIVE DISORDER

Psychiatric Differential Diagnoses	Medical/Organic Differential Diagnoses
Obsessive–compulsive personality disorder	Medical conditions
Tic disorder/Tourette disorder	Carbon monoxide poisoning
Mood disorders (depression/bipolar)	Tumors
Other anxiety disorders	Allergic reactions to wasp sting
(Panic disorder/phobias/PTSD)	Postviral encephalitis
Pervasive developmental disorders	Traumatic brain injury
Trichotillomania	Syndenham chorea
Disruptive behavior disorders (ADHD/ODD)	Prader-Willi syndrome
Eating disorders (anorexia/bulimia)	Medication side effects
Body dysmorphic disorder	Dopamine agonists (in animal studies)
Psychosis/schizophrenia	High-dose stimulants (in children)
Hypochondriasis/somatoform disorder	

PTSD, posttraumatic stress disorder; ADHD, attention deficit hyperactivity disorder; ODD, oppositional defiant disorder.

TABLE 8.4. *DIAGNOSTIC AND STATISTICAL MANUAL OF MENTAL DISORDERS,* **FOURTH EDITION, TEXT REVISION DIAGNOSTIC CRITERIA COMPARISON OF OBSESSIVE–COMPULSIVE DISORDER VERSUS OBSESSIVE–COMPULSIVE PERSONALITY DISORDER**

Obsessive–Compulsive Disorder DSM-IV-TR Diagnostic Criteria	Obsessive–Compulsive Personality Disorder DSM-IV-TR Diagnostic Criteria
Recurrent and persistent thoughts, impulses, or images that are experienced at some time during the disturbance as intrusive and inappropriate and that caused marked anxiety or distress.	Preoccupied with details, rules, lists, order, organization, or schedules to the extent that the major point of the activity is lost.
Obsessional thoughts, impulses, or images are not simply excessive worries about real-life problems.	Shows perfectionism that interferes with task completion (can't complete a task because overly strict standards are not met).
Person with obsessions attempts to ignore or suppress such thoughts, impulses, or images, or to neutralize them with some other thought or action.	Excessively devoted to work and productivity to the exclusion of leisure activities and friendships (not accounted for by obvious economic necessity).
Obsessional person recognizes that the obsessional thoughts, impulses, or images are a product of his or her own mind (not imposed from without as in thought insertion).	Overconscientious, scrupulous, and inflexible about matters of morality, ethics, or values (not accounted for by cultural or religious identification).
Repetitive behavior (e.g., hand washing, ordering, checking, praying, counting, repeating words silently) that the person feels driven to perform in response to obsession or according to rules that must be applied rigidly.	Unable to discard worn-out or worthless objects even when they have no sentimental value.
Compulsive behaviors or mental acts are aimed at preventing or reducing distress or preventing some dreaded event or situation; however, these behaviors either are not connected in a realistic way with what they are designed to neutralize or prevent or are clearly excessive.	Reluctant to delegate tasks or to work with others unless they submit to exactly his or her way of doing things.
At some point during the course of the disorder, the person recognizes that the symptoms are excessive or unreasonable (this does not apply to children).	Reluctant to delegate tasks or to work with others unless they submit to exactly his or her way of doing things.
Obsessions or compulsions cause marked distress, are time consuming (use at least 1 hour a day), or significantly interfere with the person's normal routine or usual social activities.	Rigidity and stubbornness.

DSM-IV-TR, *Diagnostic and Statistical Manual of Mental Disorders,* Fourth Edition, Text Revision.

From American Psychiatric Association. *Diagnostic and statistical manual of mental disorders*, 4th ed, Text rev. Washington, DC: American Psychiatric Association, 2000, with permission.

of tics is found in nearly 60% of children and adolescents seeking treatment for OCD, ranging from simple, mild, and transient tics up through Tourette disorder. Recent studies suggest a difference in clinical presentation, neurobiology, and responsiveness to pharmacologic interventions between tic-related versus non–tic-related OCD. Though there is significant overlap, these two possible subtypes appear to differ in gender ratio, age at onset, and the number and nature, but not severity, of symptoms. Some investigators have described these subtypes as early onset versus pubertal onset. Tic-related OCD appears to have earlier onset and to occur more frequently in boys than girls, as well as a generally less satisfactory response to treatment with an SSRI alone. While it is clearly important to assess for tics in a patient with OCD due to a high rate of comorbidity, the importance of such assessment will likely increase even further as more is learned about potential subtypes of OCD and differential treatment protocols.

ANXIETY AND MOOD DISORDERS

One third to one half of children with OCD has a current or past history of another anxiety disorder, commonly generalized anxiety disorder (GAD) or separation anxiety disorder (SAD). Children with GAD worry about many issues that are generally realistic but excessive. They do not demonstrate odd irrational thoughts, nor do they demonstrate compulsive behaviors intended to manage their intrusive irrational thoughts. GAD may coexist with OCD. Such children show baseline worry and hyperarousal in addition to their specific obsessive–compulsive symptoms. Anxiety associated with SAD is specific to separation from the attachment figure, generally the mother, and is relieved by being in that person's presence. Such youths may have major tantrums upon separation, and these tantrums may be difficult to differentiate from the tantrums associated with OCD.

Depressive disorders are also commonly comorbid with rates reported from 20% to 73%. Many depressed children demonstrate irritability as their core mood symptom rather than a depressed mood or anhedonia. As irritability is also a common symptom of OCD, other symptoms of depression should be examined to either confirm or eliminate depressive disorders in the differential.

PERVASIVE DEVELOPMENTAL DISORDERS (PDD)

Children with PDDs like Autism or Asperger disorder often have repetitive behaviors and routines, as well as unusual preoccupations with inanimate items such as fans, maps, or numbers that caregivers may describe as obsessive–compulsive. Though these characteristics can cause functional impairment or be disturbing to others, the cognitive and language delays typical of these disorders make it difficult to assess whether the child finds these symptoms distressing, that is, whether they are anxiety provoking for the child. Typically, their rigid insistence on routines is part of a larger difficulty making transitions, as well as a need for sameness and structure, or, more simply, perseveration. While the diagnosis of OCD may not be completely applicable to these children, the obsessive–compulsive symptoms appear to share common features with uncomplicated OCD, such as high rates of OCD in first-degree relatives and potential responsiveness to SSRIs. Finally, PDD and OCD can co-occur. In this case, children must demonstrate the core PDD symptom of deficits in interpersonal relatedness.

TRICHOTILLOMANIA

Trichotillomania is defined as persistent hair pulling to the point of alopecia and is classified in DSM-IV-TR as an impulse control disorder, not an anxiety disorder. However, many investigators now think of trichotillomania as part of an "obsessive–compulsive spectrum disorder" as it shares similarities with OCD in being a repetitive behavior associated with specific "urges" or "need" to perform the behavior. Many children and adolescents with trichotillomania do not manifest any other OCD symptoms, but the rate of OCD is elevated in this population and their first-degree relatives.

DISRUPTIVE BEHAVIOR DISORDERS

Most children with OCD are only neat, overly compliant, or attentive to detail within the context of their symptoms. For example, children that are perfectionistic about their schoolwork may have an extremely messy bedroom. Indeed, they may be irritable or impulsive, and as many as half of the children with OCD may meet criteria for a disruptive behavior disorder like attention deficit hyperactivity disorder (ADHD) or oppositional defiant disorder. This particular comorbidity makes it difficult to determine the relative mix of compulsiveness versus oppositionalism or inattentiveness in any particular behavioral incident. Previously well-behaved children may become defiant, demanding, and even assaultive in the desperate drive to perform their compulsions. On the other hand, children with oppositional tendencies frequently learn to claim their OCD as the basis for all their misbehavior.

OTHER DISORDERS

Obsessive–compulsive symptoms and disorder are common in patients with anorexia or bulimia nervosa. While obsessions related to food, exercise, weight, or body image would be subsumed within the eating disorder diagnosis, symptoms can extend to the full range of obsessions and compulsions including symmetry, doubting, contamination, checking, counting, and ordering. In the latter case, it would then be appropriate to make a separate diagnosis of OCD.

Body dysmorphic disorder is characterized by an obsessional preoccupation with an imagined or slight defect in appearance. This is frequently accompanied by obsessive grooming or mirror-checking rituals. It is not yet clear what relationship this disorder has to OCD.

Psychosis must be considered when children manifest bizarre behavior if they are unable to consider the possibility that their symptoms originate in their minds, that is, they lack insight, or if there is a dramatic deterioration in functioning. In most cases of OCD, thinking remains reality-based (except for the area of obsessional concern). The content of any "bizarre" thoughts is related to their obsessional theme and not generalized to other more "typical" psychiatric themes. Unless there are hallucinations, psychosis would not be an appropriate diagnosis. However, schizophrenia can also co-occur with OCD and should be considered in older children and adolescents with psychotic features.

As noted in Table 8.3, medical conditions or medication side effects can induce OCD symptoms, but this would preclude the diagnosis of OCD.

There are a large number of children with poor social skills, low frustration tolerance, cognitive unevenness, and problems with mood, anxiety, and/or attention that do not fit easily into any single diagnostic category. They are often irritable, perseverative, overfocused on specific topics, unable to shift tasks easily, and insistent that things be done "just right," with intense outbursts resulting if they are denied. Authors have used various descriptors for this group of children, depending on their theoretical or professional background. More research is needed with this group of children to delineate their relationship to OCD.

Treatment

Each child presenting with obsessive–compulsive symptoms requires an individualized, comprehensive assessment and treatment plan. The nature and severity of obsessive–compulsive symptoms, the range of comorbidities, and the functional level of each child and his or her family can vary significantly and impact treatment planning. While family members' psychopathology is neither necessary nor sufficient for the onset of OCD, they affect and are affected by the disorder. Parents or siblings can become involved in the patient's rituals; they may have difficulty dealing with the aggressive or sexual content of obsessions or have differences of opinion about how to respond to the patient's symptoms. To foster compliance in treatment, both the patient and family need to participate as much as possible in the development of the treatment plan. Family involvement can be especially important for younger patients.

Two types of treatment have been studied systematically and have shown specific efficacy for the core symptoms of OCD: cognitive-behavioral therapy (CBT) and pharmacotherapy. Although psychodynamic psychotherapy may be useful as an adjunctive treatment to teach coping skills, increase the child's sense of mastery, treat comorbid anxiety or depression, and improve peer and family relationships, it does not appear to impact the core obsessive–compulsive symptoms of OCD.

For patients with mild to moderate symptoms, CBT would ideally be the first-line treatment of choice due to potential side effects of medication. If the patient is not rapidly responsive or if symptoms are more severe or accompanied by a significant depression, then early treatment with medication would be indicated. Some patients and their families will prefer to begin with CBT in the hopes of avoiding medication and potential side effects, while others will choose medication first, trying to avoid the time, effort, and anxiety associated with cognitive-behavioral interventions. There is evidence that combination treatment is the most effective, with a larger magnitude of symptom improvement and lower relapse rates than when medication is used alone. This combination method allows use of the lowest possible dose of medication over time and may improve both short- and long-term outcome in an illness that tends to be chronic, especially for the population that requires pharmacotherapy.

PSYCHOSOCIAL INTERVENTIONS

Several good studies have systematically studied the use of CBT in children and adolescents with OCD and have found it to be an effective treatment method, either alone or in conjunction with medication. Treatment generally consists of a 3-stage approach, beginning with information gathering, then therapist-assisted exposure with response prevention (E/RP), and homework assignments. The hallmark of CBT is E/RP. This consists of real or imagined exposure to a feared object or situation without being able to perform the accompanying compulsion. The exposure portion of this treatment depends on the fact that anxiety will decrease after prolonged exposure with the feared stimulus, and repeated exposure is associated with decreased anxiety across exposure trials until the child no longer fears exposure. This can be done in a gradual way, termed *graded exposure*, or through flooding, with the process under either patient or therapist control. In graded exposure, the therapist helps the patient make a list of his or her fears using a hierarchy from easiest to hardest to tolerate, with exposure beginning at the easy end. In contrast, flooding involves prolonged exposure to the most anxiety-provoking stimulus on the hierarchy. While flooding may shorten the duration of the treatment, it is frequently not well tolerated by young people and, if failed, may reinforce their anxiety and/or disrupt the therapeutic relationship. Children and adolescents are often more compliant with a treatment if they are given as much control as possible. For this reason, it is recommended that graded E/RP be used, with targets chosen by the patient guided by consultation with the therapist, but with the understanding that the child must make progress.

Response prevention involves blocking the performance of rituals or stopping avoidance behavior. For a child with contamination fears, this would involve refraining from washing after an exposure until his or her anxiety decreases or not going out of the way to avoid exposure. Since many exposures happen naturally during the course of a day, response prevention can be selected independently of a scheduled exposure protocol. For instance, a child would normally encounter "unclean" situations in a school environment. Not avoiding bathrooms or refraining from excessive washing rituals after exposure would be noncontrived, or naturalistic, response prevention.

Probably the biggest limitation to this type of treatment remains its relative lack of availability outside of academic research centers with anxiety disorder subspecialty clinics.

However, treatment manuals developed at such academic centers are now available to assist the interested therapist.

PHARMACOTHERAPY

Of all childhood psychiatric disorders, OCD has the best evidence-based data supporting pharmacologic treatment and the largest number of Food and Drug Administration (FDA)-approved medications for use in children. Even so, the best studies find approximately 42% of patients "respond" to first-time single-agent treatment with a reduction of 25% to 40% in severity of symptoms. While this represents a significant improvement in functional level and subjective distress, the majority of patients continue to experience some symptoms of OCD, and more than half may not respond to the initial treatment trial. It is best to have a discussion of this issue during the initial treatment consent process so that the patient's expectations of treatment will not be unreasonable.

In order to decide whether a patient is a "responder," an adequate dose must be given for a sufficient time period. Several studies have shown that OCD response rates continue to increase for up to 12 weeks and that OCD may require higher doses of medication than would typically be used to treat depression. An adequate trial has been given when the patient receives the maximum allowable dose or the maximum dose the patient can tolerate for no less than 12 weeks. Response, or lack of response, to one medication does not predict response to another, nor do side effects with one agent predict side effects with another. Before moving on to polypharmacy, it is important to give adequate trials of at least two single medications for a sufficient period of time.

The most thoroughly studied medications in the treatment of childhood OCD are the selective serotonin reuptake inhibitors (SRIs/SSRIs). Blinded, placebo-controlled studies have been conducted with fluoxetine (Prozac), fluvoxamine (Luvox), sertraline (Zoloft), and clomipramine (Anafranil). The SSRIs fluvoxamine, fluoxetine, and sertraline are FDA-approved for treatment of OCD in children down to the ages of 8, 7, and 6 years, respectively. Clomipramine, an SRI, has shown efficacy in the treatment of OCD in children and is FDA-approved down to age 10, but due to its side-effect profile is generally considered a second-line treatment, for use primarily in patients with treatment-resistant OCD. Other SSRIs such as citalopram (Celexa) or escitalopram (Lexapro) are in general clinical use based on extrapolation from safety and efficacy data in adult studies of OCD or in open trials with children. Since all of the medications show similar response rates, the choice of medication is frequently based on side effect profile or the patient's comorbidities, as shown in Table 8.5. For instance, an overweight low energy child might respond best to fluoxetine (Prozac) due to its potential side effects of decreased appetite and increased energy/agitation, while a teenage boy may be more compliant with fluvoxamine (Luvox) due to its lower potential for sexual side effects.

Treatment-resistant patients are those who fail to respond to two adequate trials of a single medication or have only a partial response at the maximum tolerable dose of the medication. For these patients, consideration must be given to polypharmacy (as well as intense CBT). If the patient has a partial response to his or her current medication, the first choice would be to augment with the addition of a second SRI with a different mechanism of action. Small-scale studies have suggested that the addition of clomipramine (Anafranil) may be especially useful in these circumstances as it has noradrenergic qualities like the tricyclic medications, which makes clomipramine a unique agent among the SRIs, although it also increases the side-effect profile. The primary consideration in this instance must be avoiding potential drug–drug interactions, especially since increased side effects and even toxicity can result when mixing medications. For this reason, when adding a second agent, it is best to start with a low dose and increase carefully. For those

TABLE 8.5. PSYCHOTROPIC MEDICATIONS FOR OBSESSIVE–COMPULSIVE DISORDER

Medication	Dose Range	Pill Sizes Available	Cost (from www.drugstore.com)	Benefits	Common Potential Side Effects
Fluvoxamine (Luvox)	25–200 mg/d, once a day	25, 50, 100 mg tabs	$91–98 for 30 tabs, any strength	Lower sexual side effects	Nausea, lethargy, insomnia
Sertraline (Zoloft)	25–200 once a day	25, 50, 100 mg tabs, 20 mg/mL liquid	$70–73 for 30 tabs, any strength, liquid 60 mL for $62 mg/d	Fewer drug–drug interactions	Nausea, insomnia, agitation, tremor
Fluoxetine (Prozac)	10–60 mg/d, once a day	10, 20, 40 mg capsules, 20 mg/5 mL liquid, 10 and 20 mg tabs	Available in generic form, $34 for 30 tabs or caps 10 or 20 mg, $68 for 30 caps of 40 mg, liquid 120 mL for $73	Comes in many forms, generic available	Agitation, anorexia, insomnia, dizziness, dry mouth
Clomipramine (Anafranil)	25–250 mg/d (3–5 mg/ kg/day)	25, 50, 75 mg capsules	Available in generic form, $27 for 60 caps of 25 mg, $34 for 60 caps of 50 mg, $39 for 60 caps of 75 mg	May have higher anti-obsessional effect size	Anticholinergic: dry mouth, constipation, urinary retention, and dizziness; ECG changes, tachycardia; most toxic in overdose

ECG, electrocardiogram.

patients without a partial response to first-line treatment, clomipramine may be considered as a single agent.

For patients with Tourette disorder, tics, or a family history of tics who are refractory to single-agent treatment, several studies have shown benefit from augmentation with risperidone (Risperdal), olanzapine (Zyprexa), haloperidol (Haldol), or pimozide (Orap). These agents may also be useful as an augmentation strategy for the treatment-resistant OCD patient, especially those with lack of insight or any psychotic symptoms. α-2a agonists, such as clonidine (Catapres) and guanfacine (Tenex), may also be helpful for augmentation in patients with tics as they appear to have some benefit in reducing tics and can also be helpful with rage episodes. Clonazepam can be useful in the patient with high levels of comorbid anxiety or panic, but side effects of sedation and cognitive problems may complicate treatment with this agent. Some authors would argue that due to potential side effects, augmentation with CBT, or a change in CBT if previously initiated, should be tried prior to augmentation with medication in the case of treatment-refractory OCD. As practitioners trained to administer quality CBT become more available, this would certainly be desirable.

Treatment of children with comorbid OCD and ADHD can be particularly complicated, especially due to the risk of developing tics/Tourette disorder as a third comorbidity. Due to the high rate of comorbid tic disorders in OCD, a child with OCD should be considered at risk for the iatrogenic development of tics, especially if treated with a stimulant medication. In some children with OCD, or other anxiety disorders, stimulants can exacerbate their anxiety symptoms, especially at higher doses. This makes treating an OCD patient with ADHD somewhat more difficult. While stimulant medications are generally considered the first-line treatment for ADHD, if a child already has tics or if he has OCD and could be at risk for the development of tics, alternative medications for treating ADHD should be considered. Atomoxetine (Strattera) is a nonstimulant medication with an FDA indication for the treatment of ADHD that may be particularly relevant in the

OCD population as there has been some evidence that it may also be beneficial for the treatment of anxiety and depression, but certainly because it is unlikely to precipitate tic disorders or exacerbate anxiety symptoms. As stimulants are the most effective treatment for ADHD, some authors argue that unless there are tics currently in evidence, or a family history of tics, that stimulants are still the treatment of choice for ADHD in OCD children and that atomoxetine should be reserved for those children that cannot tolerate stimulants. There are some children with tic disorders with severe ADHD that clearly respond better to stimulants than to the alternatives. These children can sometimes use low-dose stimulants without exacerbating their tic disorders, but careful discussion of risks versus benefits must be undertaken, and the decision must be made carefully on a case-by-case basis. Bupropion (Wellbutrin) is another alternative to stimulants for treating children with comorbid ADHD and OCD. Although not as effective as stimulants, bupropion has been systematically investigated and found to be efficacious for ADHD children.

Discontinuation of medications should primarily be considered after the patient has been optimally treated and stable for 12 to 18 months. Discontinuation is best accomplished in a gradual manner, both to decrease potential withdrawal side effects and to prevent severe deterioration if symptoms reemerge with decreased doses. It would also make sense to choose a time when any symptom reemergence would be the least disruptive, that is, during school breaks. A common strategy is to reduce the maintenance dose by 25% initially and maintain this for several weeks before making further decreases to allow for any symptom reemergence. Sometimes there will be an initial mild increase in anxiety as a withdrawal side effect that calms down over time, dependent on the elimination half-life of the particular medication and its active metabolites. Long-term medication treatment should be considered if several withdrawal trials have failed. If CBT is available and the patient is motivated, a CBT "tune-up" should be considered when decreasing medications and/or prior to reinstitution of the previous dose of medications, depending on the severity of symptom reemergence. The essentials of treating OCD are summarized in Table 8.6.

TABLE 8.6. ESSENTIALS OF TREATMENT FOR OBSESSIVE–COMPULSIVE DISORDER

1. For patients with mild to moderate symptoms, CBT is the treatment of choice.
2. If the patient is not rapidly responsive to CBT or if symptoms are severe or accompanied by a significant depression, then treatment with an SRI/SSRI is indicated.
3. A combination of both medication and cognitive behavior therapies are more effective than either therapy alone.
4. As pharmacotherapy is only 50% effective in first trials, review treatment response during the consent process so that the family's expectations will not be unreasonable.
5. During the consent process, review current warnings about treating youths with SSRIs.
6. An adequate medication trial consists of the highest recommended and tolerated dose of an SSRI for at least 3 months.
7. Start with a low initial medication dose and increase as needed/tolerated until symptoms are significantly relieved or the patient experiences adverse effects.
8. If the patient has minimal response or is intolerant to the first medication trial, switch to a different SSRI.
9. If nonresponsive to a second single SSRI trial, consider a trial of clomipramine alone. If partially responsive, consider augmentation strategies based on the patient's comorbidities (clomipramine if depressed; antipsychotic if PDD, tics, or psychosis; atomoxetine or bupropion vs. stimulants if ADHD).
10. If the patient achieves only a partial response, consider further CBT, consultation with a child and adolescent psychiatrist, and/or referral to a specialty/research center.
11. If the patient achieves adequate response and is stable for 12–18 mo, consider gradual medication taper during the summertime (minimizes school disruption).

CBT, cognitive-behavioral therapy; SRI, serotonin reuptake inhibitor; SSRI, serotonin-specific reuptake inhibitor; PDD, pervasive developmental disorder; ADHD, attention deficit hyperactivity disorder.

Finally, comment is warranted regarding recent concerns about the SSRIs precipitating suicidal urges in children and adolescents. Such a reaction is a genuine concern, likely due to the "activating" effects of SSRIs. The FDA has issued a warning about the use of SSRIs at any age and now mandates such disclosure on bottles of these medications. However, the occurrence of such SSRI-related suicidality appears low (around 3% of youth taking an SSRI), and no completed suicides have been reported. Clearly, families need to be apprised of this risk. A thoughtful informed consent must be conducted with emphasis on safety as well as the relative benefits and risks of using an SSRI for OCD. Currently, most child and adolescent psychiatrists continue to judiciously use the SSRIs with appropriate monitoring.

Conclusions

Though much has been learned about OCD in the past few decades and pharmacologic and psychosocial treatment options have expanded, there is still much work to be done. Research with children and adolescents still lags behind the adult literature, where further research is also needed. Even with optimal current treatment, up to 40% of patients do not achieve adequate symptom control. Epidemiologic studies remind us that most persons with OCD have not sought treatment and continue to suffer in secret. While awareness regarding the benefit of CBT has increased, there are still far too few providers trained in its administration, especially for children and adolescents. As advocates for our patients and their families, we must continue to support ongoing research and education regarding this interesting and challenging disorder.

Case Vignettes

Case vignette #1

BD is an 11-year-old boy with an intact family. He presents to an outpatient clinic with symptoms of anxiety and school refusal. He was previously a very good student, behaviorally and academically, and a fairly compliant child in the home. Recently, his grades have decreased, he has been losing weight, and his parents have been struggling to get him ready for school on time, despite getting him up earlier every morning. Teachers describe BD as being unable/unwilling to turn in his homework because it is "not good enough," and they have observed him becoming frustrated as he repeatedly redoes his work and then destroys it. BD recently became resistant to attending school due to being upset about his inability to perform. This has resulted in conflict with the parents as they attempt to get him to school. Parents report that BD has not been eating recently because he cannot decide what to eat, and BD describes worries about eating the "right" foods. With further questioning, he describes intrusive thoughts that if he eats the "wrong" things and gains weight, his increased weight could disturb the earth's orbit and destroy the laws of gravity, ending with his family/loved ones flying off into outer space. He was hesitant to describe this thought process because he realizes that it "sounds crazy," but it still impedes his ability to eat and has led to his recent weight loss. This also involves the family in endless discussions trying to persuade the patient that various foods are "safe" or that his thoughts are illogical and his fears will not happen (which he understands but is unable to believe strongly enough to overcome his fears). BD and his parents describe past distressing intrusive thoughts and compulsive habits, but they were not overly concerned about those at the time because they had not been "severe enough" to seek treatment.

Treatment options were discussed but because of concerns with decreased nutritional status and severe disruption of school performance, medication was recommended as the first line of treatment and the patient was started on fluoxetine (Prozac) 10 mg each morning. He tolerated the medication without adverse effects, and clear benefit was seen after 1 to 2 weeks, even at the initial dose. However, in order to get optimal symptom control, his dose was gradually increased to 40 mg each morning. With each dose there was further improvement. When he was stable on 40 mg, he experienced minimal anxiety and was able to participate in activities that he was never comfortable enough to participate in previously. BD and his parents remarked that they had not realized how restricted his activities had become until he started feeling better. Over time, BD did well and remained fairly stable though he and his parents noted that if he missed a dose or two of medication (accidentally) he would experience an increase in his anxiety symptoms. On a yearly basis, the psychiatrist would discuss with the family a trial of reducing the medication. However, due to symptom recurrence with missing a dose or two, coupled with the patient's happiness with his stability and lack of adverse side effects, they were unwilling to consider this. The option of CBT was discussed as a way to reduce the medication dose, but BD and his family were unwilling to make the time commitment due to concern that it would be disruptive to their schedules. Also, they were not particularly concerned about reducing the dose of medications as he was doing so well. CBT was left as an option for the future should the patient's symptoms reemerge or his desire to reduce medication become more urgent.

BIBLIOGRAPHY

Cohen DJ, Leckman JF. Developmental psychopathology and neurobiology of Tourette's syndrome. *J Am Acad Child Adolesc Psychiatry* 1994;33:2–15.

DeVeaugh-Geiss J, Moroz G, Biederman J, et al. Clomipramine in child and adolescent obsessive-compulsive disorder: a multicenter trial. *J Am Acad Child Adolesc Psychiatry* 1992;31:45–49.

Evans DW, Leckman JF, Carter A, et al. Rituals, habit, and perfectionism: the prevalence and development of compulsive-like behavior in normal young children. *Child Dev* 1997;68:58–68.

Flament MF, Whitaker A, Rapoport JL, et al. Obsessive-compulsive disorder in adolescence: an epidemiological study. *J Am Acad Child Adolesc Psychiatry* 1988;27:764–771.

Geller D, Biederman J, Griffin S, et al. Comorbidity of juvenile obsessive-compulsive disorder with disruptive behavior disorders: a review and report. *J Am Acad Child Adolesc Psychiatry* 1996;35:1637–1646.

Grados MA, Riddle MA, Samuels JF, et al. The familial phenotype of obsessive-compulsive disorder in relation to tic disorders: the Hopkins OCD family study. *Biol Psychiatry* 2001;50:559–565.

Leckman JF, Grice DE, Barr LC, et al. Tic-related vs non-tic related obsessive-compulsive disorder. *Anxiety* 1995;1:208–215.

Leonard HL, Goldberger EL, Rapoport JL, et al. Childhood rituals: normal development or obsessive-compulsive symptoms? *J Am Acad Child Adolesc Psychiatry* 1990;29:17–23.

Leonard HL, Lenane MC, Swedo SE, et al. Tics and Tourette's disorder: a 2- to 7-year follow-up of 54 obsessive-compulsive children. *Am J Psychiatry* 1992;149:1244–1251.

Leonard HL, Swedo SE, Lenane MC, et al. A 2- to 7-year follow-up study of 54 obsessive-compulsive children and adolescents. *Arch Gen Psychiatry* 1993;50:429–439.

March JS. Cognitive-behavioral psychotherapy for children and adolescents with OCD: a review and recommendations for treatment. *J Am Acad Child Adolesc Psychiatry* 1995;34:7–18.

March JS, Leonard HL. Obsessive-compulsive disorder in children and adolescents: a review of the past 10 years. *J Am Acad Child Adolesc Psychiatry* 1996;35:1265–1273.

Pauls DL, Alsobrook JP II, Goodman W, et al. A family study of obsessive-compulsive disorder. *Am J Psychiatry* 1995;152:76–84.

Rasmussen S, Eisen J. The epidemiology and clinical features of obsessive-compulsive disorder. *Psychiatr Clin North Am* 1992;15:743–758.

Riddle MA, Scahill L, King RA, et al. Obsessive-compulsive disorder in children and adolescents: phenomenology and family history. *J Am Acad Child Adolesc Psychiatry* 1990;29:766–772.

Scahill L, Riddle M, McSwiggin-Hardin M, et al. Children's Yale-Brown obsessive compulsive scale: reliability and validity. *J Am Acad Child Adolesc Psychiatry* 1997;36:844–852.

Swedo SE, Leonard HL, Garvey M, et al. Pediatric autoimmune neuropsychiatric disorders associated with streptococcal infections (PANDAS): clinical description of the first fifty cases. *Am J Psychiatry* 1998;155:264–271.

Towbin KE, Riddle MA. Obsessive compulsive disorder. In: Lewis M, ed. *Child and adolescent psychiatry, a comprehensive textbook*, 3rd ed. Philadelphia, PA: Lippincott Williams & Wilkins, 2002:834–847.

Zohar AH, Pauls DL, Ratzoni G, et al. Obsessive-compulsive disorder with and without tics in an epidemiological sample of adolescents. *Am J Psychiatry* 1997;154:274–276.

SUGGESTED READINGS

Chansky T. *Freeing your child from obsessive-compulsive disorder: a powerful, practical program for parents of children and adolescents.* New York: Three Rivers Press, 2001.
(For parents, this volume provides both a practical understanding of and advice for children with obsessive–compulsive disorder.)

March J, Mulle K. *OCD in children and adolescents: a cognitive-behavioral treatment manual.* New York: Guilford Press, 1998.

(For clinicians, this manual outlines this current psychotherapeutic standard of care.)

Rapoport J. *The boy who couldn't stop washing: the experience and treatment of obsessive compulsive disorder.* New York: New American Library, 1997.
(A New York Times Bestseller for lay populations filled with many vignettes from the family, patient, and treating clinician.)

CHAPTER 9

Tourette Disorder

AJIT N. JETMALANI

Introduction   In 1884, the French neurologist Gilles de la Tourette described nine patients who suffered unusual repetitive motor movements and vocalizations of childhood onset, without associated cognitive impairment. Dr. Tourette's distinguished mentor, Jean-Martin Charcot, suggested the eponym "Gilles de la Tourette Syndrome" for this newly described malady. These clinicians were drawn by the profound externalizing symptoms, including profane utterances and complex motor behaviors that seemed involuntary and caused great shame and regret. Until the turn of the 19th century, victims of the syndrome were described in medical proceedings and social tabloids highlighting these externalizing effects. For many decades to follow, the disorder remained unresearched, poorly understood, and relegated to curiosity and psychogenic causation. In the late 1970s Drs. Arthur and Elaine Shapiro reinvigorated scientific inquiry into Tourette syndrome through a series of provocative papers suggesting that it was an organic disorder. Previously, Tourette syndrome had been conceptualized as a psychodynamic disorder with unconscious processes fueling the plethora of complex behaviors and offensive verbalizations. Many patients with Tourette syndrome also suffer tremendous psychological pain and remorse regarding their public symptoms and disturbing private thoughts. The Shapiros and others, however, eventually demonstrated the efficacy of haloperidol and other medications in ameliorating the motor symptoms of Tourette syndrome. In the ensuing years, intensive studies by clinicians and bench researchers led to rapid advances in knowledge and understanding of Gilles de la Tourette syndrome.

This chapter reviews tic disorders with a focus on the most severe variant, Tourette disorder. The nosology of this condition is still evolving. Scientific literature often utilizes *Tourette syndrome* (TS) rather than *Tourette disorder* (TD) to avoid the initials TD, commonly used to abbreviate tardive dyskinesia. The use of the term Tourette disorder and "TD" are consistent, however, with *Diagnostic and Statistical Manual of Mental Disorders, Fourth Edition* (DSM-IV) nomenclature and therefore used in this text, while the use of "TS" is recommended for clinical practice.

Clinical Features

The sudden repetitive muscular contractions and vocalizations catalogued by Dr. Tourette are called tics. These motoric events commonly last 1 second or less and represent *voluntary* action that can be anticipated and often suppressed. Severely affected patients, however, experience barrages of motor and cognitive impulses, which overwhelm their conscious ability to suppress. Accompanying behavioral, emotional, and academic challenges may cause great morbidity as well. The symptoms may present to the clinician cloaked in a chief complaint mimicking other conditions such as cough, dry eyes, skin irritation, or touching or pulling of genitals or other body parts suggesting disease in the affected area.

Over time, tics tend to display a rostral to caudal progression, with eye blinking as a most common beginning. At times, the anatomic origin is limited to a few muscle groups (*simple tic*: eye blinking, jaw thrusting, throat clearing) or multiple organized contractions which mimic contextual speech or movement [*complex tic*: obscene gestures such as "the finger" (copropraxia), obscene utterances (coprolalia), or repetition of others' speech and movement (echolalia, echopraxia)]. The quality of obscene utterances and behavior is that of a rapid, usually noncontextual explosion of words or actions, not to be confused with angry or antisocial statements of a frustrated or acting out child. TD patients often experience premonitory awareness of the onset of a tic. Attempts at suppression or alteration of tics may then present as a collection of odd voluntary motions or vocalizations meant to mask the underlying episode. These behaviors may phenomenologically overlap with symptoms of obsessive–compulsive disorder (OCD) as the child repetitively takes suppressive action to relieve tic tension. This is different from the pattern noted in OCD in which the action is often accompanied by thoughts related to symmetry, counting, phobic avoidance, or ritual. For patients with tic disorders without OCD, the behaviors are not associated with well formed ideas; rather, there is a feeling of physical tension resulting in an ameliorative action.

Typically, the onset of tics occurs at ages 5 or 6, with peak intensity at ages 10 to 12, and tic reduction around 15 to 17 years old. Tics tend to occur in bouts during various time increments that are clustered during the space of a few minutes periodically in a day, and/or days of intensity, and/or weeks or months of waxing and waning. Because tics are suppressible to a varying degree, some children and adults will successfully "hide" their tics at school or work and then have explosive bouts of tics at home. In addition, stress and anxiety may affect the frequency and intensity of tics. Many patients will experience substantial or near complete resolution of tics following adolescence.

Diagnostic and Statistical Manual of Mental Disorders, Fourth Edition, Diagnostic Criteria

Multiple classifications of tic disorders are available and overlapping in detail. The DSM-IV is selected for this discussion. The DSM-IV divides tic disorders into three categories: TD, chronic motor or vocal tic disorder, and transient tic disorder. The diagnostic criteria are quite simple considering the complexity of this condition and are summarized in Table 9.1. For a diagnosis of TD, vocal and motor tics must be present, although not necessarily at the same time, during 1 year of history, without a reprieve longer than 3 months. For the diagnosis of chronic motor or vocal tic disorder, symptoms should be present for 1 year or longer, without a reprieve longer than 3 months, but without both vocal and motor subtypes. For transient tic disorder, symptoms should be present for no longer than 1 year. In all categories, the onset should occur before the age of 18, and the symptoms should be severe enough to intrude on functioning.

While DSM-IV criteria focus on motor findings, TD patients frequently present with additional features of OCD and attention deficit hyperactivity disorder (ADHD). Thus, one should consider the triad of tics, OCD, and ADHD in all patients presenting with tics. These and other comorbid conditions are discussed throughout this chapter and by other authors in this book.

TABLE 9.1. COMPARISON OF *DIAGNOSTIC AND STATISTICAL MANUAL OF MENTAL DISORDERS,* FOURTH EDITION, TEXT REVISION CRITERIA FOR TIC DISORDERS

Tourette Disorder	Chronic Motor and Vocal Tic Disorder	Transient Tic Disorder
Both multiple motor and one or more vocal tics have been present at some time during the illness, although not necessarily concurrently.	Single or multiple motor or vocal tics (i.e., sudden, rapid, recurrent, nonrhythmic, stereotyped motor movements or vocalizations), but not both, have been present at some time during the disorder.	Single or multiple motor and/or vocal tics for discrete period.
The tics occur many times a day (usually in bouts) nearly everyday or intermittently throughout a period of more than 1 yr, and during this period there was never a tic-free period of more than 3 consecutive mo.	The tics occur many times a day nearly everyday or intermittently throughout a period of more than 1 yr, and during this period there was never a tic-free period of more than 3 consecutive mo.	The tics occur many times a day nearly everyday for at least 4 wk, but for no longer than 12 consecutive mo.
The disturbance causes marked distress or significant impairment in social, occupational, or other important areas of functioning.	The disturbance causes marked distress or significant impairment in social, occupational, or other important areas of functioning.	The disturbance causes marked distress or significant impairment in social, occupational, or other important areas of functioning.
The onset is before age 18 yr.	The onset is before age 18 yr.	The onset is before age 18 yr.
The disturbance is not due to the direct physiologic effects of a substance (e.g., stimulants) or a general medical condition (e.g., Huntington disease or postviral encephalitis).	The disturbance is not due to the direct physiologic effects of a substance (e.g., stimulants) or a general medical condition (e.g., Huntington disease or postviral encephalitis).	The disturbance is not due to the direct physiologic effects of a substance (e.g., stimulants) or a general medical condition (e.g., Huntington disease or postviral encephalitis).
	Criteria have never been met for Tourette disorder.	Criteria have never been met for Tourette disorder or chronic motor or vocal tic disorder.

From American Psychiatric Association. *Diagnostic and statistical manual of mental disorders*, 4th ed, Text rev. Washington, DC: American Psychiatric Association, 2000, with permission.

Epidemiology

Prevalence studies of tics and tic disorders show wide-ranging results. Tics may not be associated with functional impairment and, therefore, identification is highly variable and thresholds for diagnosis are inconsistent. Overall, approximately 0.1% of the population suffers from TD. The estimated prevalence of chronic tic disorders is much higher, ranging from 2% to 5% and 10% to 15% of children during their school years. Boys are substantially more likely to suffer tics and TD, 2 to 10 times the frequency of girls.

Etiology and Pathogenesis

GENETICS

Family studies reveal that the TD concordance rate in monozygotic (MZ) twins (TD/TD) is greater than in dizygotic (DZ) twins and reaches 100% when all tics are considered (TD/tics). Importantly, however, the rate of concordance in DZ twins is higher than in the general population, and the severity of illness within MZ pairs is variable. Researchers suggest that genetic vulnerability, interacting with positive and negative environmental influences, leads to various phenotypic outcomes (TD, tics, OCD, and ADHD). The genetics of TD suggest a major gene functioning between a dominant and recessive pattern. At this time, however, no definitive linkage studies or molecular genetic analysis have successfully identified a specific gene or genes associated with TD.

ENVIRONMENTAL FACTORS

Severe maternal nausea, low birth weight, and forceps delivery are statistically associated nonspecific findings in patients with TD, as well as with many other neuropsychiatric conditions. In addition, stimulant therapy induces earlier onset of tics in treated versus untreated MZ twins. Infection with group A β-hemolytic streptococcus leading to autoimmune disorders pose a particularly intriguing model for interaction of genetics and environment in TD. Because genetic analysis suggests a variably penetrant genetic condition, these and other environmental factors must account for the heterogeneity in presentation of vulnerable individuals.

NEUROPATHOLOGY

The neurochemical and anatomic abnormalities in tic disorders are not determined. Postmortem studies are rare, as this is not a fatal syndrome, and severe symptoms in many individuals dissipate early in life. Analysis of parallel disease models (Huntington disease, Parkinson disease, Sydenham chorea), lesion studies, neuroimaging studies, animal models, and limited neuropathologic and empiric findings support a primary disturbance in the corticostriatothalamocortical circuitry (CSTC) and limbic system. This motor limbic interphase is represented in Figure 9.1.

Cortical and subcortical structures interact normally to produce desired movement (voluntary cortical discharges), affect, and cognition. These interactions are best understood in the motor system where "pyramidal" cells in the motor cortex are modulated via input from the "extrapyramidal" system (striatum, caudate, and putamen), globus pallidus interna (GPi) and externa (GPe), substantia nigra pars reticulate (SNpr) and pars compacta (SNpc), subthalamic nucleus (STN), thalamus, cerebellum, and midbrain reticular

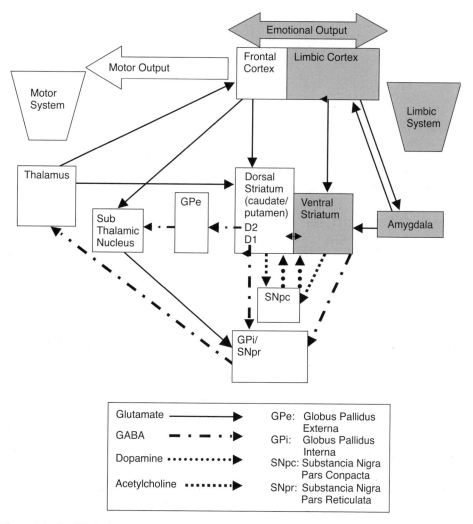

■ **Figure 9.1.** Simplified schematic diagram of the motor limbic interphase. Note that these parallel systems converge in the striatum where motor and affective discharges are interactively modified. Proposed neuropathologic models of Tourette disorder suggest anomalies in the functions of these subcortical structures which function normally to modulate desired movement (voluntary cortical discharges), affect, and cognition. Cortical structures and the substantia nigra pars compacta (SNpc) interact with D1 and D2 dopamine receptors in the striatum. D1 stimulation ("direct pathway") sends γ-amino-butyric-acid (GABA) (inhibitory) to the globus pallidus interna (Gpi)/substantia nigra pars reticulata (SNpr). These neurons are in turn inhibited in their transmission of GABA to the thalamus, which is therefore disinhibited and *increases release of glutamate* (*excitatory*) to cortical structures. D2 stimulation ("indirect pathway") sends GABA to the globus pallidus externa (Gpe) (inhibited), which diminishes GABA to the subthalamic nucleus, which increases glutamate to the GPi/SNpr. These neurons are in turn excited in their transmission of GABA to the thalamus, which is therefore inhibited and *decreases release of glutamate* (decreased stimulation) to cortical structures. These circuits are segregated via anatomic representation in all involved subcortical structures. In Tourette disorder, abnormalities in the complex cycling cascade of dopaminergic neuronal functions and influences are believed to be central in causation and potential intervention.

formation to produce wanted motor output. Primary neurotransmitters in the system include γ-amino-butyric-acid (GABA), glutamate, dopamine, acetylcholine, enkephalin, substance P, and other newly identified protein messengers.

Cortical structures and the SNpc interact with D1 and D2 dopamine receptors in the striatum. D1 stimulation ("direct pathway") sends GABA (inhibitory) to the GPi/SNpr.

These neurons are in turn inhibited in their transmission of GABA to the thalamus, which is, therefore, disinhibited and *increases* release of glutamate (excitatory) to cortical structures. D2 stimulation ("indirect pathway") sends GABA to the GPe (inhibited), which diminishes GABA to the subthalamic STN, which increases glutamate to the GPi\SNpr. These neurons are in turn excited in their transmission of GABA to the thalamus, which is, therefore, inhibited and *decreases* release of glutamate (inhibitory) to cortical structures. These circuits are segregated via anatomic representation in all involved subcortical structures. The balance of stimulation and inhibition provides smooth wanted movement. In TD, abnormalities in the complex cycling cascade of dopaminergic neuronal functions and influences are believed to be central in causation and potential intervention. Cross activation of the limbic system may account for dysregulation of affect and control of rage in some patients, as well as the premonitory sensations and subjective experiences of tic episodes and interepisode states. Dysfunction in the striatum is also associated with the pathogenesis of OCD and disorders of attention and activity regulation, hence, the often expressed triad of tics, OCD, and ADHD.

Successful pharmacologic reduction of tics appears to occur via modification of the CSTC at various levels. Antipsychotics act primarily via direct blockade of dopamine receptors. α-2a agonists, such as guanfacine and clonidine, indirectly diminish dopamine levels and stimulate cortical functions that are inhibitory. These interventions are further reviewed later in this chapter.

Assessment

CHIEF COMPLAINT

Tics may cause: (a) pain if the repetitive movements are unusually frequent; (b) cause dysfunction due to interruption of normal activity such as reading and writing; and/or (c) cause considerable social stigma. For many patients, attentional deficits, academic difficulties, depression, or obsessive–compulsive symptoms may accompany tic symptoms. The family member's chief concerns may be different from the child's because the subjective experience of tics may not correlate with the observed severity. For this reason, it is important to explore the concerns of both child and parent.

COMPREHENSIVE HISTORY

To understand a youth's tics, the clinician must characterize symptom morphology, intensity, onset, and course, as well as comorbid physical and psychiatric symptoms accompanying the tics. It is also crucial to determine whether the ticlike movements may be secondary to an underlying medical or neurologic disorder or represent some other type of movement disorder. Factors to consider in this assessment are summarized in Table 9.2.

While children with TD may have signs of neuromaturational delay such as delayed milestones and "soft signs" noted in motor overflow, the history and physical examination should not reveal a decline in functions such as motor strength, coordination, or sensation. The onset of primary tic disorders occurs in the context of normal continued developmental gains. When gathering history, parents and children may not have an adequate vocabulary to describe motor findings. The "shakes" may be tics, tremor, chorea, seizure activity, or other voluntary or involuntary abnormality. It is helpful to ask the parent or child to demonstrate the symptom or to bring a videotape if the movements are not apparent in the office. It is also difficult for a parent and child to objectively note declines in cognitive or motor functions. Questions about academic and athletic performance may reveal

TABLE 9.2. FACTORS SUGGESTING SECONDARY OR OTHER MOVEMENT DISORDER

1. Movement disorder presenting in mid to late adolescence
2. Temporal relationship of symptom onset to head injury, illness, medication, or drug use
3. Family history of neurodegenerative disorders
4. Cognitive decline
5. Rigidity
6. Tremor
7. Dysarthria
8. Dysphagia
9. Weakness
10. Lateralizing findings
11. Abnormal reflexes
12. Seizures
13. Recurrent GABHS
14. Substantial symptoms during sleep
15. Abrupt and severe onset
16. Perceived as purely involuntary
17. Nonsuppressible motor symptoms
18. No family history of tic disorder
19. Child has no premonition of tic
20. Movements are painful

GABHS, group A β-hemolytic streptococcal.

useful information regarding the child's overall symptom profile. Finally, handwriting is a sensitive measure of motor and cognitive decline, and it is helpful to obtain samples of work completed premorbidly and currently.

DEVELOPMENTAL HISTORY

There are no consistent specific findings expected in the early developmental history of children with tic disorders. Common early findings, particularly in children also diagnosed with ADHD, include sensory overstimulation noted in arching behaviors when held or tactile and auditory sensitivity. There may be delays in fine and gross motor development, although *early* gross motor development is often noted in hyperkinetic children. Later, substantial academic difficulties often accompany tic and ADHD symptoms. Learning may be impaired by developmental abnormalities in reading, math, writing, or language acquisition, or secondary to ADHD, OCD, or the interference of tics in the mechanics of reading and attention.

FAMILY HISTORY AND FUNCTIONING

Family history is often positive for ADHD, OCD, and tics in first- and second-degree relatives. Approximately 10% of TD children will have a first-degree relative with TD and a 20% likelihood of familial tics. Frequently, the clinician may also note previously undiagnosed tics in a parent or sibling of the identified patient. It is critical to ask about other movement disorders to assist in the diagnosis.

Family structure and functioning will, of course, influence symptom tolerance, management, and treatment outcome. With chaotic or highly stressed family systems, the management of this syndrome will require collaboration with mental health providers. With a highly obsessive or anxious parent, minor tics may become a major focus as the parent overattends to symptoms. In addition, these families may transfer their anxious energy or irritation to the child who may then develop increased behavioral or emotional symptoms. The pressure to use unnecessary pharmacology, or too rapidly titrate dosing, is greater under these circumstances. Education and open respectful discussion of these concerns may improve parental tolerance of symptoms. This in turn may help the child feel less anxious and may improve overall stress and tic intensity. Conversely, further discussion may clarify that the tic disorder is more severe than the clinician realized.

EXAMINATION OF THE CHILD

A screening neurologic examination should be conducted that includes assessment of co-ordination, motor overflow, strength, reflexes, tone, balance, and untoward motor movement. A mental status examination should focus on mood, affect, language, intelligence, cognitive processes, thought content, attention, orientation, insight, and judgment. In addition to a routine general examination, special attention should be paid to possible skin lesions such as café au lait spots, neurofibromas, impetigo (suggesting possible streptococcal infection), scarlatina rash, and evidence of thyroid disturbance that may suggest other etiologies.

Tics do not warrant routine serum screening, neuroimaging, or electrical studies, unless secondary tics or differential concerns are raised by history or examination. Pharmacologic intervention will also dictate possible baseline laboratory studies. Essential aspects of evaluating the child with tics are summarized in Table 9.3.

Differential Diagnosis and Comorbidity

DIFFERENTIAL DIAGNOSIS

Primary tic disorders

As noted earlier in this chapter, there are three primary tic disorders: transient tic disorder, chronic motor or vocal tic disorder, and TD. All three have an onset prior to 18 years of age, occur on a daily basis with intensity that causes marked distress or dysfunction, and are not due to ingestion of a substance or general medical condition. Patients with transient tic disorders have single or multiple motor and/or vocal tic lasting more than 4 weeks but less than 1 year. Patients with chronic motor or vocal tics disorders have single or multiple motor or vocal tics, but not both, for more than 1 year without a break of longer than 3 months. Those with TD have both multiple motor and single or multiple vocal tics for 1 year without a tic-free period greater than 3 months.

TABLE 9.3. ASSESSMENT ESSENTIALS

1. The chief complaint should be obtained from the child <u>and</u> guardian to guide a successful postevaluation discussion and treatment plan formulation.
2. History gathering should include questions that differentiate tics from other movement disorders and tics secondary to streptococcal infection.
3. A directed interview will include questions intended to reveal comorbid conditions, with particular emphasis on symptoms of OCD, ADHD, and learning problems.
4. The physical examination should focus on cutaneous abnormalities, infectious conditions, and the general neurologic exam.
5. Neuroimaging should occur in patients with movement disorder inconsistent with tics (not necessary in tic disorders).
6. Laboratory testing should occur when considering possible metabolic or infectious causes of movement disorder (not in tic disorders unless PANDAS is suspected).

OCD, obsessive–compulsive disorder; ADHD, attention deficit hyperactivity disorder; PANDAS, pediatric autoimmune neuropsychiatric disorder associated with streptococcal infection.

Other movement disorders

Other hyperkinetic movement disorders, including stereotypic behaviors, dystonias, choreiform disorders, and myoclonus, may be confused with tics.

Stereotypic Behaviors: These are repetitive actions that are complex in nature and consistent over long periods of time. There may be a ritualistic and or self-soothing quality to these behaviors. For example, autistic and mentally retarded patients often rock or pace for long periods of time. Rapid hand rubbing is a common finding in this population as well and is a prominent diagnostic finding specifically in Rett syndrome. These phenomena differ from tics in their consistency, the patient's greater ability to suppress the movement, and seemingly self-soothing quality.

Dystonias: These movements are often sustained contractions that are observed as abnormal postures of the head and neck (torticollis) or extremity and are frequently painful. As a rule, tics do not cause pain, unless the frequency and intensity cause repetitive strain. Sometimes, the movements are rapid and tic-like in quality. In dystonias, however, the anatomic location is often less fluid than in tic disorders.

Choreiform Disorders: This collection of disorders manifests as rapid motor movements, which may begin with "piano playing" finger movements evident upon finger extension. In severe syndromes (Huntington chorea, Sydenham chorea), fulminate total body jerking may render the patient incapacitated. The early presentation is easily confused with tics, family history (Huntington chorea), and streptococcal episode (Sydenham chorea), and appropriate serum and/or genetic studies assist in the differential diagnosis.

Myoclonus: This is characterized by "lightening bolt" fast muscle contractions alternating with relaxation of large muscle groups. Myoclonic movements are also common and normal during early stages of sleep.

Infectious etiology

Recent research confirms the presence of a subset of patients with tics and/or OCD who are likely suffering neurologic effects of streptococcal infection. Pediatric autoimmune neuropsychiatric disorder associated with streptococcal infection (PANDAS) should be considered if all of the following are present:

- DSM-IV diagnosis of a tic disorder or OCD
- Prepubertal onset
- Episodic presentation with abrupt onset and gradual spontaneous reduction of symptoms ("saw tooth" symptom pattern)
- Subtle neurologic findings: choreiform movements, handwriting deterioration
- Association with group A β-hemolytic streptococcal (GABHS) infection temporally or through correlation of elevated antistreptococcal antibodies during symptom exacerbation.

Further considerations in the differential diagnosis of tics are summarized in Table 9.4.

COMORBID CONDITIONS

As previously noted, children with TD have a high frequency of comorbid ADHD and/or OCD. When evaluating a child with tics, it is critical to consider the triad of tics, ADHD, and OCD as suffering multiple conditions substantially increases morbidity. Furthermore, ADHD and OCD may not be as apparent as tics in the office, requiring directed inquiry and data gathering as described in other chapters in this book.

TABLE 9.4. DIFFERENTIAL DIAGNOSIS OF TICS

Primary:
Chronic motor and vocal tics: Tourette disorder
Chronic motor or vocal tics
Transient motor or vocal tics
Secondary:
Inheritable Syndromes:
   Huntington chorea, Wilson disease, Hallervorden-Spatz, tuberous sclerosis, neuroacanthocytosis
Infections:
   PANDAS, acute viral encephalitis, chronic encephalitis (HIV, Creutzfeldt-Jakob disease)
Toxins:
   Medications and drugs of abuse (partial list): amphetamines, methylphenidate, tricyclic antidepressants, L-dopa, carbodopa, carbamazepine, cocaine, antipsychotic medication (withdrawal)
Environmental:
   Carbon monoxide, organopesticides, and volatile aromatic compounds
Other:
   Mental retardation/developmental delay, autism, head trauma, stroke, tumor, and multiple sclerosis

PANDAS, pediatric autoimmune neuropsychiatric disorder associated with streptococcal infection; HIV, human immunodeficiency virus.

Attention deficit hyperactivity disorder

Multiple studies have supported a high co-occurrence of TD and ADHD. On average, 50% of TD patients meet criteria for ADHD, and 30% to 40% of children diagnosed with ADHD have tics or TD. Children with both disorders have a much greater risk of conduct disorder, depression, and overall dysfunction than children with TD only. Children with TD and ADHD also suffer much higher rates of cognitive disturbances and learning disabilities (LD) than children with TD alone, whose rates of LD approach normal controls.

Obsessive–compulsive disorder

Phenomenologic, neurologic, and genetic overlap of TD and OCD have led many investigators to suggest that these two syndromes are part of the same illness. OCD is a condition in which patients describe unwanted disturbing, intrusive, and often nonsensical worries, accompanied by behaviors which are meant to temporarily diminish their emotional discomfort. At times, OCD patients will describe sudden intrusive thoughts and equally sudden reactive behaviors. Patients with tics often report or are aware of cognitive or emotional elements to their movement symptoms. Some TD patients will describe "thought tics," which are different from obsessions as the thoughts are instantaneous and may not be associated with anxiety or with a desire to carry out a behavior. Interestingly, selective serotonin reuptake inhibitors (SSRIs) effectively treat OCD but not tics. Conversely, α-2a agonists treat tics but not OCD. Overall, directed history gathering and examination will assist in differentiating obsessions, compulsions, and tics.

Other anxiety disorders

Children with TD may experience substantial social stigma due to the overt symptoms of their illness. For some children, social avoidance and anxiety may lead to avoidance of public places or public performance. Social phobia and performance anxiety are common in this population, either as primary or secondary conditions. In addition, older antipsychotic drugs, especially haloperidol, may induce separation anxiety as an iatrogenic condition.

Treatment

BEHAVIORAL INTERVENTION

Many older children and adolescents with tic disorders have premonitory urges and can anticipate a tic. Over time with support, they may be able to suppress or substitute alternate actions that may be more socially acceptable than the original motor event. Cataloguing and becoming aware of one's tic types and patterns may be followed by a reduction in overall tics or the ability to suppress the tics until privacy allows unrestricted expression, that is, a delay of symptoms.

Habit Reversal Training (HRT) is a specific and evidence-based behavioral technique used to reduce repetitive behavior by a cooperative and invested subject. There are a number of essential components:

- Tic description
- Awareness of tics, through feedback, video tape, and so on
- Acknowledging tics when they happen by documenting or labeling "T" verbalized after each tic
- Learning a competitive response, that is, a motor behavior that is close to the opposite of the muscle contractions that occur in the tic and rehearsing it with the therapist
- Learning relaxation techniques, such as breathing techniques and/or muscle relaxation techniques, to assist in carrying out a competitive response
- Applying the competitive response when the patient feels a tic coming or for 1 to 2 minutes after a tic or series of tics
- Great praise for the child when he/she follows through with the process; feedback to the child regarding observed improvements.

Tics and TD, like most neuropsychiatric conditions, exacerbate with stressors such as family problems, academics, environmental events, lack of adequate sleep, excessive caffeine, and so on. Stress reduction in the form of appropriate and predictable parenting, stable housing, academic support, and peer support will improve symptoms and reduce variables in management.

PHARMACOLOGIC INTERVENTIONS

General comments

The pharmacologic treatment of chronic tic disorders is a clinically challenging task. Initiation of medical intervention and assessment of medication response necessitates consideration of whether any positive change in the course of tics is due to the medication or due to the naturally waxing and waning course of the tics. The decision to treat tics and co-morbid conditions mandates a comprehensive discussion with the family about the natural course of tics and the risk of treating versus not treating the condition. The clinician and family must commit to a goal of gradual changes in dosing, up or down, and patience with exacerbation of tics. Rapid dose changes may cause excessive secondary side effects and receptor oversensitivity and reactivity. One may easily enter a complex cycle of clinically incomprehensible volatility in symptoms and medication management.

The first-line choice of medical treatment of tics varies by clinician due to the suboptimal benefits and the risks inherent in available medications. Pimazide (Orap) is the only Food and Drug Administration (FDA)-approved drug for tics in the pediatric population. The other agents noted in this chapter are not FDA-approved for children but have a range of measured efficacy under variably adequate study conditions. The clinician is encouraged to read in-depth reviews of available data in the suggested readings listed at the end of this chapter.

Most clinical studies of pharmacotherapy report average rates of tic reduction from 30% to 60%. It is rare to achieve greater than 50% *sustained* reduction in tics in a moderate to severely affected child. A baseline review of severity and use of scales developed by the clinician and family are critical in the analysis of outcome. While a number of standardized tic monitoring scales are available, they require 10 to 20 minutes to complete and may be unrealistic with various patient populations or clinical practice settings. Therefore, one might develop an individualized scale ranging from 1 to 10 to measure the number of different tics, intensity, frequency, embarrassment level, functional impairment, pain level at baseline, and follow-up titration points. Careful pretreatment goal setting will provide a stronger alliance with the family and improve satisfaction with likelihood of incomplete symptom response.

The reader is cautioned to seek the lowest effective dose when initiating psychotropic treatment of any pediatric patient. For most medications, dosage adjustment should occur at a frequency of no less than 5 days.

Treatment of tics *without* substantial comorbid condition

Clinicians and researchers have found three categories of modestly effective medications in the treatment of tic disorders: α-2a agonists (guanfacine, clonidine), typical neuroleptics (pimozide, haloperidol), and atypical neuroleptics (risperidone, olanzapine, ziprasidone, quetiapine, and aripiprazole). Risk-benefit analysis may lead most physicians and patients to begin with the α-2a agonists. These agents act at the α-2a presynaptic receptor, which diminishes release of norepinephrine. This effect is central and peripheral, impacting neurologic and cardiovascular functioning. The direct effects of agonist action, that is, diminished norepinephrine release, include vasomotor relaxation, diminished anxiety, increased sedation, and smooth muscle relaxation, which results in decreased salivation and decreased bladder outlet control. The mechanism of tic reduction is not direct manipulation of dopamine and is not completely understood. One theory is that modulation of the norepinephrine system reduces the subject's response to stress, which in turn modifies the stress-based discharge of dopamine. Stimulation of the α-2a receptor also improves the inhibitory capacity of the frontal cortex, perhaps improving voluntary control of tics.

Clonidine is more sedating than guanfacine and is often used as a sleep agent. Some patients, however, may experience midphase rebound insomnia as well as nocturnal enuresis. Clonidine is helpful in reduction of aggression and hyperactivity but is neutral or negative on measures of attention. Combined use of clonidine and methylphenidate (Ritalin, Concerta, Metadate) became a concern several years ago due to case reports of sudden death in a small number of pediatric patients taking this medication combination. It was thought that the usually mild cardiovascular effects of both medications could be cardiotoxic in combination. However, this theory was never further investigated, and stimulants and α-2a agonists continue to be widely prescribed. However, a history of ventricular or atrioventricular (AV) node dysfunction, known cardiac disease, or family history of sudden premature death probably warrants alternate pharmacology. Electrocardiogram (ECG) monitoring is required if treating patients with clonidine and methylphenidate, and some clinicians recommend baseline and periodic ECGs for patients receiving α-2a agonists alone. Guanfacine is less sedating and may be effective in the treatment of ADHD. It has a longer half-life, allowing for improved compliance. The actions of these α-2a agonists are gradual, at times causing improvement 2 to 3 weeks after each adjustment. Because sudden withdrawal of α-2a agonists may cause life-threatening rebound hypertension, families who are variably compliant with care are poor candidates for these medications.

Typical neuroleptics such as pimozide (Orap) and haloperidol (Haldol) were mainstay treatments for tic disorders prior to the discovered efficacy of α-2a agonists. The mechanism of action, postsynaptic dopamine-receptor blockade, directly addressed the presumed pathology in the basal ganglia: excessive dopaminergic activity. These agents provide the greatest tic-suppressing effect and can be quite dramatic in their impact in the medication-naïve patient. Unfortunately, dopamine blockade also leads to receptor hypersensitivity in the basal ganglia with resulting tardive dyskinesia and withdrawal dyskinesias; imbalances in the dopamine-acetylcholine pathways producing pseudoparkinsonian effects and akasthesia; excessive frontal lobe inhibition causing cognitive and affective blunting; de novo separation anxiety; pituitary dysregulation such as gynecomastia, galactorrhea, and weight gain; and cardiac conduction delays with a widened QTc. Treatment with these agents warrants pre and concurrent ECG monitoring; metabolic monitoring of glucose, triglycerides, and cholesterol; nutritional and weight counseling; and recognition of confounding disorder versus medication-related movement abnormalities. Rapid dosage adjustments increase the likelihood of dyskinesias, rendering the family and clinician unable to differentiate side effect from natural tic vacillations. Two retrospective studies have examined the use of mecamylamine (Inversine), a nicotine receptor antagonist, in treating TD. Mecamylamine was introduced as an antihypertensive in the 1950s and then reintroduced to the United States in 2000 to study its utility in the treatment of TD. The addition of mecamylamine to neuroleptics substantially reduced tic severity. However, an 8-week double-blind, placebo-controlled study of mecamylamine alone found no benefit. Therefore, mecamylamine appears to be useful only as an augmenting agent.

Many clinicians consider atypical neuroleptics such as risperidone (Risperdal), olanzapine (Zyprexa), and ziprasidone (Geodon), second-line agents after α-2a agonists and before "typical" neuroleptics. The relative advantage over typical neuroleptics is the reduced risk of tardive dyskinesias and other dopamine-receptor blockade side effects. Unfortunately, there are other substantial side effects to consider. Both olanzapine and risperidone may cause dramatic weight gain in the pediatric population. In addition and not necessarily correlated to weight gain, both of these agents may cause metabolic dyscrasias. Insulin resistance is a well-documented potential side effect of these agents. Baseline evaluation of fasting blood sugar and triglycerides is recommended. Ziprasidone is associated with QTc changes and bradycardia, especially in pediatric patients. Titration of this drug should occur slowly, with monitoring of pulse rate and consideration of ECGs. However, to date there have been no reports of cardiac fatalities or episodes of torsade de pointes with the administration of ziprasidone.

Treatment of tics *with* substantial comorbid condition

TD patients may suffer symptoms of anxiety, depression, OCD, and ADHD. With the exception of ADHD, the pharmacologic treatment of comorbid conditions is similar to treating patients without TD. Refer to specific chapters in this book for guidance as well as dosing guidelines for the drugs discussed below.

In TD patients with co-occurring ADHD, the onset of ADHD symptoms usually precedes the onset of tics. This natural history with the initial onset of ADHD, treatment with stimulants, and then the evolution of tics leads to consideration of the impact of stimulant medication on the onset or exacerbation of tic disorders. While several studies addressing this issue provide mixed data, stimulants should be considered as known to initiate or to exacerbate tics in some patients. Stimulants, therefore, should be used with caution in a patient with a family history of tics, a patient history of previous transient tic disorder, or an existing tic syndrome. Stimulant medications are the most effective drugs for ADHD, and many patients with TD have severe ADHD. When nonstimulant approaches to ADHD fail, the clinician and family must consider risk and benefit in eventually committing to stimulant use.

In addition to tic exacerbation, stimulants may cause growth suppression, loss of appetite, and sleep disturbance. Stimulants are not active for 24 hours, leaving periods of inattention or hyperactivity at both ends of a day. Some investigators suggest that long-acting stimulant preparations (Concerta, Metadate CD, Adderall XR) are less neurologically noxious in the patient with tics. These preparations are, therefore, preferred if using stimulants for a patient with tics.

The non-stimulant norepinephrine augmenting drug, atomoxetine (Strattera), is FDA approved for the treatment of children and adults with ADHD. This drug's advantage over the stimulants includes its 24-hour duration of action lower tic exacerbation risk, sleep neutral properties and lack of addictive risk/street value. Patients may experience appetite and growth suppression, as well as agitation, however. A similar but less effective drug (and not FDA approved for ADHD), buproprion (Wellbutrin), has the same advantages but less risk of agitation or appetite and growth suppression.

As noted previously, α-2a agonists such as guanfacine may benefit attention and may suppress tics. While initial interest in clonidine suggested improved ADHD symptoms, the impact is through sedation and not via improved cognition.

Tricyclic antidepressants (TCAs), now in disfavor due to case reports in the late 1980s and early 1990s of sudden death following the use of desipramine, are effective in ADHD and are thought to rarely exacerbate tics. Cautious use of tricyclic agents (other than desipramine) may yet have a role, particularly in patients for whom all else has failed.

A summary of medications used to treat patients with tics and its associated comorbidity is provided in Tables 9.5 and 9.6.

When to refer to a specialist

Uncomplicated tic disorders can be managed in the primary care office. Naturally, however, practice patterns vary by community setting, training, and interest. Specialty referral

TABLE 9.5. ESSENTIAL PHARMACOTHERAPY OF TOURETTE DISORDER

Target Symptoms	Medication

Tics	**α-2a agonists (first line)**
	 Clonidine, guanficine
	 Neuroleptics
	   Atypical (second line)
	   Risperidone, ziprasidone
	   Typical (third line)
	   Pimozide, haloperidol
	 Nicotine receptor antagonist (neuroleptic augmentation)
	 Mecamylamine

ADHD (Listed in order of risk/benefit)	Atomoxetine, buproprion, guanficine **Stimulants: long acting** Adderall XR, Concerta, Ritalin LA, Metadate CD, Adderall **Stimulants: short acting** Dextroamphetamine, Methylphenidate, Dexmethlyphenidate **Tricyclic antidepressants:** Imipramine, nortriptyline inversine?
OCD	**SSRIs:** fluoxetine, fluvoxamine, sertraline (escitalopram, citalopram, and paroxetine not approved under 18) **TCAs:** clomipramine

Note: Refer to Chapter 22 for precautions and dosage recommendations.

ADHD, attention deficit hyperactivity disorder; OCD, obsessive–compulsive disorder; SSRIs, selective serotonin reuptake inhibitors; TCA, tricyclic antidepressant.

TABLE 9.6. TREATMENT ESSENTIALS

1. Inform the family and child of the waxing and waning course of tics.
2. Support acceptance of tics in the family through reassurance and education.
3. Treat tics with medication only if there is pain, physical dysfunction, or marked social impact.
4. Set realistic targets and goals prior to beginning medical treatment.
5. If medication is used, start low and go slow; consider the natural flux in tics and medication side effects when evaluating titration outcomes (including discontinuation rebound symptoms).
6. Comorbid conditions or psychological issues may cause greater dysfunction than tics and should be weighted accordingly in the treatment plan.

is frequently required in moderate to severe TD and in tic syndromes with substantial co-morbid conditions.

Neurology

Referral for neurologic evaluation is recommended if the patient presents with findings suggesting a secondary movement disorder or if the patient has a tic syndrome not responsive to an initial trial of an α-2a agonist.

Psychotherapist

Family systems in chaos will limit the already complex management challenges of treating tic disorders, supporting referral for a family therapy approach. Children with comorbid conditions may warrant individual and family approaches for effective and potentially nonmedical management of symptoms. The therapies most effective for ADHD and OCD are structural and cognitive behavioral in approach. Open-ended insight therapies are not effective in the treatment of tic disorders. The referring primary care provider (PCP) should request regular consultation with the psychotherapist, especially if the PCP is prescribing medication for the TD child.

Psychologist

Referral to a psychologist is recommended for cognitive and academic testing or for *cognitive-behavioral therapy* (CBT). Asking the psychologist whether he or she is proficient in CBT will preclude unintended referral to a therapy that is psychodynamic in nature and not appropriate to the treatment of the tics or ADHD. Diagnosis of LDs is made primarily through psychometric testing of cognitive potential and academic performance. Wide variation in subscales of these tests suggests LDs. Differential in potential versus actual performance also suggests a secondary learning problem caused by ADHD, other major psychopathology, a medical problem, stress, or environmental problems.

Child and adolescent psychiatrist

Child and adolescent psychiatrists provide comprehensive evaluation and clarification of diagnostic issues, comorbid conditions, and treatment recommendations. Child and adolescent psychiatrists often provide ongoing care, including psychotherapy and medication management, or are useful for periodic consultation supporting primary care management.

Occupational therapy

Occupational therapy (OT) referral is helpful if the child has prominent handwriting deficits, sensory defensiveness, or late gross motor development. In particular, sensory motor integration therapy may provide substantial relief of irritability and inflexibility in affected children.

Conclusions

Children with tic disorders present clinical challenges that require a combined approach of patient and family education, behavioral therapies, and medical intervention. Successful outcomes depend on attention to alliance building as well setting realistic goals for the family and clinician. These disorders overtly bridge neurology and the behavioral sciences, undermining the artificial split of brain and mind while encouraging an integrated conceptualization and treatment approach.

Case Vignettes

Case vignette #1

Tony was a 6-year-old boy brought to his pediatrician for evaluation of a dry cough. His mother, in particular, was initially concerned and then annoyed with his repetitive coughing that seemed different from an ordinary cough ("it's as though he's forcing it to happen or something"). This had been going on for weeks at a time and then he would quiet down for a while. There did not seem to be an association with febrile illness or other upper respiratory infection (URI) symptoms. Tony was also very active. He had visited the pediatrician for a laceration to his occiput when he fell off a stool (no concussion observed) 1 month earlier. A long string of mild injuries, family exasperation, and complaints from his kindergarten led the pediatrician and family to consider medical treatment of hyperactivity, but they decided to wait until first grade. Sometimes Tony got stuck on projects and would protest at times of transition. He wore sweats at all times and was very annoyed with tags on his clothing. He flapped his arms when he was excited about something but had no other repetitive behaviors or movements. Tony loved to tell "knock–knock" jokes and enjoyed pretending that he was a dog or a Power Ranger.

He was the product of a normal pregnancy and delivery and met developmental milestones on time or early. His past medical history included recurrent otitis media with bilateral tubes, two episodes of streptococcal pharyngitis, chronic intermittent rhinitis, and multiple injuries without loss of consciousness or concussion. He had no other history of surgery, seizure, hospitalization or ongoing medication, or exposure to heavy metals. No history of psychiatric evaluation or exposure to psychotropic medications was noted.

His family history was positive for ADHD in his father and paternal uncle, but negative for tics. His paternal grandmother was a "control freak" who did not let anyone sit on the white furniture in the living room. No psychiatric diagnoses were noted in the maternal family.

On examination, Tony was a well developed and nourished 6-year-old who was curious about many things in the office and had a knack for precarious acrobatics in the waiting room and the examination room. He had a difficult time leaving a toy in the waiting room. He had no overt genetic stigmata. He seemed to have normal articulation and language development and appeared to have at least a normal intelligence. He displayed a forceful dry cough of which he appeared oblivious. He also displayed frequent bilateral eye blinking in spurts. He had a normal skin examination. He denied sore throat or eye irritation. He was afebrile. Tympanic membranes were scarred but not inflamed, and his oropharnyx revealed enlarged tonsils bilaterally, with clear postnasal excretions, without erythema or exudates. Lung and cardiac exams were normal, as was the remainder of his general examination. Neurologically, he showed normal strength, reflexes, and gross motor coordination. He did display substantial motor overflow and mirroring during rapid alternating hand movements. The examiner noted that the father displayed subtle sniffing and eye blinking tics.

Discussion

Tony was a hyperkinetic and impulsive little boy presenting with waxing and waning motor and vocal tics. While he was developing normally, he had tactile defensiveness and had a typical history of frequent upper respiratory illnesses, including streptococcal infection. Motor overflow and mirroring movements are normal until the age of 8 or 9. Tony's arm flapping with excitement appeared to be motor overflow not associated with autistic spectrum disorder as he had the capacity for interpersonal engagement, fantasy play, joke telling, and normal language development.

The examiner should further detail the history of tic exacerbation to rule out correlation with streptococcal infection and a diagnosis of PANDAS. In this case, careful history taking did not reveal injury, illness, or medications temporally related to the course of illness. His father's apparent tics, the family history positive for ADHD, school problems, and obsessive traits fit with probable TD. At this stage, with less than 1 year of symptoms, Tony's diagnosis is transient tic disorder. He also meets criteria for ADHD, predominantly the hyperkinetic type.

While Tony's family is troubled by his coughing behaviors, his greatest functional difficulties are hyperkinesis, attentional deficits, and inflexibility. The family's concerns may respond to education regarding the waxing and waning nature of tics, the risk of escalation with stimulant medication, and indications for treatment of tics (social and academic dysfunction) that are not met in this case. A treatment plan might include the following:

1. Education about TD if tics persist beyond a 12-month period; possible referral to the local chapter of the *Tourette Syndrome Association* (TSA).
2. Recommend school-based evaluation and educational support, possibly with an Individual Education Plan (IEP) or a 504 plan, based on the diagnosis of tic disorder and ADHD and to rule out specific learning disabilities. Recommend school evaluation for occupational therapy (OT) services based on sensory defensiveness and soft neurologic signs.
3. Behavioral structure and support plan at home for ADHD symptoms including diminishing overstimulation and providing organized and predictable schedules, clear social rules and expectations, and opportunities for "noncontingent" positive regard and engagement.
4. Pharmacologic intervention: guanfacine or clonidine, which may address hyperkinesis and tics, or atomoxetine for the treatment of ADHD (as it has not been reported to exacerbate tics). The use of stimulants warrants caution as exacerbation of tics must be weighed against the potential benefit and alternatives.

BIBLIOGRAPHY

Leckman JF, Zhang H, Vitate A, et al. Course of tic severity in Tourette syndrome: the first two decades. *Pediatrics* 1998;102:14–19.

Pauls DL. An update on the genetics of Gilles de la Tourette syndrome. *Psychosom Res* 2003;55:7–12.

Peterson BS, Leckman JF. The temporal dynamics of tics in Gilles de la Tourette syndrome. *Biol Psychiatry* 1998;44:1337–1348.

Swedo SE, Leonard HL, Garvey M, et al. Pediatric autoimmune neuropsychiatric disorders associated with streptococcal infections: clinical description of the first 50 cases. *Am J Psychiatry* 1998;155: 264–271.

Wilhelm S, Deckersbach T, Coffey BJ, et al. Habit reversal versus supportive psychotherapy for Tourette's disorder: a randomized controlled trial. *Am J Psychiatry* 2003;160:1175–1177.

SUGGESTED READINGS

Cohen D, Jankovic J, Goetz C, eds. *Tourette syndrome, Advances in neurology, Vol. 85.*
Philadelphia, PA: Lippincott Williams & Wilkins, 2001.
(A comprehensive and technical review of Tourette disorder for the clinician.)

Haerle T, Eisnreich J. *Children with Tourette Syndrome: a parent's guide (special needs collection).* Bethesda, MD: Woodbine House, 2003.
(A compact guide for families and useful for clinicians as well.)

Martin A, Schahill L, Charney D et al., eds. *Pediatric psychopharmacology, principles and practice.* New York: Oxford University Press, 2003.
(State of the art and science.)

Robertson M, Baron-Cohen S. *Tourette syndrome: the facts.* Oxford: Oxford University Press, 1998.
(A good overview for families.)

www.tsa-usa.org. Accessed 2005.
(Official website of the Tourette Syndrome Association: clinician, family and educators.)

CHAPTER 10

Depressive Disorders

DAVID A. JEFFERY
D. BIANCA SAVA
NANCY C. WINTERS

Introduction

Mood disorders are among the most common psychiatric disturbances in children and adolescents and are considered to be a leading cause of morbidity and mortality in this population. The spectrum of mood disorders includes depression and mania. This chapter will focus on the depressive disorders, including major depressive disorder (MDD), dysthymic disorder (DD), depressive disorder not otherwise specified, and adjustment disorder with depressed mood. Mania and bipolar disorder are covered in Chapter 11. Although case reports of depression in children date back to the 17th century, until the 1970s many investigators doubted that preadolescent children were capable of experiencing depression. Psychoanalytic theory held that their immature superego would not allow children to become depressed. Cultural attitudes held that children were largely a product of their environments and could not develop what was thought to be an autonomous disorder. Children and adolescents who were not able to articulate their internal emotional states might instead act out, engendering use of such terms as *masked depression* or *depressive equivalent* to describe behavioral problems for which depression was suspected to be the underlying cause. With the advent of systematic research diagnostic criteria for children and adolescents consistent with the nomenclature for adults and data from large-scale epidemiologic studies, it was found that children and adolescents experience depressive symptoms comparable to adult depression. By 1987, the *Diagnostic and Statistical Manual of Mental Disorders*, Third Edition (DSM-III) included MDD and DD as disorders of childhood and adolescence.

Clinical Features

One of the most common questions facing the clinician in evaluating a child or adolescent with mood difficulties is how to differentiate depression as a disorder from normal sadness or transient depressed mood states that many children and adolescents experience periodically. The key differences are in the extent, severity, and impact of the symptoms. In a depressive disorder, the child's or adolescent's mood is depressed (or irritable) most of the day, more days than not, and the symptoms result in significant impairment in his or her ability to function in the important developmental tasks, including school, peer, and family relationships, and maintenance of general health.

Symptoms of MDD, the most severe depressive disorder (see Table 10.1) must be present for 2 weeks. Several associated features that have important treatment implications are specified in the diagnosis, including: (a) psychotic features, (b) melancholic features, (c) atypical features, and (d) seasonal pattern. DD is a less severe, but more chronic, disorder that must be present for at least 1 year in children and adolescents (Table 10.1). Adjustment disorder with depressed mood or with mixed anxiety and depressed mood occurs in relation to an identified psychosocial stressor within 3 months of the onset of the stressor (Table 10.1). The diagnosis of depressive disorder not otherwise specified is used when there are significant depressive features that do not meet the criteria for the above diagnoses, for example, an episode lasting for 2 weeks, but not meeting the full symptom criteria for MDD. This diagnosis can also be made when it is not possible to determine whether the depression is substance induced or related to a medical condition. Substance-induced mood disorder or mood disorder due to a general medical condition can be diagnosed when these factors are determined to be causing the depression.

DEVELOPMENTAL DIFFERENCES IN SYMPTOM PRESENTATION

Depression in children and adolescents resembles adult depression in its core features, albeit with some important developmental variations. Similar to adults, depressed children and adolescents may feel sad, lose interest in typically enjoyable activities, and neglect their appearance and hygiene; they often have disturbed sleep patterns, such as difficulty with sleep onset, early morning awakening, or hypersomnia. They may be indecisive, have problems concentrating, and may lack energy and motivation, resulting in poor school performance (which may be an early warning sign of depression). They may feel pessimistic and even hopeless about the future and have suicidal ideation and/or suicidal behaviors. Unlike adults, however, children and adolescents who are depressed may display a primarily irritable rather than sad mood, and their irritability may at times lead to aggressive behavior, especially in those children with poor impulse control.

Specific clinical manifestations vary across developmental stages. Infant forms of depression have been described over the years in circumstances of emotional deprivation or loss of a mother figure. Such infants and toddlers may present with distress, withdrawal, weight loss, sleep disturbance, and developmental delay. Preadolescent children tend to present more often with irritability, boredom (anhedonia), psychomotor agitation, and have cormorbid somatic complaints (such as stomachaches or headaches), anxiety symptoms (such as separation anxiety or phobias), and conduct problems. Adolescents are more likely to report a depressed mood and suicidal thoughts, although it should be kept in mind that preadolescent children with depression can also be at risk for suicide. Adolescents may also present with irritability, conduct problems, and report boredom. They may attempt to treat themselves with alcohol or drugs. Adolescents often have atypical symptoms such as hypersomnia, increased appetite, rejection sensitivity, and lethargy.

TABLE 10.1. CHARACTERISTICS OF *DIAGNOSTIC AND STATISTICAL MANUAL OF MENTAL DISORDERS,* FOURTH EDITION, TEXT REVISION, DEPRESSION DIAGNOSES

Disorder	Chronologies	Salient Findings	Differentiating Findings
Major depression	Symptoms must be present for at least 2 wk	Nearly everyday throughout most of the day: presence of depressed mood or irritability, markedly diminished interest or pleasure in all or almost all activities, feelings of worthlessness or excessive or inappropriate guilt, diminished ability to think or concentrate, fatigue or loss of energy, psychomotor retardation or agitation, recurrent thoughts of death, recurrent suicidal ideation or a suicide attempt or plan for committing suicide, significant weight loss or failure to make expected weight gains, or insomnia or hypersomnia	The most severe depressive disorder; psychotic features may not be present in the other depressive disorders
Dysthymia	Symptoms must be present for at least 1 yr in children and adolescents	Poor appetite or overeating, insomnia or hypersomnia, low energy or fatigue, low self-esteem, poor concentration or difficulty making decisions, feelings of hopelessness	Less severe but more chronic than major depression
Adjustment disorder with depressed mood	Considered acute if the disturbance lasts less than 6 mo; considered chronic if the disturbance lasts for 6 mo or longer; symptoms occur in relation to an identified psychosocial stressor within 3 mo	Marked distress that is in excess of what would be expected from exposure to the stressor; significant impairment in social, academic, or occupational functioning	The depressive symptoms do not persist for more than an additional 6 mo if the stressor (or its consequences) has terminated
Depression NOS	Variable	Used when there are significant depressive features that do not meet the criteria for the above diagnoses	This diagnosis can be also be made when it is not possible to determine whether the depression is substance induced or related to a medical condition

NOS, not otherwise specified.

From American Psychiatric Association. *Diagnostic and statistical manual of mental disorders*, 4th ed, Text rev. Washington, DC: American Psychiatric Association, 2000, with permission.

Adults are more likely to have psychotic features, although this can also occur in children and adolescents. Children are more likely to have auditory hallucinations than delusions when psychotically depressed. Adults more often have the melancholic form of depression (e.g., loss of pleasure in almost all activities, depression worse in the morning, psychomotor agitation or retardation, and weight loss). However, some adolescents do present with a more adultlike picture of anhedonia, hopelessness, and weight change. In contrast, depressed children more rarely have anhedonia. Even when depressed, their mood may improve temporarily during pleasurable activities, although they may initiate them less frequently. They often criticize themselves and feel that others criticize them. Several developmental variants have been incorporated in the diagnostic criteria for MDD and DD: (a) children and adolescents with MDD may present with a primarily *irritable,* as opposed to a *depressed,* mood, (b) in children and adolescents failure to make expected weight gains is taken into consideration, and (c) children and adolescents may be diagnosed with DD after having symptoms for 1 year, as opposed to the 2 years required for adults.

Epidemiology

The prevalence of MDD is approximately 2% in preadolescent children with a roughly equal prevalence in boys and girls. In adolescents, the prevalence is approximately 6%, with a female-to-male ratio of 2:1, similar to the adult population. Population-based studies estimate lifetime prevalence rates of MDD by age 19 to be 28% (35% in young women and 19% in young men), again comparable to the lifetime prevalence seen in adults with MDD. Prevalence rates for DD are similar to MDD: 0.6% to 1.7% in children and 1.6% to 8.0% in adolescents. There are fewer data about the prevalence of adjustment disorder with depressed mood and depressive disorder not otherwise specified.

A number of trends seen over the past five to six decades has been noted in the literature, and these trends inform our overall understanding of depression in youths. Each successive generation since 1940 appears to have been at greater risk for developing depressive disorders, and these disorders are being recognized at an earlier age. This trend applies to mild-moderate depression, probably not severe depression or DD. The etiology is not clear for this trend. Of particular note is the shift in psychiatric knowledge and medical practice over the past 25 years that has increasingly grasped the biologic basis of depression and the ability of a child to experience a depressive episode.

With the increased rates of depressive disorders has come an increased rate of suicide. We have witnessed a threefold increase in the suicide rate among young people over the past four decades. The incidence of suicide attempts reaches a peak during the late adolescent years. As with adults, adolescent boys are twice as likely as girls to complete suicide, whereas adolescent girls attempt suicide two to three times more often than boys. MDD is the most significant risk factor for completed suicide in this age group. Other risk factors include a previous suicide attempt, alcohol or drug abuse, stressful life events (e.g., getting into trouble at school, breakup with significant other), poor communication between parents and children, exposure to a close friend or relative who commits suicide, poor coping skills, an impulsive personality style, and access to lethal means of suicide. In completed suicides, firearms are the most commonly used method in the United States, followed by hanging and ingestions.

Course and Outcomes of Depression

The average duration of an untreated major depressive episode in a child or adolescent is 7 to 9 months. Ninety percent of patients will have recovered within 18 months. Less favorable is that 50% of youths relapse (i.e., become symptomatic again before full recovery), and recurrence (i.e., a new episode of depression after recovery) rates are high. Forty percent will have another episode within 2 years, 70% within 5 years, and 6% to 10% will have a chronic course. Having the first episode of MDD during adolescence seems to increase the risk of developing a recurrent disorder in adulthood. DD can last for many years, with the unfortunate consequence that the youth and his or her family may not recognize the depression as different from his or her baseline. Increasingly, it is clear that depression is a chronic, recurrent disorder likely to continue into adulthood, and, therefore, educating the youth and family about the course of the illness is a critical part of treatment.

Factors that increase the risk of less favorable outcomes in MDD include comorbid psychiatric disorders, exposure to negative life events, and family history of recurrent MDD. The overall prognosis is also worsened by comorbidity with conduct disorder and by conflict within the youth's family. There is an increased risk of developing other psychiatric disorders, especially for patients who had their first episode of MDD during childhood. Twenty to forty percent of patients with the following risk factors will develop bipolar disorder in 5 years: (a) psychotic features or psychomotor retardation at presentation, (b) a family history of bipolar disorder, or (c) the patient developed a hypomanic episode as a result of antidepressant treatment.

Depression can result in many serious complications in the academic, interpersonal, and family spheres of the child's or adolescent's life. During the depressive episode, school attendance and performance often diminishes, peer and family relationships can be drastically impaired, and there is a significant increase in the risk of suicide and substance abuse (drugs, alcohol, and nicotine). Following an episode of depression, poor self-image and continuing subclinical depression can occur.

One of the most difficult aspects of depression in childhood and adolescence is that psychosocial impairments tend to continue even after the core symptoms of the disorder have improved. For example, the youth may not be socially reintegrated into a peer group, may not be caught up in schoolwork, or may continue to be overly dependent on his or her family. These ongoing psychosocial difficulties become continuing stressors interfering with the youth's self-esteem and complicating full recovery. Although the symptoms of DD are less severe than those of MDD, there is evidence that the psychosocial impairments may be comparable. Thus, it is critical to treat depressive disorders early and target not only depressive symptoms, but also associated problems in functioning.

Etiology

Although the etiology of depression is not completely understood, the evidence is strongest for a transaction between biologic, personality, and environmental factors. Postulated biologic factors include genetic heritability, dysregulation of central serotoninergic or noradrenergic systems, hypothalamic–pituitary-adrenal (HPA) axis dysfunction, and the influence of pubertal sex hormones. Personality factors such as a negative cognitive style have been implicated both as possible causes of depression and markers for a constitutional vulnerability to depression. Individuals with negative cognitive styles have a distorted view of themselves, the world, and the future. They tend to feel responsible for any negative events in their lives and have negative expectations for the future. Evidence points to a stress-diathesis model in which a negative cognitive style results in hopelessness and depression in the context of negative life events such as rejection, perceived failure, and interpersonal losses. Environmental adversities such as abuse and neglect, stressful life events (e.g., significant losses, family divorce), and family dysfunction (e.g., high levels of conflict, parental substance abuse and psychiatric illness) also appear to play significant roles in increasing the risk of depression.

Assessment

When assessing the child or adolescent who may be depressed, it is important to perform a comprehensive psychiatric evaluation that considers all possible psychiatric disorders as symptoms of depression overlap with other disorders such as attention deficit hyperactivity disorder (ADHD) and anxiety disorders. One should also be alert to the possibility of mania as juvenile bipolar disorder frequently presents with a mixed state of depressive and manic symptoms (see Chapter 11).

The psychiatric assessment of children and adolescents requires obtaining information from multiple sources, including the child or adolescent himself or herself, his or her parents, and review of all other relevant ancillary information. It is important to interview the child or adolescent separately to obtain accurate information about depressive symptoms, suicidal thinking and behavior, and other potentially harmful behaviors. In the clinical interview, one must take into consideration the developmental differences not only in the manifestation of depression but also in the child or adolescent's capacity to provide history and make accurate self-observations. Several rating scales and laboratory studies are also available to assist in screening, diagnosis, and assessment of symptom severity. The essential aspects of assessment are summarized in Table 10.2.

THE CLINICAL INTERVIEW

The key aims of the interview are to obtain a detailed history of symptom onset, duration, and intensity; perform a developmentally appropriate mental status examination, including assessment of parent–child interactions; and review the developmental and psychosocial matrix of the patient's life. This includes the child's or adolescent's functioning at home, school, and with peers; developmental and social history; current and past stressors; and examination of the environmental context in which the symptoms occur. Children and adolescents are often reactive to family and environmental stressors, including the mental state and level of functioning of important adults in their lives. There is substantial data indicating that very young children are negatively (and potentially irreversibly) impacted by maternal depression. It is thus paramount to identify parental mental health issues during the child's assessment and recommend appropriate interventions.

Important aspects of the mental status examination include: (a) appearance (e.g., hygiene, facial expression, appropriateness of attire); (b) motoric activity (e.g., psychomotor agitation or retardation); (c) affect (including types and range of affect) and mood; (d) language (including organization of thought process); (e) presence of psychotic symptoms; (f) suicidal

---

TABLE 10.2. ASSESSMENT ESSENTIALS FOR DEPRESSION

- The clinical interview remains the most accurate method for assessing the presence of depression.
- It is important to interview the child or adolescent separately to obtain accurate information about depressive symptoms.
- Rating scales may be helpful for more information about the child's or adolescent's symptoms but should not be relied on to make a diagnosis.
- Assessment of suicidality is an essential component of the assessment of depression.
- Both the parent and the youth should be asked about the presence of any suicide risk factors, including the availability of guns, large quantities of medications, or other potential methods of suicide.
- Comorbid conditions such as anxiety disorders, substance abuse, and disruptive disorders should be evaluated.
- Physical examination, review of systems, and laboratory testing should be done to rule out medical causes (e.g., anemia, infectious illness, hypothyroidism, effects of illicit substances or medications).

or homicidal ideation/plans; (g) developmental/cognitive status; (h) thought content (including self-image, preoccupations, and goals for the future); (i) insight into the problem; and (j) judgment (relative to age). (See Chapter 3.)

In general, children younger than age 7 have limited ability to provide information through verbal interviews, as their language, self-observational capacity, and understanding of time are not well developed. Attention should thus be paid to their physical appearance, affect, and nonverbal communication such as facial expression (e.g., appearing sad, tearful), body posture, agitation or psychomotor retardation, and preoccupation with specific themes relating to trauma or other psychosocial stressors. A combination of play and verbal exchange may facilitate the interaction. Depressed children may appear whiny, clingy, irritable, and have difficulty separating from parents. These observations will need to be integrated with history obtained from the parents, again taking into account the parent's own mental state.

School-aged children are better able to describe their emotional states, often reporting sadness, anger, sleep disturbances, and thoughts of suicide. They may describe themselves in negative terms (e.g., "I'm stupid," "nobody likes me"). School-aged children will frequently have a sad appearance and might have slow movements and monotone voice or be restless and agitated. Some children will endorse low self-esteem, apathy, difficulty concentrating, and anxiety. There is great variation of verbal abilities in this age group. When interviewing school-aged children, asking directly about symptoms may be less helpful than first inquiring about the child's favorite activities and gradually introducing questions about mood in the context of a friendly discussion. Children with impulsive personality styles or comorbid disruptive behavior disorders may be less able to describe their emotions and may present with an irritable mood. Some children of this age may disclose more symptoms when filling out a depression questionnaire (e.g., Child Depression Inventory).

School-aged children are not yet accurate reporters of differences between their current state and baseline or the time course of their symptoms. This is especially true of children with longstanding depression who do not recognize their state as different. The interview with the child's parents helps to clarify these issues, as well as to obtain accurate information on the child's peer relationships, school functioning, and behavior at home. When observing the child with the parent, note whether the child is clingy or immature in his behavior and whether there is overt hostility in the interaction or pejorative language used toward the child. Tensions at home may be present if the child is more relaxed in the individual interview than when seen with the parent.

Assessment of adolescents should rely heavily on the individual interview as adolescents are generally more willing to supply information that they may not wish to share with their parents when speaking in private. Some developmental variations should be kept in mind when interviewing adolescents. Older adolescents tend to be more reliable historians than younger adolescents, and there is considerable variation in the extent of adolescents' insight into their symptoms. Some adolescents may describe their difficulties obliquely, for example, feeling bored rather than depressed. The clinician may need to provide openings for them to discuss their moods, such as inquiring about the extent of their involvement in social and extracurricular activities. Adolescents are frequently brought to an evaluation by their parents due to behavioral concerns. As a result, they may be somewhat defensive initially and reluctant to share personal information, uncertain whether the clinician is more allied with them or with their parents. The clinician may need to reassure the adolescent that information he or she shares will be kept confidential, with the exception of anything posing a risk of harm. As trust is established, the adolescent is more able to disclose symptoms such as depressed mood, low self-esteem, hopelessness, and feeling that things will never change. The interviewer should make sure to learn about suicidal thoughts and behavior, other risky or dangerous behaviors, stressful events, sexual activity, and use of alcohol, drugs, and tobacco. Signs of depression in adolescents include a pale and tired appearance, sad or irritable affect, psychomotor retardation or agitation, impaired concentration, and diminished abstract reasoning ability for their age.

Interviewing the child's or adolescent's parents is an essential component of the assessment. Children and adolescents may not be aware that they are depressed, especially if they have been depressed for a long time. The parents are more likely to report changes in the child's or adolescent's behavior such as irritability, moodiness, loss of interest, and dropping out of extracurricular activities. Parents might often describe preadolescent children as very demanding. Adolescents, on the other hand, might be described as withdrawing from family and peers or associating themselves with a negative peer group. Parents are better than children at estimating the duration of symptoms and are usually able to describe changes in school performance. It should be kept in mind that it is very likely that the parents of depressed children or adolescents are themselves depressed. This may lead them to overreport symptoms (especially behavioral symptoms) in their children due to their negative perceptions or to underreport symptoms as they might be less aware of what is going on around them.

It can be challenging to tease apart symptoms of anxiety and depression, especially in children with comorbid disorders. In younger children, a page of drawings of different facial expressions that the child may point to may be useful. Strategies to learn about anxious versus sad affects in the school-aged child include offering them different words for sadness (e.g., feeling blue, disappointed, lonely, or like crying) and anxiety (e.g., nervous, tense, worried, or scared). Another strategy is to describe situations in which unhappy feelings might occur and inquire about their feelings. For example, being the only child not invited to a birthday party is likely to engender sadness, whereas leaving home to go to school is likely to engender anxiety in the child with separation anxiety disorder. It may also be helpful to inquire about physical sensations of anxiety, for example, butterflies in the stomach, tight chest, or sweaty palms. The child or adolescent with conduct disorder may benefit from an empathic interviewing style (e.g., "it must be difficult when your friends don't treat you the way you feel you deserve," "I can imagine how hard it is when your mother won't get you the toy you want").

ASSESSMENT OF SUICIDALITY

Assessment of suicidality is an essential component of the clinical assessment. Children and adolescents should be asked in a separate interview about thoughts of dying, preoccupation with death, prior suicide attempts, whether they have a current plan for suicide, and whether they have access to lethal means such as large quantities of medications or guns (either in the home or another place they frequent). They should be asked about other self-harming behaviors (e.g., cutting, burning), risky behaviors that might result in death, stressful life events, and their perceived level of family and peer support.

Information should be gathered from the parents and child or adolescent about the presence of risk factors for suicide, including previous suicide attempts, substance abuse, stressful life events, poor parent–child communication, exposure to a close friend or relative who attempted or completed suicide, an impulsive personality style, poor coping skills, and access to lethal means of suicide.

Using this information, the clinician must then assess the seriousness of the risk, weighing suicidal intent, severity of depressive symptoms (especially if psychotic features are present), degree of stress and support in the environment, and capacity to comply with treatment and form a therapeutic alliance. The youth and parents should be counseled about safety, including locking up medications and removal of firearms from the home.

USE OF ADJUNCTIVE MEASURES

Although the clinical interview remains the most accurate method for assessing the presence of depression, there are a number of rating scales that may add additional information in the evaluative process, as summarized in Table 10.3. While these measures should not be relied on to make a diagnosis, there are several benefits to their use during the diagnostic process and treatment course: (a) some children and adolescents may endorse a symptom in writing that they might not disclose in an interview; (b) questionnaires may cover areas not included in the clinical interview; and (c) they provide some quantification of symptoms that may be especially useful when monitoring treatment response. They may also be useful to the adolescent in serving as a self-assessment measure. Types of adjunctive measures include brief rating questionnaires completed by the child or adolescent and structured clinician-administered instruments that require training. Some of the more easily completed rating scales may also be useful for screening purposes.

LABORATORY STUDIES

To rule out medical disorders or substance exposure that may present with depressive symptoms, it is helpful to perform a physical examination, obtain a medical review of systems, obtain a history of all medications used, learn the extent of alcohol and drug use, and obtain a sexual history. The following laboratory tests may also be considered depending on findings in the history and physical examination. Useful tests include a complete blood count (CBC) with differential to rule out infections and anemia; thyroid function tests [T3, T4, and thyroid stimulating hormone (TSH)]; electrolytes; drug and alcohol screens if substance use is suspected; Blood, urea, nitrogen (BUN), creatinine, creatinine clearance, and urine osmolality to rule out renal dysfunction; and liver function tests when hepatitis or other liver dysfunction is suspected. An electroencephalogram (EEG) may be performed if the history suggests seizure disorder. Head computed tomography (CT) or magnetic resonance imaging

---

TABLE 10.3. ADJUNCTIVE MEASURES FOR EVALUATION OF DEPRESSION

Self-report questionnaires:
- *Childhood Depression Inventory (CDI):* a self-report scale used in children from 7 to 17 years old. It is useful in rating the severity of depression but less so for diagnosis since children tend to answer based on what they think adults expect from them.
- *Beck Depression Inventory (BDI):* a 21-item self-report inventory that can be used in adolescents; has good reliability and validity.
- *Center for Epidemiologic Studies-depression Scale (CES-D):* a 20-item self-report inventory that can be used in adolescents; in the public domain; has good reliability and validity.
- *Center for Epidemiologic Studies-depression Scale for Children (CES-DC):* a 20-item childhood version of the CES-D that can be used in children from ages 7-13.

Semistructured measures for more precise evaluation:
- *Childhood Depression-Rating Scale-Revisited (CDRS-R):* a semistructured clinician-administered interview that rates the severity of depression based on information obtained from child, parent, teacher, and clinician.
- *Diagnostic Inventory for Children and Adolescents (DICA):* a computerized structured or semistructured diagnostic interview with child/adolescent and parent versions. It contains 266 items, takes 1–2 h to administer, generates 14 diagnoses, and has good validity and reliability.
- *The Diagnostic Interview Schedule for Children (DISC)* (youth- and parent-report versions): A structured diagnostic interview. A recent computerized version (C-DISC) allows youngsters to hear the interview questions over headphones and to respond in privacy at a computer keyboard. Provides a feasible and cost-effective approach for screening of youths for depression and other emotional/behavioral disorders.
- *The Kiddie Schedule for Affective Disorders and Schizophrenia (K-SADS):* a comprehensive, semistructured interview that is a tool for assessing current, past, and lifetime diagnostic status in children and adolescents ages 6–17; it requires a substantial rater training for reliable administration. K-SADS is considered the gold standard for depression research.

(MRI) may be indicated if there are neurologic abnormalities on history or physical examination. The Dexamethasone Suppression Test (DST) has been studied, but its results are less consistent in children and adolescents and it is generally not considered useful for diagnosis.

Differential Diagnosis and Comorbidity

DIFFERENTIAL DIAGNOSIS

It is important to consider a broad differential diagnosis, including both medical and psychiatric conditions. The most common medical conditions presenting with depression are summarized in Table 10.4. They may include common illnesses such as anemia, hypothyroidism, and infectious diseases such as infectious mononucleosis. If the child or

TABLE 10.4. MEDICAL CONDITIONS ASSOCIATED WITH DEPRESSION IN CHILDREN AND ADOLESCENTS

Medication- or substance-induced	**Infectious**
Antihypertensives (e.g., clonidine, β-blockers)	Infectious mononucleosis
Corticosteroids	Influenza
Benzodiazepines	Encephalitis
Oral contraceptives	AIDS
Acutane	Subacute bacterial endocarditis
Anticonvulsants	Pneumonia
Cimetidine	Hepatitis
Aminophylline	Syphilis (CNS)
Digitalis	
Thiazide diuretics	
Interferon therapy	
Barbiturates	
Some chemotherapeutic agents	
Alcohol abuse and withdrawal	
Drug abuse and withdrawal (e.g., cocaine, amphetamine, opiates)	
Endocrine or metabolic	**Neurologic**
Hypothyroidism or hyperthyroidism	Epilepsy
Diabetes	Traumatic brain injury
Hypopituitarism	Postradiation/chemotherapy
Cushing disease	Cerebrovascular accident
Addison disease	Subarachnoid hemorrhage
Hyperparathyroidism	Migraine headaches
Electrolyte abnormality (hypokalemia, hyponatremia)	Temporal lobe epilepsy
Uremia	Multiple sclerosis
	Huntington disease
Other	
Anemia	
Malnutrition/failure to thrive	
Lupus	
Wilson disease	
Porphyria	
Malignancies	
Cardiac disease	
Irritable bowel syndrome	

AIDS, acquired immunodeficiency syndrome; CNS, central nervous system.

From Weller EB, Weller RA, Rowan AB, Svadjian H. Depressive disorders in children and adolescents. In: Lewis M, ed. *Child and adolescent psychiatry: a comprehensive textbook*. Philadelphia, PA: Lippincott Williams & Wilkins, 2002.

adolescent presents with somatic symptoms (e.g., stomachaches, headaches) or overall health concerns (e.g., low weight), it is important to rule out medical illnesses that might explain these symptoms. Additionally, the possibility that medical conditions are present in addition to depression needs to be considered.

The clinician should be alert to disorders with symptoms or signs that overlap with depressive symptoms. For example, decreased concentration may also be seen in ADHD, anxiety disorders, and mania. Children with chronic depression can be misdiagnosed as having ADHD due to their chronic problems with concentration, motivation, and resulting difficulty with school performance. Sleep disturbances may also occur in mania, anxiety disorders, and ADHD. A blunted affect may be seen in children with pervasive developmental disorders (PDD), psychotic illnesses, and reactive attachment disorder. In such cases, a history of mood disturbance or loss of interest in usual activities is needed from the youth or parents to differentiate depression from these conditions. Weight loss or failure to make expected weight gain may signal an eating disorder rather than depression if the depressed mood follows the weight loss and if the youngster has a disturbed body image.

Developmental stage of the child or adolescent is also important to consider. In preschoolers, depressed mood might be a symptom of neglect, abuse, separation anxiety disorder (these children are usually unhappy when separated from their parents but not when with the parents), or adjustment disorder with depressed mood (in this case there are not enough symptoms to fulfill the criteria for MDD and the symptoms last less than 6 months). In school-aged children one must rule out adjustment disorder and anxiety disorders (including separation anxiety disorder, generalized anxiety disorder, and post-traumatic stress disorder). Adolescents with substance abuse disorders may present with symptoms of depression but these usually diminish after detoxification. It must be noted, though, that substance abuse in adolescents may be caused by depression, be comorbid with depression, or cause depression. Prodromal symptoms of schizophrenia can also mimic depression and the differential diagnosis is often difficult. In this case, the family history might be helpful, and careful examination of the patient's thought process is warranted. The underlying dysphoria in prodromal schizophrenia may be a response to the disordered thought process and growing isolation from others. It may be necessary to assess the presence of mood symptoms after resolution of the psychotic episode to determine whether a separate diagnosis of depression is warranted. Dysphoria in higher functioning individuals with PDD may also result from social isolation.

Bipolar disorder should also be included in the differential diagnosis, considering the fact that in children symptoms of a manic episode and depressive episode might be difficult to differentiate (irritability, aggressive behavior, and agitation can be seen in both); children with an initial major depressive episode are at high risk of developing a subsequent manic or hypomanic episode. Many children with MDD or ADHD display symptoms such as hyperactivity sleep disturbance and irritability that overlap with mania. In 1988, Geller in found that the symptoms of elation and grandiosity best differentiate mania from other related conditions.

COMORBIDITY

MDD in children and adolescents is highly comorbid with other psychiatric conditions. The rates of comorbidity vary across different types of samples, depending on whether the sample is clinical or epidemiologic, outpatient or inpatient, and includes children, adolescents, or both. Forty to seventy percent of depressed children and adolescents have comorbid psychiatric disorders; 20% to 50% have two or more comorbid diagnoses. The most frequent comorbid diagnoses are DD (30%–80%) and anxiety disorders (40%–90%), followed by disruptive behavior disorders (10%–80%) and substance use disorders

(20%–30%). MDD is more likely to occur *after* the onset of other psychiatric disorders, with the exception of substance abuse, which is more likely to precede (and likely increases the risk for) depression.

Youths with DD who develop superimposed MDD episodes ("double depression") have been found to have more severe and chronic depression, higher comorbidity, more suicidality, and greater social impairment than youths with either MDD or DD alone. Children and adolescents with comorbid anxiety disorders appear to have longer episodes of depression and less favorable responses to psychotherapy. Separation anxiety in elementary school appears to be a risk for MDD in early to later adolescence.

Children and adolescents with ADHD are at increased risk for comorbid depression, which may complicate their course and prognosis. Depression itself, however, may be the cause of behavioral and attentional difficulties, especially if these symptoms are recent in onset. Although opinions have differed as to treatment for comorbid ADHD and depression, recent practice algorithms recommend treatment of the ADHD first. Youths with conduct disorder are more likely to have comorbid bipolar disorder than unipolar depression. However, conduct disturbances are frequent in prepubertal-onset MDD and in MDD with comorbid anxiety. Conduct disorder may persist or remit after treatment of mood disorders.

Finally, some investigators have estimated that over 60% of depressed adolescents fulfill criteria for comorbid personality disorders (borderline personality disorder being 30% of those). As these personality disorder symptoms may no longer be evident after the depression is treated, a diagnosis of personality disorder should not be made during an acute depressive episode. Comorbid psychiatric disorders pose a significant problem in that they appear to increase the risk for recurrent depression, lengthen the duration of the depressive episode, increase the number of suicide attempts or behaviors, worsen functional outcome, decrease response to treatment, increase the risk of medical problems, and, finally, decrease the likelihood of utilizing mental health services.

Treatment

Psychosocial therapies and pharmacotherapy each have a role in the treatment of children and adolescents with depressive disorders. Treatment of depression is generally most effective when *multimodal*. When treating youths with depression, medication is rarely, if ever, indicated as the sole treatment strategy in isolation of psychosocial interventions. The initial acute therapy choice depends on the weighing of various clinical issues such as symptom severity and chronicity, exposure to family conflict and negative life events, previous response to treatment, compliance with treatment, and the patient's and family's motivation for treatment. For example, medication may be indicated as an initial acute therapy in an adolescent with MDD whose symptoms are disabling, or who has had a prior episode of MDD, or if the symptoms are chronic. If the youth is seriously suicidal, has psychotic symptoms, or if there is a strong family history of MDD with good medication response, early pharmacotherapy would also be warranted. The benefit of combining medication and psychosocial treatment was demonstrated in a recent multisite randomized controlled trial, the Treatment for Adolescents with Depression Study (Treatment for Adolescents With Depression Study [TADS] Team, 2004), which found that fluoxetine combined with cognitive–behavioral therapy (CBT) was superior to either placebo or fluoxetine alone in reducing symptoms of MDD.

Psychosocial treatment is indicated as a first-line treatment in preschool and school-aged children, in cases of mild-moderate depression, in a first (mild-moderate) episode of depression, in cases where there are identifiable psychosocial stressors implicated in the development of symptoms, and where the patient has had previous response to psychosocial interventions. The essential aspects of treatment are summarized in Table 10.5.

TABLE 10.5. TREATMENT ESSENTIALS FOR DEPRESSED YOUTH

- Treatment begins with psychoeducation about depression as a disease, the nature of the treatment available, the prognosis, and, ultimately, how depression has affected or can affect the life of the patient and the family.
- Treatment of depression is generally most effective when *multimodal*.
- Medication is rarely, if ever, indicated as the sole treatment strategy in isolation of psychosocial interventions.
- Given the lack of data on antidepressant medication use in preschool children, psychosocial interventions, including parent guidance and therapy, are the treatment of choice.
- There is no evidence that "no-harm" contracts protect against suicide.
- In developing a treatment plan, the clinician must also treat any comorbid conditions, especially addressing substance abuse that may be contributing to the depression and also increases the risk of suicide.
- The treatment plan should address safety issues and provide a level of intensity to ensure the patient's safety.
- Before starting treatment with an antidepressant, the patient and family should be informed about the FDA's new warnings and precautions. The patient should be monitored (weekly for the first 4 wk and then biweekly for the next 8 wk) for adverse events such as activation, restlessness, manic switching, or suicidal, or self-harm thoughts or behavior.
- It is important to target not only depressive symptoms, but also associated problems in functioning that may persist after core symptoms are resolved.
- Family intervention is important to ameliorate difficulties in family functioning and to increase available psychosocial support.

FDA, Food and Drug Administration.

The first consideration in developing a treatment plan should always be the patient's safety. If the youth is suicidal or engaging in self-destructive behaviors, hospitalization needs to be considered. Although no-harm contracts may help develop a therapeutic alliance, there is no evidence that they protect against suicide. Consultation with a mental health specialist may be needed to fully evaluate the risks and develop a safe and comprehensive treatment plan.

In developing a treatment plan, the clinician must also treat any comorbid conditions, especially addressing substance abuse that may be contributing to the depression and also increases the risk of suicide. It has been found, for example, that untreated anxiety predicts a poorer response to depression treatment. Also important is to attend quickly to social and environmental stressors that are precipitating or exacerbating the episode. For example, initial goals of a multimodal treatment approach might be to attend to social isolation, harassment at school, or exposure to domestic violence in the home. These factors often complicate the treatment of depression, and attention to these issues early can prevent or at least lessen the impact and severity of the depressive episode. Finally, to successfully treat a child, especially a younger child, the physician should assess the parents and refer them to appropriate mental health treatment, as untreated parental illness is often present in children with depression. For example, the depressed young child of a depressed mother will have significant barriers to achieving wellness if the mother's depression is not also attended to.

PSYCHOSOCIAL TREATMENTS

Psychosocial treatments are especially effective for mild to moderate uncomplicated depression and include multiple modalities. Often treatment begins with psychoeducation about depression as a disease, the nature of the treatment available, the prognosis, and, ultimately, how depression has affected or can affect the life of the patient and the family. This education may include referring the patient and family to supporting literature, web sites, and consumer organizations for further support (e.g., National Alliance for the Mentally Ill, especially helpful for family members). (See resources at the end of the chapter.)

Upon engaging in psychosocial treatment selection, one must consider psychotherapeutic treatment interventions with demonstrated effectiveness. For depression, CBT has the strongest evidence base. Therapeutic intervention in CBT occurs through identifying the patient's cognitive distortions and consequently the patient's emotions. Behavioral strategies include mood monitoring, increasing pleasant activities, relaxation, problem solving, and social skill development. CBT may be conducted individually or in a group format; it may be highly structured or part of a more eclectic approach. CBT manuals are widely available and can help provide a template for this structured approach (see list of resources at the end of the chapter). CBT is often very useful in late elementary school-aged children, preadolescents, and adolescents in helping identify and utilize connections among thoughts, feelings, and behaviors. CBT appears to be the most effective psychotherapeutic modality for MDD with comorbid anxiety.

There are a number of other psychosocial modalities that appear to be useful for depressed children and adolescents. Interpersonal therapy (IPT) focuses on problematic styles of interaction that may be a symptom of or a contributor to depression. Behavior therapy focuses on changing the depressed person's behaviors that may be exacerbating or even fueling the depression. Aspects of behavior therapy are applicable to all ages and may help to further engage parents in the treatment. Family therapy is often a requisite component of treating a depressed youth as family difficulties can play a role in both etiology and resistance to treatment, especially in suicidal youths.

Supportive psychotherapy involves helping patients return to their previous level of functioning, including helping them reconnect with their previous coping skills and ego strengths. This may include the patient utilizing the ego strength of the therapist to restore his or her sense of hopefulness and personal strength and can be applied to most age groups. Psychodynamic psychotherapy is reserved for those who can commit to a course of psychotherapy that requires some level of psychological insight and stability as well as motivation to change. Many higher functioning adolescents are able to benefit greatly from psychodynamic therapy. Play therapy can provide a route of nonverbal communication in younger children and is generally provided by therapists in an individual or group setting. Often play therapy provides the route to therapeutic exploration of the child's concerns that would otherwise be unreachable in the preschool or elementary school-aged child.

Specific interventions provided to parents to help them effectively manage their child's irritability, defiance, isolation, and other behavior problems and are often performed under the rubric of psychoeducation, family therapy, or parent guidance. Dyadic therapy is a form of therapy that focuses distinctly on the relationship between the primary caregiver and the child as there can be specific problematic ways of relating between the two that are cause for clinical concern in treating a depressed child. Group therapy also has a place and can often be helpful in a community setting with fewer resources or for patients who are not motivated, ready, or capable of engaging in individual treatment.

Clinicians often utilize an individualized eclectic approach, integrating CBT, IPT, psychodynamic psychotherapy, family therapy, and other psychosocial treatments. Primary care physicians can also apply some of the principles of these modalities in their offices. Examples include contracting with the youth to increase pleasurable activities, making a schedule of small steps for each week to activate the youth away from his or her lethargy and isolation, brief sessions with the parent and youth to rehearse communication and negotiating strategies (e.g., each talks for 5 minutes with no interruption, use of non-blaming statements), and helping the youth rehearse positive cognitions to offset negative ones (e.g., "my strongest points are..."). It is helpful for the primary care physician to develop clinical collegial relationships with mental health specialists trained in these modalities.

Safety of the self-harming or suicidal youth needs to be ensured in the initial stages of treatment. Suicidality and self-harming behaviors usually indicate the need for a more intensive treatment approach involving the child or adolescent and his or her family. Successful interventions for suicidal behavior in youths target three domains: (a) treatment of current psychopathology; (b) remediation of social, problem solving, and affective regulation deficits; and (c) family psychoeducation and intervention. One example is SNAP (Successful Negotiation Acting Positively) described by Rotheram-Borus, a structured intervention that includes the youth and family in learning problem-solving skills, improving communication, and creating a more positive family atmosphere. Hospitalization needs be considered when the youth has serious suicidal intent and the possibility of acting on it, when the suicidal youth is in a hostile or unsupportive environment, or when psychotic symptoms are present in the context of depression and suicidality. These can be difficult clinical judgments, and erring on the side of safety is recommended.

PSYCHOPHARMACOLOGICAL TREATMENT

Pharmacotherapy has assumed a more prominent role in the treatment of MDD in children and adolescents since the advent of the selective serotonin reuptake inhibitors (SSRIs). Although their use has become controversial due to the recent Food and Drug Administration (FDA) decision to add black box warnings to all antidepressant package inserts regarding use with children and adolescents (see further discussion under Adverse Effects), they continue to benefit many youths with MDD. Table 10.6 summarizes important aspects of antidepressant use with youths.

The SSRIs have the advantage of low lethality in overdose and are generally well tolerated. They do not show a therapeutic antidepressant dose-response relationship, but the side effects are dose dependent. None of the SSRIs, except fluoxetine, has official FDA approval for treatment of youths with MDD. Thus, their use in children or adolescents is considered "off label," and this should be explained to the patient and parents. There are some randomized, placebo-controlled studies that lend some support to the use of SSRIs in children and adolescents, most notably the fluoxetine study conducted by Emslie; the paroxetine study by Keller et al., the recent multisite TADS study with fluoxetine; and controlled trials reporting the efficacy of sertraline and citalopram. Although these studies lend support to the use of SSRIs for adolescents, there have also been questions about the relatively small effect sizes found and some methodologic issues raised. For example, only one symptom of the primary outcome measure showed paroxetine to be superior to placebo. In the fluoxetine studies, self-reports did not show improvement, and there were high rates of relapse over 1 year. Many of the studies do not show full remission of symptoms. In general, placebo response rates are high. The paucity of clearly supportive data regarding the currently available antidepressants indicates that they should not be used as sole treatments for MDD in children and adolescents.

When contemplating treating preschool children with antidepressants, it is important to recognize that none of the randomized controlled trials have included preschool-aged children. Little is known about the effects of these medications on the developing brain. Thus, psychosocial interventions should be the first line of treatment. Parent guidance or therapy is often needed in these cases and should be recommended before medications are contemplated. If MDD persists in preschoolers after appropriate psychosocial interventions, referral should be made to a psychiatrist before initiating antidepressant treatment.

TABLE 10.6. ANTIDEPRESSANTS AND FOOD AND DRUG ADMINISTRATION APPROVAL

Medication Generic (Brand Name)	Approved Age	Dose Ranges	Start Dose	Class/Comments
Buproprion (Wellbutrin) (Wellbutrin SR) (Wellbutrin XL)	18 and older	75–150 mg tid 100–200 mg bid 150–300 mg qd	75–100mg/d or bid 100–150 mg/d (SR) 150 mg/d (XL)	Dopamine-norepinephrine reuptake inhibitor
Citalopram (Celexa)	18 and older	10–40 mg/d	10–20 mg/d	SSRI
Clomipramine (Anafranil)	8 and older (OCD)	50–250 mg/d (or 2–3 mg/kg)	25 mg/d	TCA; only useful for OCD; treatment requires ECG and serum monitoring
Escitalopram (Lexapro)	18 and older	5–20 mg/d	5–10 mg/d	SSRI
Fluoxetine (Prozac)[a]	8 and older (MDD, OCD)	10–80 mg/d	10–20 mg/d	SSRI; only FDA-recommended agent for MDD in children and adolescents
Fluvoxamine (Luvox)[a]	8 and older (for OCD)	25–300 mg/d	25–50 mg QHS	SSRI
Mirtazapine (Remeron)	18 and older	7.5–45 mg QHS	7.5–15 mg QHS	Norepinephrine-serotonin modulator
Nefazadone (Serzone)	18 and older	50–600 mg/d	50 mg QHS or bid	Serotonin modulator; Black box advisory
Paroxetine (Paxil)	18 and older	10–50 mg/d	10–20 mg/d	SSRI; banned in the United Kingdom
Sertraline (Zoloft)	6 and older (for OCD)	25–200 mg/d	25–50 mg/d	SSRI
Trazodone (Desyrel)[a]	18 and older	50–300 mg/d	25–50 mg QHS	Serotonin modulator w/ prominent sedative properties
Venlafaxine (Effexor) (Effexor XR)	18 and older	25–125 mg tid 37.5–375 mg/d	25–75 mg bid or tid 37.5–75 mg/d (XR)	Serotonin-norepinephrine-reuptake inhibitor; manufacturer recommends no use in children and adolescents

SSRI, selective serotonin reuptake inhibitors; OCD, obsessive–compulsive disorder; *FDA, Food and Drug Administration,* TCA, tricyclic antidepressant; ECG, electrocardiogram; MDD, major depression.
[a]generic available.

ADVERSE EFFECTS

The most frequent adverse effects of SSRIs (in all populations) include gastrointestinal symptoms (e.g., nausea, diarrhea), decreased appetite, decreased or increased weight, headaches, restlessness, jitteriness, tremor, insomnia or hypersomnia, increased diaphoresis, vivid dreams, and sexual dysfunction (delayed or painful ejaculation and anorgasmia). Clinicians must be aware that all antidepressants, including SSRIs, may induce hypomania or mania in vulnerable patients (note the importance of obtaining family psychiatric history of bipolar disorder). "Activation," as it has been called, comprised of agitation and disinhibition, can occur as a behavioral complication of SSRIs. Activation appears to be more common in children and is distinct from hypomania and/or mania. Serotonin syndrome bears mentioning as a possible complication of severe serotonin blockade that can occur when an SSRI is given with other serotonergic agents (e.g., lithium, trazodone, tryptophan, sumatriptan). Key symptoms of the syndrome are agitation, confusion, and hyperthermia. This can be a medical emergency and can be fatal if not adequately treated. Lastly, effects of SSRIs on the cytochrome P450 enzyme system make it necessary for the clinician to be aware of the common metabolic pathways of other medications/herbals the patient may be taking. Briefly, among their many sites of hepatic action, paroxetine and fluoxetine are moderate inhibitors of 2D6, whereas sertraline, fluvoxamine, and citalopram are mild inhibitors of 2D6. Fluvoxamine also inhibits at 1A2, 3A4, and 2C19. Citalopram has the least effect on the P450 system and may, therefore, be preferred for medically ill youths on other medications. Use of the SSRIs at high doses should be avoided. At high doses, they can affect the dopamine system and have resulted in extrapyramidal symptoms.

There has been much recent controversy about the use of SSRIs and non-SSRIs (e.g., venlafaxine, mirtazapine, nefazodone, and buproprion) in children and adolescents. Wyeth Pharmaceuticals issued a letter to health professionals recommending against use of venlafaxine in children and adolescents due to its lack of efficacy and increased reports of "hostility and suicide-related adverse events." The FDA added a black box warning against use of nefazodone due to reports of liver toxicity.

In the fall of 2003, the United Kingdom banned the use of paroxetine and venlafaxine in children and adolescents following an analysis of aggregated data that suggested an increased risk of suicidal ideation and self-harming behaviors. The rate was approximately 1% to 2% in the placebo group and about 2% to 3.5% in the group taking the medicine. They also issued a strong advisory against use of antidepressant agents other than fluoxetine in individuals younger than 18. In the United States, the FDA followed by initially strongly recommending against use of agents other than fluoxetine for children and adolescents based on the data on adverse effects and their assessment of lack of demonstrated efficacy of agents other than fluoxetine. In October 2004, based on a reanalysis of 4,400 patients receiving nine antidepressant drugs (SSRIs and others) for MDD, obsessive–compulsive disorder, or other psychiatric disorders, the FDA decided to add black box warnings to all antidepressants regarding use with children or adolescents. This decision was based on the finding of antidepressants posing a 4% risk, versus a 2% risk in placebo, of suicidal thinking or behavior. Notably, there were no suicides in the sample of 4,400 patients. They also determined that only fluoxetine showed a significant advantage over placebo in terms of efficacy.

The FDA's decision to issue black box warnings is controversial, and competing interpretations of the data have been offered. Lack of efficacy may be related to high placebo response rates typically seen in child and adolescent studies. Even in adult studies, effect sizes diminish when mild depression is included since these individuals are more likely to respond to placebo. Child and adolescent antidepressant studies generally enroll subjects with mild MDD to achieve the needed sample size. While it appears possible that these medicines increase the risk of suicidal or self-harming behaviors in the initial treatment period for a subgroup of youths (possibly through activation), this may not be unique to children and adolescents. Most importantly, there are also clear risks of leaving depression untreated. Many children and adolescents do not improve with psychosocial treatment alone and will need the help of pharmacotherapy. It is clear that antidepressants will continue to have a significant role in the treatment of child and adolescent MDD, but with added caution and need for careful monitoring of activation, manic switching, and suicidal thinking and behavior. In any case, antidepressants that are working should be continued and should not be discontinued abruptly as this may result in a discontinuation syndrome.

Figures 10.1 and 10.2 provide suggested algorithms for the acute and maintenance pharmacotherapy of MDD. In general, it is recommended to begin with agents that have had successful randomized trials with children and adolescents. Once undertaking an antidepressant trial, a minimum of 4 to 6 weeks on a therapeutic dose is necessary. If after 4 to 6

Acute Treatment of MDD
Mild-Moderate Episode
(few if any symptoms in excess to make diagnosis, mild to moderate functional impairment)

---

1. Start with psychoeducation and psychotherapy (for 4–6 weeks).
2. If only partial or no response, continue psychoeducation, psychotherapy, and start SSRI (continue for 6–12 weeks).
3. If no response after 6–12 weeks, switch to another SSRI (continue for 6-12 weeks).
4. If no response after 6–12 weeks of second SSRI, recheck diagnosis/comorbidities (especially ADHD and anxiety), adherence/compliance, medical illnesses, family functioning, negative life events, parent/sibling illness. Consider referral to specialist. May switch to a second-line antidepressant (buproprion, venlafaxine, nefazodone, mirtazapine).
5. Continue medication for 6–12 months after a response, then, if no relapse, progressively discontinue treatment.
6. If a second uncomplicated episode, then continue medication for 1–3 years.

Acute Treatment of MDD
Severe Episode
(several symptoms in excess of those to make diagnosis and symptoms markedly interfere with functioning, suicidality, psychotic features, bipolar, and/or recurrent)

---

1. Start with psychoeducation, psychotherapy, and an SSRI (for 4–6 weeks). If suicidality is present, consider safety issues and level of care.
2. If no response after 6–12 weeks, switch to another SSRI (continue for 6–12 weeks).
3. If no response after 6–12 weeks, consider referral to specialist or switch to a second-line antidepressant (buproprion, venlafaxine, nefazodone, mirtazepine).
4. Continue medication for 1–3 years.
5. If two or more complicated depressive episodes, three or more uncomplicated episodes, or chronic depression, then continue medication for 3 years to lifelong.

■ **Figure 10.1.** Suggested algorithm for acute treatment of major depression.

weeks on an SSRI the patient has had only a partial response, the clinician may consider increasing the dose. If no response is obtained after 6 weeks, the clinician may consider switching antidepressants. In children, in particular, the clinician must often wait 8 to 10 weeks for a full antidepressant response. Often, another SSRI is chosen after an inadequate partial response or nonresponse and a new trial commenced. If the second SSRI trial is not effective, the clinician should look to alternate classes of antidepressants. Newer antidepressants (e.g., bupropion, mirtazapine) may have their place as second-line agents for treatment of MDD, but only a few open-label studies have been completed in children and adolescents. Tricyclic antidepressants (TCAs) are not first-line agents for treatment of MDD in youths due to the lack of efficacy shown in available studies and are generally left for treatment-resistant cases. They also require electrocardiogram (ECG) and serum monitoring due to the risk of cardiac toxicity. Once a patient has not responded to two successive trials of SSRIs, the clinician should consider referral to a specialist in child and adolescent psychiatry.

Once efficacy has been established, antidepressant treatment should generally continue for at least 9 to 12 months given the high rate of relapse and recurrence. Follow-up should be at least monthly in the clinic setting. If the patient has had a single but complicated episode of MDD or two noncomplicated episodes, then maintenance should be for 1 to 3 years on the antidepressant. If the patient experiences three or more episodes, two or more complicated episodes, or chronic depression, then maintenance antidepressant

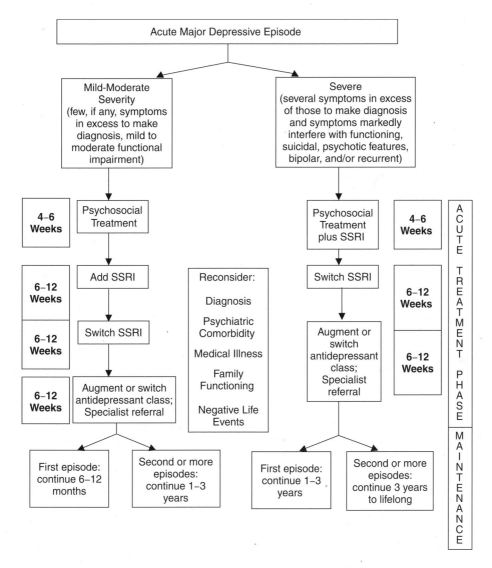

■ **Figure 10.2.** Suggested algorithm for acute and maintenance treatment of major depression.

treatment should continue for 3 years to lifelong. Discontinuation of antidepressants should be effected with a taper over a 2-month period. A discontinuation syndrome may occur if the SSRI is tapered too rapidly and is more likely to occur in short half-life agents (e.g., paroxetine, venlafaxine). Symptoms of discontinuation include dizziness, irritability, lethargy, nausea, vivid dreams, lowered mood, and paresthesia. When discontinuing antidepressant treatment, it is important to recall that MDD is likely to recur, and symptoms should be monitored closely for a period of time.

Treatment of sleep problems complicating depression may warrant use of a medication such as melatonin, diphenhydramine, or trazodone. These agents may be used before undertaking an antidepressant trial (to determine whether resolution of the sleep problem improves mood symptoms) or may be added to an antidepressant that has been effective for mood but not sleep symptoms.

Conclusions

Depression is a serious and frequently chronic disorder, with onset often beginning in childhood. It is associated with increased risk of other psychiatric disorders; poor academic, social, and work functioning; substance abuse; and suicide. It is important to screen children and adolescents routinely for depression and to provide treatment at the earliest stage possible. Multimodal treatment is most effective and should address not only the depressive symptoms but also problems in functioning. Early and comprehensive treatment may lower the risk of chronic psychosocial impairment.

BIBLIOGRAPHY

American Academy of Child and Adolescent Psychiatry. Practice parameters for the assessment and treatment of children and adolescents with depressive disorders. *J Am Acad Child Adolesc Psychiatry* 1998;37(10 Suppl.):4S–20S.

Birmaher B. Depressive disorders. *Proceedings of the annual meeting of the American Academy of Child and Adolescent Psychiatry*. Miami, FL: 2003.

Birmaher B, Arbelaez C, Brent D. Course and outcome of child and adolescent major depressive disorder. *Child Adolesc Psychiatr Clin N Am* 2002;11:619–637.

Birmaher B, Ryan ND, Williamson DE, et al. Childhood and adolescent depression: a review of the past 10 years. Part I. *J Am Acad Child Adolesc Psychiatry* 1996a;35(11):1427–1439.

Birmaher B, Ryan ND, Williamson DE, et al. Childhood and adolescent depression: a review of the past 10 years. Part II. *J Am Acad Child Adolesc Psychiatry* 1996b;35(12):1575–1583.

Brent DA. Assessment and treatment of the youthful suicidal patient. *Ann N Y Acad Sci* 2001;932:106–131.

Brent DA, Holder D, Kolko D, et al. A clinical psychotherapy trial for adolescent depression comparing cognitive, supportive, and family therapy. *Arch Gen Psychiatr* 1997;54:877–885.

Emslie GJ, Heiligenstein JH, Wagner KD, et al. Fluoxetine for acute treatment of depression in children and adolescents: a placebo-controlled, randomized clinical trial. *J Am Acad Child Adolesc Psychiatry* 2002;41:1205–1215.

Emslie G, Rush AJ, Weinberg WA, et al. A double-blind, randomized, placebo-controlled, trial of fluoxetine in children and adolescents with depression. *Arch Gen Psychiatry* 1997;54:1031–1037.

Geller B, Williams M, Zimerman B, et al. Prepubertal and early adolescent bipolarity differentiate from ADHD by manic symptoms, grandiose delusions, ultrarapid or ultradian cycling. *J Affect Disord* 1998;51:81–91.

Hughes CW, Emslie GJ, Crismon ML, et al. The Texas children's medication algorithm project: report of the texas consensus conference panel on medication treatment of childhood major depressive disorder. *J Am Acad Child Adolesc Psychiatry* 1999;38(11):1442–1454.

Keller MB, Ryan N, Strober M, et al. Efficacy of paroxetine in the treatment of adolescent major depression: a randomized, controlled trial. *J Am Acad Child Adolesc Psychiatry* 2001;40:762–772.

Kovacs M, Askikal S, Gatsonis C, et al. Childhood onset dysthymic disorder. *Arch Gen Psychiatry* 1994;51:365–374.

Lewinsohn PM, Clarke GN. Psychosocial treatments for adolescent depression. *Clin Psychol Rev* 1999;19:329–342.

Lewinsohn PM, Joiner TE Jr, Rohde P. Evaluation of the cognitive diathesis-stress models in predicting major depressive disorder in adolescents. *J Abnorm Psychol* 2001;110:203–215.

Pliszka SR, Greenhill LL, Crismon ML, et al. The Texas children's medication algorithm project: report of the Texas consensus conference panel on medication treatment of childhood attention-deficit/hyperactivity disorder. Part II: tactics. Attention-deficit/hyperactivity disorder. *J Am Acad Child Adolesc Psychiatry* 2000;39:920–927.

Rotheram-Borus MJ, Piacentini J, Van Rossem R, et al. Enhancing treatment adherence with a specialized emergency room program for adolescent suicide attempters. *J Am Acad Child Adolesc Psychiatry* 1996; 35(5):654–663.

Treatment for Adolescents With Depression Study Team. Fluoxetine, cognitive-behavioral therapy, and their combination for adolescents with depression: Treatment for Adolescents With Depression Study (TADS) randomized controlled trial. *JAMA* 2004;292:807–820.

Wagner KD, Ambrosini P, Rynn M, et al, Sertraline Pediatric Depression Study Group. Efficacy of sertraline in the treatment of children and adolescents with major depressive disorder: two randomized controlled trials. *JAMA* 2003;290:1033–1041.

Weller EB, Weller RA, Rowan AB, et al. Depressive disorders in children and adolescents. In: Lewis M, ed. *Child and adolescent psychiatry: a comprehensive textbook*. Philadelphia, PA: Lippincott Williams & Wilkins, 2002.

SUGGESTED READINGS

Clarke G, De Bar L, Ludman E, et al. Steady Manual for Adolescent Depression. Can be downloaded at: http://www.kpchr.org/public/acwd/acwd.html, 2001. *[An individual cognitive-behavioral therapy (CBT) manual for clinicians treating depressed adolescents; it was developed by Clarke and his colleagues, whose group CBT depression intervention has been shown to be effective in several research studies.]*

Fristad MA, Golberg Arnold JS. *Raising a moody child: how to cope with depression and bipolar disorder.* New York: Guilford Press, 2004. *(Written by a well-known researcher, this book provides a very clear overview of mood disorders—including bipolar disorder—and a helpful toolkit of coping strategies for parents and youths coping with mood difficulties.)*

Koplewicz H. *More than moody: recognizing and treating adolescent depression.* New York: G.P. Putnam's Sons, 2002. *(A well written and up-to-date book covering the topic comprehensively.)*

Seligman MP. *The optimistic child: a revolutionary program that safeguards children against depression and builds lifelong resilience.* New York: Houghton Mifflin Co, 1995. *(A very original book by one of the seminal writers in cognitive psychology; provides insight into the relationship between depression and thinking style and how changing these patterns of thinking can protect against depression.)*

CHAPTER 11

Early Onset Bipolar Disorder

CAROL M. ROCKHILL
STEFANIE A. HLASTALA
KATHLEEN M. MYERS

Introduction

HISTORIC BACKGROUND

It has long been recognized that many individuals with bipolar disorders (BD) had the onset of their pathognomonic manic symptoms during adolescence. More controversial has been whether BD can onset before puberty. Prominent psychiatrists throughout the 19th and early 20th centuries sporadically published reports of mania in children. However, from 1930 to 1960 psychoanalytic theory postulated that melancholia and mania could not occur in children due to inadequate superego development. This perspective changed in the 1980s when investigators showed that major depressive disorder (MDD) does occur during prepuberty but is masked by comorbid disruptive behaviors that are common in all childhood disorders. Careful work over the next decade delineated the syndrome of prepubertal onset MDD and noted that such early onset marks a more severe form of MDD.

The first empiric research documenting BD in children emerged from longitudinal studies of these MDD youths. By early adulthood these youths had "switched" from MDD to mania at rates 3 to 5 times higher than the rate for adult-onset MDD. Their MDD represented the first stage or "pole" of BD with the next "pole" of mania emerging in young adulthood. The second wave of research came in the 1990s when investigators working with children diagnosed with attention deficit hyperactivity disorder (ADHD) hypothesized that a subset with severe symptomatology who did not respond to stimulant medication actually suffered from BD. Ensuing research has focused on documenting the syndrome of BD in children. Many investigators now postulate a scenario for BD similar to that for MDD, that is, that BD can onset prepubertally but is masked by other comorbid disruptive behaviors, and such early onset marks a severe form of BD.

CURRENT STATUS

The past 5 years have seen systematic investigations of early onset BD, including the recognition of developmentally relevant expressions of manic symptoms, comorbidities that mask mania, an emerging consensus on definitions, and development of instruments to document criterion symptoms and monitor their course. Current studies focus on children whose presentations are marked by irritability, disruptiveness, and ADHD. There is a rich debate on this controversial issue.

Clinical Features

DEFINITIONS

The *Diagnostic and Statistical Manual of Mental Disorders,* Fourth Edition, Text Revision (DSM-IV-TR) documents two major categories of mood disorders: depressive disorders and BD. The pathognomonic feature distinguishing BD from depressive disorders is the experience of a manic or hypomanic episode, as shown in Table 11.1.

In depressive disorders, patients experience a change from their normal mood (euthymia) to depression; while in BD patients experience moods that alternate between two poles, depression and mania. These episodes may vary in the severity of the manic symptoms and be separated by months, weeks, days, or hours, in part defining the subtypes of BD described in Table 11.2.

As noted in Table 11.2, bipolar-I disorder (BD-I) requires the occurrence of at least one manic or mixed episode with marked psychosocial impairment of *at least 1 week* or requiring hospitalization. Per DSM-IV-TR, the presence of psychotic symptoms during mania necessitates a diagnosis of BD-I. This is the most common form of BD in youths, in part due to the frequent presence of psychotic symptoms during mania in children. Bipolar-II disorder (BD-II) differs from BD-I in that the manic symptoms are of shorter duration and less severe and, therefore, termed *hypomanic.* An episode of hypomania does not result in marked psychosocial impairment, although it is sufficiently severe to constitute a departure from normal functioning and to be noted by others. Some investigators conceptualize BD-II as a recurrent depressive disorder with intermittently superimposed hypomania. In youths, the hypomania may be a more frequent occurrence.

When criteria for a manic, or hypomanic, episode and a depressive episode occur concurrently for at least 1 week, the mood episode is termed a mixed episode. This is difficult to identify in children due to the co-occurrence of elation, irritability, and depression with disruptiveness as the youth quickly cycles between moods but seems to adults to be having a severe tantrum. Additionally, if an individual experiences more than four episodes of depression or mania/hypomania in 1 year, a rapid cycling specifier is used. The term *ultradian*

TABLE 11.1. CHARACTERISTICS OF MANIC AND HYPOMANIC EPISODES PER THE *DIAGNOSTIC AND STATISTICAL MANUAL OF MENTAL DISORDERS*, FOURTH EDITION, TEXT REVISION

Type of Episode	Duration	Salient/diagnostic Symptoms	Differentiating Features
Manic episode	At least 1 wk, or any length if hospitalized	A *distinct period* of abnormally and persistently elevated, expansive, or irritable mood, which includes 3 or more of the following symptoms (4 if mood is mostly irritable): • Increased self-esteem or grandiosity • Decreased *need for* sleep • More talkative or pressure to keep talking • Flight of ideas or racing thoughts • Distractibility • Increased goal-directed activity or psychomotor agitation • Involvement in pleasurable activities with increased potential for harm	• Sufficiently severe to cause *marked* impairment in social or occupational function, or to necessitate hospitalization • May have psychosis • Should have at least one cardinal symptom of elation, euphoria, or grandiosity • In children, there are fewer distinct episodes, more rapid cycling, and/or a more chronic course
Hypomanic episode	At least 4 d	A distinct period of elevated, expansive, or irritable mood along with 3 of the diagnostic symptoms described above for a manic episode (4 symptoms if mood is mostly irritable)	• Change in functioning, which is less severe than in mania • Shorter duration than mania • No psychosis • Often perceived to be a personality style, not an illness
Mixed episode	Nearly everyday for at least 1 wk; may occur for mania or hypomania	Criteria are met for both a manic episode and a major depressive episode, but duration of each is very short or episodes are concurrent; term sometimes used interchangeably with "ultradian rapid cycling"	• Sufficiently severe to cause impairment in social or occupational function or to require hospitalization • May have psychosis; can be difficult to distinguish from other conditions with severe irritability or other forms of affective dysregulation

From American Psychiatric Association. *Diagnostic and statistical manual of mental disorders*, 4th ed., Text rev. Washington, DC: American Psychiatric Association, 2000, with permission.

rapid cycling has been unofficially used to describe multiple cycles within a day and is difficult to distinguish from mixed episodes. Ultradian cycling has been posited to predominate in early onset BD.

Cyclothymia is another subtype. Cyclothymic individuals experience numerous periods of hypomanic and depressive symptoms that do not meet criteria for either a full manic or depressive episode but do cause psychosocial distress. These symptoms must occur over a period of at least 1 year (2 years for adults) without any symptom-free intervals lasting longer than 2 months. Individuals with BD may return to a baseline of cyclothymia much as individuals with MDD may return to a baseline of dysthymia.

Bipolar disorder, not otherwise specified (BD, NOS) is the final subtype and allows the diagnosis of BD for individuals with more heterogeneity in presentation. For example,

TABLE 11.2. CHARACTERISTICS OF BIPOLAR DISORDERS PER THE *DIAGNOSTIC AND STATISTICAL MANUAL OF MENTAL DISORDERS*, FOURTH EDITION, TEXT REVISION

Diagnosis	Time Course and Relationship to Depressive and Manic Episodes	Differentiating Features
BD-I	<ul><li>At least one manic episode or mixed episode</li><li>May or may not have had prior major depressive episode</li></ul>	<ul><li>Thought to be the most severe form of the illness due to extremes of the mania</li><li>Cycling less evident in youths as depressive episodes may be less well developed or short</li><li>Cycling may not be evident as children may sustain chronic manic states</li><li>The mania may be "masked" by comorbid ADHD and other disruptive behaviors</li><li>Must document the pathognomonic features of BD, such as grandiosity and hypersexuality, to distinguish from ADHD and ODD</li></ul>
BD-II	<ul><li>At least one major depressive episode and at least one hypomanic episode</li><li>May have multiple recurrent major depressive episode with only intermittently superimposed hypomanic episodes</li><li>No manic episodes</li><li>No psychosis</li></ul>	<ul><li>Hypomania not as severe as mania</li><li>Major depressive episodes as severe as in BD-I and can be more difficult to treat, increasing overall severity</li><li>May be more susceptible to antidepressant-induced "switching"</li><li>Differentiation from personality disorders with affective dysregulation may be difficult, e.g., borderline, narcissistic, histrionic</li></ul>
Cyclothymic disorder	<ul><li>Numerous cycles of lower grade depression and hypomania</li><li>Symptoms ongoing for at least 1 yr in children</li><li>During symptomatic period, no remission of hypomania or depression for more than 2 mo at a time</li><li>No major depressive episode or mixed episode occurs during the first year of the disturbance</li></ul>	<ul><li>May exist as a distinct disorder, may be prodromal to later BD-I or BD-II, or may exist intermorbidly between cycles of major depressive episode and manic episode</li><li>May be perceived more as a personality style</li><li>Diagnosis not often used in children or adults</li></ul>
BD, NOS	<ul><li>Diagnosis for individuals who have manic-like and depressive symptoms that do not meet criteria for BD-I or BD-II</li><li>Criteria for change in functioning not indicated</li><li>Variable time course</li><li>Heterogeneous samples in studies</li></ul>	<ul><li>Examples include recurrent hypomanic episodes without apparent interepisode depressive symptoms</li><li>Diagnosis has been applied to children with severe affective instability of uncertain relationship to BD-I and BD-II</li><li>Most controversial of early onset BD diagnoses; be cautious when using this diagnosis</li></ul>

BD-I, bipolar-I disorder; BD-II, bipolar-II disorder; ADHD, attention deficit hyperactivity disorder; BD, bipolar disorders; ODD, oppositional defiant disorder; BD, NOS, not otherwise specified.

From Amercian Psychiatric Association. *Diagnostic and statistical manual of mental disorders*, 4th ed., Text rev. Washington, DC: American Psychiatric Association, 2000, with permission.

some youths who do not meet full DSM-IV-TR criteria for BD-I or BD-II because of severity or duration criteria but are impaired by their mood instability could be diagnosed with BD, NOS. Unfortunately, the resulting heterogeneity introduces considerable laxity in the construct of BD and apparent overdiagnosis of BD, especially for youths.

SUSPECTING/ESTABLISHING THE DIAGNOSIS OF BIPOLAR DISORDER

Irritability and *Diagnostic and Statistical Manual of Mental Disorders, Fourth Edition, Text Revision* criteria for bipolar disorder

According to the DSM-IV-TR, the same criteria are used to diagnose BD irrespective of age, so that children and adolescents must show the same core symptoms as adults. Early studies have been criticized for focusing on BD, NOS due to the heterogeneous samples that result using BD, NOS criteria. Also, past studies based on BD, NOS emphasized irritability, rather than elation, as the primary indication of mania. This is an especially important issue during childhood when most psychiatric disorders present with irritability. Thus, while most manic youths experience irritability, the majority of irritable youths are likely to have more common psychiatric disorders such as MDD, ADHD, or oppositional defiant disorder (ODD). Geller et al. emphasize that the diagnosis of BD in youths should be based on the cardinal symptoms of mania, that is, elation, euphoria, or grandiosity, to optimally discriminate BD from other diagnoses. The problem is that among the most common prodromal symptoms in youths who later demonstrate BD are mood changes, irritability, anger, and vegetative symptoms. So, many primarily irritable youths with evolving BD would be missed if considering only the cardinal symptoms. One approach with good sensitivity but low specificity would be to include primarily irritable youths in the first iteration, then to look more carefully for underlying elation, euphoria, or grandiosity. However, cross-sectional evaluation can be misleading. A diagnosis of BD is best validated by following youths over time.

Understanding cardinal symptoms of mania: elation and grandiosity

Geller notes that mania evidenced by adults is rarely seen in children due to developmental differences. For example, adults might overspend on their credit cards, become sexually promiscuous, take on multiple new businesses, drive their cars at high speeds, and show other high-risk behaviors. Equivalent childhood behaviors might include trying to use their parents' credit card or stealing money and giving it away, expressing age-inappropriate sexual interest, speaking in an unusually loud and rapid manner, starting unusual activities and not completing them, and disdainfully acting superior to adults.

Obfuscating the diagnosis of bipolar disorder: mixed episodes

The other major hurdle in identifying BD in youths is the greater occurrence of mixed episodes in which the cardinal symptoms of mania co-occur with depression showing a youth who is tearful, sad, laughing, feeling on top of the world, and desperate all at the same time. When they cannot express themselves appropriately, they become frustrated and act out aggressively. These youths may appear angrily disdainful to adults or cry while retelling how good their lives are. In addition, mixed episodes in youths generally include comorbid psychotic symptoms and/or ADHD, further contributing to a moody, hostile, erratic, disruptive, and generally idiosyncratic presentation. Typically, these disruptive behaviors, not mood variability, lead to clinical referral. By adolescence, substance abuse further masks the underlying mood swings.

Epidemiology

The prevalence of BD in childhood has not been established, and rates during adolescence have been estimated from relatively small community surveys and retrospective data. Retrospective data indicate that 40% to 60% of bipolar adults report that their symptoms began prior to 19 years old. In community-based studies of adolescents, Carlson and Kashani found a 0.6% point prevalence of mania among 14- to 16-year-olds, while Costello et al. and Lewinsohn et al. independently found a lifetime prevalence (primarily BD-II) of approximately 1%.

Rates of BD in children can only be indirectly estimated. Early onset BD often begins with an episode of depression, not mania. Birmaher et al. have noted that the prevalence of MDD ranges from 0.4% to 2.5% in children and 0.4% to 8.3% in adolescents. Of these youths, 20% to 40% will "switch" to BD within 5 years of their initial depression. Features associated with this "switch" include early onset of depression, psychomotor retardation, psychosis, mood lability, seasonal pattern, family history of BD or heavy loading of all mood disorders, and pharmacologically induced hypomania. The rate of BD onsetting with symptoms of ADHD has not been established.

Gender rates for BD are also not well established, although prepubertal boys appear to outnumber girls 3.85 times more often. This gender pattern is typical of that noted for other early onset psychiatric disorders. It is not clear whether this finding reflects a true gender difference or a difference in presenting symptoms that more readily bring boys to clinical attention. Gender rates are equal for BD occurring during later adolescence and adulthood.

Clinical Course

When depression is the initial presentation of BD, the "switch" into mania is obvious due to rapid resolution of the depression and the emergence of manic features. However, if irritability is a primary presenting symptom, adults may think that the youth is just getting more moody or aggressive as part of a worsening depression or due to ADHD that may be comorbid with depression. The eventual emergence of elation, grandiosity, racing thoughts, pressured speech, lack of need for sleep, and erratic behavior clarifies the diagnosis. However, if a manic episode or a mixed episode comprises the first presentation in a prepubertal child, the clinical picture is murky. It is difficult to identify the discrete depressed and manic episodes due to the frequent cycling, and this cycling drives behavioral disruptions that lead to disciplinary crises.

Accumulating evidence suggests that early onset BD portends a poorer course. For example, Geller et al. have found a high occurrence (59%) of psychosis, 28.6 weeks to recovery, low rates of recovery (37.1% at 1 year and 65.2% at 2 years; defined by having an 8-week period in which they did not meet DSM-IV-TR criteria for mania or hypomania), and for those youths who did recover, a relapse rate of 55.2% before their second year of follow-up. These youths are very ill.

Etiology and Pathogenesis

HERITABILITY

Inheritance studies over 30 years with adult twins, adoptees, and family aggregation support a genetic contribution to BD with a polygenic transmission. Early inheritance studies of youths by Strober et al. and by Todd et al. are consistent with adult studies showing increased loading for all mood disorders in family members of BD children, some specificity for increased loading of BD, and family loading that is higher for childhood-onset than for adolescent-onset BD. Family loading for mood disorders not only increases the likelihood that young people will develop BD, but also pushes forward the age of onset, and perhaps increases severity of symptoms. Chang et al. further suggest that earlier onset of BD in adults increases the risk of BD in offspring during childhood or adolescence.

NEUROBIOLOGY

Recently, in work with bipolar adults, the serotonin transporter gene has been linked to mood disorders with the long (l) allele, and to a lesser extent the short (s) allele, producing transcriptional and functional activities of the serotonin transporter. These findings seem relevant given the selective serotonin reuptake inhibitors' (SSRIs) proposed therapeutic effects through inhibition of the serotonin transporter, reducing synaptic serotonin. The "l" allele has also been associated with the prophylactic antidepressant response to lithium. The "s" allele has been identified as a risk factor for suicidal behavior, which is so common in BD, and for pharmacologically induced mania.

Two neurotransmitter hypotheses have been proposed from work with adults. One hypothesis posits that a sodium and potassium ATPase pump deficiency increases neuronal excitability. The other posits that lithium's therapeutic benefits result from attenuation of guanine nucleotide binding protein and, thus, dampening of the oscillatory system. Neither hypothesis has been tested.

Steingard et al. have documented decreased frontal lobe volume and increased ventricular volume on magnetic resonance imaging (MRI) scans of depressed children, similar to findings with depressed adults. Additionally, Blumburg et al. found volume reduction in the amygdala upon neuroimaging of a small sample of bipolar adolescents. By contrast, bipolar adults have not consistently shown volume differences in these medial temporal lobe structures, but have shown abnormalities of the corpus collosum. It is unclear whether these structural abnormalities represent a genetic vulnerability, developmental differences, or a consequence of illness.

ENVIRONMENTAL FACTORS

While environmental factors do not cause BD, they may potentiate a genetic vulnerability. Indeed, behavioral genetic research suggests that genetically vulnerable individuals are also at greatest environmental risk. Hlastala has shown that either acute (e.g., death of a loved one) or chronic (e.g., chaotic family) stressors may worsen the course of illness in bipolar adults. For example, patients who live with families characterized by high levels of "expressed emotion" marked by intrusiveness, hostility, and overinvolvement experience higher rates of relapse and hospitalization than patients in families with lower "expressed emotion." Geller has found similar patterns for bipolar youths, noting that youths in homes with low "maternal warmth" relapse sooner. Thus, the home environment may affect the course of illness.

Assessment

The essentials of assessment for BD in youths are summarized in Table 11.3 and discussed below.

HISTORY GATHERING

The American Academy of Child and Adolescent Psychiatry notes that the aims of the clinical interview are to obtain a detailed history of symptom onset, duration, and intensity;

TABLE 11.3. ESSENTIALS OF ASSESSMENT FOR EARLY ONSET BIPOLAR DISORDER

- Physical examination, review of systems, and laboratory testing are included to rule out suspected medical etiologies including neurologic, systemic, and substance-induced disorders.
- The clinical interview of the youth is the cornerstone of assessment for BD. Although many young patients lack insight regarding their manic symptoms, they can often describe their internal states.
- A longitudinal perspective with a timeline of symptom evolution is needed to demonstrate cyclicity and understand the youth's illness.
- No clear role for rating scales at this time.
- The child or adolescent interview should include open-ended questions and discussion of unrelated topics in order to assess thought processes.
- Always inquire about psychotic symptoms.
- Always inquire about suicidality, which is a risk during both depressed and manic stages due to impaired judgment.
- For older children and adolescents, part of the interview should occur without parental presence in order to assess risk-taking behavior such as substance abuse, sexuality, and legal transgressions.
- Family members' behavioral observations provide corollary information regarding the patient's range of difficulties and comorbidity.
- School performance and interpersonal relationships should be assessed to determine the youth's functional impairment and educational needs.

BD, bipolar disorder.

develop a timeline of symptoms; perform a developmentally appropriate mental status examination; and review the child's functioning across settings. A timeline of mood symptoms using holidays and important events as anchors to assess the chronology of symptoms can help to delineate a pattern of some cyclicity. It is important to cue the family and child regarding periods of increased goal-directed activity, irritability, amount or rate of speech, excessive involvement in pleasurable activities, delusions or hallucinations, and decreased need for sleep. In addition, major changes in function, such as worsening performance at school or social isolation, may elucidate mood changes. It is also important to interview the child alone about substance use.

A developmental history includes a chronologic picture of the child's growth and development, including early temperament that may be prodromal to BD, the need for sleep and disrupted sleep, stressors that may exacerbate temperamental features, and emotional milestones that vary in different childhood disorders. Determining patterns in peer relationships and academic performance helps to determine the degree of impairment. In addition, the parents' view of the family dynamics provides context that may relate to comorbidity or the differential diagnosis and sets the tone for interventions. Of course, a family history of mood disorders increases the suspicion of BD in the youth.

MENTAL STATUS EXAMINATION

The mental status examination of the bipolar child in a depressed state is consistent with that of unipolar depression as described in Chapter 10, with the exception that there may be more psychotic symptoms. Motor function is hyperactive and, unlike the ADHD youth, the manic youth may describe a subjective need to move. Speech will show an increased production, rate, and volume. Typically, these youths become verbally intrusive, may demonstrate flight of ideas, and are very difficult to redirect. The manic child will seem to want to be the center of attention, but also seems truly unable to control himself or herself and is difficult to redirect. Affect is elated although this may not be initially evident, especially if the child is also irritable. The elation may be evident as the youth discusses topics that should not evince elation. Inappropriate sexual themes may arise in a way that suggests pleasure for the child.

Evaluation of the youth's mood should include observation, the parent's report, and the youth's own description. Youths with mood disorders, including mania, are better able to describe their moods than are youths with disruptive behavior disorders. Manic youths will not show concern about their situation appropriate to the difficulty they are experiencing. They may talk about being outside societal rules, knowing more than relevant adults, and describe grandiose, unrealistic plans. In the setting of a clinical interview, excessive joking, especially the use of puns or metaphoric thinking, is an indicator of manic symptoms. If the youth is in a mixed state, there may be shifts between such euphoria and irritability during the course of the interview, with the youth becoming demanding or confrontational.

BD youths will not spontaneously discuss their hallucinations unless they are ego dystonic. Parents are often unaware of these psychotic symptoms. Thus, it is important to query the youth about hallucinations and any other odd or intrusive ideation. Delusional thinking is not common in children, but when present is generally grandiose with tales of great plans or feats, making the diagnosis simple. However, their delusions may be bizarre, like those in schizophrenia. Manic youths display self-aggrandizement and may appear narcissistic. They may also display impulse dyscontrol and can be threatening or assaultive when crossed. Obviously, their insight and judgment are impaired, the degree of which will help to determine disposition, that is, the need for hospitalization.

Suicide risk must be ascertained, no matter how young the child, as bipolar youths are at risk for suicide whether in the depressed or manic phase of illness. In a clinical follow-up study, Strober et al. found that 20% of their adolescent patients made at least one medically significant suicide attempt over 5 years; in a community-based study, Lewinsohn et al. found that an astounding 44% of bipolar teens had attempted suicide. The combination of suicidal behavior with psychosis and mood lability is dangerous and such youths are not appropriate for management at home.

RATING SCALES

Rating scales have not yet been widely used in work with bipolar youths. However, two scales are being investigated. The General Behavior Inventory (GBI) was developed by Depue and is in the public domain. Youngstrom and Findling have modified it as the General Behavior Inventory-parent Version (GBI-P) to screen clinically referred youths for BD. The GBI-P contains 76 items and is rated by the parent on a Likert type scale from 0 to 3. There are two mood-related subscales: one for depression and one for hypomania/biphasic. The original GBI can be used as a self-report by adolescents. Reportedly, the GBI-P shows good sensitivity in detecting cases that meet criteria for BD during subsequent diagnostic evaluation. Further psychometric evaluation is in progress.

Another scale is the Young Mania Rating Scale (Y-MRS) that documents the presence and severity of manic symptomatology. The Y-MRS was developed in the 1970s as a brief clinician-administered scale that integrates data from various sources, such as staff on an inpatient unit. Gracious et al. have modified this scale into a parent-report version (YMRS-P). The YMRS-P has only 11 items, rated on a 0 to 4 or 0 to 8 scale. Initial examination of its psychometric properties by Youngstorm et al. are encouraging, but much more work is needed before the Y-MRS can be routinely used in research or in practice.

Due to the evolving nature of rating scales specific to mania or BD, many investigations rely on structured diagnostic interviews, carefully constructed time lines of symptom course, and then use a global rating scale, such as the Children's Global Assessment Scale (CGAS), to rate overall symptomatology at baseline and during treatment. While informative regarding the youth's overall status, such global scales do not provide information specific to mania. The YMRS-P may eventually provide the needed specificity.

MEDICAL WORKUP

The first consideration is the potential medical causes for the youth's presentation. Any youth with manic symptoms and fever should be emergently referred for medical workup, including neuroimaging and lumbar puncture. The presence of risk factors for human immunodeficiency virus (HIV) mandates testing. If the patient is taking antidepressant medication, stimulants, steroids, or less common medications such as isoniacid and sympathomimetics, these medications should be stopped. A period of observation off of potentially causal agents may elucidate the diagnosis. A urine toxicology screen will detect amphetamines, cocaine, and phencyclidine (PCP); however, methylenedioxymethamphetamine (Ecstasy) and inhalants are not tested in urine toxicology screens. A noncontrast head computed tomography scan (CT) or an MRI is generally recommended for patients with a first episode of mania. As temporal lobe and partial complex seizures can rarely cause manic symptoms, an electrencephalogram (EEG) should be considered but not routinely completed, particularly if the patient reports visual perceptual distortions. Thyroid studies, electrolytes, and blood urea nitrogen (BUN)/creatinine are part of a standard medical workup for any first-episode mood disorder and to establish a baseline for monitoring. Further testing is individualized to the clinical findings.

Differential Diagnosis and Comorbidity

The differential diagnosis of BD in youths cannot be discussed separately from comorbidity. Not only must BD be differentiated from other disorders presenting with affective dysregulation, but comorbidity is the rule rather than the exception.

MOOD DISORDER DUE TO A GENERAL MEDICAL CONDITION

It is important to consider that a clinical presentation of any mood disorder may be secondary to a general medical condition, some of which are summarized in Table 11.4.

After medical etiologies have been ruled out, other psychiatric disorders must be considered, either as alternative diagnoses to BD or as comorbidities that mask the underlying bipolarity. For example, some youths with comorbid severe conduct problems cause so much chaos and are in so much legal trouble that the underlying mood swings, particularly

---

TABLE 11.4. DIFFERENTIAL DIAGNOSES: MEDICAL CONDITIONS

Neurologic disorders
- CNS infections (encephalitis, HIV)
- Head trauma
- Multiple sclerosis
- Seizures (temporal lobe or partial complex seizures)
- Tumors (thalamic, gliomas, meningiomas)
- Other CNS insult

Medication/substance induced
- Medications (steroids, isoniazid, sympathomimetics, antidepressants)
- Substances of abuse (e.g., cocaine, methamphetamine, Ecstasy)

Systemic illness
- Hyperthyroidism
- Uremia, hemodialysis
- Wilson disease
- Infections (influenza. encephalitis)

CNS, central nervous system; HIV, human immunodeficiency virus.

TABLE 11.5. DIFFERENTIAL DIAGNOSIS: PSYCHIATRIC DISORDERS

- Mood disorder due to general medical condition
- Major depressive disorder
- Major depressive disorder with psychosis
- Anxiety disorders
  Separation anxiety
  Panic disorder
  Posttraumatic stress disorder
- Disruptive behavior disorders
  Attention deficit hyperactivity disorder
  Oppositional defiant disorder
  Conduct disorder
- Schizophrenia and other psychotic disorders
- Substance use disorders
- Pervasive developmental disorders
- Personality disorders
  Borderline
  Narcissistic
  Histrionic

the mania, are not evident. In other situations, a child may be so anxious that the mood swings are thought to be part of anxiety attacks. It takes considerable clinical skill to diagnose bipolarity in the face of other such disabling symptoms and behaviors. The primary clinician or general psychiatrist encountering these youths in the outpatient setting may not feel comfortable in trying to diagnose the bipolarity but can establish an index of suspicion that leads to further evaluation. Relevant differential diagnoses and comorbidities are summarized in Table 11.5.

DISRUPTIVE BEHAVIOR DISORDERS

ADHD is the most common differential diagnosis as well as the most common comorbidity for prepubertal youths with BD. Most children who meet criteria for prepubertal BD also meet criteria for ADHD, while the converse is not true. Age of onset may help to discriminate these two disorders. By definition, ADHD begins before 7 years old, while BD usually becomes evident after 9 years old. However, many children with prepubertal-onset BD actually have prodromal symptoms very early in life, and age of onset is not easily determined. ADHD and BD have considerable overlap of symptoms, including increased motor activity, hyperactivity, impulsivity, irritability, dysphoria, loquaciousness, poor attention, easy distractibility, and sleep disturbances. However, bipolar youths demonstrate greater severity of these symptoms and have additional symptoms that cannot be attributed to ADHD, such as the quality of their mood lability, euphoria, grandiosity, racing thoughts, pressured speech, sexual inappropriateness, and psychosis. If ADHD is present, symptoms should persist after mood stabilization.

Youths with conduct disorders (CD) may have underlying BD that fuels their disruptive behaviors and sensation seeking. In such cases, the CD would occur in the context of a manic episode and should resolve with mood stabilization. Of course, it is possible to have independent CD and BD, in which case the CD may appear deliberate and predetermined rather than reactive or sensational.

ODD is a common comorbidity in early onset psychiatric disorders. Bipolar youths may demonstrate considerable irritability with explosive tantrums, often called "rages."

Similarly, ODD youths may show "rages" when they do not get their way, are frustrated by authority figures, or feel overwhelmed. This may be especially likely for children with fetal alcohol exposure or pervasive developmental disorders (PDD), who have deficits in self-regulation. Bipolar youths are more likely to demonstrate their symptoms across multiple settings, often without provocation. Also, it is unlikely that BD youths will show the deficits in interpersonal relatedness demonstrated by PDD youths. Rather, BD youths seek interpersonal contact.

SUBSTANCE ABUSE DISORDERS

Substance abuse may mimic BD. Cocaine and stimulants have "activating" effects and can precipitate a manic episode. Amphetamine "highs" and "crashes" can mimic the cycling of BD, and hallucinogens can mimic a manic psychosis. In these cases, the differential must be delayed until the youth has been detoxified. A timeline can determine whether the bipolar symptoms started after the use of substances, in which case the diagnosis would be a substance-induced mood disorder, bipolar type; or whether the bipolar symptoms started first and the youth "self-medicated" to treat mood symptoms, in which case diagnoses of BD and comorbid substance use disorder would be appropriate.

SCHIZOPHRENIA AND OTHER PSYCHOTIC DISORDERS

Youths often exhibit psychotic symptoms during a manic episode and are thus often misdiagnosed with schizophrenia. Manic youths are more likely to experience mood congruent or grandiose delusions and do not exhibit "negative symptoms" (e.g., flat affect, paucity of speech and thought) that characterize schizophrenia. Of course, such symptoms must be distinguished from depressive cycles of BD. Depressed youths are better able to describe their subjective distress than schizophrenics, whose negative symptoms are generally egosyntonic. Also, negative symptoms would not be evident during euthymic periods. Schizophrenic youths often show prodromal schizoid traits, whereas bipolar youths intrusively seek out others but are unsuccessful due to their behavioral disturbances.

ANXIETY DISORDERS

Anxiety disorders are important comorbidities with all mood disorders, including BD, at any age. Certain anxiety disorders may also be misdiagnosed as BD. In particular, youths with posttraumatic stress disorder may show affective dysregulation with reexposure to traumatizing stimulus and may also describe psychotic-like symptoms. The history of trauma and of symptom expression in relation to reactivation of that trauma are important features to determine in teasing out the diagnosis. During panic attacks, youths experience autonomous surges of anxiety with concomitant cognitive symptoms (decreased concentration, feelings of losing control) and irritability that can result in tantrums. The differential from mania is based on the physiologic arousal during panic attacks. Generally, the quick escalation and defervescence of panic also distinguishes it from mania. However, this may be more difficult in rapid cycling subtypes of BD. Separation anxiety disorder (SAD) is one of the most common misdiagnoses due to the sudden onset of irritability, irrational anger, and rages. Also, these youths often have depressive symptoms and sleep disturbances that suggest the cycling of BD. The appropriate diagnosis becomes evident when the dysregulation is linked to separation or anticipated separation and by the lack of core manic symptoms. Additionally, the sleep disturbance in SAD is due to worrying that precludes falling asleep, and the youth is tired the next day; whereas the sleep disturbance in mania is due to a *decreased need* for sleep and the child is not fatigued the next day. BD youths also frequently awaken in the middle of the night, a pattern not seen in most other disorders unless accompanied by nightmares.

BORDERLINE PERSONALITY DISORDER

Affective instability, impulse dyscontrol, and interpersonal difficulty characterize patients with both BD and borderline personality disorder (BPD). Furthermore, early onset BD may show a chronicity and persistence similar to BPD. Thus, there may be considerable difficulty in differentiating these diagnoses. Youths with BPD traits may be more likely to have abuse histories, to exhibit self-mutilation, and to show a more malignant pattern of unstable interpersonal relationships and pervasively disturbed self-images. This is another example of the importance of a longitudinal perspective in diagnosing BD youths.

Treatment

Like most early onset disorders, a multimodal approach to treatment is needed. In BD, all domains of a youth's functioning are impaired and spill over to the family's functioning. Parents may find their employment jeopardized due to having to be at home with their depressed child or having to take their disruptive child home from school. Bipolar youths are so dysregulated that everyone around them needs to be vigilant for aggression and self-harming behaviors. For these reasons, optimal treatment involves structured psychosocial interventions and pharmacologic containment of symptoms.

PHARMACOTHEARPY

Pharmacotherapy is the cornerstone of treatment for BD at any age. However, guidelines for treating youths are limited. Furthermore, the emerging literature suggests that bipolar youths respond more slowly and/or less adequately to pharmacotherapy than do bipolar adults. Despite the lack of clear guidelines, clinicians need strategies now to treat their young patients. Thus, the following guidelines are derived from the adult literature, complemented when possible by juvenile studies, and comprise current clinical practice. For information on pharmacokinetics, dosages, side effects, laboratory monitoring, and available preparations, please refer to Chapter 22. Treatment essentials focusing on pharmacotherapy are summarized in Table 11.6.

Mood stabilizers

Davanzo and McCracken have summarized the role of mood stabilizers as the first line of treatment for both acute stabilization and maintenance in BD, including children and adolescents. However, only 40% to 60% of youths have an adequate response, which often leads to polypharmacy. Furthermore, relapse rates are high even when youths consistently comply with taking mood stabilizers.

Lithium is approved by the Food and Drug Administration (FDA) approved for acute treatment of mania and for maintenance therapy in bipolar individuals over 12 years old. Geller et al. have published the only prospective controlled study of lithium in adolescents. In 25 outpatients with comorbid BD and substance use disorders, 46% responded to lithium. In a recent open-label trial of 100 manic adolescents, Kafantaris et al. found

TABLE 11.6.   TREATMENT ESSENTIALS FOR EARLY ONSET BIPOLAR DISORDER

- Mood stabilizers are the cornerstone for treatment of bipolar disorder.
- Among the mood stabilizers, lithium and divalproex sodium are the first-line treatment for episodes of euphoric mania. Divalproex may be more effective for mixed or rapid cycling episodes, but take caution in using with women of childbearing age. Oxcarbazepine is gaining acceptance.
- Adjunctive antipsychotic medication can be used during acute mania to rapidly stabilize the youth, ensure safety, and provide sleep. Chronic use may be needed.
- If using antipsychotic medications, establish baseline and then monitor for "hypermetabolic syndrome" due to hyperphagia and weight gain. Establish dietary plan and exercise regimen at the start of pharmacotherapy.
- Antidepressants should be avoided; but if the youth becomes depressed and is not responsive to other pharmacotherapy, cautious use of antidepressants may be necessary. Carefully monitor for manic "activation" or "switch."
- Stimulants may be used to treat comorbid ADHD once the patient has been stabilized on a mood stabilizer.
- Adjunctive psychosocial treatments (e.g., psychoeducation, family therapy, individual therapy) are always indicated in the treatment of early onset BD. At a minimum, treatment should include psychoeducation about BD, its risks, treatment, prognosis, and complications associated with medication noncompliance.
- Constant vigilance about suicide potential during any phase of BD is indicated.
- Ongoing collaboration with the school should focus on education about BD, development of an appropriate individualized education plan, and assistance with behavioral management planning.

ADHD, attention deficit hyperactivity disorder; BD, bipolar disorder.

that 63% responded, but only 26% achieved remission by week 4. Sometimes clinicians are fearful of using lithium with youths and, therefore, do not prescribe adequate doses. However, treatment with youths follows the same guidelines established for adults, as summarized in Chapter 22.

Divalproex sodium is also a first-line agent approved by the FDA as a mood stabilizer in adults. As reported by Muller-Oerlinghausen et al., divalproex and lithium are equivalent in the treatment of euphoric mania, but divalproex may afford a better response when the manic episode includes two or more depressive symptoms or if the patient experiences rapid cycling episodes or a mixed state. In addition, divalproex may be useful for the management of behavioral dyscontrol and anxiety that are comorbid with BD. While antimanic response is reportedly associated with serum levels above 45 mg per L, the serum level needed to achieve anticonvulsant effects, in practice serum levels of 75 mg per L to 125 mg per L are indicated to consider a trial adequate for BD. The earlier concern about a relationship between divalproex and polycystic ovarian syndrome is unclear and should be discussed when obtaining consent from the patient and parent for the use of this medication. Divalproex is a teratogen associated with neural tube defects, another reason for caution in using this medication with any woman of childbearing age. Supplementary folic acid may be given to protect against teratogenic effects with unanticipated pregnancy.

Carbamazepine has been recommended when lithium and divalproex effects are suboptimal. Serum levels between 6 and 12 mg per L are associated with therapeutic effects. Oxcarbazepine, which is related to carbamazepine, is gaining acceptance as a first-line mood stabilizer although there are minimal data even with adults. The major advantage for youths is that no blood monitoring is needed.

Several other anticonvulsants are used as adjunctive mood stabilizers with lithium, divalproex, or carbamazepine. One of their advantages for youths is the lack of needed serum monitoring. Lamotrigine's major advantage appears to be effectiveness for BD patients with a predominantly depressive course and treatment-refractory rapid cycling. Such antidepressant effects are appealing since the use of antidepressants with any form of BD, but especially with rapid cycling and mixed states, is relatively contraindicated. Concerns with the use of lamotrigine include the risk of the potentially lethal Stevens–Johnson syndrome. Slow titration of lamotrigene can reduce this risk but also reduces effectiveness in acute mania. Topiramate has been widely used for acutely manic adults based upon predominantly open-label studies. In a retrospective chart review of 26 bipolar youths 5 to 20 years old, DelBello et al. found that topiramate was an effective adjunctive treatment. Advantages of topiramate include the lack of hyperphagic properties. In fact, weight loss is a potential side effect. Unfortunately, topiramate may exacerbate cognitive deficits in attention, concentration, and overall academic abilities. While gabapentin continues to be widely used as an adjunctive mood stabilizer, recent evidence suggests that it is ineffective and should be avoided.

Antipsychotic agents

Antipsychotics are commonly used for the acute and maintenance treatment of mania and for concomitant psychotic symptoms. Some of the atypical antipsychotic medications have shown mood stabilizing effects and are starting to be used alone without a primary mood stabilizer, particularly olanzapine, as recently reported by Tohen et al. Published algorithms indicate treatment with antipsychotic medications in acute mania after two to three mood stabilizers have failed. The role of antipsychotics in maintenance treatment is not well addressed. In clinical practice, atypical antipsychotics are commonly used as adjunctive acute and maintenance treatments well before a second or third mood stabilizer is considered. Their rapid onset of action in controlling mania and psychosis improves safety, relieves youth's distress and the burden on the family, and allows quicker integration back into school. DelBello recently showed such effects in a randomized, double-blinded, placebo-controlled trial of quetiapine in combination with divalproex in 15 adolescents with acute mania compared to 15 controls treated with divalproate alone. These results will likely extend further the role of quetiapine and other antipsychotics in the routine treatment of bipolar youths. Indeed, Pavuluri et al. recently published an algorithm for the use of atypical antipsychotics in conjunction with mood stabilizers for BD youths, including those who present with a predominantly irritable mood and those with psychotic symptoms. While awaiting further studies on the efficacy of antipsychotics as single and adjunctive agents, clinicians must weigh the risks of using antipsychotics without empiric studies against the risks associated with mania.

A major side effect and increasing concern of using atypical antipsychotics with youths is severe hyperphagia with potentially tremendous weight gain over 3 to 12 months. This should be discussed during the consent process with the youth and family. Also, recommendations are made to monitor serum glucose, lipids, and cholesterol, to alter eating habits, and to increase exercise. These interventions should be implemented at the beginning of treatment and should not wait until the youth starts to gain weight. The newer atypical antipsychotics, ziprasidone and particularly aripiprazole, appear to be less likely to cause this hypermetabolic syndrome. Nevertheless, these youths are at risk for weight gain from most medications used to control BD. Thus, weight-controlling interventions should be implemented concurrently with prescribing any of these medications.

Antidepressant medications

Antidepressants should be used cautiously in BD individuals due to the risks of accelerating mood cycling and worsening the long-term course of illness, particularly for patients with rapid cycling or mixed states. However, the depression associated with BD can be incapacitating and life threatening. Therefore, current practice standards for adults recommend the use of antidepressants on top of a mood stabilizer in patients with treatment-refractory depression. Another option is lamotrigine, which has shown efficacy in the acute and prophylactic treatment of bipolar depression in adults.

Stimulant medications

The potential of stimulants to "activate" youths and/or to precipitate a manic state is well known. Nevertheless, ADHD is a common comorbidity in prepubertal-onset BD, and residual ADHD symptoms may persist after stabilization of the BD. A stimulant may improve academic and social performance of BD youths beyond the advantages of mood stabilizers but only after adequate mood stabilization has been achieved. An alternative is atomoxetine, a nonstimulant medication that has found considerable success in treating ADHD youths. Both the stimulants and atomoxetine have been successfully prescribed with mood stabilizers and/or with atypical antipsychotics for bipolar youths.

PSYCHOSOCIAL INTERVENTIONS

According to the Practice Parameters of the American Academy of Child and Adolescent Psychiatry, a combination of pharmacology and psychosocial therapy is "almost always indicated" for early onset BD. Recently, several adjunctive psychotherapies for BD in adults have been developed including Family Focused Treatment by Miklowitz et al., Interpersonal and Social Rhythm Therapy by Frank et al., and Cognitive Behavioral Therapy by Newman et al. These therapies have been shown to improve the psychosocial factors implicated in the onset and maintenance of BD, speed recovery, delay relapse, and decrease symptoms between episodes in adults with BD. Unfortunately, no empirically validated psychosocial interventions for bipolar youths have yet been developed. Clinicians must adapt these evidence-based treatments for adults to their young bipolar patients.

General psychosocial interventions that are indicated for early onset BD include psychoeducation, mood monitoring, social skills training, and strategies aimed at increasing lifestyle regularity and decreasing activities/situations that are overstimulating to the child. Parent training in behavioral interventions for dealing with problematic behaviors may also be helpful. The therapist plays an important role in helping to resolve factors in the family that might exacerbate the youth's course, such as high expressed emotion and other negativity. The therapist is also often an important liaison with school personnel and may assist in the development of an individualized education plan or other school accommodations.

As in adult treatment, psychosocial interventions should always include a strong and consistent focus on medication adherence. Strober et al. found that 35% of bipolar adolescents were nonadherent with their lithium regimen over 18 months. The relapse rate of youths who were nonadherent (92.3%) was nearly three times that of adolescents who continued to take their lithium (37.5%). These researchers also stated that levels of "ambient stress and interpersonal discord" were increased in the families of nonadherent patients. Therefore, psychosocial interventions that focus specifically on medication adherence, interpersonal functioning, and family stress could potentially improve the long-term outcome in bipolar youths.

Miklowitz et al. have shown that family psychoeducation is an effective adjunct to medication in the treatment of adults with BD and is currently being adapted for use with bipolar adolescents (D.J. Miklowitz, personal communication, 2004). Fristad et al. are applying this intervention with bipolar children. The goal of family psychoeducation is to increase knowledge about BD and its treatments, increase medication adherence, and decrease the levels of familial expressed emotion. Preliminary findings from Fristad suggest that family psychoeducation helps to increase parental knowledge about BD and decrease levels of parental expressed emotion, helping families to cope with their child's illness overall.

Conclusions

The onset of BD early in life is now well accepted. However, controversy continues as to which youths meet criteria for BD. The debate focuses on whether a predominantly irritable mood is adequate to establish mania or whether core symptoms such as elation and grandiosity must also be evident. Thus, at this point, it is not clear whether investigators at different centers are describing the same patient population. These uncertainties have impeded our optimal understanding of this illness in youths and the development of effective treatments. Nevertheless, clinicians are increasingly treating youths with a diagnosis of BD. While pharmacotherapy forms the cornerstone of treatment, there are pitfalls. Youths are often noncompliant. Many of the medications cause hypermetabolic syndrome and severe weight gain. Also, even in the absence of evidence-based psychosocial interventions to treat BD, clinicians must adapt from adult interventions to help their young patients through their many challenges of life and to assist their distressed families in containing their "high expressed emotion," which could lead to a more malignant course for the BD youth. The coming decade should bring better understanding and newer interventions to help these needy families.

Case Vignette

Case vignette #1

Michael is a 14-year-old white male patient. He was diagnosed at 4 years old with severe ADHD and ODD. His parents worked with a therapist to develop behavioral programs to little avail. He became increasingly aggressive and impulsive. At 7 years old he impulsively but unintentionally choked his cat to death. He was then prescribed stimulant medication which helped him to stay on task for school work. However, his impulsivity and aggression continued and seemed to be more and more bizarre, including throwing a trash can across the classroom, assaulting his mother, and talking of "another Michael" making him do these things. He started to have middle of the night awakening. Addition of an α-2a agoinst, clonidine, at bedtime was somewhat helpful and was eventually added during the daytime to control his impulsivity. During this time, he got in trouble for inappropriate sexual remarks, for sexually harassing a girl, and then for exposing himself. A referral for evaluation of sexual abuse was inconclusive.

At age 13, Michael began having symptoms of depressed mood, poor energy and concentration, social withdrawal, and suicidal ideation. On interview, he endorsed vague auditory hallucinations of a "man telling me to do bad things." He was placed on an antidepressant medication. Two weeks later the police were called due to his wielding a knife and threatening to kill his mother and himself. He was admitted to an inpatient psychiatric hospital and found to be grossly psychotic, possibly manic.

His psychiatrist developed a timetable of symptom evolution since 4 years of age. It appeared that Michael's impulsivity and anger were episodic, maybe cyclical, and typically followed by much briefer periods of remorse, guilt, and suicidality. He also episodically would sit in a dark room due to feeling sad. Depression seemed evident although episodes were fleeting. Michael revealed that he had been having auditory hallucinations for as long as he could remember, but they waxed and waned and only sometimes bothered him, although increasingly so as he aged. His parents further revealed periods of possible pressured speech, racing thoughts, and goal-directed activity which he found pleasurable but which his parents found hectic and unproductive. He seemed "narcissistic" to the staff, which later was recognized as grandiosity. Michael stated that he wanted to stop his inappropriate behaviors and not get into trouble, but that he could not stop. Finally, in considering the mix of both elevated and depressed symptoms, along with hallucinations and some cyclicity, he was diagnosed with BD-I.

Michael had a rocky 2-month hospitalization during which prior medications were stopped, and then multiple medications were tried alone and in combination. Finally, he was stabilized with sodium divalproex, lithium carbonate, and an atypical antipsychotic at moderate doses. He was sufficiently stable to be stepped down to partial hospitalization for 2 months. Academic work was reintroduced, and more normative experiences at home and in the community were instituted. His parents were offered family therapy to work on the negative home environment, particularly the conflict regarding how to manage Michael. They refused, thinking that the medications had sufficiently treated their son. At discharge he was stable, but slowed down due to medication side effects. Over 6 months of treatment, Michael gained 60 pounds. His cholesterol and triglycerides were slightly elevated. An attempt was made to slowly decrease his dosage of atypical antipsychotic, which was responsible for his weight gain. After decreasing the dosage, and poor medication compliance, Michael was rehospitalized for violence at home and was placed in a residential treatment center due to safety concerns. In residential treatment, he transitioned to a different atypical antipsychotic with good improvement of symptoms and started a diet and exercise program, which helped him achieve gradual weight loss. He also participated in family therapy, with a focus on decreasing hostility at home and increasing his ability to cope with negative emotions expressed by family members. Finally, due to some persistent difficulties in attention and concentration, a low-dose stimulant was resumed with good results in treating residual ADHD symptoms.

BIBLIOGRAPHY

American Academy of Child and Adolescent Psychiatry. Practice parameters for the assessment and treatment of children and adolescents with bipolar disorder. *J Am Acad Child Adolesc Psychiatry* 1997;36:138–157.

American Psychiatric Association. *Diagnostic and statistical manual of mental disorders,* 4th ed., Text rev. Washington, DC: American Psychiatric Association, 2000.

Blumberg HP, Kaufman J, Martin A, et al. Amygdala and hippocampal volumes in adolescents and adults with bipolar disorder. *Arch Gen Psychiatry* 2003;60:1201–1208.

Birmaher B, Ryan ND, Williamson DE, et al. Childhood and adolescent depression: a review of the past 10 years. Part I. *J Am Acad Child Adolesc Psychiatry* 1996;35:1427–1439.

Carlson GA. Mania and ADHD: comorbidity or confusion. *J Affect Disord* 1998;51:177–187.

Carlson GA, Kashani JH. Manic symptoms in a nonreferred adolescent population. *J Affect Disord* 1988;15:219–226.

Chang KD, Steiner H, Ketter TA. Psychiatric phenomenology of child and adolescent bipolar offspring. *J Am Acad Child Adolesc Psychiatry* 2000;39:453–460.

Costello EJ, Pine DS, Hammen C, et al. Development and natural history of mood disorders. *Biol Psychiatry* 2002;52:529–542.

Davanzo PA, McCracken JT. Mood stabilizers in the treatment of juvenile bipolar disorder: advances. *Child Adolesc Clin North Am* 2000;9:159–182.

DelBello MP, Kowatch RA, Warner J, et al. Adjunctive topiramate treatment for pediatric bipolar disorder: a retrospective chart review. *J Child Adolesc Psychopharmacol* 2002a;12:323–330.

DelBello MP, Schwiers ML, Rosenberg HL, et al. A double-blind, randomized, placebo-controlled study of quetiapine as adjunctive treatment for adolescent mania. *J Am Acad Child Adolesc Psychiatry* 2002b;41:1216–1223.

DelBello MP, Simmerman ME, Mills NP, et al. Magnetic resonance imaging analysis of amygdala and other subcortical brain regions in adolescents with bipolar disorder. *Bipolar Disord* 2003;6:43–52.

Depue RA, Krauss S, Spoont MR, et al. General behavior inventory identification of unipolar and bipolar affective conditions in a nonclinical university population. *J Abnorm Psychol* 1989;98:117–126.

Findling RL, Youngstrom EA, Danielson CK, et al. Clinical decision-making using the General Behavior Inventory in juvenile bipolarity. *Bipolar Disord* 2002;4:34–42.

Frank E, Swartz HA, Kupfer DJ. Interpersonal and social rhythm therapy: managing the chaos of bipolar disorder. *Biol Psychiatry* 2000;48:593–604.

Fristad MA, Gavazzi SM, Mackinaw-Koons B. Family psychoeducation: an adjunctive intervention for children with bipolar disorder. *Biol Psychiatry* 2003;53:1000–1008.

Geller B, Cooper TB, Sun K. Double-blind, placebo-controlled study of lithium for adolescent bipolar disorders with secondary substance dependency. *J Am Acad Child Adolesc Psychiatry* 1998;37:171–178.

Geller B, Craney JL, Bolhofner K. Phenomenology and longitudinal course of children with a prepubertal and early adolescent bipolar disorder phenotype. In: Geller B, DelBello MP, eds. *Bipolar disorder in childhood and early adolescence.* New York: Guilford Press, 2003.

Geller B, Williams M, Zimerman B, et al. Prepubertal and early adolescent bipolarity differentiate from ADHD by manic symptoms, grandiose delusions, ultra-rapid or ultradian cycling. *J Affect Disord* 1998;51:81–91.

Gracious BL, Youngstrom EA, Findling RL, et al. Discriminative validity of a parent version of the Young Mania Rating Scale. *J Am Acad Child Adolesc Psychiatry* 2002;41:1350–1359.

Hlastala SA. Stress, social rhythms, and behavioral activation: psychosocial factors and the bipolar illness course. *Curr Psychiatry Rep* 2003;5:477–483.

Kafantaris V, Coletti DJ, Dicker R, et al. Lithium treatment of acute mania in adolescents: a large open trial. *J Am Acad Child Adolesc Psychiatry* 2003;42:1038–1045.

Lewinsohn PM, Klein D, Seeley JR. Bipolar disorders in a community sample of older adolescents: prevalence, phenomenology, comorbidity, and course. *J Am Acad Child Adolesc Psychiatry* 1995;34:454–463.

Miklowitz DJ, George EL, Richards JA, et al. A randomized study of family-focused psychoeducation and pharmacotherapy in the outpatient management of bipolar disorder. *Arch Gen Psychiatry* 2003;60:904–912.

Muller-Oerlinghausen B, Retzow A, Henn FA, et al., European Valproate Mania Study Group. Valproate as an adjunct to neuroleptic medication for the treatment of acute episodes of mania: a prospective, randomized, double-blind, placebo-controlled, multicenter study. *J Clin Psychopharmacol* 2000;20:195–203.

Newman CF, Leahy RL, Beck AT, et al. *Bipolar disorder: a cognitive therapy approach.* Washington, DC: American Psychological Association, 2002.

Pavuluri MN, Henry DB, Devineni B, et al. A phamcotherapy algorithm for stabilization and maintenance of pediatric bipolar disorder. *J Am Acad Child Adolesc Psychiatry* 2004;43:859–867.

Steingard RJ, Renshaw PF, Yurgelun-Todd D, et al. Structural abnormalities in brain magnetic resonance images of depressed children. *J Am Acad Child Adolesc Psychiatry* 1996;35:307–311.

Strober M. Bipolar disorders: natural history, genetic studies, and follow-up. In: Shafii M, Shafii SL, eds. *Clinical guide to depression in children and adolescents.* Washington, DC: American Psychiatric Press, 1992:251–268. pp

Strober M, Schmidt-Lackner S, Freeman R, et al. Recovery and relapse in adolescents with bipolar affective illness: a five-year naturalistic, prospective follow-up. *J Am Acad Child Adolesc Psychiatry* 1995;34:724–731.

Tappia PS, Ladha S, Clark DC, et al. The influence of membrane fluidity, TNF receptor binding, cAMP production and GTPase activity on macrophage cytokine production in rats fed a variety of fat diets. *Mol Cell Biochem* 1997;166:135–143.

Todd RD, Reich W, Reich T. Prevalence of affective disorder in the child and adolescent offspring of a single kindred: a pilot study. *J Am Acad Child Adolesc Psychiatry* 1994;33:198–207.

Tohen M, Baker RW, Altshuler LL, et al. Olanzapine versus divalproex in the treatment of acute mania. *Am J Psychiatry* 2002;159:1011–1017.

Youngstrom EA, Findling RL, Danielson CK, et al. Discriminative validity of parent report of hypomanic and depressive symptoms on the General Behavior Inventory. *Psychol Assess* 2001;13:267–276.

Youngstrom EA, Gracious BL, Danielson CK, et al. Toward an integration of parent and clinician report on the Young Mania Rating Scale. *J Affect Disord* 2003;77:179–190.

Youngstrom EA, Findling RL, Calabrese JR, et al. Comparing the diagnostic accuracy of six potential screening instruments for bipolar disorder in youth aged 5 to 17 years. *J Am Acad Child Adolesc Psychiatry* 2004;43:847–858.

Youngstrom EA, Findling RL, Calabrese JR. Effects of adolescent manic symptoms on agreement between youth, parent, and teacher ratings of behavior problems. *J Affect Disord* 2004;82:S5–S16.

SUGGESTED READINGS

Jamison KR. *An unquiet mind: a memoir of moods and madness.* New York: AA Knopf, 1995.
(*An excellent, best selling autobiography of a leading investigator of bipolar disorder chronicling her own struggle with this disorder.*)

Miklowitz DJ. *The bipolar disorder survival guide: what you and your family need to know.* New York: Guilford Press, 2002.
(*For families living with an individual with bipolar disorder, geared to the adult, but the principles apply*)

at all ages. The author is an investigator of family processes contributing to mental illness.)

Papolos DF, Papolos J. *The bipolar child: the definitive and reassuring guide to childhood's most misunderstood disorder*. New York: Broadway Books, 2002.
(A popular reading for families with a child diagnosed with bipolar disorder. It is controversial due to overinclusiveness in identification of this diagnosis in youths.)

Additionally, patients and families can benefit from information and connection with support groups some of which can be found on the following websites:

The Depression and Bipolar Support Alliance, www.dbsalliance.org

National Association for the Mentally Ill, www.nami.org

CHAPTER 12

Early Onset Schizophrenia

STEFANIE A. HLASTALA
JON MCCLELLAN

Introduction   Early onset schizophrenia (EOS), with an onset prior to age 18, is a serious, often debilitating, disorder characterized by deficits in affect, cognition, and the ability to relate socially with others. EOS is often associated with significant morbidity, chronicity, and psychosocial impairment. Although schizophrenia and other severe psychotic disorders are rarely found in children, the profoundly negative effects of these illnesses and the necessity for intensive intervention require that clinicians who work with youths be familiar with their phenomenology, course of illness, assessment, and treatment. This chapter will review current research findings on the etiology, illness course, diagnostic considerations, and treatment of schizophrenia and related psychotic disorders in children and adolescents.

HISTORIC NOTES

Until relatively recently, physicians were reluctant to diagnose schizophrenia and other psychotic disorders in children and adolescents. Indeed, the existence of an early onset form of schizophrenia has been debated since Kraepelin's early groundbreaking work on psychotic disorders. Although Kraepelin's early descriptions of childhood onset schizophrenia were similar to the adult form of the disorder, other descriptive psychopathologists lumped early onset psychosis into a broader range of childhood syndromes that were defined by developmental deficits in language, social relations, perception, and movement. Psychotic speech and thought were believed to be important components of early onset psychosis, but hallucinations and delusions were not required for a diagnosis. As a result, childhood psychoses often included a broader rubric of neurodevelopmental disorders, including autism.

It was not until the 1970s that EOS was demonstrated to be distinct from other developmental disorders found in children such as autism and pervasive developmental disorders (PDD). In 1980, the *Diagnostic and Statistical Manual of Mental Disorders,* Third Edition (DSM-III) revised the diagnostic criteria so that EOS was diagnosed using the same criteria as those used for adult onset schizophrenia. This practice has been maintained in subsequent DSM iterations and is widely accepted as valid. Because a large portion of past research used the term childhood onset schizophrenia overinclusively to describe a broader range of severely disturbed children, older studies of EOS need to be interpreted with caution.

Clinical Features

Although EOS is a syndrome consisting of a group of varied symptoms including social withdrawal, self-care deficiencies, and bizarre behaviors, hallucinations and delusions are the characteristic symptoms of schizophrenia. Schizophrenia is usually categorized as having two broad sets of clusters, positive and negative. Positive symptoms are those that are traditionally considered to be the disorder's hallmark—florid hallucinations, delusions, and thought disorder. Negative symptoms include flat affect, anergia, and paucity of speech and thought. A third cluster, including disorganized speech, bizarre behavior, and poor attention, has been more recently discussed in the literature. In a study of youths with early onset psychotic disorders (including schizophrenia and bipolar disorder), McClellan et al. found four symptom domains: positive symptoms, negative symptoms, behavioral problems, and dysphoria. Only negative symptoms were specifically associated with a diagnosis of schizophrenia. In descriptive studies, hallucinations, thought disorder, and flattened affect have been consistently found in EOS, whereas systematic delusions and catatonic symptoms are less frequent. Caplan found that children with EOS exhibit low rates of incoherence and poverty of speech. When assessing a child's thinking, it is important to distinguish between psychotic thought processes and developmental delays or language disorders.

DIAGNOSTIC AND STATISTICAL MANUAL OF MENTAL DISORDERS, FOURTH EDITION, TEXT REVISION CRITERIA

According to the DSM-IV-TR, at least two of the following are needed for a diagnosis of schizophrenia, each present for a significant period of time during a 1-month period: (a) delusions, (b) hallucinations, (c) disorganized speech, (d) grossly disorganized or catatonic behavior, and/or (e) negative symptoms, that is, affective flattening, alogia, or avolition. Only one of the following symptoms is needed for the diagnosis of schizophrenia: the delusions are bizarre, hallucinations consist of a voice keeping a running commentary on the child's behavior or thoughts, or two or more voices are conversing with each other. For a significant amount of time since the onset of the disorder, one or more areas of social functioning, such as school functioning, interpersonal relationships, and/or self-care are noticeably below the preonset level or the expected level of age-appropriate social and academic achievement. The disturbance must persist for at least 6 months including at least 1 month of active psychotic symptoms. If the duration criterion of 6 months is not met, a diagnosis of schizophreniform disorder is made.

Several different subtypes of schizophrenia are described in the DSM-IV-TR including paranoid, disorganized, catatonic, undifferentiated, and residual. Studies on schizophrenic children and adolescents report that the paranoid and undifferentiated subtypes are the most commonly found.

DIAGNOSTIC AND STATISTICAL MANUAL OF MENTAL DISORDERS LIMITATIONS (HOW PRESENTATION IN YOUTHS DIFFERS FROM ADULT)

Because it can be difficult to distinguish true psychotic symptoms in young children, clinicians should be very careful when making a diagnosis in these patients. Overactive imaginations, developmental delays, language problems, posttraumatic phenomena, and/or misperceptions of the questions being asked all may lead to misinterpretations of psychotic symptoms in youths. Furthermore, very young children's inability to apply logical reasoning to their perceptions can make it difficult to identify delusions in children younger than age 5.

Russell has noted that in school-aged children with psychosis, the delusional content often revolves around ideas of reference, somatic preoccupations, or delusions of persecution. Compared to psychotic adults, delusions are less likely to be richly detailed or elaborate and are often nonsystematized. In fact, more elaborate descriptions of suspected psychotic phenomena should raise questions as to the validity of the report.

Studies in the 1980s indicate that most children who report psychotic symptoms do not actually have a psychotic disorder. In particular, McClellan's group notes that many youths with conduct and other nonpsychotic emotional disorders may report psychoticlike symptoms and are at risk of being misdiagnosed. In these cases, the psychotic symptom reports are often atypical in nature in the following manner: (a) the reports are inconsistent, and there is no other documented evidence of a psychotic process (e.g., thought disorder, bizarre disorganized behavior); (b) the qualitative nature of the reports were not typical of psychotic symptoms, (e.g., greatly detailed descriptions or reports more suggestive of fantasy or imagination); and/or (c) the reported symptoms only occurred at specific times, (e.g., only hearing voices after an aggressive outburst). Atypical psychotic symptoms may represent a number of phenomena, including posttraumatic stress disorder, factitious or conversion disorders, or developmental delays that interfere with the accurate reporting of internal experiences, difficulty distinguishing fantasy from reality, and/or misunderstanding the questions being asked by the clinician. Children with a history of abuse, especially those with posttraumatic stress disorder (PTSD), often report higher rates of psychoticlike symptoms than do control children. In these children, atypical psychotic symptoms may actually represent dissociative phenomena or anxiety symptoms, including intrusive thoughts/worries, derealization, and/or depersonalization. In general, it is reasonable to assume that an older adolescent presenting with psychotic symptoms is more likely to have a primary psychotic illness than a young child, although the validity of the reports in either age group needs to be carefully assessed.

Another complicating factor is the presence of developmental delays. Ten to twenty percent of children with EOS have intelligence quotients (IQs) in the borderline to mentally retarded range as noted by Kenny et al. and other groups. Because many research studies have excluded patients with mental retardation, rates may actually be higher in clinical populations. Although youths with schizophrenia are at risk for cognitive deficits, the presence of developmental delays also creates diagnostic difficulties. In these cases, reported psychotic symptoms may simply represent misunderstanding of the concepts and/or misinterpreted normal sensory phenomena.

Epidemiology

Because EOS is relatively uncommon, few studies have examined incidence rates in the population. Available evidence suggests that the prevalence of schizophrenia in children is significantly lower than in adults, which is estimated to be approximately 1%. The onset rate rises precipitously during the age range of 15 to 30 years. Although the timing of disorder suggests a relationship with pubertal status, puberty has not been specifically associated with this trajectory.

Beitchman notes that the prevalence in children less than 15 years of age is approximately 14 per 100,000. Prepubertal EOS (VEOS—prior to age 13) is extremely rare, perhaps as low as 1.6 cases per 100,000 in the general population and 1% of hospitalized schizophrenic youths, as reported by Thomsen. VEOS occurs predominantly in boys with ratios of approximately 2:1, but several investigators have noted that this ratio becomes closer to 1:1 as age increases. Russell notes that the youngest age of onset reported in the scientific literature is 3 years, although any case below age 8 years needs to be carefully scrutinized.

Course of Illness

Although often characterized as a chronic condition, schizophrenia is a phasic illness, with the course and duration of the phases varying dependent on the illness and treatment response. The phases include: (a) prodrome, (b) acute, (c) recuperative/recovery, and (d) residual. The prodromal phase involves general deterioration in functioning before the onset of psychotic symptoms in the active phase. Social withdrawal, idiosyncratic or bizarre preoccupations, unusual behaviors, academic decline, deteriorating self-care, increasing anxiety, depression, somatic complaints, and/or changes in appetite and sleep are common disturbances that occur during the prodromal phase. Children in the prodromal phase of illness may also exhibit increased behavioral problems, including aggression, deceitfulness, and/or substance abuse. Such symptoms may represent a significant change from baseline functioning or a worsening of premorbid personality characteristics, which may make it difficult to identify the onset of the disorder in some children. Prodromes can vary from an acute change (days to weeks) to a more insidious, chronic impairment. Children (VEOS) tend to have more insidious onsets, whereas both acute (less than 1 year) and insidious onsets have been noted in adolescents. The acute phase is marked by a predominance of positive psychotic symptoms (i.e., hallucinations, delusions, disorganized thinking and behavior) that often shift to negative symptoms (i.e., affective flattening, avolition, paucity of thought or speech) over time. This phase usually lasts between 1 and 6 months, however, it may last longer if the child does not respond adequately to treatment. As the acute psychosis remits, there is often a recuperative/recovery phase lasting several months where the patient continues to experience a significant degree of impairment. This is most often due to negative symptoms (flat affect, anergia, social withdrawal), although it is common for some positive symptoms to persist. In addition, some patients will develop a postpsychotic depression characterized by dysphoria and flat affect.

The residual phase is characterized by the overall improvement of active psychotic symptoms. Generally, there is some persistence of negative symptoms, including social isolation, poverty of speech, odd beliefs/perceptions, and/or anergia. Individuals may continue to display peculiar behavior (e.g., poor hygiene, blunted or inappropriate affect) and disordered thinking (tangentiality, circumferentiality). The residual phase may last for several months or more.

Several investigators such as Eggers et al. have noted that some patients exhibit significant symptoms that do not respond to adequate pharmacologic and psychosocial treatment. These chronically ill patients exhibit the most severe impairment over time and require the most comprehensive treatment resources (e.g., medications combined with individual, family, and school interventions).

Etiology and Pathogenesis

EOS is a heterogeneous disorder with multiple potential causes. A neurodevelopmental model is generally proposed, whereby underlying vulnerabilities interact with environmental/biologic risk factors leading to neurologic damage that ultimately results in the disorder. It is evident that there is no single unique cause and that the timing of the neurodevelopmental injury may be just as important as the source. Three primary mechanisms have been identified in the research literature so far: (a) genetics, (b) viral exposure, and (c) neurodevelopmental insults. Psychological factors have also been a focus of research attention. While psychological factors have not been found to cause schizophrenia, chronic interpersonal stress within the family has been found to influence the onset and exacerbation of acute psychotic episodes and relapse/rehospitalization rates. Below are brief summaries of the most commonly hypothesized etiologic factors for schizophrenia.

GENETIC FACTORS

Genetic factors appear to play a significant role in the development of schizophrenia, for which Owen et al. have estimated a heritability rate of approximately 80%. Tsuang has noted that the lifetime risk of developing schizophrenia is approximately 10 times higher in first-degree biologic relatives of affected individuals when compared to the general population. The early onset variant of schizophrenia may have an even higher genetic risk than adult onset schizophrenia. Although a great deal of evidence suggests the importance of genetic factors in the etiology of schizophrenia, the existence of a relatively substantial discordance rate in monozygotic twins indicates that environmental factors also play an etiologic role. Unfortunately, the specific genes for schizophrenia and other psychotic disorders remain elusive. Because schizophrenia is a heterogeneous disorder, no single model of genetic inheritance has been identified in the research literature. As recently presented by Harrison and Owen, current theories conceptualize schizophrenia in the context of a multifactorial polygenic model where susceptibility genes act in conjunction with epigenetic processes and environmental factors to cause the disorder.

VIRAL EXPOSURE

Individuals with schizophrenia are more likely to have been born during the winter months or soon after an influenza epidemic than expected by chance, as noted by Huttunen et al., suggesting that viral exposure during gestation may be a risk factor for the later development of schizophrenia. Some research studies have found that birth cohorts who were in the second trimester of pregnancy during an influenza epidemic were shown to have an increased risk of schizophrenia, although this result has not been consistently noted. Some investigators, such as Gaughran, have also found that schizophrenic patients exhibit an increase in viral titers and/or immunologic markers. Yet, these findings are inconsistent as well. The equivocal findings are likely due to the complexity and heterogeneity of schizophrenia and methodologic inadequacies of previous research.

NEURODEVELOPMENTAL FACTORS

Early neurodevelopmental problems, such as obstetric complications, minor physical irregularities, and disruption of fetal neural development during the second trimester, have been associated with the eventual development of schizophrenia. Children who ultimately develop schizophrenia display a variety of subtle behavioral abnormalities that often remain undetected until the full onset of the disorder. Davidson et al. have noted that these children exhibit delayed motor milestones, speech problems, lower educational test scores, and/or poor social adjustment before the onset of the disorder. These developmental delays have been hypothesized to represent the early neuropathologic manifestations of schizophrenia.

NEUROIMAGING FINDINGS

In the adult literature, neurobiologic theories of schizophrenia have focused on the prefrontal cortex, heteromodal association cortex, thalamus, and hippocampal structures, including the cingulate cortex, as the primary sites of brain abnormalities in schizophrenic patients. Numerous neurobiologic abnormalities have been found in EOS, including deficits in smooth pursuit eye movements and autonomic responsivity, as well as anatomic and functional changes in neuroimaging as documented by Jacobsen et al. Gilmore et al. have summarized studies documenting that first-episode schizophrenic patients tend to have increased lateral ventricular volumes, increased third ventricular volumes, abnormal hemispheric asymmetries, asymmetries of the planum temporale, reduced temporal limbic structure volumes, reduced size in specific regions of the thalamus, and/or abnormal morphology of the lateral ventricle, medial temporal lobe, and frontoparietal cortex. Since these abnormalities were found in young first-episode patients, the findings are less likely to be caused by long-term exposure to medications or environmental factors secondary to the illness, such as substance abuse or chronic institutionalization.

An investigation of EOS at the National Institute of Mental Health (NIMH) Child Psychiatry Branch by Frazier et al. found similar results to research conducted on older first-episode patients. Total cerebral volume and the midsagittal thalamic areas were significantly smaller in schizophrenic children than in normal controls. Also, the caudate, putamen, globus pallidus, and lateral ventricles were larger in schizophrenic children. Rapoport et al. found that when rescanned 2 years later, ventricular volume increased and the midsagittal thalamic area decreased in schizophrenic children. Furthermore, the schizophrenic children with the greatest increase in ventricular volume had the lowest levels of premorbid adjustment and highest levels of clinical symptoms at follow-up. Additional research by the same group suggests that patients with EOS have progressively smaller temporal lobe structures and progressive cortical differences in the temporal, frontal, and parietal regions over time. Overall, the data provide compelling evidence of the neurobiologic continuity between early and adult onset schizophrenia. Moreover, these findings are in concordance with other research indicating that brain development is altered in some individuals with schizophrenia.

Assessment

A complete history and physical exam are necessary to provide an accurate assessment of psychosis in children and adolescents. A careful and systematic assessment of the child's current and previous psychiatric symptoms, psychosocial functioning, and family psychiatric history is a vital source of information when making a diagnosis. Whenever possible, the history should be gathered from all available sources, including the child, his or her parents, other caregivers, teachers, treatment providers, and community support persons (e.g., case workers, probation officers, peers). The psychiatric history should focus on the presenting symptomatology, the longitudinal timeline of symptom development, and associated features and/or confounding factors (e.g., mood disorders, developmental problems, substance abuse). Because of the many phases of psychotic disorders, it is important to obtain a longitudinal understanding of the child's illness. Certain core aspects of psychotic disorders may be missed if the clinician conducts only a cross-sectional checklist of symptoms.

A thorough physical examination is also necessary to rule out any medical causes of psychotic symptoms. Drug or alcohol intoxication, delirium, central nervous system lesions, tumors, bacterial or viral infections, metabolic disorders, and seizure disorders are potential organic conditions that can cause psychosis. Neuroimaging, electroencephalographs (EEGs), and laboratory tests are not required to diagnose primary psychotic conditions. However, such tests are often indicated based on information obtained from the history and physical examination to rule out other organic illnesses and/or to serve as a baseline for medication therapy monitoring.

An assessment of the child's current and past psychosocial functioning is also extremely important given the role of family support and stressors in modulating the course of illness and treatment response. Because cognitive deficits may influence the presentation and/or interpretation of psychotic symptoms, an intellectual assessment may also be helpful when there is evidence of developmental delays. However, neuropsychological testing is not indicated as a method for differentiating schizophrenia from other psychiatric psychotic disorders (see Table 12.1).

TABLE 12.1. EVALUATION ESSENTIALS FOR EARLY ONSET SCHIZOPHRENIA

1. A systematic psychiatric history focusing on a longitudinal understanding of the patient's current and past symptomatology should be obtained.
2. A thorough psychosocial history including current and past academic and interpersonal functioning and current and past abuse should be obtained.
3. A comprehensive physical examination is necessary to rule out organic causes of psychotic symptoms.
4. Multiple historic informants (e.g., child, parents, teachers, past treatment providers) should be included in the evaluation process.
5. There are no specific laboratory tests, neuroimaging procedures, rating scales, or psychological tests that have been established to be individually diagnostic of EOS. These tests are used primarily to rule out other disorders such as organic psychoses.
6. Baseline and follow-up rating scales that assess positive and negative symptoms and psychosocial functioning are helpful in monitoring the effectiveness of treatment interventions.

EOS, early onset schizophrenia.

Differential Diagnosis and Comorbid Diagnoses

Several other psychiatric disorders manifest themselves with the expression of symptoms that either overlap or are easily mistaken for the primary symptoms of schizophrenia. If the symptoms of schizophrenia have not persisted for a 6-month period, a diagnosis of schizophreniform disorder should be made. In youths, this often ultimately develops into schizophrenia. Schizoaffective disorder and mood disorders with psychotic features need to be ruled out when diagnosing a child or adolescent presenting with psychotic symptoms. This is especially important for adolescents with bipolar disorder because, as McClellan et al. note, manic episodes during adolescence often include psychotic symptoms during the acute phase of illness. In fact, early onset bipolar disorder is associated with higher rates of psychosis than bipolar disorder of adult onset. As a result, bipolar youths are often misdiagnosed as schizophrenic when seen during an acute manic or mixed episode.

Psychotic symptoms during the acute phase of illness in EOS and early onset bipolar disorder have considerable overlap. However, Pavuluri et al. have recently noted that bipolar youths tend to have more mood congruent delusions and a lower percentage of hallucinations, loosening of associations, and negative symptoms than schizophrenic children. In addition to differences during the acute phase of illness, a thorough understanding of the child's symptomatic and psychosocial history will aid in the differential diagnosis of schizophrenia and bipolar disorder. Youths with schizophrenia also tend to have higher rates of premorbid social withdrawal and global impairments than bipolar youths. Further, psychotic symptoms must only present during active periods of depression or mania for a diagnosis of bipolar disorder. During euthymic periods, the bipolar patient will not experience psychotic symptoms.

Calderoni notes that schizoaffective disorder and major depression with psychotic features may be the most difficult disorders to distinguish from schizophrenia. Negative symptoms of EOS are sometimes mistaken for depression, especially since dysphoria is commonly experienced as a part of the illness. Although an accurate picture of the temporal overlap between mood episodes and psychotic symptoms can be extremely difficult to obtain, this retrospective understanding is necessary to distinguish EOS from other psychotic disorders. For a diagnosis of depression with psychotic features, psychosis will only be present in the context of a severe major depressive episode. For a diagnosis of schizoaffective disorder, positive and negative psychotic symptoms must occur in the absence of significant mood episodes. The diagnosis of schizoaffective disorder appears to be somewhat unreliable in community settings, due in part to the tendency to use this diagnosis when mood and psychotic episodes co-occur (which may represent a primary mood disorder) or when an individual with schizophrenia has mood symptoms (i.e., dysphoria, grandiosity) without meeting the prerequisite mood episode criteria. Moreover, it is not uncommon in clinical settings that youths with emotional and behavioral dysregulation problems, often with traumatic histories, report psychotic-clike symptoms and are diagnosed with schizoaffective disorder even though they may not actually have true psychosis.

Youths with traumatic histories, including physical, sexual, and/or emotional abuse, may report symptoms suggestive of auditory or visual hallucinations and/or paranoid delusions. However, these symptoms are generally either brief or atypical in nature, and the child does not demonstrate the other hallmark symptoms of schizophrenia. Further, some children with abuse histories may report psychotic symptoms in the context of reinforcement that occurs in a chaotic environment. Therefore, potential environmental reinforcers of psychotic behaviors should be assessed. For example, a child who reports hearing voices telling her to kill herself only when her parents are arguing (which, as a result, stops the parents from arguing because they are concerned with her behavior) is unlikely to have a primary psychotic condition such as EOS. Conversely, as McClellan et al. have noted, children with schizophrenia may also have suffered abuse and, therefore, a history of trauma does not rule out a primary psychotic illness.

Some psychoses are caused by substance intoxication or delirium. Patients with substance-induced psychosis, generally present with an acute onset of psychotic symptoms that are temporally related to the intake of the drug. Psychostimulants can produce paranoid delusions and disorientation, whereas hallucinogens may produce vivid hallucinations and delusions. Substance intoxication and/or withdrawal can also induce delirium, which is associated with fluctuating mental status, varied levels of consciousness, and altered short-term memory. Therefore, it is important to identify if the psychosis is attributable to delirium or substances because psychoses of these etiologies often have a different clinical course and require different treatment strategies than psychosis due to EOS. Some youths may present with a psychotic illness in the context of substance/alcohol abuse, leading to an uncertain diagnosis. Because substance-induced psychosis generally clears within hours to days, psychotic symptoms that persist after a significant period of detoxification indicate the possibility of an underlying primary psychotic illness that may have been precipitated or exacerbated by substance abuse.

There are other psychotic disorders that are generally rare in youths and have not been studied. Delusional disorder presents with nonbizarre delusions (e.g., isolated paranoid belief) without the other accompanying symptoms of schizophrenia. Brief psychotic disorder consists of schizophrenic symptoms lasting less than 1 month in duration. Such presentations warrant careful evaluation, including the possibility of an acute response to stress, intoxication, or misreporting (or misinterpretation) of psychotic symptoms. Brief psychotic episodes may also be harbingers of developing schizophrenia or a psychotic mood disorder.

Developmental disorders, especially PDD, may overlap in symptomatology with EOS. Behavioral oddities, restricted interests, and significant interpersonal deficits are often present in both EOS and PDD. However, frank psychosis is evidence of a primary psychotic condition, regardless of developmental disabilities or autistic-spectrum disorders.

A significant number of patients with transient psychotic symptoms who fail to meet full criteria for any of the primary psychotic disorders discussed above are often given a diagnosis of psychotic disorder not otherwise specified (PDNOS). Kumra et al. note that PDNOS children have been found to exhibit significant overall impairment and similar risk factor profiles and neurobiologic abnormalities to EOS children. Follow-up studies ranging from 2 to 17 years by several investigators including Nicolson et al. indicate that many PDNOS patients continue to have hallucinations or delusions over the long-term, are chronically impaired, require residential placement, or have significant work and social difficulties as adults. Only a very small number of these children (1/57) received a follow-up diagnosis of schizophrenia. Half of the patients in the study by Nicolson et al. received a later diagnosis of a psychotic mood disorder (e.g., schizoaffective disorder, bipolar disorder, major depressive disorder with psychotic features). It is questionable whether some of the individuals actually have true psychoses, and it is likely that some have personality disorders and/or posttraumatic phenomena. These issues have been addressed by McClellan in the United States and Thomsen in Scandinavia (see Table 12.2).

TABLE 12.2. DIFFERENTIAL DIAGNOSIS FOR EARLY ONSET SCHIZOPHRENIA

Psychiatric
Psychotic disorder due to a general medical condition
Bipolar disorder
Major depressive episode with psychotic features
Schizoaffective disorder
Psychotic disorder NOS
Delusional disorder
Posttraumatic stress disorder
Obsessive compulsive disorder
Pervasive developmental disorder
Conduct disorder
Evolving borderline personality disorder

Psychosocial
Abuse
Traumatic stress
Chaotic family environment

Medical
Substance intoxication
Delirium
Brain tumor
Head injury
Seizure disorder
Meningitis

NOS, not otherwise specified.

Treatment

PHARMACOTHERAPY

The efficacy of antipsychotic agents for the treatment of schizophrenia in adults is well established. These medications reduce psychotic symptoms, help prevent relapse, and improve general functioning. Atypical antipsychotic medications are now considered the drugs of first choice given their efficacy for both positive and negative symptoms, mood stabilizing properties, and more favorable side effect profile in comparison to the traditional neuroleptic agents. However, these agents also cause some difficulties with weight gain, and metabolic changes are a significant concern. Finally, a newer agent, aripiprazole, which works by mechanisms somewhat different from the other agents, is Food and Drug Administration (FDA) approved for adults and available for use with children.

There are only four randomized controlled trials examining the efficacy and safety of antipsychotics in youths with EOS, three of which examined typical agents. Together these studies involved only 132 children and adolescents. Spencer found that haloperidol was superior to placebo in reducing symptoms of thought disorder, hallucinations, and persecutory ideation in 15 children, and Pool found similar effects in 75 adolescents with schizophrenia. Loxapine was also examined in the latter study and found to be superior to placebo but not different from haloperidol. In another small study (n = 21) that did not include a placebo arm, Realmuto found that both thiothixene and thioridazine improved psychotic symptoms in about 50% of youths diagnosed with chronic schizophrenia. Youths appear to have the same spectrum of side effects noted in adults, for example, extrapyramidal symptoms, sedation, tardive dyskinesia, and neuroleptic malignant syndrome, and may be especially sensitive to extrapyramidal side effects.

More recently, an open trial with clozapine by Frazier et al. showed much promise in the treatment of positive and negative symptoms of childhood onset schizophrenia and paved the way for the only randomized controlled trial of an atypical antipsychotic in youths. In that systematic study, Kumra et al. examined 21 youths with treatment-resistant childhood onset schizophrenia and found clozapine to be superior to haloperidol. However, an extremely high rate of serious side effects was associated with clozapine. Five of the 21 subjects developed significant neutropenia, and two had seizures. Therefore, although potentially more efficacious, clozapine's apparent increased risk for adverse reactions in youths raises concerns.

In another open label study of eight treatment-resistant schizophrenic children, Kumra found that olanzapine was efficacious [defined as more than 20% improvement in Brief Psychiatric Rating Scale (BPRS) scores] in two children. Increased appetite, constipation, somnolence, insomnia, tachycardia, and transient increases in liver function tests were the main side effects observed. Other open label trials by Findling et al. of olanzapine and by Shaw et al. of quetiapine suggest effectiveness for EOS. In a controlled trial comparing olanzapine, risperidal, and haloperidol in youths with more broadly defined psychotic disorders, Sikich found that subjects maintained treatment on olanzapine significantly longer than the other two agents. Weight gain due to atypical antipsychotics appears to be an even greater problem for youths than for adults.

Treatment varies depending on the phase of illness and the patient's history of medication response and side effects. Since the literature regarding the use of antipsychotic medications for psychosis in children and adolescents is sparse, the most recent American Academy of Child and Adolescent Psychiatry (AACAP) treatment guidelines extrapolate from the adult literature. In these practice parameters, the AACAP laid out the following general guidelines for the psychopharmacologic management of schizophrenia:

Acute Phase: Antipsychotic therapy should be implemented for at least 4 to 6 weeks, using adequate dosages, before any judgment of efficacy can be made. Large medication doses instituted very early in the course of treatment do not necessarily hasten recovery and may result in excessive doses and increased side effects. The short-term use of benzodiazepines as adjuncts to neuroleptics may help in stabilizing acutely psychotic and agitated patients. A trial of a different neuroleptic should be undertaken if no results are apparent or if side effects are not manageable after 4 to 6 weeks. For those patients who do not respond adequately, clozapine should be considered. Clozapine has been found to be effective for treatment-resistant cases. However, given clozapine's potential serious side effects (e.g., neutropenia, seizures), it is generally used only in patients who have not responded to two or more adequate trials of different antipsychotic agents, including at least one atypical agent.

Recuperative Phase: As positive symptoms improve, usually after 4 to 12 weeks of treatment, patients may have persistent confusion, disorganization, and dysphoria. Antipsychotic medication should be maintained during this period because additional improvement may be obtained over the 6 to 12 months following the acute psychotic phase. To decrease side effects, a gradual dosage taper may be indicated, especially if high dosages were necessary to control the acute psychotic phase. However, when lowering the dose, the patient may be at increased risk for relapse and, therefore, should be monitored carefully. Persistent dysphoria may benefit from an antidepressant trial, although this has not been systematically studied and raises concerns over polypharmacy.

Recovery/residual Phase: Maintenance antipsychotic medications have well-documented efficacy in preventing relapse in adults and are indicated for the vast majority of schizophrenic patients. Without maintenance therapies, Robinson et al. found that approximately 65% of adult patients relapse within 1 year and a striking 80% relapse at least once over 5 years. While still far from ideal, the 1-year relapse rate drops to approximately 30% in patients maintained on antipsychotic agents. Because the adult literature has documented a small percentage of patients who do not relapse,

TABLE 12.3. PSYCHOTROPICS TO TREAT EARLY ONSET PSYCHOSES

First line:
Atypical antipsychotics: olanzapine, risperidone, quetiapine, aripiprazole, ziprasidone

Second line:
Typical antipsychotics: haloperidol, thiothixene, chlorpromazine, trifluoperazine, molindone

Considered for treatment-resistant cases:
Clozapine
Electroconvulsive therapy

Note: Recommendations are drawn from the adult literature and clinical consensus as controlled trials are not yet available justifying the atypical agents as first-line treatments in youths.

a medication-free trial may be considered in newly diagnosed youths who have been symptom free for at least 6 to 12 months. During maintenance treatment, physician contact should be maintained on a regular basis to adequately monitor symptoms, side effects, and medication adherence, while also directing or referring out for any necessary psychosocial interventions (see Table 12.3).

PSYCHOSOCIAL INTERVENTIONS

Adjunctive psychosocial interventions are almost always indicated in the treatment of EOS. While EOS is certainly an illness mediated by genetic and neurodevelopmental factors, psychosocial factors often play a powerful role in the expression of the illness course, treatment response, and prognosis. In turn, the illness and its various manifestations can wreak havoc on the child's psychosocial world. Psychotherapy as a stand-alone treatment has not proven to be effective for treating schizophrenia. However, adjunctive psychosocial treatments including psychoeducation described by Rund et al., behaviorally based family therapy described by Goldstein and Miklowitz, and cognitive-behavioral therapy (CBT) described by Rector and Beck have been shown to reduce relapse rates and improve positive and negative symptoms in schizophrenic patients.

Psychoeducational therapy can be extremely helpful for the patient and his or her family to learn how to cope better with effects of the illness and enhance the long-term outcome. Psychoeducation for the patient should include ongoing education about the illness, treatment options, social skills training, relapse prevention, basic life skills training, and problem-solving strategies. Psychoeducation for the family should include information to increase their understanding of their child's illness, treatment options, short- and long-term prognosis, and for developing strategies to cope with their child's symptoms and behavioral manifestations of the disorder. Rund's work with schizophrenic adolescents suggests that psychoeducational treatment leads to lower rates of rehospitalization and greater cost-effectiveness than usual or standard treatment.

Family therapies for schizophrenia evolved from research examining the effects of "expressed emotion" in families on the long-term illness course in schizophrenic patients. Expressed emotion refers to attributes of hostility, overprotectiveness, and/or criticism expressed toward the patient by his or her family members. Relapse rates have been shown to be consistently higher for schizophrenic patients who live in families with high levels of expressed emotion. Therefore, it is not surprising that Goldstein and Miklowitz's work with adjunctive family interventions aimed at educating the family about schizophrenia and the medications used to treat the disorder, improving problem solving, and increasing communication skills has decreased relapse rates.

CBT for schizophrenia developed by Rector and Beck focuses on challenging and testing key beliefs associated with hallucinations and delusions, teaching problem-solving skills,

TABLE 12.4. TREATMENT ESSENTIALS FOR EARLY ONSET SCHIZOPHRENIA

1. Antipsychotic medications are the frontline treatment for psychosis, with the atypical antipsychotic agents generally considered the drugs of first choice.
2. A trial of antipsychotic medication should be implemented for at least 4–6 wk before any judgment about effectiveness can be made. After 4–6 wk, if significant improvement is not apparent and/or side effects are unmanageable, then a different neuroleptic should be tried.
3. Other medications, such as antidepressants, mood stabilizers, and/or benzodiazepines can be used to manage mood and anxiety symptomatology once antipsychotic agents have been given the appropriate time to exert effects.
4. Some form of adjunctive psychosocial treatment (e.g., psychoeducation, family therapy, cognitive-behavioral therapy) is always indicated in the treatment of EOS.
5. It is important to educate and collaborate with the child's teachers and school counselors to formulate appropriate expectations and goals to ensure academic success.

EOS, early onset schizophrenia.

enhancing coping strategies, and increasing medication adherence. In adults, adjunctive CBT has been found to produce large clinical effects on both positive and negative symptoms of schizophrenia. However, there are no published research studies examining the effects of CBT on symptomatic or functional outcomes in patients with EOS. Certainly, the effectiveness of CBT would depend on the developmental level of the patient and whether the patient possesses the metacognitive abilities to "think about one's thinking," which may be beyond what the majority of EOS individuals are capable of during childhood and early adolescence.

Behavioral interventions for weight management may also be indicated in children who gain a significant amount of weight on antipsychotic medications. Traditional behavioral interventions focus on self-monitoring of weight, food intake, and exercise. Unfortunately, research on the effectiveness of behavioral interventions for antipsychotic-induced weight gain is virtually absent. The research literature on nonpsychotic overweight children and adolescents indicates that a comprehensive, multidisciplinary program including a dietician, physical therapist, psychologist, and physician is needed to produce significant weight loss. Clearly, more research on weight management in youths with medication-induced weight gain is greatly needed.

Specialized educational programs and/or vocational training may be indicated for some children or adolescents to address the cognitive and functional deficits associated with the disorder. Some children will require more intensive community support services, including day programs and/or community caseworkers. In more chronic and/or severely ill children, long-term placement in a residential facility may be warranted (see Table 12.4).

Conclusions

EOS is a rare, but very severe, disorder. Because these youths often demonstrate prodromes across multiple domains of functioning for many years prior to the onset of frank psychotic symptoms, they have received multiple other diagnoses and treatments prior to formal diagnosis and enrollment in treatment. During this time, these youths fall farther behind in life. Thus, it is important for clinicians who treat youths with odd ideation, decreased affective expression, and lack of appropriate socialization to seek formal comprehensive evaluation as soon as possible. The evidence base for treating these youths is limited, although evolving, as clinicians become more attuned to diagnosing this chronic disorder. Usual and customary care focuses on pharmacotherapy to decrease the more impairing symptoms such as hallucinations and bizarre ideation, as well as to improve mood and school performance. Adjunctive psychosocial interventions include psychoeducation of families, reduction of negative home environments, collaboration with schools, and individual cognitive-behavioral strategies to help youths optimize their functioning and enjoyment of life.

Case Vignette

Case vignette #1

Jennifer presented as a 13-year-old girl who had been acting increasingly bizarre at home and in school for the past year. Her parents reported that her grades and school attendance had worsened significantly that year. She was not completing her homework, and she had been spending excessive amounts of time in the evenings on tarot card and astrology websites trying to predict her future. She had become increasingly oppositional at home and often refused to get out of bed until late afternoon. Her self-care had deteriorated significantly over the past 8 months, so that she would only shower once a week at the insistence of her parents. She had become increasingly socially odd and exhibited significant blunting of her affect with sudden periods of inappropriate laughter. Her best friend refused to spend time with Jennifer anymore because of her behavioral oddities and obsessive interest in the supernatural realm.

During the initial interview, Jennifer complained of seeing ghosts in her house and believed that evil spirits were haunting her. She stated that the devil tried to kill her when she was asleep and, therefore, she was trying to stay awake at night. Her affect was blunted with virtually no eye contact. She denied any significant symptoms of mania or depression (past or current). Her developmental milestones were slightly delayed, with onset of speech at age 18 months and walking at 15 months. Neuropsychological testing indicated a full-scale IQ within the normal range. There was no documented history of physical, emotional, or sexual abuse. An in-depth physical including laboratory tests, an EEG, and computed tomography (CT) scan of the head all indicated that she had no significant medical problems. Her family psychiatric history consisted of schizoaffective disorder (maternal grandfather), depression (mother), drug-induced psychosis (paternal uncle), and alcoholism and drug abuse (father, paternal grandfather).

Jennifer was diagnosed with schizophrenia and started on an atypical antipsychotic agent. She also met with a psychologist weekly for support, psychoeducation, and social skills training. Within several months, her hallucinations, delusions, and disorganized thinking were improving significantly. She was attending school on a regular basis and trying to make new friends. Although she had improved significantly, she was still complaining of seeing ghosts at times and continued to exhibit blunted affect with moderate psychomotor retardation. Her concentration in school, ability to complete her homework, and grades had improved, but she remained far below her premorbid level of academic functioning. She participated in an individualized education program in school, which helped her considerably. Jennifer's supportive family environment was a huge asset for her and, ultimately, contributed to her successful completion of high school at age 19. After high school, she continued to live at home with her parents who supported her financially and were helping her to find appropriate employment.

BIBLIOGRAPHY

American Psychiatric Association. Practice guideline for the treatment of patients with schizophrenia. *Am J Psychiatry* 1997;154(Suppl. 4):1–63.

Beitchman JH. Childhood schizophrenia: a review and comparison with adult-onset schizophrenia. *Psychiatr Clin North Am* 1985;8:793–814.

Calderoni D, Wudarsky M, Bhangoo R, et al. Differentiating childhood-onset schizophrenia from psychotic mood disorders. *J Am Acad Child Adolesc Psychiatry* 2001;40:1190–1196.

Caplan R, Guthrie D, Gish B, et al. The Kiddie Formal Thought Disorder Scale: clinical assessment, reliability, and validity. *J Am Acad Child Adolesc Psychiatry* 1989;28:408–416.

Davidson M, Reichenberg A, Rabinowitz J, et al. Behavioral and intellectual markers for schizophrenia in apparently healthy male adolescents. *Am J Psychiatry* 1999;156:1328–1335.

Eggers C, Bunk D. The long-term course of childhood-onset schizophrenia: a 42-year follow-up. *Schizophr Bull* 1997;23:105–117.

Findling RL, McNamara NK, Youngstom EA, et al. A prospective, open-label trial of olanzapine in adolescents with schizophrenia. *J Am Acad Child Adolesc Psychiatry* 2003;42:170–175.

Frazier JA, Giedd JN, Hamburger SD, et al. Brain anatomic magnetic resonance imaging in childhood-onset schizophrenia. *Arch Gen Psychiatry* 1996;53:617–624.

Frazier JA, Gordon CT, McKenna K, et al. An open trial of clozapine in 11 adolescents with childhood-onset schizophrenia. *J Am Acad Child Adolesc Psychiatry* 1994;33:658–663.

Gaughran F. Immunity and schizophrenia: autoimmunity, cytokines, and immune responses. *Int Rev Neurobiol* 2002;52:275–302.

Gilmore JH, Sikich L, Lieberman JA. Neuroimaging, neurodevelopment, and schizophrenia. *Child Adolesc Psychiatr Clin N Am* 1997;6:325–341.

Goldstein MJ, Miklowitz DJ. The effectiveness of psychoeducational family therapy in the treatment of schizophrenic disorders. *J Marital Fam Ther* 1995;21:361–376.

Harrison PJ, Owen MJ. Genes for schizophrenia? Recent findings and their pathophysiological implications. *Lancet* 2003;361:417–419.

Huttunen MO, Machon RA, Mednick SA. Prenatal factors in the pathogenesis of schizophrenia. *Br J Psychiatry* 1994;164(Suppl. 23):15–19.

Jacobsen LK, Giedd JN, Castellanos FX, et al. Progressive reduction of temporal lobe structures in childhood-onset schizophrenia. *Am J Psychiatry* 1998;155:678–685.

Kenny JT, Friedman L, Findling RL, et al. Cognitive impairment in adolescents with schizophrenia. *Am J Psychiatry* 1997;154:1316–1325.

Kraepelin E. *Dementia praecox and paraphrenia* (trans by RM Barclay of the 8th German edition of the Textbook of Psychiatry, vol. III, part ii). Edinburgh: E & S Livingstone.

Kumra S, Frazier JA, Jacobsen LK, et al. Childhood-onset schizophrenia: a double-blind clozapine-haloperidol comparison. *Arch Gen Psychiatry* 1996;53:1090–1097.

Kumra S, Jacobsen LK, Lenane M, et al. Childhood-onset schizophrenia: an open-label study of olanzapine in adolescents. *J Am Acad Child Adolesc Psychiatry* 1998;37:377–385.

McClellan J, McCurry C. Early onset psychotic disorders: diagnostic stability and clinical characteristics. *Eur Child Adolesc Psychiatry* 1999;8(Suppl. 2): 1S–7S.

McClellan J, McCurry C, Snell J, et al. Early onset psychotic disorders: course and outcome over a two year period. *J Am Acad Child Adolesc Psychiatry* 1999;38:1380–1389.

McClellan JM, Werry JS, Ham M. A follow-up study of early onset psychosis: comparison between outcome diagnoses of schizophrenia, mood disorders and personality disorders. *J Autism Dev Disord* 1993;23:243–262.

Nicolson R, Lenane M, Singaracharlu S, et al. Premorbid speech and language impairments in childhood-onset schizophrenia: association with risk factors. *Am J Psychiatry* 2002;157:794–800.

Owen MJ, O'Donovan M, Gottesman II. *Psychiatric genetics and genomics*. Oxford: Oxford University Press, 2003:247–266.

Pavuluri MN, Herbener ES, Sweeney JA. Psychotic symptoms in pediatric bipolar disorder. *J Affect Disord* 2004;80:19–28.

Pool D, Bloom W, Mielke DH. et al. A controlled evaluation of loxitane in seventy-five adolescent schizophrenia patients. *Curr Ther Res Clin Exp* 1976;19:99–104.

Rapoport JL, Giedd JN, Blumenthal J, et al. Progressive cortical change during adolescence in childhood-onset schizophrenia: a longitudinal magnetic resonance imaging study. *Arch Gen Psychiatry* 1999;56:649–654.

Realmuto GM, Erikson WD, Yellin AM, et al. Clinical comparison of thiothixene and thioridazine in schizophrenic adolescents. *Am J Psychiatry* 1984;141:440–442.

Rector NA, Beck AT. Cognitive behavioral therapy for schizophrenia: an empirical review. *J Nerv Ment Dis* 2001;189:278–287.

Robinson D, Woerner MG, Alvir JM, et al. Predictors of relapse following response from a first episode of schizophrenia of schizoaffective disorder. *Arch Gen Psychiatry* 1999;56:241–247.

Rund BR, Moe L, Sollien T, et al. The psychosis project: outcome and cost-effectiveness of a psychoeducational treatment programme for schizophrenic adolescents. *Acta Psychiatr Scand* 1994;89: 211–218.

Russell AT, Bott L, Sammons C. The phenomenology of schizophrenia occurring in childhood. *J Am Acad Child Adolesc Psychiatry* 1989;28:399–407.

Shaw JA, Lewis JE, Pascal S, et al. A study of quetiapine: efficacy and tolerability in psychotic adolescents. *J Child Adolesc Psychopharmacol* 2001;11: 415–424.

Sikich L, Hamer RA, Bashford RA, et al. Comparative efficacy and effectiveness of risperidone, olanzapine, and haloperidol in psychotic youth. *Neuropsychopharmacology* 2004;29:133–145.

Spencer EK, Kafantaris V, Padron-Gayol MV, et al. Haloperidol in schizophrenic children: early findings from a study in progress. *Psychopharmacol Bull* 1992;28:183–186.

Thomsen PH. Schizophrenia with childhood and adolescent onset: a nationwide register-based study. *Acta Psychiatr Scand* 1996;94:187–193.

Tsuang MT, Stone WS, Faraone SV. Schizophrenia: a review of genetic studies. *Harv Rev Psychiatry* 1999;7:185–207.

CHAPTER 13

Autism Spectrum Disorders

E. GENE STUBBS
KEITH CHENG

Introduction

In 1943, Kanner described 11 children who manifested "extreme affective aloneness" and gave them the label of "autism," meaning "withdrawn into the self," a term derived from Bleuler's initial use of the word in describing schizophrenia. For a period of time, childhood schizophrenia and autism were thought to comprise the same disorder. Subsequently, these severe disorders have been conceptualized as two different syndromes based upon research showing that schizophrenia and autism do not aggregate in the same families, have different core symptomatology, and have different times of onset. In the *Diagnostic and Statistical Manual of Mental Disorders,* Fourth Edition, Text Revision (DSM-IV-TR), autism is one of five disorders that fall under the broad category of pervasive developmental disorders (PDD). The other disorders include Asperger disorder, pervasive developmental disorder not otherwise specified (PDD, NOS), childhood disintegrative disorder, and Rett disorder. The term "pervasive developmental disorder" is used synonymously with "autism spectrum disorder" (ASD) in different settings. As the term ASD is commonly used in school settings and in the recent pediatric literature, it will be preferentially used in this chapter instead of the DSM-IV-TR diagnostic term PDD.

Clinical Features

The essential feature of ASD is abnormal relatedness and social development. In infancy and toddlerhood, this is manifested by abnormal eye contact, failure to orient to name, failure to use gestures to point or show things, aloofness, lack of sharing or seeking comfort, and lack of interest in peers. Parents usually express concern about social development between the ages of 18 months and 4 years. However, Osterling and Dawson's research shows that videotapes made as early as 1 year of age and viewed later in life show that these abnormalities in communication and relatedness are evident in the first year of life. The other essential feature of ASD is a delay in language acquisition and communication. With the exception of Asperger disorder, ASDs always present with abnormal language development, or in severe cases, the lack of any language. When delays or regression of both language and social relatedness are present, prompt evaluation and early intervention are indicated.

By preschool, the hallmark features of ASD are well developed with a marked lack of interest in others and absent or severely delayed speech and communication. These children also show marked resistance to change, restricted range of interests, and stereotyped repetitive behaviors.

The cognitive function of children with ASDs varies widely. Intelligence quotient (IQ) varies from severe mental retardation to genius. Typically, children with autism show severe cognitive deficits and mental retardation. By contrast, children with Asperger disorder, which is considered a milder form of autism, are often described as having average or above average cognitive abilities with language skills intact.

AUTISM

The cardinal features of autism include marked deficits in relatedness and social abilities and problems with communication. At 6 months, concerns regarding autism are raised by the infant's lack of babbling, not making eye contact with parents during interaction, and not smiling reciprocally when parents smile. Parents should not have to touch the baby to elicit a smile. Autistic infants do not participate in vocal "turn-taking," in which the baby makes a sound, the parent imitates the baby, the baby makes the sound again, and so on. They also do not consistently respond to playing "peekaboo." By 14 months, autistic children show no attempts to speak or to communicate in other ways such as pointing, waving, or grasping, and they show no response when called by name. These young children are already showing their indifference to others. They also show motor abnormalities, especially repetitive body motions such as rocking and hand flapping. They may fixate on a single object and show a strong resistance to changes in routine. They are also oversensitive to certain textures, sometimes termed "tactile defensiveness," as well as to smells or sounds. Some autistic children engage in severe self-injurious behaviors and, in rare instances, may even lose their eyesight due to repeated trauma to their heads and eyes.

ASPERGER DISORDER

The clinical description of Asperger disorder has been evolving over the past several decades. The validity of Asperger disorder as a distinct diagnostic subtype of ASD continues to be controversial in academic and clinical centers. At this time, the DSM-IV-TR and the International Statistical Classification of Diseases and Related Health Problems (ICD-9) have conceptualized Asperger disorder as a subtype of ASD in which individuals do not demonstrate the severe cognitive and language abnormalities of autism but do show deficits in relatedness and social development, albeit milder than that shown in autism. Thus, these children are not able to adequately read social cues and understand the gist of social situations. Individuals with Asperger disorder often appear self-centered and odd as they do not appropriately engage in or enjoy reciprocal social interactions and have difficulty with daily living because of a lack of "common sense." Although they express interest in developing social relationships and like to be with their peers, they are unable to successfully negotiate everyday social interactions due to their self-centeredness, their inability to read social cues, their inflexibility, and their individual idiosyncrasies. They often possess unusual circumscribed interests in such things as cars, government, war, or mechanical objects, sometimes to the point of virtuosic abilities in areas such as math, music, art, or history. In contrast to autism, children with Asperger disorder usually have average intellect and normal language, and thus they often like to talk. Because of this, the diagnosis is frequently not made until the child starts school. Many developmental experts conceptualize Asperger disorder as a mild variant of autism in relatively bright children. Any research regarding the diagnostic criteria for Asperger disorder needs to be carefully considered because, until recently, most studies did not separate subjects with Asperger disorder from those with "high functioning autistics."

RETT DISORDER

In contrast to autism, a period of normal development prior to the onset of ASD symptoms is required to make the diagnosis of Rett disorder. In the original study of 22 cases, it was noted that after about 5 months of normal physical development, these children demonstrated deceleration in head growth between 5 to 48 months of age. One distinctive diagnostic feature of Rett disorder is cessation in the functional use of the child's hands and the onset of stereotypical wringing, washing, twisting, clapping, or rubbing motions. Other cardinal features of Rett disorder include the appearance of uncoordinated gait, severe impairment of language skills, psychomotor retardation, and loss of social connections.

CHILDHOOD DISINTEGRATIVE DISORDER

Childhood disintegrative disorder is the current DSM-IV-TR diagnosis used to describe a group of youths previously described as having "Heller syndrome," "dementia infantalis," and "disintegrative psychosis of childhood." Diagnostic criteria include apparent normal language and social development for the first 2 to 4 years of life; then, there is clinically significant loss of previously acquired abilities such as expressive or receptive language or other communication skills, social skills or adaptive behavior, bowel or bladder control, play, and motor skills. Other problems include the development of restrictive, repetitive, or stereotypic patterns of behavior.

PERVASIVE DEVELOPMENTAL DISORDER, NOT OTHERWISE SPECIFIED

The DSM-IV-TR diagnosis of PDD, NOS is used for a heterogeneous group of children who show ASD symptoms but who do not meet the criteria for the other ASDs, schizophrenia, or schizotypal and avoidant personality disorders. In fact, there are no diagnostic criteria for PDD, NOS. The diagnosis is often used for children with atypical signs of autism, for example, children who have the onset of autistic features after 3 years of age or children who initially met criteria for autism in their early years but then improved sufficiently so that they no longer meet the criteria for autism, although some core features persist. More commonly, PDD, NOS is diagnosed for children with social awkwardness, odd behaviors,

TABLE 13.1. CHARACTERISTICS OF THE AUTISM SPECTRUM DISORDERS

Disorder	Clinical Findings
Autism	• Clinical picture varies depending on the child's age and severity of symptoms • All children with autism manifest some degree of severe impairment of reciprocal social interaction and communication • Restricted, repetitive, and stereotypic patterns of behavior, interests, and activities commonly present
Asperger syndrome	• Impaired social relatedness always present, but milder than in autism • Cognitive skills are relatively intact • Language is intact but may be "stilted" or like a "little professor" • Perseveration preoccupations, obsessions, or compulsions common • Motor clumsiness, sensory regular deficits (hypo- or hyperresponsiveness) common
Childhood disintegrative disorder	• Normal development for at least 2 yr after birth • Clinically significant loss of skills before age 10 in at least two areas of development including language, social or adaptive skills, bowel or bladder control, play, or motor skills • Prognosis is considered to be worse than autism
Rett disorder	• Predominantly found in girls • Appears to have normal prenatal and perinatal development • Normal head circumference at birth followed by deceleration of head growth between ages of 5 and 48 mo • Loss of previously acquired purposeful hand skills and development of nonpurposeful, repetitive movements
Pervasive developmental disorder, not otherwise specified	• This category is frequently described as "atypical autism" • Criteria include the presence of some but not sufficient symptoms, or insufficiently severe symptoms, to meet criteria for autism or Asperger disorder • Must have some difficulty with relatedness and socialization

and emotional immaturity. Children with severe neurologic disorders that affect social and communication skills are also often diagnosed with PDD, NOS. Core features of the five ASDs are summarized in Table 13.1.

Epidemiology

Prevalence estimates vary, with the highest estimate for all ASDs being 1%. Only about 25% of this group would fall under the category of "classic" autism. According to Fombonne, ASD is no longer considered a rare disorder. The number of children diagnosed with ASD has increased rapidly in the last 10 years. The reason for the rapid increase is hotly debated. Some investigators note that there has been a broadening of the diagnosis of ASD to include diagnoses such as PDD, NOS, and Asperger disorder, while others suggest that clinicians are more aware of ASD, thus increasing their rate of detection. Others posit environmental contributions, such as mercury in vaccines. When girls have ASD, it appears to manifest in a more severe form. ASDs present in equal prevalence across race, ethnicity, and nationality.

AUTISM

The DSM-IV-TR states that the prevalence of autistic disorder in the United States is 2 to 5 per 10,000. A review of the literature from the United States as well as Asian and European countries reveals a prevalence range of 0.15 to 34 cases per 10,000. This very broad range of prevalence is probably secondary to the lack of consensus regarding the definition of autism. Earlier studies reported a lower prevalence than more recent research, probably reflecting both changes in definitions and improved diagnostic awareness. The gender ratio is 3 to 4 boys per girl, a consistent finding across national boundaries. In addition, autistic girls tend to have a greater symptom severity than autistic boys.

ASPERGER DISORDER

Data on the prevalence of Asperger disorder is somewhat limited in both quality and quantity in part due to the variability of definitions across studies. In a study conducted in the United Kingdom by Wing and Gould, the prevalence was reported to be 0.6 per 10,000 for children with a combination of Asperger disorder and mental retardation. In two Swedish studies, the prevalence ranged from 10 to 26 per 10,000 in one study and 36 per 10,000 in another study. Boys outnumber girls in all prevalence studies of Asperger disorder with 4 to 10 boys per girl.

RETT DISORDER

Rett disorder is a rare disorder when compared to autism and Asperger disorder. Epidemiologic studies from both Europe and the United States have estimated a prevalence from 0.44 to 2.1 cases per 10,000. Initially, Rett disorder was thought to only occur in girls. However, there are now several case reports with boys. This disorder is now known to exist in all races. Worldwide, over 2,000 cases have been recognized.

CHILDHOOD DISINTEGRATIVE DISORDER

Although the prevalence of childhood disintegrative disorder has not been well established, it appears to be even more rare than Rett disorder. In 1989 Burd et al. reported a prevalence of 0.11 per 10,000 population. Volkmar and Cohen found 10 cases of childhood disintegrative disorder in a group of 160 children initially diagnosed with ASD. They concluded that childhood disintegrative disorder may be about one-tenth as common as autism. Boys are afflicted about 8 times more frequently than the girls.

PERVASIVE DEVELOPMENTAL DISORDER, NOT OTHERWISE SPECIFIED

Similar to autism and Asperger disorder, the imprecise definition of PDD, NOS has led to broad prevalence estimates ranging from 2 to 16 cases per 10,000 population. Most studies indicate that boys outnumber girls.

Clinical Course

All ASDs follow a chronic course as the symptoms generally do not fully remit with time. The life expectancy for most children with ASDs is normal with the exception of Rett disorder, for which life expectancy is shortened. In general, children with no to mild mental retardation have a better prognosis. With intensive intervention, a minority of children with ASD improve sufficiently to be declassified, that is, they no longer meet criteria for ASD as they mature. However, all investigators agree that the majority will continue to manifest symptoms of ASD into adulthood, though often to a lesser degree. Without any intervention, these children may die early because of the lack of supportive and medical interventions. Children with Rett disorder and childhood disintegrative disorder are at particular risk. However, with the exception of these two disorders, most children with ASDs do improve with intervention. Even in Rett disorder, intervention may produce moderate improvement.

AUTISM

Autism shows two modes of onset, or perhaps more precisely, shows two modes for age of recognition. The first age of recognition occurs in early infancy, and the second occurs after a period of "normal" development, followed at 1 to 3 years of age by loss or plateau of the development of language and relatedness. More severely affected individuals also have a higher occurrence of seizures, up to 25% by adolescence. This also leads to higher mortality and morbidity. While the majority of autistic children continue to experience social and communication difficulties well into adulthood, some do improve with communication skills progressing more than social abilities. Early studies showed that between 39% and 74% of autistic individuals were eventually placed in institutions. However, more recently, Schopler reported that only 8% were institutionalized, probably due to more effective interventions. Up to 11% of autistic individuals obtain employment in menial jobs, and an additional 16% may be employed in sheltered workshops. Higher IQ, greater amounts of time spent in school, and development of some language are associated with better prognosis.

ASPERGER DISORDER

Asperger disorder tends to be diagnosed at an older age, usually after age 3. Children with Asperger disorder seem to improve as they mature. Compared to autism cohorts, children with Asperger disorder have better outcomes. They reach higher educational levels, are employed more often, and are more likely to live unassisted, to marry, and to have children. However, the abnormalities in relatedness exhibited during childhood persist in some form during adolescence and adulthood. A minority will enter higher education, obtain consistent employment, and live independently. Most live with their parents, and a few are institutionalized. About one third of children diagnosed with Asperger disorder later develop a comorbid psychiatric disorder.

RETT DISORDER

The child with Rett disorder appears fine at birth and develops normally for several months, but by 6 months to 2 years old, the child begins to show less social interaction, uses speech less appropriately, and even loses motor skills. The regression may plateau or may continue until the child dies. A mortality rate of 1.2% per annum has been reported. Most early deaths occur in individuals who become physically debilitated by their disorder.

CHILDHOOD DISINTEGRATIVE DISORDER

Childhood disintegrative disorder also has a period of normal development followed by a loss of skills. The regression occurs between 2 and 10 years of age in the areas of cognition, social skills, play, self-help, language, and motor skills. What is striking about the regression of these skills is that they seem to uniformly occur over a 6- to 9-month period, followed by a plateau, and then some limited improvement. Despite the limited improvement period, the prognosis for childhood disintegrative disorder is very poor. These individuals require assistance with activities of daily living throughout their lives as they are moderately to severely mentally retarded.

PERVASIVE DEVELOPMENTAL DISORDER, NOT OTHERWISE SPECIFIED

At present, there are only limited and equivocal data regarding the course of PDD, NOS. Because of the heterogeneous nature of this disorder, follow-up studies indicate that a child initially diagnosed with PDD, NOS will eventually be diagnosed with some other comorbid disorder during adolescence or adulthood.

Etiology and Pathogenesis

The cause of autism and all ASDs is unknown. Autism is the best studied of the ASDs. The consensus is that autism originates in a genetic diathesis, but many investigators posit an environmental component or trigger. Folstein and Rutter note that estimates of heritability depend upon whether narrow or extended criteria are used. Extended criteria include subtle signs of the ASD phenotype, such as difficulty with language pragmatics and being socially aloof. Within this variability, identical twins have a 60% to 90% concordance for autism while fraternal twins have a 3% to 10% concordance. A polygenetic model of inheritance is suggested with 3 to 20 gene loci contributing. There are several chromosomes of interest including 1p, 2, 7q, 15, and 16p and 17p, but no gene has been isolated. The genes responsible for Rett disorder have been identified, and, thus, this disorder has been categorically separated from autism. Causative genes for fragile X syndrome, which has overlapping symptoms with autism, have also been identified leading to its categorization as a separate disorder.

The environment may play an etiologic role in ASDs. For example, intrauterine infections of rubella, cytomegalovirus, or herpes simplex and exposure to drugs such as thalidomide have been associated with autism. There is controversy as to whether mercury (thimerosal) in vaccines and/or fish may contribute to autism. Even more controversial is a potential role of the trivalent MMR (measles, mumps, and rubella) vaccine. Finally, faulty immune regulation has been theorized. There is no scientific evidence to support these interesting theories.

Neuroimaging has shown some important abnormalities in autism. The most consistent findings involve the cerebellum where cells are reduced in size and number along with stunted dendritic arbors. Bauman and Kemper have demonstrated that the limbic system, especially the amygdala and the hippocampus, show increased cell packing density. Using positron emission tomography (PET) scans, Chugani et al. have shown decreased serotonin synthesis in the thalamus and frontal lobes, but an increase in the dentate nucleus. A distinct neural pathway connects these three areas. Studies of the fusiform gyrus, the section of the brain that recognizes human faces, have shown lack of appropriate activation in autistic individuals; that is, the autistic child shows the same level of activation in the fusiform gyrus whether looking at a human face or at an object. However, other studies have found that although the fusiform gyrus does not activate when looking at the face of a stranger, the area has a burst of activation when the child is looking at a familiar face, like a parent.

There are quantitative abnormalities in the glutamate, serotonin, dopamine, opioid, and γ-aminobutyric acid (GABA) neurotransmitter systems. Additionally, children with autism and mental retardation, in contrast to typically developed children and children with cerebral palsy, have shown elevated neuropeptides and neurotrophins at birth. Courchesne et al. report that children with autism have relatively smaller brain sizes at birth, and then within several months have larger brains than typically developing children. This growth in brain size apparently precedes the development of symptoms of autism. The relationship between these abnormal growth factors and the abnormal growth of the brain needs further clarification.

Assessment

There are multiple components to an assessment for ASD including careful clinical history focused on early social and language development; mental status examination of the child with his or her family members as well as in the home or school environment if possible; pediatric assessment to rule out treatable medical illnesses that are suggestive of ASDs; psychological testing to determine baseline cognitive level and possible comorbid mental retardation; assessment of adaptive functioning to determine deficits and areas of need; and academic assessment to develop an individualized education plan (IEP). Speech and language therapy, occupational therapy, and physical therapy assessments should also be completed as indicated for the individual child. The essentials for ASD evaluation are summarized in Table 13.2.

Rating scales are also frequently incorporated into a comprehensive evaluation of ASDs. Rating scales may be helpful to screen for the presence of ASDs but are particularly valuable to monitor treatment progress. The Checklist for Autism in Toddlers (CHAT), developed by Baron-Cohen et al., offers the advantage of screening by primary care providers of children down to 18 months of age. Other frequently used scales for children with ASD and mental retardation that have been reviewed by Sevin et al. and South et al. include the Autism Behavior Checklist (ABC), the Gilliam Autism Rating Scale (GARS), and Schopler Childhood Autism Rating Scale (CARS). Additionally, two structured instruments comprise the gold standards for diagnosing autism: the Autism Diagnostic Observation Scale (ADOS) and the clinician-administered Autism Diagnostic Interview (ADI) that has been revised by Lord et al. [Autism Diagnostic Interview-Revised (ADI-R)]. Both of these instruments have been reviewed by DeBildt et al., who note their established reliability and validity. These instruments require extensive training until the examiner meets interrater-reliability criteria. Additionally, administration of the ADI-R is both labor intensive and time consuming, requiring 2 to 4 hours. As an alternative, many clinicians use the DSM-IV criteria and ask specific questions to elicit whether criteria symptoms are present. The questions in Table 13.3 are used by the author along with clinical observations of the child to confirm or refute a diagnosis of autism. Questions can be asked of the parents or other primary caretaker. Additional questions may need to be asked to determine whether the child meets criteria. Answers may be scored with (a) definitely positive, (b) plus/minus for meeting criteria, (c) questionable for meeting criteria, or (d) definitely negative for meeting criteria.

TABLE 13.2. EVALUATION ESSENTIALS FOR AUTISM SPECTRUM DISORDERS

- Clinicians should have a high index of suspicion for ASD in infant/toddlers with abnormal relatedness, especially with primary caregiver; delayed language and communicative development; unusual sensitivities to sounds, bright lights, or smells; and/or odd repetition behaviors.
- All children suspected of having an ASD should receive a medical and neurologic assessment to identify medical illnesses that mimic ASDs and to identify medical illnesses that are comorbid with ASDs.
- Referral to audiologist to evaluate hearing. Some children will need evoked response brainstem audiometry to accurately assess their hearing.
- A comprehensive evaluation should include developmental evaluation, an adaptive functional assessment, speech/language assessment, and cognitive assessment.

ASD, autism spectrum disorders.

TABLE 13.3. *DIAGNOSTIC AND STATISTICAL MANUAL OF MENTAL DISORDERS,* **FOURTH EDITION, TEXT REVISION-BASED QUESTIONS TO ESTABLISH A DIAGNOSIS OF AUTISM**

Symptom Category	Diagnostic Questions
Social interaction	• How would the parents describe their child's use of nonverbal behaviors such as eye contact, facial expression, body postures, and gestures to communicate? • How would the parents describe their child's ability to relate to other children? Does he/she have friends? Does he/she show interest in other children? In all of these questions, response should be assessed in relation to the age of the child. • Does the child share enjoyment, interests, or achievements with parents or other people, such as showing things, bringing things to them, or pointing to objects of interest? • Does the child show social-emotional give and take? For example, does the child show or receive affection? If someone cries or if a child is hurt, does the child show concern or provide comfort?
Communication	• How does the child communicate? Was there a delay in talking? When did the child have first words? When did the child use two word combinations? Did the child use alternative forms of communication if he/she could not talk? Did the child lose previously established speech and language skills? • Does the child initiate and carry on a conversation? Is it limited to his/her interests, or is there reciprocity? • Does the child have unusual language such as echolalia, pronoun reversal repetitive speech, or a stilted quality to his speech? • How does the child play? Does he/she have pretend, make-believe play appropriate to his/her developmental level?
Other behaviors	• Does the child have preoccupations with objects, restricted patterns of interest that are abnormal in intensity, or focus stereotypes? • Does the child have difficulty with change of routine, perseveration, rituals, or obsessive–compulsive traits? • Does the child have any unusual movements such as hand flapping, spinning, or toe walking? • Does the child have preoccupations with parts of objects rather than playing with the whole object? • Does the child play with toys in a nonsymbolic manner atypical for age?

For a diagnosis of autism, six criterion symptoms must be positive, with at least two from the first category (social interactions) and at least one item from each of the following two categories (communication and restricted or stereotypical behaviors). The onset must be before 3 years of age. For a diagnosis of Asperger disorder, at least four criteria must be positive with language or communication relatively intact (category two) and cognitive abilities in the normal range. For a diagnosis of PDD, NOS, the criteria for autism and Asperger disorder are not met, but some of the criterion items are present, especially social difficulties. PDD, NOS is a subthreshold diagnosis (meets some, but not all of the criteria for autism). This is the most difficult diagnosis to make because the criteria are not delineated. By contrast, lack of established criteria can lead to inappropriate use of the diagnosis.

The Vineland Adaptive Behavior Scales (VABS) created by Sparrow et al. is the standard assessment of adaptive functioning and assesses the child's abilities in four domains of daily living: personal skills such as hygiene, social skills, communication skills, and motor skills. The author's recommendations for the non–autism-specialists is to have a high index of suspicion relying on the key symptoms. If there are any doubts, refer to an experienced interdisciplinary team or to a specialist in autism for a confirmation of diagnosis and treatment recommendations.

Differential Diagnosis and Comorbidity

The differential diagnosis for ASD is broad. Autism is differentiated from the other ASDs by its more severe deficits in social relatedness and language skills. Often conceptualized as a milder form autism, Asperger disorder can be distinguished from autism by relatively intact language skills that approximate that of children without developmental delays. Asperger disorder is rarely diagnosed before age 3, while the signs of autism are usually present by 1 year of age. Autism and Asperger disorder can be differentiated from childhood disintegrative disorder because of the latter's presence of normal development during the first several years of life followed by regression. Rett disorder can be differentiated from childhood disintegrative disorder by the characteristic deceleration of head growth and pathognomonic hand rubbing stereotypes. The core features of the ASDs are summarized in Table 13.1.

More common psychiatric disorders that may be misdiagnosed as an ASD are compared in Table 13.4 and include mental retardation, particularly in combination with hearing or vision loss; severe learning disabilities; selective mutism; social anxiety disorder; obsessive–compulsive disorder (OCD); attention deficit hyperactivity disorder (ADHD); schizoid and avoidant personality disorders; and childhood schizophrenia.

Other developmental disorders commonly occur with ASDs. Fombonne has noted that the majority of children with autism are also mentally retarded, with 50% of children with classic autism having severe to profound mental retardation, 30% mild to moderate mental retardation, and 20% normal range IQ. Most nonretarded autistic children have obsessive, ritualistic, or perseverative behaviors, some of sufficient severity to warrant a diagnosis of OCD. Up to 25% of children with the chromosomal disorders fragile X syndrome

TABLE 13.4. DIFFERENTIAL DIAGNOSIS FOR AUTISM SPECTRUM DISORDERS

Non-ASD Disorders	Comments
Selective mutism	• Child speaks in familiar situations with intimate family members, but does not speak or whispers to parent in unfamiliar social situations such as school • The disturbance interferes with educational achievement and social communication • May be coupled with a language disorder • History supports normal relatedness and social interactions with familiar individuals, and with family at home
Verbal apraxia/dyspraxia	• Child communicates by gesture, pantomime, and intermittent and variable speech and relates much better than children with ASDs, i.e., wants to communicate even if difficult to do so • Often coupled with an anxiety disorder, further impeding communication
Developmental language disorders	• Even though these children have difficulty with language, they relate much better than children with ASD • Difficult if coupled with an anxiety disorder; developmental language disorders can be hard to distinguish from ASD
Attention deficit hyperactivity disorder	• Although these children have social problems, they are usually able to make friends, but rapidly lose them because of their aggressive and dominating behavior not due to core deficits in relatedness • Frequently have learning disabilities, but have much better language skills than children with ASDs • Coupled with learning disorders, ADHD can be difficult to distinguish from Asperger syndrome
Mental retardation	• Severe mental retardation in combination with hearing loss can be difficult to distinguish from ASD

ASD, autism spectrum disorders; ADHD, attention deficit hyperactivity disorder.

TABLE 13.5. COMMON COMORBIDITIES WITH AUTISM SPECTRUM DISORDERS

Psychiatric Disorders	Genetic Syndromes	Infectious/Metabolic/Medical
ADHD	Fragile X syndrome	Rubella embryopathy
Tourette disorder		Landau–Kleffner syndrome
Obsessive–compulsive disorder	Moebius syndrome	Intrauterine cytomegalo-viral infection
Anxiety disorders	Goldenhar syndrome	Herpes encephalopathy
Selective mutism	Hypomelanosis of Ito	Lactic acidosis
Psychosis NOS	Neurofibromatosis	Hypothyroidism
Schizophrenia	Tuberous sclerosis	Phenylketonuria
Schizotypal personality	Duchennes muscular dystrophy	Seizure disorders

ADHD, attention deficit hyperactivity disorder; NOS, not otherwise specified.

and tuberous sclerosis are found to have autistic-like features. A Wood's lamp examination should be used to examine for hypopigmented "ash leaf" macules characteristic of tuberous sclerosis. Later, facial angiofibromas become evident. In fragile X syndrome, dysmorphic features include long faces, large ears, and large testes (postpubertal). In Angelman syndrome, an ataxic gait and a broad persistent smile are found. Severe lead poisoning from pica can lead to symptoms similar to ASDs in very young children. From a technical standpoint, ADHD is never comorbid with ASD, as the DSM-IV-TR states that the diagnosis of ADHD should not be made in the presence of a PDD. However, in clinical practice ADHD is often diagnosed and treated as a comorbidity of ASDs. Psychosocial deprivation, failure to thrive, and reactive attachment disorders (RAD) often present with signs and symptoms that are highly suggestive of ASDs. A history of abuse and neglect distinguishes these diagnoses from the ASDs. Of course, they could occur together comorbidly. For example, an ASD child might be very difficult for young parents who might then neglect or abuse the child, leading to comorbid diagnoses of RAD or even posttraumatic stress disorder.

Psychiatric, neurologic, and medical disorders are also frequently comorbid with ASDs, as shown in Table 13.5. In particular, seizure disorders have been noted in 4% to 42% of autistic individuals. Seizures are more likely to occur early in childhood rather than later in adolescence. Girls are at greater risk. The neurologic disorder Landau-Kleffner syndrome is associated with PDD, NOS. Children with this disorder develop language deficits at an older age than in autism. Recently, there has been endoscopic evidence of gastrointestinal pathology in autistic children including esophagitis, gastritis, duodenitis, and colitis. The significance of these findings remains unclear.

Treatment

As noted in Table 13.6, treatment is multidisciplinary and multimodal. The primary goals of treatment are to promote communication development, enhance and support social and academic skills, decrease behavioral difficulties, and decrease stress in the family. Indicated interventions should include parental education, family support, parent training in behavior management, special education planning, and referral for rehabilitative therapies and disability services as indicated.

There is no specific pharmacologic treatment for ASD. The use of psychotropic medications is aimed primarily at treating comorbid psychiatric disorders. Pharmacotherapy may also be helpful in augmenting psychosocial interventions by reducing anxiety and thereby improving flexibility and interpersonal relations and by reducing stereotypes and other nonsensical behaviors.

TABLE 13.6. TREATMENT ESSENTIALS FOR AUTISM SPECTRUM DISORDERS

- Treatment should start as soon as the diagnosis is established. Early interventions improve prognosis. Most communities have early intervention programs for children under 3 yr.
- Because of multiple special needs of ASD youths, a team of clinicians and educators is needed to provide optimal care. It is important for all the team members to have a shared vision of their roles, the problems being addressed, and the interventions being utilized to ensure coordination of services and prevent clinical conflicts.
- Treatment should be multidimensional as well as multimodal. Because ASD affects many domains of development, a comprehensive treatment plan must address the multiple areas of developmental delay. Treatment takes place in the home, at school, and in the community by collaboration of educational, medical, and psychiatric professionals.
- To maximize the effectiveness of psychosocial interventions, any comorbid medical or psychiatric conditions should be identified and treated.
- Treatment for ASD will be ineffective if parental needs are not met. Clinicians should emphasize the need for support services, such as respite care and community resources.

ASD, autism spectrum disorders.

EDUCATIONAL INTERVENTIONS

The primary intervention for ASDs is education. Public Law 94-142, the Individuals With Disabilities Educational Act (IDEA), stipulates that every child, regardless of his or her disability, has a right to a free and appropriate public education in the least restrictive environment. A primary care physician or psychiatric clinician can make the referral to the school system or assist the parent in the process of obtaining needed educational services. The majority of an ASD child's treatment occurs in the school setting. According to Osterling and Dawson, elements considered important to the success of a child include: (a) teaching the child to pay attention to other people, imitate others, use preverbal and verbal communication, play, and socially interact; (b) a teaching environment that is highly supportive of the child's learning needs and involves systematic teaching of skills in a one-to-one setting with trained personnel; (c) a program that is predictable and routine; (d) a functional approach to problem behaviors; (e) a thoughtful strategy for transition from the specialized preschool classroom to the kindergarten class; and (f) family involvement.

Several educational approaches to improve the child's behavioral compliance and learning have been proposed and are summarized in Table 13.7. Some parents prefer one over the other, and not all have empiric support. Applied Behavioral Analysis (ABA), the best example of which is Discrete Trial Analysis, focuses upon the acquisition of compliance behavior, imitation activities, language acquisition, and integration with peers using repeated discrete behavioral trials supported by positive reinforcement to accomplish goals. Pivotal response training (PRT) focuses on motivation. Incidental learning focuses on teaching around "natural incidents" that occur. Structured teaching focuses on visual strengths using pictures, color-coding, physical arrangements, sequences, and templates. "Floortime," or Developmental Individual Difference Relationship Model (DIR), developed by Stanley Greenspan, is a relational approach involving sensory modulation and processing, motor planning, effective integration, and the child's interaction with the family. The parents are taught to "open and close" circles of communication with the child, that is, initiate communication with the child and encourage the child to communicate back to the adult, thus, making a "circle" of communication. DIR is implemented by the parents following the child's lead in play. Perhaps the most well known curriculum for ASD children is the Treatment and Education of Autistic and Communication Handicapped Children (TEACCH) program developed by Eric Schopler in North Carolina during the 1970s. TEACCH is based on the intervention philosophy that autism is not caused by pathologic parents, but that collaboration between mental health, educational professionals, and parents of ASD children forms the cornerstone of effective education and treatment planning.

TABLE 13.7. EDUCATIONAL APPROACHES TO AUTISM

Educational Approach	Comments	Reference
Applied behavioral analysis (ABA)	Recognized by the surgeon general of the United States as the preferred method of treating children with autism. Based on learning theory, ABA is an overarching behavioral plan that teaches behaviors that are to be generalized to all domains of a child's environment.	Rosenwasser and Axelrod; Lovaas
Discrete trial training (DTT)	Not synonymous with ABA, DTT is also based upon principles of learning theory but focuses on teaching skills in specific situations. These skills may then be used in an overall ABA plan.	Grindle and Remington
Pivotal response training (PRT)	Addresses the subject of pivotal behaviors such as motivation and responsiveness to multiple cues, which produce widespread positive effect on many other behaviors.	Koegel
Incidental learning	Incidental learning is unintentional or unplanned learning that results from nontraditional school activities. It occurs many ways: through observation, repetition, social interaction, and problem solving.	McGee
Structured teaching	Structured teaching is a system for organizing environments, developing appropriate activities, and helping people with autism understand what is expected of them. Structured teaching describes the conditions under which a person should be taught rather than "where" or "what" (i.e., "learning how to learn").	Schopler
Developmental individual difference relationship model (DIR)	Also known as "Floortime," this approach to teaching youths with ASD is based on a relationship method that emphasizes being observant of the feeling states and following the child's lead.	Greenspan
Treatment and education of autistic and communication-handicapped children	Based on the intervention philosophy that autism is not caused by pathologic parents but that collaboration between mental health and educational professionals with parents of ASD children forms the cornerstone for developing any effective education and treatment plan.	Schopler
Social stories	This technique is aimed at helping higher functioning children with ASD understand and behave in basic social situations through the use of stories.	Carol Gray

ASD, autism spectrum disorders.

The use of "Social Stories" as developed by Carol Gray can be very helpful in enabling families to deal with transitions, to prepare for important activities such as dentist and doctor appointments, and for handling problematic behavior including change of routine.

PSYCHOSOCIAL INTERVENTIONS

In addition to education, several psychosocial interventions can augment the child's development. The speech therapist assists with language and overall communication development including the use of alternative functional communication such as gestures, sign language, or the use of augmentative devices when the child has not developed any speech. The occupational therapist can help the child to deal with adverse sensory experiences such as hypersensitivity to touch, smell, sound, taste, and visual stimuli. The occupational therapist also assists the parents in developing strategies for improving motor planning, such as horseback riding lessons for children with disabilities. Psychotherapists can help higher functioning ASD youths who are capable of improving their social relatedness or are susceptible to depression and anxiety. Social skills groups facilitate the youth's interpersonal and social skills. Support groups and resources can be helpful to families in finding services, advocating, and assisting in dealing with difficult behaviors.

Developmental disability case managers usually located at the county level are crucial resources for families. They can assist with the coordination of care, the development of individualized services, out of home placements, or respite care later in life. They may also assist in finding residential services, which include independent living arrangements, supervised apartments, and group homes. Vocational rehabilitation counselors are helpful in finding work placements. Job coaches are used to identify available jobs, provide training for work placements, track progress, and provide crisis management to maintain employment placements. Some agencies broker services for individuals and families who want to design their own services and find their own providers of service. These psychosocial interventions are summarized in Table 13.8.

PSYCHOPHARMACOLOGY

While there is no specific pharmacologic treatment that substantially changes the course of the ASDs, psychotropic medications can ameliorate some core symptoms, prevent harmful behaviors such as aggression and self-injurious behavior, facilitate access to intervention programs, maximize beneficial effects of nonmedical interventions, and improve the quality of life for the ASD child and family. They are also useful for treating comorbid conditions that impact these children's lives. Children with ASD are at increased risk for developing other comorbid disorders such as depression, anxiety, hyperactivity, obsessions, and compulsions. The National Institutes of Health (NIH) funded "Centers of Excellence" are investigating several medications aimed at symptomatic treatment. These medications are used much as they would be for nonautistic children with comparable symptoms. Usual pharmacologic options, their target symptoms, and related issues are summarized in Table 13.9. It should be noted that there is no solid evidence base supporting their effectiveness. Rather, their inclusion here derives from their use in customary clinical practice. Specifics regarding the use of these medications with youths are presented in the Chapter 22.

The selective serotonin reuptake inhibitors (SSRIs) are the most popular psychotropic agents used in this population. The SSRIs are thought to decrease ASD youths' anxiety, thereby improving their flexibility and tolerability of new experiences. They may also reduce compulsive, repetitive, or perseverative behaviors. Antipsychotics, such as the traditional

TABLE 13.8. PSYCHOSOCIAL INTERVENTIONS FOR AUTISM SPECTRUM DISORDERS

Interventions	Comments
Family support	• Support to families should begin as soon as the child is diagnosed with ASD • Diagnosing clinician provides time for counseling the parents or caretakers • Support groups provide parents with resources, advocacy, and practical strategies
Parental psychoeducation	• Providing up-to-date information about ASD is essential • Need to teach parents of ASD children the acceptance of developmental deficits, the limitations of medical treatments, and the need for behavioral interventions • Treatment is individualized • Parent and professional/educational collaboration is critical
Parent training in behavioral management	• Parents should be trained to employ behavior management protocols based on a comprehensive individualized behavioral analysis of the child in his school and home environments • Use of positive reinforcements should be the primary intervention used in the behavior protocol • Extinction or punishment should be limited to very specific situations and used only in consultation with a behavioral specialist or other treating clinician
Public education systems	• The public education system is usually the primary source of interventions for the ASD child between 3 and 21 yr of age • Medical and psychiatric collaboration with the school systems to provide adequate comprehensive care individualized to the child
Referral to rehabilitative therapies (speech, occupational, and physical therapies)	• Significant speech and language delays need referral to speech and language therapist • Occupational therapy referral for sensory processing and fine motor deficits • Physical therapy referral for gross motor coordination deficits • These therapies should be integrated into the overall treatment plan with parent approval
Referral for disability services and support	• Many children with ASD meet state eligibility requirements for monetary and specific program supports • Most states have specific agencies that help coordinate services for children with developmental disabilities • Respite, educational, and community programs can be accessed from the state if a child meets criteria for disability services

ASD, autism spectrum disorders.

haloperidol and thioridazine, were the mainstays of treatment for aggression and self-injurious behaviors for many years. More recently, they have been replaced with the atypical antipsychotics, such as aripiprazole, olanzapine, quetiapine, risperidone, and ziprasidone. In addition to reduction of harmful behaviors, the antipsychotics may improve relatedness somewhat, thereby facilitating social interventions. They may also help youths with serious sleep disturbances to stay in bed throughout the night when the rest of the family is sleeping. Stimulants are also very frequently used to decrease hyperactivity and impulsive behavior. However, stimulants are not as successful in treating the increased motor activity and poor concentration of youths with ASD as they are in treating youths with ADHD. In fact, stimulants may increase aggressiveness, insomnia, irritability, and stereotypic behaviors. They should not be considered first-line treatment for disruptive symptoms exhibited by ASD youths. The α-2a agonists, clonidine and guanfacine, are used to treat the physiologic arousal that can lead to impulsive aggression. However, the side effects of sedation and decreased physical activity in the ASD population may decrease their usefulness for long-term use. Anticonvulsants are often used with ASD patients who demonstrate abnormal electroencephalogram (EEG) findings without overt seizure activity. Recent studies of small sample sizes have reported positive and sustained behavioral improvement with anticonvulsants in decreasing affective lability, impulsivity, and aggression. Naltrexone and amantadine

TABLE 13.9. PHARMACOLOGIC INTERVENTIONS

Medication	Target Symptoms	Comments
Selective serotonin reuptake inhibitors: fluoxetine, sertraline, citalopram, escitalopram, fluvoxamine	Anxiety, perseveration, compulsions, depression, and social isolation	• SSRIs are becoming more popular because of their effectiveness and low adverse effects • Some studies have demonstrated more global effects on behavior, language, cognition, and social relatedness; positive response is often correlated with a family history of an affective disorder • Adverse reactions in ASD populations are uncommon but may include restlessness, hyperactivity, agitation, insomnia, and mania
Antipsychotics: risperidone, olanzapine, quetiapine, aripiprazole, ziprasidone, haloperidol, thioridazine	Aggression, agitation, irritability, hyperactivity, and self-injurious behavior	• Thioridazine and haloperidol have been the most extensively investigated for use in ASD • Atypicals antipsychotics are now the primary drug used for treating behavioral disturbance in ASD • Atypical antipsychotic complications of severe weight gain, hypertension, and hyperlipidemia may cause clinicians to reconsider employing atypicals in the treatment of ASD aggression and SIB
Stimulants: methylphenidate, dextroamphetamines, amphetamine salts	Hyperactivity	• Stimulant effectiveness in decreasing hyperactivity and increasing attention span is variable in ASD youth population • Stimulants may increase agitation and stereotypic behaviors including SIB • More likely to be effective in Asperger disorder than other ASDs
α-2a agonists: guanfacine, clonidine	Hyperactivity, aggression, and sleep dysregulation	• Sometimes effective in treating hyperactivity • Clonidine used more often when sleep dysregulation is prominent
Anticonvulsants and lithium	Aggression and SIB	• Also may be useful for cyclical behavior patterns • Need for blood monitoring for lithium, carbamazepine, and valproate limits their use in ASD children without epilepsy
Naltrexone	SIB	• Naltrexone has been shown to be effective to decrease SIB • Overall usefulness has never been robust • Hepatic monitoring
Amantadine	Hyperactivity, irritability, and aggression	• Recent studies show amantadine effective in treating behavioral disturbances in ASD children
Melatonin	Sleep dysregulation	• May be effective in treating insomnia in ASD youths

(Continued)

TABLE 13.9.   CONTINUED

Medication	Target Symptoms	Comments
Fenfluramine	Once thought to be effective for treating core symptoms of autism	• A popular treatment in the past • Subsequent controlled studies showed no efficacy • Currently considered contraindicated according to the AACAP treatment guidelines for ASD

SSRIs, selective serotonin reuptake inhibitors; ASD, autism spectrum disorders; SIB, self-injurious behavior; AACAP, American Academy of Child and Adolescent Psychiatry.

may decrease some of the disruptive behaviors, particularly when the aforementioned medications fail. Several pharmacologic agents that initially seemed effective in decreasing core autistic features but were later shown to be ineffective include secretin, dimethylglycine, and fenfluramine. These pharmacologic interventions are summarized in Table 13.9.

COMPLEMENTARY AND ALTERNATIVE TREATMENTS

Families often feel desperate to help their children and frequently try many alternative interventions, some of which are summarized in Table 13.10.

TABLE 13.10.   ALTERNATIVE THERAPIES

Alternative Treatment	Comments
Nutritional supplements	• High-dose pyridoxine, magnesium supplementation, and dimethylglycine have been cited as effective treatments for ASD. • Controlled studies have not shown efficacy.
Elimination diets	• Popular to identify food allergies as an aggravating factor in ASD. • Lack of controlled studies to support these notions. • Recent studies have failed to show that children with ASD have higher rates of hypersensitivities to common food allergens.
Immune globulin therapy	• Several small-scale studies show this therapy to be efficacious, however, these studies did not use standard outcome measures nor control for other concomitant treatments. • Larger controlled research is needed. • AAP strongly believe that there is no scientific evidence to justify the use of infusions of immune globulin to treat ASD.
Auditory integration therapy	• Treatment is based on the unproven theory that ASD is caused by auditory perception deficits. • Consists of presenting sounds with a machine called the Audiokinetron. • Controlled studies have not shown efficacy. • AAP refutes this treatment based on the lack of data.
Secretin	• Anecdotal reports touted amelioration of autistic symptoms; subsequent controlled studies failed to show efficacy.
Chelation therapy	• Treatment was developed due to concern about environmental toxins, such as mercury, as etiology of ASD. • Chelators used include succimer, penicillamine, and *N*-acetylcysteine. • Treatment is titrated based on urine mercury levels. • To date there is no evidence that chelation therapy improves neurodevelopmental function.
Facilitated communication	• A trained communication facilitator helps a nonverbal ASD child by supporting his or her arm and hand while the child types on a keyboard attached to another communication device. • Many claims of its success in improving expressive communication from prominent academic center. • Despite the lack of empiric support, there is apparent widespread use of this intervention.

ASD, autism spectrum disorders; AAP, American Academy of Pediatrics.

In taking a history it is important to query the family about nontraditional approaches including any herbal remedies the child is currently taking. Examples of alternative treatments include: (a) casein-free, gluten-free, soy-free diet; (b) removal of mercury and other heavy metals if present; (c) checking for yeast (candida) overgrowth and treating if present; (d) probiotics to help with abnormal bacterial and yeast overgrowth; and (e) vitamins and nutrient supplements if tests show deficits. None of these treatments has been systematically investigated, nor approved by the Food and Drug Administration (FDA) for treatment of ASD. The American Academy of Pediatrics (AAP) warns that these interventions frequently distract families from using evidence-based interventions. Clinicians working with parents of ASD children can be most helpful by offering compassionate and open-minded care. Parents who are criticized for suggesting controversial treatments may be less likely to comply with recommended medical treatments. These families can be greatly assisted by open discussions about placebo effects, evidence-based practice, and current standard of care for ASDs. Allowing adequate time for discussing alternate treatments and for ensuring understanding about recommended treatment is recommended.

Conclusions

The diagnosis of ASDs is usually made in early childhood based on the core deficits in relatedness and communication. Later in early childhood comorbidity with other psychiatric, medical, and developmental disorders may be evident. Therefore, assessment is ongoing at each developmental stage, and treatment planning is multimodal at each stage. The primary interventions focus on educational programs and behavioral modification. School is the primary site and source of interventions for youths with ASDs. Psychotropic medications may augment educational and psychosocial interventions by minimizing core symptoms, preventing aggression and self-injurious behaviors, and increasing youths' flexibility and ability to benefit from treatment. These families' desperation may lead them away from evidence-based treatments to unproven and potentially harmful alternative treatments. Medical and psychiatric clinicians help to guide to appropriate interventions throughout the child's development. With the available interventions, the quality of life for many youths can improve.

Case Vignettes

Case vignette #1

Jon presented at age 3 with multiple problems including decreased and unusual language (echolalia, pronoun reversal), lack of interest in other children, poor eye contact, impaired relatedness with adults other than parents, and preoccupation with bus schedules. Despite multiple interventions in special education with small classes using behavioral intervention, a modified educational curriculum, and advocacy from parents, Jon did not show any improvement in his language or relatedness as he transitioned into adolescence. His new pediatrician decided to order an audiogram. Test results showed significant hearing loss. After being fitted with a hearing aid, Jon began to develop language skills. As an adult, he now works in a medical clinic cleaning equipment, and he lives in an apartment nearby, while supervised by his parents.

Case vignette #2

Rick was diagnosed with ASD at 3 years. Now, as a first grader he showed severe hyperactivity. It appeared he had no time for interacting with others or learning. He was not interested in being cuddled by his parents or playing with other children. Rick had limited language. He constantly repeated phrases he heard on the television. Unfortunately, he also had a proclivity for repeating the obscenities of his teenage brother. Rick would tantrum for 1 to 2 hours if not allowed to do as he pleased. His parents were exhausted and decided to relent on their commitment to avoid using medication. Rick had a cousin whose nonstop whirlwind behavior was effectively treated with Ritalin. Thus, Rick's parents agreed to a trial of Ritalin to facilitate learning and to improve daily life. However, Rick became more aggressive and less manageable with the initiation of stimulant medication, and it was discontinued. Treatment goals were expanded from control of hyperactivity to also include his inflexibility and relatedness. An atypical antipsychotic was initiated at a low dose. Rick's motor activity decreased to a more age-appropriate level, tantrums decreased dramatically, and he was amenable to a new curriculum. His parents were then sufficiently encouraged to implement a previously recommended behavior modification program.

BIBLIOGRAPHY

Baron-Cohen S, Wheelwright S, Cox A, et al. Early identification of autism by the Checklist for Autism in Toddlers (CHAT). *J R Soc Med* 2000;93:521–525.

Bauman M, Kemper T, eds. Neuroanatomic observations of the brain in autism. *The neurobiology of autism*. Baltimore, MD: The Johns Hopkins University Press, 1994:119–145.

Burd L, Fisher W, Kerbeshian J. Pervasive disintegrative disorder: are Rett syndrome and Heller dementia infantilis subtypes? *Dev Med Child Neurol* 1989;31:609–616.

Chugani DC, Muzik O, Rothermel R, et al. Altered serotonin synthesis in the dentatothalamocortical pathway in autistic boys. *Ann Neurol* 1997;42:666–669.

Courchesne E. Brain development in austim: early overgrowth followed by premature arrest of growth. *Ment Retard Dev Disabil Res Rev*, 2004; 10:106–111.

De Bildt A, Sytema S, Ketelaars C, et al. Interrelationship between Autism Diagnostic Observation Schedule-Generic (ADOS-G), Autism Diagnostic Interview-Revised (ADI-R), and the Diagnostic And Statistical Manual of Mental Disorders (DSM-IV-TR) classification in children and adolescents with mental retardation. *J Autism Dev Disord* 2004;34:129–137.

Folstein S, Rutter M. Infantile autism: a genetic study of 21 twin pairs. *J Child Psychol Psychiatry* 1977;18:297–321.

Fombonne E. The epidemiology of autism: a review. *Psychol Med* 1999;29:769–786.

Gillberg IC, Gillberg C. Asperger syndrome—some epidemiological considerations: a research note. *J Child Psychol Psychiatry* 1989;30:631–638.

Gray CA, Garand JD. Social stories: improving responses of students with autism with accurate social information. *Focus Autistic Behavr* 1993;8:1–10.

Greenspan S, Wieder S. Developmental patterns and outcomes in infants and children with disorder of relating and communicating: a chart review of 200 cases of children with autistic spectrum diagnoses. *J Dev Learn Dis* 1997;1:87–141.

Grindle CF, Remington B. Discrete-trial training for autistic children when reward is delayed: a comparison of conditioned cue value and response marking. *J Appl Behav Anal* 2002;35:187–190.

Koegel L, Koegel RL, Shoshan Y, et al. Pivotal response intervention II: preliminary long-term outcomes data. *J Assoc Pers Sev Handicaps* 1999;24:186–198.

Lord C, Rutter M, Le Couteur A. Autism Diagnostic Interview-Revised: a revised version of a diagnostic interview for caregivers of individuals with possible pervasive developmental disorders. *J Autism Dev Disord* 1994;24:659–685.

Lovaas OI. Behavioral treatment and normal educational and intellectual functioning in young autistic children. *Consul Clin Psychol* 1987; 55:3–9.

McGee GG, Almeida MC, Sulzer-Azaroff B, et al. Promoting reciprocal interactions via peer incidental teaching. *J Appl Behav Anal* 1992;25:117–126.

Osterling J, Dawson G, Munson J. Early recognition of 1-year-old infants with austim spectrum disorder versus mental retardation. *Dev Psychopathol* 2002;14: 239–251.

Rett A. On an unusual brain atropic syndrome with hyperammonemia in childhood. *Wien Med Wochenschr* 1966;116:723–726.

Rett A. Über ein eigenartiges hirnatrophisches syndrom bei hyperamonaemie im kindesalter. *Wien Med Wochenschr* 1966;116:723–728.

Rosenwasser B, Axelrod S. The contribution of applied behavior analysis to the education of people with autism. *Behav Modif* 2001;25:671–677.

Schopler E. Implementation of the TEACCH philosophy. In: Cohen DJ, Volkmar FR, eds. *Handbook of autism and pervasive developmental disorders*, 2nd ed. New York: Wiley, 1997:767–795.

Schopler E, Reichler RJ, Renner BR. *The Childhood Autism Rating Scale (CARS)*. Los Angeles, CA: Western Psychological Services, 1988.

Sevin JA, Matson JL, Coe DA, et al. A comparison and evaluation of three commonly used autism scales. *J Autism Dev Disord* 1991;21:417–432.

South M, Williams BJ, McMahon WM, et al. Utility of the Gilliam autism rating scale in research and clinical populations. *J Autism Dev Disord* 2002; 32:593–599.

Sparrow SS, Balla DA, Cicchetti DV. *Interview edition survey form manual: Vineland adaptive behavior scales*. Circle Pines, MN: American Guidance Service, 1984.

Volkmar FR, Cohen DJ. Disintegrative disorder or "late onset" autism. *J Child Psychol Psychiatr* 1989;30:717–721.

Wing L, Gould J. Severe impairments of social interaction and associated abnormalities. *J Autism Dev Disord* 1979;9:11–29.

SUGGESTED READINGS

American Academy of Child and Adolescent Psychiatry, Working Group on Quality Issues. Practice parameters for the assessment and treatment of children, adolescents, and adults with autism and other pervasive developmental disorders. *J Am Acad Child Adolesc Psychiatry* 1999;38(12 Suppl.):32S–54S.
(These are standards of care for children with autism spectrum disorder from the field of child psychiatry.)

American Academy of Pediatrics, Committee on Children with Disabilities. Technical report: the pediatrician's role in the diagnosis and management of autistic spectrum disorder in children. *Pediatrics* 2001;107(5):e85.
(This report is a comprehensive update of recommendations for the management of children with autistic spectrum disorders for primary care physicians.)

Autism Society of America 7910 Woodmont Avenue, Suite 300 Bethesda, MD 20814; Phone: 1-800-328-8476; Fax: 1-301-657-0869; Website: http://www.autism-society.org

McCandless Jacquelyn. *Children with starving brains—a medical treatment guide for autism spectrum disorder*. Canada: Bramble Books, 2002.
(For clinicians and families to update information about recent alternative approaches.)

Siegel B. *Help children with autism learn: a guide to treatment approaches for parents and teachers*. Oxford: Oxford University Press, 2003.
(A comprehensive text written for parents and teachers with much practical information.)

The Association for Severely Handicapped (TASH) 29 W. Susquehanna Avenue, suite 210 Baltimore, MD 21204; Phone: 410-828-8274; Fax: 410-828-6706; Website: http://www.tash.org

CHAPTER 14

Eating Disorders

LAWRENCE A. MAAYAN
JOSEPH L. WOOLSTON

Introduction   Anorexia nervosa and bulimia nervosa are two of the most challenging disorders afflicting children and adolescents, with the potential for serious impact on both physical and psychological development. Anorexia nervosa has been documented as far back as the medieval period when historians coined the phrase *Holy Anorexia* to describe the drastic fasting and self-initiated purging among those aspiring to sainthood. This was best exemplified in the life of Catherine of Sienna (Italy), a 13th century woman who fasted and purged from age 12 until her death at age 33 in a quest for sainthood and, as historians have speculated, in order to gain control over the circumstances of her life. In modern medical history there is debate regarding first descriptions of currently defined anorexia nervosa. In England in the late 1600s, John Reynolds wrote of an 18 year old who had lost her menses after restricting food, commenting "most of these damsels fall into this abstinence between the age of 14 and 20." In 1688, the British philosopher Thomas Hobbes described a syndrome of weight restriction. Richard Morton also wrote of a psychological anorexia, calling it "nervous consumption" in contradistinction to the wasting that was a common and fatal sequel to tuberculosis. In 1873, Sir William Gull wrote a paper on "Hysterical Anorexia," in which he made the recommendation that "the patients should be fed at regular intervals, and surrounded by persons who would have moral control over them."

Bulimic activity has been described for an even longer time than anorectic behavior. The ancient Egyptians purged for "health" reasons, and binge eating and purging by the Roman upper class is well documented, most notably by Emperors Claudius and Vitellius. In modern times, Gerald Russell, a British psychiatrist, first described bulimia nervosa as a distinct syndrome in 1979. He suggested three criteria for the disorder: a powerful and irresistible urge to overeat, an avoidance of fattening effects of food by vomiting or abusing purgatives, and a morbid fear of becoming fat.

Clinical Features

ANOREXIA NERVOSA

There are three core features that define anorexia nervosa as described in the *Diagnostic and Statistical Manual of Mental Disorders*, Fourth Edition, Text Revision (DSM-IV-TR), which are summarized in Table 14.1.

First, the patient must fall below 85% of ideal body weight for age and height. In childhood, this may be accomplished by weight loss or by failing to gain weight commensurate with height. Second, there is an intense fear of gaining weight or becoming fat. Indeed, this is often the greatest source of anguish for many patients. They feel that they should not eat and that anything but the most stringent control of their food intake will result in an explosive weight gain. The primary distortion in anorectics' self-perception is viewing their emaciated state and still perceiving themselves as overweight. Even those youths who achieve remission often still experience the discomfort of feeling overweight. The third core feature includes amenorrhea, defined as three consecutive missed menstrual cycles, in postmenarchal women. Obviously, this last core feature does not apply to premenarchal girls or to boys.

Patients with anorexia nervosa are further divided into those who are primarily restricting, meaning that they achieve their weight loss by limiting caloric intake, and those who both restrict and engage in binge eating and/or purging. The binging and purging subtype of anorexia nervosa is distinct from the binge eating and purging of bulimia nervosa in that it is associated with being at least 15% underweight and amenorrheic.

Typically, the patient with anorexia nervosa will initially present to a primary care clinician, will be an adolescent girl, and will often conceal her condition by wearing loose fitting clothes and will be reluctant to undress. Her general appearance is likely to show perfectionistic attention to her physical appearance. She is commonly found to be in good physical condition, due to excessive exercise. A disproportionate number of these patients are involved in activities that focus on weight and physique such as ballet or gymnastics.

Less commonly afflicted are boys and younger children. In younger children, there may be a more guileless presentation. They will appear thin but may be more likely to reveal their eating habits and bodily concerns. There may also be a greater degree of family pathology, which will be helpful to note for later treatment planning. Younger children with anorexia nervosa tend to have even less insight into and often have more significant pathology in social functioning with peers and siblings.

BULIMIA NERVOSA

Individuals with bulimia nervosa share many diagnostic characteristics with anorexia nervosa as noted in Table 14.1. Indeed, many bulimic youths have been anorectic in the past. The chief differentiating factor between these disorders is the absence of severe weight loss, that is, bulimics are above 85% of their ideal weight. The DSM-IV-TR criteria for bulimia nervosa focus primarily on two components: binge eating and an inappropriate compensatory

TABLE 14.1. *DIAGNOSTIC AND STATISTICAL MANUAL OF MENTAL DISORDERS,* **FOURTH EDITION, TEXT REVISION, DIAGNOSTIC COMPARISONS FOR ANOREXIA NERVOSA AND BULIMIA**

Anorexia	Bulimia
A. Refusal to maintain body weight at or above a minimal normal weight for age and height (e.g., weight loss leading to body weight less than 85% of ideal body weight or failure to make expected weight gain during period of growth, leading to less than 85% of ideal body weight)	A. Recurrent episodes of binge eating an episode of binge eating is characterized by both of the following: 1. Eating, in a discrete period of time (e.g., within any 2-h period), an amount of food that is definitely larger than most people would eat during a similar period of time and under similar circumstances 2. A sense of lack of control over eating during the episode (e.g., a feeling that one cannot stop eating or control what or how much one is eating)
B. Intense fear of gaining weight or becoming fat, even though underweight	B. Recurrent, inappropriate compensatory behavior in order to prevent weight gain, such as self-induced vomiting; misuse of laxatives, diuretics, enemas, or other medications; fasting; or excessive exercise
C. Disturbance in the way in which one's body weight or shape is experienced, undue influence of body weight or shape on self-evaluation, or denial of the seriousness of the current low body weight	C. The binge eating and inappropriate compensatory behaviors both occur, on average, at least twice a week for 3 mo
D. In postmenarcheal women, amenorrhea (i.e., the absence of at least three consecutive menstrual cycles)	D. Self-evaluation is unduly influenced by body shape and weight
E. Restricting type: during the current episode of anorexia nervosa, the person has *not* regularly engaged in binge-eating or purging behavior (i.e., self-induced vomiting or the misuse of laxatives, diuretics, or enemas)	E. The disturbance does not occur exclusively during episodes of anorexia nervosa Specify type:
Binge-eating/purging type: during the current episode of anorexia nervosa, the person has regularly engaged in binge-eating or purging behavior (i.e., self-induced vomiting or the misuse of laxatives, diuretics, or enemas)	Purging type: during the current episode of bulimia nervosa, the person has regularly engaged in self-induced vomiting or the misuse of laxatives, diuretics, or enemas Nonpurging type: during the current episode of bulimia nervosa, the person has used other inappropriate compensatory behaviors, such as fasting or excessive exercise, but has not regularly engaged in self-induced vomiting or the misuse of laxatives, diuretics, or enemas

From American Psychiatric Association. *Diagnostic and statistical manual of mental disorders*, 4th ed, Text rev. Washington, DC: American Psychiatric Association, 2000, with permission.

action to prevent weight gain. Binge eating is defined as eating more than a regular person would eat in a 2-hour period on at least two occasions per week for 3 months. The binges may consist of any food, but tend to be of high-sugar and high-carbohydrate content, for example, cake and ice cream. These episodes of binge eating are typically associated with a sense of loss of control and often occur following an unpleasant experience involving an injury to self-esteem. The individual usually feels ashamed during a binging episode and immediately afterward. Engagement in some other activity to "undo" the previous binge is common, such as self-induced vomiting and, less commonly, misuse of laxatives, enemas, or diuretics. For individuals with the nonpurging subtype, compensatory behaviors may include further restricting food intake, the misuse of appetite suppressants or thyroid hormone (to speed metabolism), or, in diabetics, deliberately missing insulin doses in order to avoid weight gain. Other compensatory behaviors may include excessive exercise.

A typical bulimic presentation is a young woman in late adolescence who is mildly overweight. She may have poor dentition or halitosis from repeated self-induced emesis. She may be engaged in other pathologic behaviors that will become apparent on examination or during interview, such as substance abuse, which may be identified only on urine toxicology, or self-mutilation, which may be evident as scarring on the arms, abdomen, hips, or thighs. Bulimics are often guarded about their condition and may dissimulate to avoid detection. When younger preadolescents present with bulimia, it is often part of broader psychopathology. Most often, these girls are engaged in other maladaptive activity that is more common in older aged peers, such as sexual activity and substance abuse. They may be 11 or 12 years old chronologically but act and appear as if they are 16 or 17 years old.

DIAGNOSTIC ISSUES

In the *Diagnostic and Statistical Manual of Mental Disorders,* Third Edition, Revised (DSM-III-R), anorexia nervosa and bulimia nervosa were categorized under "Disorders Usually Diagnosed in Infancy, Childhood and Adolescence," along with pica and rumination. In the DSM-IV, anorexia nervosa and bulimia nervosa were given their own diagnostic section: Eating Disorders. This delineates them from other disorders diagnosed in early childhood. In addition, the distinction between anorexia nervosa, binge-eating type and bulimia nervosa was clarified. Individuals below 85% of their normal weight were classified solely as anorectic. In the DSM-III-R, such an individual could receive both diagnoses, thus clouding the picture for research and treatment.

In examining the distinctions between the restricting and the binge-eating/purging types of anorexia nervosa, there are several points worthy of mention. Overall, the binge-eating/purging anorectics are more similar to bulimics in terms of behavior, history, and comorbidity. These youngsters tend to have a higher prevalence of self-mutilation. They are more likely to have had prior episodes of obesity and to have obesity in their family. Their personality structure is more likely to include "Cluster B" personality traits, specifically traits from narcissistic, borderline, histrionic, or antisocial personality disorders. Such youths most frequently present with a lack of empathy, unstable self-image, and unstable relationships.

Bulimia nervosa also contains two subtypes in the DSM-IV. There is a purging type, in which the patient must binge and purge (i.e., misuse laxatives, diuretics, enemas, or self-induce vomiting) at least twice a week for 3 months, and a nonpurging type, in which the patient has utilized fasting or exercise but has not purged. It is interesting to note that anorexia nervosa, binge-eating type and bulimia nervosa are separated solely by the fact of the anorectic patient being underweight. Indeed, with the trend toward rethinking of psychiatric disorders on a continuum, it is likely that these categories will undergo further adjustment for the DSM-V, scheduled for publication in 2010.

Epidemiology

Eating disorders are among the most serious psychiatric disorders in terms of morbidity and mortality. Over a 30-year period, approximately 15% to 20% of individuals with anorexia nervosa will die from the disorder. The prevalence of eating disorders has been increasing since the 1950s. These disorders typically begin in adolescence, with onset by age 20 in over 85% of patients. Among women, the lifetime prevalence of anorexia nervosa is approximately 0.5% to

1%, and the lifetime prevalence of bulimia nervosa is approximately 2%. When anorexia nervosa occurs in younger children, it is usually as part of more severe psychopathology. Individuals who are afflicted at a young age, however, tend to have a better prognosis in terms of remission of the disorder. Bulimia nervosa has a slightly older profile, affecting 1% to 3% of girls during adolescence and up to 4% in young adulthood. These statistics underscore the well-known gender component. Both anorexia nervosa and bulimia nervosa are 10 times more prevalent in women than in men. There is also a strong cultural component. Both disorders are more common in Western postindustrialized nations, and, in the United States, whites are more often affected than African Americans or Hispanic Americans. Immigrants to Western countries tend to be afflicted at a rate similar to their new society.

Course of Illness

ANOREXIA NERVOSA

Anorexia nervosa typically onsets in mid to late adolescence (age 14–18 years) and rarely onsets after 40 years of age. Its onset is often associated with a stressful life event. The course and outcome of anorexia nervosa are highly variable. Some individuals recover fully after a single episode, some exhibit a fluctuating pattern of weight gain followed by relapse, and others experience a chronically deteriorating course over many years. With time, particularly within the first 5 years of onset, up to 50% of individuals with the restricting type of anorexia nervosa develop binge eating, indicating a change to the binge-eating/purging subtype. A sustained shift in clinical presentation to weight gain plus binge eating and purging may eventually warrant a change in diagnosis to bulimia nervosa. Of the remainder who do not show such a shift in presentation, many have a chronic course with high likelihood of depression. Mortality is high. Approximately 10% of chronic anorectics die from complications of malnutrition and electrolyte abnormalities, and another 5% die from suicide.

BULIMIA NERVOSA

Bulimia nervosa usually onsets in late adolescence. Dieting often precedes the first binge-eating episode. Typically, the course is chronic, although there may be interspersed periods of remission. As the individual passes from early into middle adulthood, symptoms tend to decrease. Periods of remission longer than 1 year are associated with better long-term outcome. Mortality is rare and is related to underlying pathology that was exacerbated by the rigors of frequent purging.

Etiology and Pathogenesis

There is no known etiology for either anorexia nervosa or bulimia nervosa. A combination of biologic, psychological, environmental, and social factors have been implicated in their pathogenesis. Once a pattern of disordered eating begins, multidetermined factors maintain and promote the dysregulated eating patterns.

While no candidate gene has been identified for either disorder, data from family and twin studies suggest heritable factors. Anorexia nervosa has a concordance rate of nearly 70% for identical twins and 20% for nonidentical twins. Bulimia nervosa also shows a higher concordance in monozygotic twins than dizygotic twins. First-degree relatives of anorectics are more likely to be anorectic, and there is an increased prevalence of mood disorders among the first-degree relatives of anorectics, particularly among the binge-purging type. Bulimics share this same heritability profile but have the additional vulnerability of higher rates of substance use disorder and substance dependence disorders in first-degree relatives.

There is evidence of neurochemical and functional abnormalities in eating disorders. The weight gain caused by atypical antipsychotics that antagonize dopamine and serotonin receptors suggest that these neurotransmitters affect the regulation of hunger and satiety. Children's greater susceptibility to these hyperphagic effects suggests neurodevelopmental aspects of these disorders. The hypothalamus contains the anatomic and neurochemical structures regulating appetite and satiety. These structures are rich in serotonin activity. Thus, recent studies showing elevated metabolite of serotonin (5HIAA) levels in the cerebral spinal fluid (CSF) of anorectic patients after they have regained weight suggest a role for dysregulated serotonin in anorexia nervosa. By contrast, bulimia nervosa has been associated with low CSF 5-HIAA levels, again suggesting a role for serotonin. Early neuroimaging research of anorectics suggests hypoperfusion in the temporal lobe and increased ventricular size, although the latter finding may be secondary to semistarvation.

Several theories have been postulated to explain the psychological underpinnings of eating disorders. While most of these theories are based on case studies of anorexia nervosa, they appear applicable to bulimia nervosa as well. Disturbance in the mother–child relationship is a commonly cited contributor to eating-disordered behaviors. It is hypothesized that mothers of eating-disordered youths lack affective attunement with their children. In this situation, maternal needs are imposed on the child. This lack of maternal sensitivity leads to the inability of young children to decode external and internal stimuli. In order not to alienate their mothers, who are the key to their survival, young children feel compelled to constantly comply with maternal needs. Children in this situation feel misunderstood and become confused, frustrated, and exploited. Combined with other attachment and separation predicaments, this situation leads to subsequent disturbed body image, cognitive misinterpretations, and impulsivity in gratifying needs. In later years, the child who feels constantly controlled develops intense anger. However, to avoid breaking the fragile maternal connection, anger is turned inward, resulting in self-loathing and, ultimately, self-starvation. Disturbances in psychosexual development are also thought to lead to anorectic behaviors. Adolescents with conflicted feelings about emerging sexuality, either due to difficulties with individuation or sexual abuse, halt their menses or minimize secondary sexual characteristics such as increased breast and hip size by not eating. The resulting stunted sexual characteristics help them to avoid the anxiety associated with sexual development. These theories are part of the psychological understanding of eating disorders but have not been empirically tested.

While heritable factors appear important, sociocultural factors may further facilitate the development of eating disorders. The large national and cultural differences in these disorders support an important role of societal preferences. Specifically, it has been hypothesized that the high rates of eating disorders in young women pursuing professional acting, modeling, and dancing careers is secondary to the emphasis on an excessively lean appearance as a standard of attractiveness. Similarly, in athletic activities requiring a low weight, such as gymnastics and wrestling, there is also an increased occurrence of abnormal eating behaviors. The most powerful factors may be the difference between boys and girls in terms of body image.

Assessment

The essentials of assessment for eating disorders are summarized in Tables 14.1 and 14.2.

The diagnoses of anorexia nervosa and bulimia nervosa are based on the history, physical examination, and mental status examination. Standardized assessment instruments are

TABLE 14.2. ESSENTIALS OF ASSESSMENT OF EATING DISORDERS

- Medical illnesses should be ruled out, as many medical illnesses may include decreased appetite, electrolyte imbalances, and weight loss.
- Historic data should be collected from multiple sources. Expect the eating-disordered youth to minimize his or her symptoms and the parents to have significant gaps in their observations of pathologic eating patterns.
- Clinicians suspecting anorexia nervosa should look for physical findings such as cachexia, dry skin, lanugo, bradycardia, and hypotension; and when suspecting bulimia nervosa should look for calluses on the backs of hands, decreased gag reflex, chipped teeth (moth eaten in appearance), and hypertrophy of the parotids.
- Screening tools such as the "SCOFF" questions may be useful in identifying eating-disordered youths when reviewing mental health status.
- Psychiatric comorbidity should be identified as eating-disordered patients commonly suffer from comorbid depressive disorders, substance abuse, anxiety disorders, and personality disorders.
- Family dynamics should be assessed as eating-disordered behaviors tend to exacerbate pathologic family interactions, and such interactions impede recovery.

also helpful adjuncts to the evaluation. The physical examination provides the first clues regarding the patient's compromised health. A flow chart should be started to determine the youth's actual growth compared to expected height and weight for age.

HISTORY AND PHYSICAL EXAMINATION

Anorexia nervosa

The challenge of accurate diagnosis and evaluation of anorexia nervosa is compounded in youths by several factors. At the most concrete level, a young patient may be gaining weight, however, not at a rate appropriate to height. Anorexia nervosa in prepubertal children is complicated by the fact that prepubertal youths have less body fat, are more prone to volume depletion, are more likely to fluid restrict, and are more difficult to engage in the interview, and in later treatment, because of their cognitive limitations. Girls may not have a well-established pattern of menses. Therefore, the third diagnostic criteria of missing three menstrual periods may not always apply. Thus, a developmental framework is needed when dealing with youths.

Because of the special circumstances presented when assessing youths for eating disorders, parents are a particularly valuable resource. Questions to keep in mind include: How much do you actually see your son/daughter eat? Is he or she on a particularly restrictive diet (vegan, vegetarian) and willing to find nutritious options within these parameters? Does he or she appear to spend long times in the bathroom immediately after meals (purging)? Do food items (e.g., tubs of ice cream) disappear without explanation (binge eating)? Does your child exercise inordinately on a regular basis? Affirmative answers to any of these questions should guide further clinical exploration.

A body weight less than 85% of ideal body weight establishes the first criteria for anorexia nervosa. This information is needed to make decisions about medical and nutritional management. Physical complaints and findings on examination are consistent with those of acute malnutrition. Obviously, these individuals appear cachectic, and they may complain of decreased cold tolerance, dysregulation in sleep/wake cycle, low energy, and constipation. There may be hypotension and bradycardia with associated vertigo. In terms of dermatologic findings, individuals with anorexia nervosa often exhibit dry skin, sometimes with lanugo (fine hair) on their trunks and rarely a yellowing of the skin associated with hypercarotenemia. Head and neck examination may exhibit hypertrophy of the parotid glands and erosion of the dental enamel in those inducing emesis. A comprehensive

TABLE 14.3. COMMON LABORATORY FINDINGS IN ANOREXIA NERVOSA

Hematologic Studies	Anemia
	Leukopenia
Blood Chemistries	Hypercarotenemia
	Hypoproteinemia
	Hypercholesterolemia
Endocrine Studies	Decreased estrogens
	Decreased testosterone (in men)
	Immature LH pattern
	Decreased T3
	Increased corticoids
	Increased growth hormone
Urine Analysis	Increased or decreased osmolality
	Proteinemia
ECG Findings	QTC prolongation

LH, luteinizing hormone; T3, triiodothyronine; ECG, electrocardiogram; QTC, corrected QT interval.

evaluation of anorexia nervosa includes consideration of medical conditions that may cause weight loss. These may include metabolic, infectious, neoplastic, and endocrine illnesses. Physiologic monitoring includes complete blood count (CBC), electrolytes with glucose, liver function tests, and thyroid function tests. While anorexia nervosa is typically accompanied by a normal laboratory profile, some laboratory findings may be abnormal due to malnutrition. Typical abnormalities are included in Table 14.3.

Hematologic studies reveal occasional leukopenia and/or anemia (normochromic, normocytic). Blood, urea, nitrogen (BUN) may be increased due to of dehydration. Increased bicarbonate (HCO_3) and decreased potassium result from repeated emesis. In contrast, a drop in HCO_3 and a rise in potassium occur with laxative abuse. Low levels of zinc, magnesium, phosphate, and serum amylase can be found as well as a slight increase in liver function tests (LFTs). Endocrine findings may include slightly decreased serum thyroxine (T4) and triiodothyronine (T3) levels, despite a normal thyroid stimulating hormone (TSH). Hyperadrenocorticism and abnormal responsiveness to a variety of neuroendocrine challenges are common, indicating dysfunction of the hypothalamic-pituitary-adrenal axis. In women, low serum estrogen levels are present, whereas men have low levels of serum testosterone. In young adults, there is also a regression of the hypothalamic-pituitary-gonadal axis in both sexes, evidenced in decreased 24-hour secretion of luteinizing hormone (LH) typical of that normally seen in prepubertal individuals. Electrocardiogram (ECG) studies usually show sinus bradycardia, and, rarely, arrhythmias are observed which can be particularly malignant in the presence of hypo- or hyperkalemia. These laboratory values generally remain normal until the late stages of illness. Therefore, these values should not independently influence decisions about the intensity of treatment. Finally, bone loss is common due to anorectics' starvation, placing them at risk for osteoporosis. This risk persists even after normal weight has been restored.

Bulimia nervosa

Bulimia nervosa is more easily hidden on initial examination; however, the malignant effects of repeated vomiting and laxative abuse could be pernicious and affect multiple systems. Repeated emesis may cause alkalotic conditions with low potassium and high bicarbonate levels, while laxative abuse may cause acidotic conditions with high potassium and low bicarbonate levels. Amylase levels are occasionally high and are almost always due to increased salivary, rather than pancreatic, amylase. Frequent purging can also cause hypokalemia, hyponatremia, and hypochloremia.

The physical examination of bulimic individuals may also reveal markedly eroded tooth enamel that can predispose to frequent chipping. There is often swelling of the parotid glands. Other telltale signs of self-induced emesis include calluses on the dorsum of the hand. More rare but serious complications include cardiac and skeletal myopathy in those patients who abuse ipecac to induce emesis, esophageal tears due to repeated vomiting, and rectal prolapse due to abuse of laxatives.

MENTAL STATUS EXAMINATION

During the mental status exam, these youths are not likely to have an open discussion of body image and eating habits. Indeed, in both adults and adolescents, individuals with eating disorders actively conceal their symptoms. Frequently, they feel their appearance is inadequate, and they hide their bodies by wearing layers of oversized clothes. Poor self-esteem and feelings of insecurity are often noted to be very intense. Bulimic youths in particular often report feeling depressed and empty. The affective states of eating-disordered youths may range from being subdued and dysphoric when depressed to bright and giddy when feeling good about recent success in losing weight. These youths, when presenting to mental health professionals, however, are usually sad and present with a restricted range of affect and psychomotor retardation. They frequently feel annoyed for being forced to see a mental health professional and respond with irritation and aloofness. It is important to check for suicidal ideations, which are frequently present. Obsessions with appearance or a tendency to perfectionism are almost always present. Most eating-disordered youths are preoccupied with their body size and shape, weight, and food. Cognitive function is often impaired from starvation states. Therefore, poor concentration, short-term memory impairment, and diminished attentional abilities are prominent. Insight and judgment are usually poor. The absence of self-awareness is particularly glaring in anorectics as they defend against the reality of their true body appearance. Without the capacity for insight, self-observation, or psychological mindedness, the body image distortions of eating-disordered youths are quite striking, sometimes appearing almost psychotic in nature.

ASSESSMENT INSTRUMENTS

Assessing eating disorders is complicated by the heterogeneity of the presentation. Several questionnaires and assessment tools may aid in diagnosis and establishing a baseline for monitoring. The most facile is the SCOFF, a group of basic screening questions that can be asked during a clinical interview.

The SCOFF consists of 5 general questions and a clever mnemonic:

- Do you make yourself *Sick* because you feel uncomfortably full?
- Do you worry that you have lost *Control* over what you eat?
- Have you lost more than *One* stone (14 pounds) in a 3-month period?
- Do you believe yourself *Fat* when others say you are thin?
- Would you say that *Food* dominates your life?

An affirmative response to *any* of these questions should raise concern about an eating disorder and lead to in-depth evaluation.

Specific structured interviews, such as the eating disorder examination, are available but are of limited clinical utility with youths. Self-report questionnaires include the eating disorder inventory (EDI), which has normative data for youths as young as 14 years, and the eating attitude test (EAT), which has a version applicable to school-aged children.

These screening questionnaires have been tested and used predominantly with nonclinical, young adult samples. Their applicability to children and adolescents is untested.

Differential Diagnosis and Comorbid Conditions

Ruling out medical illness is an important diagnostic issue as anorexia and weight loss can be a presenting symptom of many medical illnesses including neoplasms, acquired immunodeficiency syndrome (AIDS) and other infectious diseases, vascular disease (e.g., the superior mesenteric artery syndrome characterized by postprandial emesis caused by gastric outlet obstruction), metabolic abnormalities, and endocrine disease.

Other psychiatric disorders should also be evaluated both as etiologies for weight loss and as relevant comorbidities. The loss of appetite or weight occurs in major depressive disorder (MDD). The depressed individual without an eating disorder, however, will not want to lose weight and will often complain of the loss of appetite. The weight loss, therefore, should abate with successful treatment of the MDD. Treatment of MDD comorbid with anorexia nervosa may make the patient more amenable to treatment; up to 60% of anorectics will develop MDD.

Changes and idiosyncrasies in eating behavior can occur in schizophrenia; however, these individuals rarely have the distorted body image demonstrated in anorexia nervosa. Obsessive–compulsive disorder (OCD), body dysmorphic disorder, and social phobia share features with anorexia nervosa regarding repetitive behaviors, need for perfection, or social avoidance, but they do not usually involve weight loss. Anxiety disorders are also highly comorbid, particularly OCD, which may afflict up to 30% of anorectics. A diagnosis of OCD should be made only if the compulsive behaviors extend beyond those related to food and eating.

Both anorexia nervosa and bulimia nervosa show an association with personality disorders. Features of avoidant personality disorder are especially common in anorectics, while features of borderline personality disorder including impulsivity and substance use disorders are common in bulimics and in anorectics with binging and purging. Anorectics also show a strong need to control their environment, maintain inflexible thinking, and to strive for perfectionism. Like bulimics, they eschew eating in public.

Treatment

The treatment of eating disorders usually occurs in an outpatient setting, though medically comprised patients will periodically need hospitalization. Treatment plans use both psychosocial and pharmacologic interventions in conjunction with careful medical monitoring. Flow charts documenting ideal body weight, body mass index (BMI), and vital signs are used to guide both medical and psychiatric interventions and track treatment progress. The essentials of treatment are summarized in Tables 14.4, 14.5, and 14.6.

PSYCHOSOCIAL INTERVENTIONS

The goal for psychosocial interventions is to help eating-disordered patients develop the ability to self-regulate their eating patterns and improve their body image. This is challenging as these patients generally lack interest in and willingness to change their eating patterns. This lack of motivation and deceitful attempts to sabotage their treatment commonly result in patients evoking reactions of anger and helplessness in treating

TABLE 14.4. TREATMENT ESSENTIALS FOR EATING DISORDERS

- Medications are of limited value in treating anorexia nervosa. The presence of comorbid psychiatric conditions is the most compelling indication for psychopharmacotherapy in youths with anorexia nervosa or bulimia nervosa.
- Medications appear to be more effective in the treatment of bulimia nervosa than in anorexia nervosa. Fluoxetine has shown efficacy in reducing bulimic symptoms in both mental health and primary care settings. Furthermore, it has been shown to increase treatment compliance in bulimia.
- In anorexia nervosa, fluoxetine may be helpful in maintaining weight gain after refeeding goals have been achieved.
- Antipsychotic medications may be considered for treating persistent body image distortions and to combat poor appetite and insomnia in treatment-resistant anorectics.
- In contrast to most psychosocial interventions, family therapy has been shown to be effective in the treatment of anorexia nervosa, particularly with younger patients.
- CBT has been shown to be effective in the treatment of bulimia and should be used first before medications in bulimic youths without significant comorbid psychiatric disorders.
- Therapists should be mindful of developing countertransference reactions to eating-disordered patients who are often not insightful, manipulative, and unmotivated in treatment.
- Hospitalization may be utilized for severe and life-threatening medical complications.
- Nutrition should be applied at a judicious pace so as to avoid "refeeding syndrome."

CBT, cognitive-behavioral therapy.

clinicians. Divisive family processes that may precede or result from eating-disordered behaviors are often recapitulated in treatment teams through contradictory communications among team members. As a team approach is crucial to the treatment of eating disorders, careful attention to team dynamics and process is needed to avoid "splitting" among team members themselves as well as "splitting" of the team by the patient and family. Another pathologic process that treatment teams must address is the use of starvation and/or binging to force others to take control of eating patterns, which paradoxically is the very process against which an eating-disordered youth struggles. These youths often use isolation, passive-aggression, and even overt hostility in control struggles with family and treatment providers. Psychosocial interventions then rely on psychological awareness of pathologic dynamics, empathy with the patient's struggle, respect of the patient and family, and consistent adherence to safety and treatment goals to move patients toward healthy eating, realistic body image, and individuation with respect to the family.

Anorexia nervosa

Psychosocial approaches to anorexia nervosa have been myriad in number but moderate to equivocal in success. Few evidence-based treatments for anorexia nervosa exist. There have been two major foci for treatment. First, family therapy has focused on decreased enmeshment and parental control while facilitating the youth's individuation. Second, cognitive-behavioral therapies (CBTs) have focused on techniques to alter an eating-disordered youth's perceptions of food, eating, and his or her body, and to tolerate weight gain as proper eating is restored. However, there is little empiric support for the efficacy of these treatments. CBT approaches have not been consistently successful, probably due to the intractable nature of anorexia nervosa and the reluctance of anorectics to analyze and challenge their behaviors. Thus, CBT appears more effective for younger anorectics. Families of anorectic patients may also be less able to support the patient. In the absence of evidence-based treatments, "best practices" emphasize: (a) psychoeducation to help patients and families understand that anorexia nervosa is a multifactorial problem; (b) setting behavioral goals for improving medical and nutritional status; (c) reestablishing

TABLE 14.5. PSYCHOTROPIC MEDICATIONS USED IN THE TREATMENT OF ANOREXIA

Psychotropic	FDA Indication	Dosage	Target Symptoms	Comments
Risperidone	No current pediatric indication	0.5–8 mg/d; give once or twice daily	Persistent distortions in body image Appetite stimulant May assist with insomnia	May cause extrapyramidal symptoms at doses above 6 mg/d May cause hyperprolactinemia
Olanzapine	No current pediatric indication	2.5–20 mg/d; usually given once at night	Persistent distortions in body image Appetite stimulant Insomnia	Often sedating; occasional anticholinergic effects like constipation
Quetiapine	No current pediatric indication		Persistent distortions in body image Appetite stimulant Insomnia	Daytime doses may be sedating
Fluoxetine	Major depressive disorder	5–20 mg/d; FDA may go up to 80 mg/d in clinical practice	Assists in treating depressive symptoms and in prevention of relapse	Available in generic form
Sertraline	OCD	25–200 mg/d	Research suggests improvement in depressive symptoms and perfectionism, but no difference in weight compared with controls	SSRI warnings, FDA
Fluvoxamine	OCD	25–200 mg/d	Little research in anorexia, however, may help with obsessive symptomatology	SSRI warnings, FDA

FDA, Food and Drug Administration; OCD, obsessive–compulsive disorder; SSRI, selective serotonin reuptake inhibitor.

eating as a process based on hunger and satiety cues as well as nourishment needs; (d) family therapy for minimizing dynamics that promote disordered eating and for maximizing support for the patient's progress; (e) developing the patient's and family's tolerance for negative emotions including the use of anxiety management skills; (f) developing adaptive cognitive techniques for addressing the distortions regarding weight and body image; and (g) developing a balanced lifestyle including work, play, and social relationships. These goals make up the major parts of a comprehensive treatment plan for anorexia nervosa.

One model that incorporates these goals and treatment components is meal support therapy (MST), variations of which are used in both acute and residential treatment programs. Rose Calderon, PhD, the Director of the Eating Disorders Program at Children's Hospital and Regional Medical Center (CHRMC) in Seattle, Washington, notes that MST can be defined as a combination of social modeling, psychoeducation, and cognitive-behavioral techniques that are aimed at stabilizing and normalizing eating behaviors in individuals with eating disorders. Additionally, MST is a present-oriented intervention to be used "in the moment" during a meal with adolescents suffering from eating disorders. Hall et al. regard the supervision, emotional support, reassurance, and education offered

TABLE 14.6. PSYCHOTROPICS USED IN THE TREATMENT OF BULIMIA

Psychotropic	Pediatric Indication	Dosage	Target Symptoms/Comments	Comments
Fluoxetine	Major depressive disorder	10–80 mg/d given in a.m. or p.m.; depression (children 5–18 yr): 5–10 mg/d orally or 10 mg orally 3 times weekly may increase to a max dose of 20 mg/d if needed	Depressed mood Purging and binge eating Increased compliance with treatment in primary care setting	Safety and effectiveness in pediatric patients younger than age 7 have not been established
Sertraline	OCD	20–200 mg/d	Depressive symptoms Obsessive symptoms	FDA approved for PTSD in adults
Citalopram	No current pediatric indication	10–40 mg/d	Depressive symptoms Obsessive symptoms	Has advantage over others of having minimal cytochrome p-450 interactions

OCD, obsessive–compulsive disorder; FDA; Food and Drug Administration; PTSD, posttraumatic stress disorder.

in order to help the teen complete each meal or snack as the key therapeutic elements of MST. Thus, the rationale of MST is to provide this structure and encouragement through modeling, CBT, and family therapy approaches to stabilize and normalize eating behaviors in order to facilitate further treatment and recovery.

Bulimia nervosa

The best evidence for psychosocial treatments of bulimia nervosa comes from CBT, as described by Wilson et al. Most CBT approaches use a 20-session program over three stages to decrease binge eating and purging. Throughout each stage, the therapist takes an advice-giving stance. In the first stage, the therapist discusses the CBT-based theory of eating disorders and helps the patient to analyze his or her disturbed eating behaviors. The second stage builds on the first. The patient looks at his or her range and types of eating-disordered behaviors and works with the therapist to change the patterns. Some therapists utilize an exposure-response prevention (E/RP) model of treatment at this point (e.g., having the bulimic patient eat a regular meal without allowing purging). The third stage is focused on consolidating gains and developing relapse prevention strategies. Such CBT approaches have been particularly helpful in reducing the frequency of binge-eating and self-induced vomiting in adults. Empiric support with adolescents is not yet available. However, studies with adults have shown that the response to CBT is more rapid than that of other therapies, indicating a specific therapeutic effect, not just a nonspecific result of starting treatment or establishing a relationship with a therapist. The rapid effects of CBT have been attributed to behavioral homework assignments such as self-monitoring. Homework is thought to validate the specific CBT rationale and enhance self-efficacy in eating behavior, negative affect, body shape, and weight by fostering a sense of control over behavior previously experienced as out of control.

Other psychotherapies show promise in the treatment of bulimia nervosa. Interpersonal psychotherapy (IPT), initially developed for the treatment of depression, has recently been shown by Fairburn et al. to be as effective as CBT in normal weight bulimic youths. In contrast to CBT, the focus is on interpersonal problems instead of binging and purging behaviors. Dialectical behavior therapy (DBT), the preferred treatment for borderline personality disorder, is also being used in the treatment of bulimia nervosa, perhaps a natural application as bulimics share many characteristics with borderline patients. Psychodynamic psychotherapies may be most successful in treating older bulimics, perhaps due to greater maturity and to less concern with body image at older ages, allowing greater self-reflection and motivation. Younger patients may also benefit from psychodynamic approaches when used in combination with family, group, and psychotropic interventions. Family therapy is indicated in addition to or instead of CBT for bulimic patients who are resistant to CBT or other individual therapies.

PSYCHOPHARMACOLOGIC MANAGEMENT

Studies of psychopharmacology for treating eating disorders have been mixed. In adults, bulimic symptoms appear to respond to both tricyclic antidepressants (TCAs) and selective serotonin reuptake inhibitors (SSRIs). In particular, fluoxetine is associated with a decrease of binge eating and purging activity in both mental health and primary care settings. Furthermore, fluoxetine appears to increase bulimic patients' compliance with primary care appointments. The data for anorexia nervosa are more equivocal, and no clear benefit from antidepressant treatment during active illness has been documented. There is some suggestion, however, that SSRIs help prevent relapse in anorectics whose illness is in remission. Furthermore, both bulimic and anorectic patients with comorbid depressive disorders and anxiety disorders, in particular, OCD, benefit from treatment of these comorbid illnesses. SSRIs should be used with caution due to recent concerns about precipitating suicidal tendencies. The risks of SSRIs are described in Chapter 22.

Two other antidepressants deserve mention because of their unique characteristics with respect to eating disorders. Bupropion (Wellbutrin) is contraindicated for two reasons. First, bupropion lowers the seizure threshold, thus placing youths at risk for a seizure, reportedly in 25% of bulimics. Second, initial studies and anecdotal reports suggest that bupropion may curb appetite and occasionally cause weight loss.

Although mirtazepine (Remeron) is poorly studied in children and adolescents, its side effect profile makes it attractive for treating eating disorders. Mirtazepine is a centrally acting α-adrenergic antagonist, which has shown efficacy in treating depression in adults. Weight gain is a common side effect that may be beneficial for youths with eating disorders. One caveat regarding mirtazepine treatment is the report of agranulocytosis in adults. Hematologic monitoring is variably recommended.

The atypical antipsychotics have found a special niche in the pharmacologic management of eating disorders. "Atypicals" such as olanzapine, risperidone, and quetiapine stimulate appetite, particularly in children and adolescents, which may aid weight gain by stimulating their caloric intake. They also have sedating properties that improve the insomnia that often accompanies the semistarvation of anorexia nervosa. These atypical antipsychotics may also alleviate the body image distortions that characterize anorexia nervosa, perhaps due to the near delusional nature of these distortions. Because anorectics are vulnerable to hypotension, caution is warranted with the administration of all atypical antipsychotics, particularly quetiapine.

The opiate blockers naltrexone and naloxone have been successfully used to treat bulimia nervosa. One theory postulates that the anxiety experienced by alcoholics and opiate abusers is similar to the anxiety experienced by bulimics who share personality character-istics with substance abusers. Unfortunately, the high risk of hepatotoxicity in the doses needed to treat bulimia nervosa has discouraged routine use of opiate blockers.

Stimulants, the most commonly prescribed psychotropics for children, do not have a role in the treatment of eating disorders but warrant mention as they cause appetite sup-pression. Thus, they may be subject to abuse by youths with either anorexia nervosa or bu-limic nervosa.

LEVELS OF CARE

As in many other areas of medicine and psychiatry, the role of hospitalization in the treat-ment of eating disorders is limited, particularly for bulimia nervosa. Bulimic patients are usually hospitalized only for severe electrolyte imbalance such as life-threatening hy-pokalemia or volume depletion. By contrast, anorectic patients may be so medically and psychiatrically compromised that mortality from starvation, electrolyte imbalance, or sui-cide is increased, up to 10%. When the eating-disordered patient is hospitalized, inpatient treatment requires a multimodal team approach. The team usually includes a pediatrician, psychiatrist, nutritionist, family therapist, and nursing staff all specifically trained to treat eating disorders. Inpatient treatment should include a comprehensive psychiatric and medical evaluation with appropriate laboratory monitoring. Severe cases of anorexia ner-vosa may require rapid refeeding. Anorectic individuals who are discharged from the hos-pital at lower weights tend to have a poor prognosis as they are less psychologically amenable to psychosocial interventions.

One option that can be particularly useful for anorectic patients with a history of re-peated acute hospitalizations is a "partial hospitalization program (PHP)." These programs allow patients to receive hospital-based treatment during the day and then return home in the evenings. Attendance is individualized from 4 to 7 days per week. PHP is often under-taken as an intermediate step between inpatient and outpatient care. PHP may be used to prevent acute hospitalizations or to step patients down from inpatient to outpatient treat-ment. Similar to inpatient programs, most PHPs provide multimodal treatments including individual, family, and group therapy, usually with a behavioral or cognitive-behavioral orientation. Medication management and nutritional counseling are also included. Pa-tients are typically ready for discharge to outpatient care when they are within 5% of their target weight.

Long-term residential programs have fallen out of favor as a treatment intervention for eating disorders. These programs traditionally have lengths of stay of several months and, in some cases, over 1 year. Because of their high cost and lack of an evidence-base to sup-port their effectiveness, these programs are reserved for the most treatment-resistant cases but are generally not financially covered by commercial insurance.

MEDICAL CONSIDERATIONS

Writing for the American Academy of Child and Adolescent Psychiatry, Stevenson recom-mends medical hospitalization for the following indications: weight less than 75% of ideal body weight, hypoglycemic syncope, severe electrolyte imbalances, cardiac arrhythmias, and severe volume depletion. Other complications that may require medical attention in-clude recalcitrant vomiting, bradycardia, hypotension, hypothermia, amenorrhea, vasomo-tor instability, nutritional anemia, impaired renal functioning, and intestinal atony. Refeeding in the inpatient or outpatient setting should not be too rapid: no more than

1 pound per week for outpatients and 2 to 3 pounds per week for inpatients. Refeeding diets usually start at 500 to 1,000 kcal per day, with an increase of 200 to 300 kcal per day, as tolerated, in order to reach these targets. Care should be taken to avoid an overly aggressive approach that may result in "refeeding syndrome." This syndrome is caused by a drop in phosphate levels, which depletes intracellular adenosine triphosphate (ATP), with resulting delirium and cardiovascular collapse. Phosphate levels should be closely monitored in the first 2 to 3 weeks of weight gain.

Bone density is often lost in the malnourished state. In addition to a well-balanced diet, bone density can be increased through exercise. However, exercise is often overused by anorectics to reduce their weight or by bulimics to compensate for binges. Studies are equivocal as to whether exercise can benefit the recovery from anorexia nervosa. Therefore, only moderate levels of exercise should be part of the treatment plan and should be monitored. Other nonconventional approaches include oral contraceptives and dihydroepiandosterone (DHEA). Both have been used with some success in promoting bone formation.

Conclusions

Anorexia nervosa and bulimia nervosa are associated with potentially life-threatening medical conditions. In particular, anorexia nervosa has the highest mortality rate of all psychiatric disorders. However, these disorders are easier to diagnose than to treat. While there is some evidence to support the use of psychosocial interventions and psychotropic medications in the treatment of bulimia nervosa, success with anorexia nervosa remains unclear. Further research is needed to develop more effective treatments for these disorders. Meanwhile, community standards of care emphasize multimodal and multidisciplinary treatments designed to restore and maintain optimal health status as much as possible.

Case Vignettes

Case vignette #1

Jane is a 13-year-old girl in the ninth grade of a suburban high school. She has always excelled academically, is involved in ballet, and is a talented musician. While she appears attractive to her peers, she has always disparaged her appearance while striving to be more perfect in her many activities. During the course of a viral illness, she lost 5 pounds. Her friends commented about how good she looked and she perceived more attention from boys. She began to cut back on her food intake, initially insisting on a strict vegetarian diet and then on a vegan diet. Mealtime became a time of anxiety for her and she avoided eating in public. Over the next 4 months she lost an additional 15 pounds and stopped menstruating. Some friends asked if she were anorectic, but she usually humorously replied, "I wish." Secretly, though, she sometimes felt as though the other students in the cafeteria were watching her eat. At those times she could almost hear them thinking "Jane is such a pig." Her parents repeatedly confronted her about her weight loss, but she could not quite believe their concern. She trusted their sincerity but also believed that she would be better off losing more weight and that she would "balloon up" if she ate the regular family diet.

Jane was referred by her family practitioner to a child and adolescent psychiatrist. Initial CBT was unsuccessful; therefore, family therapy was initiated focusing on the parents' difficulty in allowing individuation of their children, Jane's frenetic attempts to excel and to please her parents, and the family's intolerance of negative emotions. In family sessions, Jane revealed that she had occasionally purged. After several months of family therapy and the initiation of low dose risperidone to aid her eating patterns and to alleviate body distortions and insomnia, Jane experienced a decrease in eating-disordered symptoms. She maintained her vegan diet but was able to eat on a regular basis. As her eating and weight normalized, a depression was evident. Prozac was added to her regimen and titrated to 20 mg per day over 2 months. Jane became increasingly more comfortable with her appearance, felt less guilty and self-conscious about her food intake, and was able to tolerate return of her menses. She has been able to maintain within 5% of her ideal body weight for 6 months.

Case vignette #2

Vicki is a 17-year-old high school junior. She comes from an upper middle-class family and is a good student with success in both athletics (gymnastics) and academics, with aspirations to attend an Ivy League college. Last year, she lost her spot in the gymnastics line up. Her coach told her that her technique needed improvement and that she "may want to trim down a little." She began a crash low-calorie diet. She soon regained her spot in the line up, but her weight continued to drop from the initial of 120 pounds to 108 pounds. Her parents became concerned and discussed the matter with Vicki at length, but she denied any problem. She began to eat more at meals but also started to sneak boxes of cookies into her room and gorge them in one sitting at night. She felt anxious and disgusted after these episodes and began to induce emesis. Over the next few months, she binged and purged 6 to 8 times per day. She withdrew from her friends and became depressed. She was finding school increasingly unpleasant and felt bored much of the time. Her relationship with her boyfriend deteriorated, and he broke up with her. In a fit of anger, she cut her upper arm several times.

During a visit to her primary care physician, the light scars on Vicki's arm, calluses on the back of her hand, enlarged parotid glands, halitosis, and precipitous weight loss aroused her physician's suspicions. He asked about her mood. She reluctantly admitted to being depressed and to hating her body. After consultation with a child and adolescent psychiatrist, Vicki was prescribed Prozac, 10 mg per day. She also began psychotherapy and adopted some behavioral techniques to help her curb her binge eating, purging, and self-mutilation. Later she developed techniques to tolerate the discomfort of eating and to reduce the anxiety leading to binging. She developed a therapeutic alliance with her psychiatrist and was eventually able to explore her feelings of emptiness, alienation, and need for others' approval. Her parents engaged in family therapy to examine the role that parental conflict and eating styles played in Vicki's difficulties. After 12 months of treatment, Vicki's depression abated. She still binges intermittently, feels guilty afterwards, but does not purge. She remains in psychotherapy but now is focusing on individuation as she prepares to transition to college.

BIBLIOGRAPHY

Attia E, Haiman C, Walsh BT. Does fluoxetine augment the inpatient treatment of anorexia nervosa? *Am J Psychiatry* 1998;155:548–551.

Bergh C, Sodersten P. Anorexia nervosa: rediscovery of a disorder. *Lancet* 1998;351:1427–1429.

Chowdhury U, Gordon I, Lask B, et al. Early-onset anorexia nervosa: is there evidence of limbic system imbalance? *Int J Eat Disord* 2003;33:388–396.

Crichton P. Were the Roman emperors Claudius and Vitellius bulimic? *Int J Eat Disord* 1996;19:203–207.

Ercan ES, Copkunol H, Cykoethlu S, et al. Olanzapine treatment of an adolescent girl with anorexia nervosa. *Hum Psychopharmacol* 2003;18:401–403.

Fairburn CG, Jones R, Peveler RC. Three psychological treatments for bulimia nervosa: a comparative trial. *Arch Gen Psychiatry* 1991;48:463–469.

Gordon I, Lask B, Bryant-Waugh R, et al. Childhood-onset anorexia nervosa: towards identifying a biological substrate. *Int J Eat Disord* 1997;22:159–165.

Hall D, Leichner P, Calderon R, eds. *Meal support introduction for parents, friends, and caregivers. instruction manual.* Seattle, WA: British Columbia Children's Hospital and Children's Hospital and Regional Medical Center, 2004.

Halmi KA. Models to conceptualize risk factors for bulimia nervosa. *Arch Gen Psychiatry* 1997;54:507–508.

Halmi KA. Anorexia nervosa and bulimia nervosa. In: Lewis Melvin, ed. *Child and adolescent psychiatry, a comprehensive textbook*, 3rd ed. Philadelphia, PA: Lippincott Williams & Wilkins, 2002:692–699.

Hirano H, Tomura N, Okane K, et al. Changes in cerebral blood flow in bulimia nervosa. *J Comput Assist Tomogr* 1999;23:280–282.

Jordan J, Joyce PR, Carter FA, et al. Anxiety and psychoactive substance use disorder comorbidity in anorexia nervosa or depression. *Int J Eat Disord* 2003;34:211–219.

Kaye WH, Frank GK, Meltzer CC, et al. Altered serotonin 2A receptor activity in women who have recovered from bulimia nervosa. *Am J Psychiatry* 2001;158:1152–1155.

Keel PK, Mitchell AB, James E. Outcome in bulimia nervosa [special article]. *Am J Psychiatry* 1997;154:313–321.

Kotler LA, Devlin MJ, Davies M, et al. An open trial of fluoxetine for adolescents with bulimia nervosa. *Child Adolesc Psychopharmacol* 2003;13:329–335.

Kuikka JT, Tammela L, Karhunen L, et al. Reduced serotonin transporter binding in binge eating women. *Psychopharmacol* 2001;155:310–314.

Liles EG, Woods SC. Anorexia nervosa as viable behaviour: extreme self-deprivation in historical context. *Hist Psychiatry* 1999;10:205–225.

Mehler P. Diagnosis and care of patients with anorexia nervosa in primary care settings. *Ann Intern Med* 2001;34:1048–1059.

Olfson M, Shaffer D, Marcus S, et al. Relationship between antidepressant medication treatment and suicide in adolescents. *Arch Gen Psychiatry* 2003;60:978–982.

Rosenblum J, Forman S. Evidence-based treatment of eating disorders. *Curr Opin Pediatr* 2002;14:379–383.

Rosenblum J, Forman S. Management of anorexia nervosa with exercise and selective serotonergic reuptake inhibitors. *Curr Opin Pediatr* 2003;15:346–347.

Steiner H, Lock J. Anorexia nervosa and bulimia nervosa in children and adolescents: a review of the past 10 years. *J Am Acad Child Adolesc Psychiatry* 1998;37:352–359.

Stevenson K. Guidelines for peer review of child and adolescent psychiatric treatment including substance abuse disorder and eating disorders. In: DuPrat MM, Stevenson K, eds. *Child and adolescent psychiatric illness: guidelines for treatment resources, quality assurance, peer review and reimbursement.* Washington, DC: American Academy of Child and Adolescent Psychiatry, 1989.

Walsh B, Fairburn T, Christopher G, et al. Treatment of bulimia nervosa in a primary care setting. *Am J Psychiatry* 2004;161:556–561.

Wells LA, Sadowski CA. Bulimia nervosa: an update and treatment recommendations. *Curr Opin Pediatr* 2001;13:591–597.

Wilson GT, Fairburn CG. Cognitive treatments for eating disorders. *J Consult Clin Psychol* 1993;61:261–269.

Wilson GT, Fairburn CC, Agras WS, et al. Cognitive-behavioral therapy for bulimia nervosa: time course and mechanisms of change. *J Consult Clin Psychology* 2002;70:267–274.

Wonderlich S, Brewerton T, Jocic Z. Relationship of childhood sexual abuse and eating disorders. *J Am Acad Child Adolesc Psychiatry* 1997;36:1107–1115.

Woolston J. Eating and growth disorders in children and adolescents. In: Lewis M, ed. *Child and adolescent psychiatry, a comprehensive textbook*, 3rd ed. Philadelphia, PA: Lippincott Williams & Wilkins, 2002:681–691.

SUGGESTED READINGS

Brumberg J. *Fasting girls: the history of anorexia nervosa.* New York: Vintage Books, 2000.
(For both clinicians and interested families, a fascinating historic look at anorexia nervosa.)

Kinoy BP. *Eating disorders: new directions in treatment and recovery.* New York: Columbia University Press, 2001.

(A valuable compilation of findings for clinicians and families.)

Levenkron S. *Anatomy of anorexia.* New York: W.W. Norton, 2001.
(Description of thought processes of anorectics; nice clinical examples).

Marcontell D, Michel SG, Willard A. *When dieting becomes dangerous: a guide to understanding and treating anorexia and bulimia.* New Haven: Yale University Press, 2003.
(For patients and family members. Discusses presentations and what to expect in the assessment and treatment process.)

Nash JD. *Binge no more: your guide to overcoming disordered eating.* Oakland, CA: New Harbinger Publications, 1999.
(Handbook divided into five sections discussing etiologies and treatments for families and patients.)

Rhodes C. *Life inside the "thin" cage: a personal look into the hidden world of the chronic dieter.* Colorado Springs, Colorado: Shaw Books, 2003.
(For families and adolescents, entertaining and informative discussion of subclinical weight issues.)

Website: www.nationaleatingdisorders.org, 2004.

CHAPTER 15

Pediatric Sleep Disorders

KYLE P. JOHNSON

Introduction

Pediatric sleep disorders have long been recognized, as any parent or pediatrician will attest; however, systematic study has only recently been applied. Nineteenth and early twentieth-century clinicians were primarily interested in sleep-related breathing problems. Some of the earliest descriptions of pediatric sleep disorders are in the literary works of Charles Dickens, most famously the depiction of Joe in the Pickwick Papers published in 1836. Joe was an obese boy who was always excessively sleepy. He snored loudly and likely had right-sided heart failure as a result of severe obstructive sleep apnea syndrome (OSAS). In 1892, William Osler described childhood OSAS in his classic textbook, *The Principles and Practice of Medicine*. Over 60 years passed before there was further study, linking OSAS to adenotonsillar hypertrophy and cardiac failure.

In the second half of the 20th century, as adult sleep medicine was developing into a medical science, a systematic study of children and adolescents started at Stanford University under the direction of Mary Carskadon, PhD. For 10 years beginning in 1976, Dr. Carskadon and her colleagues ran the Stanford Summer Sleep Camp. The same cohort of preadolescents and adolescents returned each summer allowing for the systematic collection of data. This information provided the first objective description of pediatric sleep and how it changes with development. During the same time span, other pioneers in the field such as Dr. Richard Ferber and Dr. Thomas Anders concentrated on sleep in infants, toddlers, and school children.

More recently, studies have documented the deleterious effect of persistent sleep disturbance on various areas of functioning in children and adolescents. Sleep loss in adolescents is associated with excessive daytime sleepiness, depressed mood, and poor school performance. OSAS can result in serious sequelae such as failure to thrive and cor pulmonale, as well as neurocognitive deficits such as learning problems and disruptive behavior. In young children who are at particular risk for adenotonsillar hypertrophy, these neurocognitive deficits present similarly to attention-deficit hyperactivity disorder (ADHD). Treatment for OSAS often improves daytime functioning and school performance. Chronic sleep deprivation can impair the secretion of growth hormone and subsequently, physical growth.

Review of Normal Sleep in Children and Adolescents

In simple behavioral terms, sleep is a reversible state of perceptual disengagement from and unresponsiveness to the environment, typically occurring while lying down with closed eyes. Although the exact purpose of sleep still eludes investigation, it appears necessary for healthy functioning as persistent disturbance causes psychological and often physical impairments.

There are two states within sleep, non-rapid eye movement sleep (NREM) and rapid eye movement (REM) sleep, which are distinct from one another as well as from wakefulness based on a myriad of physiologic parameters. NREM sleep is divided into four stages (stages 1, 2, 3, and 4) that correspond with depth of sleep. The combination of stages 3 and 4 is called slow-wave sleep (SWS), or δ sleep. Fragmented mental activity occurs in NREM and bodily movement is possible. REM sleep is defined by electroencephalogram (EEG) activation, muscle atonia, and periodic bursts of REMs. Mental activity is more continuous in REM sleep and is associated with dreaming. In adults, approximately 20% of sleep is REM sleep and 80% is NREM, and these stages alternate in 90 to 120 minute cycles. Sleep changes over the course of development with the most pronounced changes occurring in the first 5 years of life, as outlined in Table 15.1.

At birth, normal full-term newborns spend 16 to 20 hours out of 24 hours asleep. As any new parent knows, sleep in the first month of life is not consolidated at night, instead

TABLE 15.1. AVERAGE SLEEP NEEDS OVER DEVELOPMENT

Age	Duration of Sleep Over 24 Hours (h)
Newborn	16–20
Infant (0–1 yr)	14
Toddler (1–3 yr)	12
Preschooler (3–5 yr)	11–12
School age (6–12 yr)	10–11
Adolescent (>12 yr)	9
Young adult (19–22 yr)	8–8.5

occurring in 3- to 4-hour cycles throughout a 24-hour period of time. After the first month, the infant starts adapting to the light–dark cycle and regularly recurring time cues. By 6 months of age, most infants have a continuous sleep period of 6 hours during the night. At 1 year, the infant is sleeping 14 to 15 hours per day with the majority of sleep at night and two naps during the day. In the second year, sleep decreases to about 12 hours and the morning nap usually ceases. The afternoon nap tends to drop out by 4 to 5 years of age. Infants spend more time in REM sleep compared with adults and actually enter sleep through REM, a phenomenon considered pathologic in adults. REM and NREM cycles are 50 to 60 minutes in infants and young children and progressively increase until adult cycle lengths are reached in adolescence.

School-aged children demonstrate excellent sleep as evidenced by high sleep efficiencies and considerable daytime alertness compared to other age groups. Sleep efficiency is the ratio of total sleep time to time in bed expressed as a percentage. Problems with sleep or daytime alertness at this age is reason for concern. School-aged children typically need 9.5 to 11 hours of sleep, usually consolidated at night. Adolescents' sleep requirements do not decrease significantly, if at all, compared with school-aged children. However, they tend to delay preferred sleep times, going to bed on school nights an average of 1 hour later than school-aged children. Teenagers tend to have lower levels of alertness during the day, particularly during the morning and early afternoon, and this seems to correlate more with pubertal development (Tanner Stages) than with age. This appears to be a normal part of development as level of daytime sleepiness correlates more with pubertal development than age when adequate amounts of sleep are ensured. Adolescents also have more irregular sleep patterns, delaying sleep onset even longer on weekend nights and then sleeping later the next morning.

Epidemiology

Sleep problems in children and adolescents are very common. It has been estimated that at least 20% to 30% of this group has sleep disturbances sufficient to warrant concern. Population studies of toddlers demonstrate bedtime settling or frequent awakening problems occurring most nights or every night at rates of 20% to 25%. Once these sleep problems are established in toddlers, they tend to persist into early childhood at rates ranging from 25% to 84% over a 3-year period. Obstructive sleep apnea occurs in approximately 2% of the pediatric population. Narcolepsy, which occurs in one in 2000 people, usually has its onset during adolescence.

Insufficient sleep and irregular sleep patterns are particularly common in adolescents, with the majority of students getting inadequate sleep during school nights. Children with developmental and neurologic disabilities are at high risk for severe sleep disturbances. Up to 80% of children with mental retardation, Down syndrome, brain damage, and blindness suffer with clinically significant sleep disorders. Sleep disturbance is often comorbid with psychiatric disorders including depression, anxiety, trauma-related pathology, and disruptive behavior disorders. Thus, sleep problems are common but probably inadequately considered or evaluated in clinical practice.

Sleep Disorder Syndromes

OVERVIEW AND GENERAL ISSUES

Sleep disorders in children and adolescents differ from those occurring in adults. Some sleep disorders are specific to childhood while others occur across the developmental spectrum but may have different presentations and etiologies in early life. In pediatric sleep medicine, the parents are often the ones to complain, not the child, making parental perception an important part of the picture. Often the complaint is more consistent with a problem rather than a true disorder. What is defined as a sleep problem will vary from family to family and culture to culture. Therefore, pediatric sleep disturbances need to be considered within the specific psychosocial context of the child being assessed.

Sleep disorders are classified into four major categories in the *Diagnostic and Statistical Manual of Mental Disorders,* Fourth Edition (DSM-IV): Primary Sleep Disorders; Sleep Disorder Due to a Medical Condition; Sleep Disorder Due to Another Mental Disorder; and Substance Induced Sleep Disorder. These DSM-IV categories appropriately describe sleep disorders in adults but are inadequate for categorizing sleep disorders in children. Instead, it is easier to conceptualize pediatric sleep problems in three broad categories: sleeplessness, excessive daytime sleepiness, and disturbed behavior during sleep. Some of the more common pediatric sleep disorders are summarized in Table 15.2.

SLEEPLESSNESS

Sleeplessness is a broad category that can be broken down into three basic types: problems of settling and initiating sleep, frequent awakenings during the night, and awakening too early in the morning. These particular forms can occur in isolation or combination. It is important to determine the specific type of sleeplessness as etiologies will differ and, subsequently, so will treatment. In addition, potential causes of sleeplessness change according to the age of the child or adolescent.

Infants and toddlers often experience problems with settling and frequent awakenings. Potential medical causes need to be considered, particularly in infants. Etiologies can include "colic," middle ear disease, gastroesophageal reflux, or milk allergies. Difficult temperaments can also manifest as sleeplessness. Behavioral issues are often the cause, specifically inappropriate sleep associations, clinically described as "sleep-onset association disorder." Sleep onset is a learned behavior and therefore is assisted or inhibited by certain environmental stimuli. If a child learns to fall asleep at bedtime in his or her mother's arms, it will be difficult for the child to initiate sleep independently during a nighttime awakening. These children will signal care providers to aid in sleep transition.

Family expectations can play a part in "sleeplessness" in toddlers. Often, parents expect a child to sleep more than is biologically necessary. When total sleep time is added up, including daytime naps, expected sleep is excessive, leading to a decrease in homeostatic sleep drive. A sleep diary can help determine this cause. Inadequate limit setting and sleep routines are often the culprits, especially in overwhelmed or chaotic families.

School-aged children (5–12 years) have the best sleep efficiency of any age group, so sleeplessness is of concern when it happens. Psychiatric disorders such as anxiety and depression become more common at these ages as well as circadian rhythm disturbances. Children can develop into either "larks" or "owls" based on their tendency to advance or delay their sleep schedules. The intrinsic, biologically driven sleep/wake rhythms may be in conflict with parental and societal expectations, leading to a perception of sleeplessness, particularly problems of falling asleep or arising either too late or early in the morning. If these children are allowed to sleep their own schedule, they sleep soundly and are rested during waking hours. Behavioral sleep disorders continue to be prevalent in this age group. More recently, restless leg syndrome (RLS) has been described in children. RLS is thought to be an autosomal-dominant condition and therefore shows strong familial trends. Manifestations include uncomfortable sensations in the legs associated with urges to move the legs and motor restlessness. These symptoms are experienced during times of

TABLE 15.2. COMMON PEDIATRIC SLEEP DISORDERS

Disorder	Typical Age	Prevalence	Symptoms/Signs	Evaluation	Treatment
OSAS	3 to 8 yr olds and adolescents	1%–2% of children	Habitual snoring, noisy breathing, pauses in breathing, nocturnal sweating, mouth breathing	Full PSG is gold standard; limited channel cardiopulmonary study; home oximetry	Adenotonsillectomy; CPAP/BIPAP
DSPS	Adolescents	5%–10% of adolescents	Delayed sleep onset (usually after midnight) with difficulty awakening in AM; sleep very late on weekends; normal sleep quality	Detailed sleep history; sleep diaries; actigraphy	Chronotherapy; behavioral interventions; light therapy; motivational counseling; potentially melatonin
Narcolepsy	Adolescents	0.05%	Cataplexy, hypnogogic hallucinations, sleep paralysis, sleep attacks	PSG and MSLT	Modafinil or stimulants for EDS; SSRIs or TCAs for cataplexy; scheduled naps
Sleep terrors	Toddlers and school-aged children	3%	Occur in first third of the night; autonomic arousal with tachycardia, tachypnea, sweating; inconsolable screaming; amnesia for event	Detailed sleep history with attention to timing of episodes; family history of parasomnia; video taping	Reassurance of parents; avoid sleep deprivation; benzodiazepines for severe cases
Sleep walking	4 to 8yr olds	15%–40% have one episode; 3%–4% have weekly/monthly episodes	Usually occur 1–2 h after sleep onset; walks for a few min up to 1/2 h; confusion; incoherence; difficult to awaken; amnesia for event	Detailed sleep history; video taping; family history	Reassurance of parents; safety measures (lock outside doors and windows, alarm on bedroom door); benzodiazepines for severe cases
Sleep-onset association disorder	Infants and toddlers	25%–50% of 6 to 12 mo olds; 15%–20% of 1 to 3 yr olds	Frequent signaling of parents after nightwakings; initiation of sleep requires parental involvement; inappropriate sleep associations (falls asleep in parent's arms)	Detailed sleep history with attention to reinforcing behaviors of parents; charting of sleep associations; sleep diaries; video taping	Behavioral interventions (put to bed awake but sleepy); parental guidance to establish new routines that help the child to fall asleep on own

OSAS, obstructive sleep apnea syndrome; PSG, polysomnogram; CPAP, continuous positive airway pressure; BIPAP, bi-level positive airway pressure; DSPS, delayed sleep phase syndrome; MSLT, multiple sleep latency test; EDS, excessive daytime sleepiness; SSRI, selective serotonin reuptake inhibitor; TCA, tricyclic antidepressant.

rest, particularly in the evening when recumbent. The discomfort is relieved when the legs are moved. RLS tends to cause sleep-onset problems.

Adolescents experience sleeplessness for reasons similar to those described for school-aged children. In addition, substances such as caffeine and illicit drugs can disrupt sleep. Social and academic pressures may cause worry and anxiety and, subsequently, sleep disturbance. Other psychiatric disorders to consider in this age group are bipolar disorder and psychotic illnesses such as schizophrenia, both of which can cause sleeplessness. Delayed sleep phase disorder is a circadian rhythm disturbance often manifesting at puberty. Adolescents with this problem have sleep-onset insomnia and excessive daytime sleepiness during the first half of the day.

EXCESSIVE DAYTIME SLEEPINESS

Sleepiness differs from tiredness. Tiredness is similar in nature to fatigue, lethargy, or exhaustion and typically has a medical cause such as depression or endocrine dysfunction. Sleepiness describes an actual urge to fall asleep which tiredness does not entail, although the two conditions can simultaneously exist. Daytime sleepiness in children and adolescents has long been ignored, only recently supported by systematic research. Sleepiness can range from mild to severe and can present differently with age. Preschoolers and school-aged children usually do not manifest the behavioral signs seen in adolescents and adults, that is, difficulty in initiating or sustaining motor activity, droopy eyelids, or head nodding. Instead, they often present with hyperactivity, increased impulsivity, and aggressiveness as well as impaired concentration and irritability. The behavioral complications associated with excessive daytime sleepiness (EDS) in children are listed in Table 15.3.

EDS is often unrecognized in children because it presents similarly to other conditions such as learning disabilities or ADHD. A standard way to objectively measure daytime sleepiness is the multiple sleep latency test (MSLT). The patient is asked to try to take a nap on four or five separate occasions separated by 2 hours during the day. The time it takes to fall asleep (sleep latency) is recorded as well as sleep stages, most importantly sleep-onset REM periods. Research using the MSLT has demonstrated that school-aged children tend to be very alert during the day (longer sleep latencies during MSLT) compared with adolescents.

There are multiple causes for EDS in the pediatric population with leading causes differing among age groups. The most frequently encountered etiologies will be reviewed here. The reader is referred to textbooks in the suggested readings for a more detailed discussion.

Obstructive sleep apnea syndrome

It has been estimated that 2% of children from infancy through adolescence have some degree of sleep-related upper airway obstruction. Children between the ages of 3 to 8 years

---

TABLE 15.3. BEHAVIORAL COMPLICATIONS OF SLEEP DISORDERS

- Poor attention span
- Hyperactivity
- Irritable mood
- Poor judgment
- Use of substances
- Motor vehicle and other accidents
- Poor school performance

are most commonly afflicted with OSAS due to higher rates of the main etiology, adenotonsillar hypertrophy. Adolescents who are obese or have craniofacial abnormalities are also at risk.

Snoring is a major symptom of OSAS. Approximately 10% of children habitually (almost every night) snore to some degree, with about 20% of this group meeting criteria for OSAS when formally studied in a sleep lab. Since snoring alone does not predict OSAS, other risk factors need to be considered in determining who undergoes a formal sleep study. Other symptoms of OSAS include witnessed apnea, snorting or gasping for breath while asleep, excessive sweating or restlessness, and unusual extension of the neck during sleep. Daytime functioning is often affected, including sleepiness, mood instability, and poor attention and concentration with associated poor school performance. Findings on physical examination include enlarged tonsils, deviated nasal septum, large tongue, abnormal palate or uvula, and craniofacial abnormalities such as midface hypoplasia or micrognathia. Obesity is not a common risk factor for OSAS in children as compared to adolescents and adults.

When these symptoms and signs are present, further evaluation is warranted. Specialists in this area include sleep medicine clinicians, pediatric otolaryngologists, and pulmonologists. A sleep study may be needed, preferably an overnight, full-channel polysomnogram (PSG). A PSG is the gold standard for assessing OSAS. It measures electrical activity in the brain (EEG) and movements of eyes allowing staging of sleep. The PSG also measures airflow, effort of breathing, and oxygen saturation. Once OSAS is diagnosed, treatment is highly successful.

Narcolepsy

Narcolepsy is a neurologic syndrome that afflicts about 1 in 2,000 persons. Its chief symptoms, apart from daytime sleepiness, are cataplexy (sudden loss of muscle tone induced by strong emotions) and daytime sleep attacks. Other symptoms include sleep paralysis (inability to move although fully conscious during the onset of sleep or while waking) and hypnagogic hallucinations (dreamlike auditory or visual hallucinations at the onset of sleep). These symptoms arise when REM sleep intrudes into waking periods. The diagnosis is confirmed with a PSG and MSLT. The time it takes to fall asleep (sleep latency) is measured and sleep stages are determined. An average sleep latency of less than 5 minutes and the presence of REM sleep in two or more naps are diagnostic of narcolepsy. The sleep latency criteria may change depending on the age of the patient. Narcolepsy has a strong genetic component, although the pattern of hereditary transmission is not yet known. In recent research, it has been linked to decreased numbers of the neurons in the hypothalamus that produce a neuropeptide called hypocretin (also known as orexin). An autoimmune etiology has been proposed.

Insufficient sleep

Inadequate amount of sleep is the most common cause of EDS, particularly in adolescents. In young children, parents may underestimate the amount of sleep needed by a child of a certain age. Adolescents face other impediments to getting adequate sleep. As noted previously, adolescents delay their sleep schedule by an average of 1 hour over the course of puberty, while overall sleep needs remain essentially the same as for latency-aged children. Coupling this biologically driven delay in sleep onset with earlier school schedules in high school and increasing social, occupational, and academic demands leads to chronic sleep deprivation and EDS. Although most adolescents need approximately 9 hours of sleep, surveys indicate that during the school week, average sleep times are closer to 7.5 hours. Only 15% of adolescents sleep as long as 8.5 hours on school nights, and 26% say they usually sleep 6.5 hours or less. Teenagers generally compensate on weekends by sleeping nearly 2 hours longer. This "catch-up" sleep is a normal response in adolescents.

Circadian rhythm disorders

Disorders of circadian rhythms may take the form of delayed sleep phase syndrome (DSPS) or irregular sleep–wake schedules. Children with blindness are particularly at risk for irregular sleep–wake cycles. Blind children and adolescents may be unable to consistently consolidate sleep at night due to underlying circadian rhythm pathology. Research demonstrates that many blind youths and adults, especially those with no light perception, have circadian rhythms that progressively drift later and later over time or "free run." Free-running rhythms lead to episodes of insomnia and EDS when the endogenous rhythm for sleep is out of phase with preferred nighttime sleep schedules.

DSPS is most common among adolescents due to the normal delay in circadian rhythms, which occurs with puberty. This is a disorder defined by society, as sleep quality and quantity is normal if the patient is left to sleep his or her own schedule. Adolescents with DSPS have a delay in sleep onset of at least 3 to 4 hours. They then have difficulty waking up in the morning, often causing conflict with parents. Patients with DSPS have severe sleep deprivation, which impairs academic and social functioning. This syndrome should be suspected if EDS resolves when the patient is allowed to sleep on his or her own biologic schedule, for example, 2 AM until 12 PM. Teens with DSPS often develop poor sleep habits such as using the bed for purposes other than sleep. DSPS may be an unrecognized cause of behavior that looks like delinquency or depression.

DISTURBED SLEEP BEHAVIORS (PARASOMNIAS)

Parasomnias are recurrent undesirable physiologic or mental phenomena that occur during sleep, such as autonomic arousal, skeletal muscle activity, emotions, thoughts, and images. The etiology is thought to be state dissociation involving aspects of sleep impinging on wake, essentially getting caught between the two states. Children are at particular risk given developmental differences in sleep architecture, namely, greater amounts of SWS.

Parasomnias can be primary sleep phenomena or secondary to medical or psychiatric disorders (Table 15.2) and may develop out of different sleep states (REM versus NREM). The most concerning medical cause is nocturnal seizures. An EEG is not routinely ordered in the workup of a parasomnia but should be considered when the problem is refractory or associated with atypical features. EEG telemetry is often needed to capture an event.

The most common parasomnias seen in clinical practice are the arousal disorders, including sleep terrors, confusional arousals, and sleepwalking. These disorders arise out of NREM SWS and, therefore, occur in the first third of the night. They tend to run in families. Children with arousal disorders will have amnesia for the events. Sleep terrors are usually the most disturbing to parents because the child experiences autonomic arousal and appears terrified. Sleep terrors occur most frequently in 4 to 12 year olds and usually disappear by adolescence. The event typically lasts 3 to 5 minutes and may recur during the night. Sleepwalking is prevalent, occurring in as many as 20% of children. Usual onset is between the ages of 4 and 6 years and events typically last 5 to 15 minutes. Sleepwalking can potentially be dangerous if a child falls down stairs or wanders outside. Confusional arousals are more common in infants and toddlers and typically last longer than sleep terrors with less autonomic arousal. Arousal disorders can be precipitated by sleep deprivation, stress, or medical illnesses.

Nightmares are another common form of parasomnia. Nightmares are dream phenomena arising out of REM sleep. They are differentiated from sleep terrors in that they tend to occur in the second half of the night when REM sleep is frequent. Another differentiating feature is that the child recalls the perceptual phenomena in dreams.

Rhythmic movement disorder is a stereotyped parasomnia characterized by purposeless, repetitive movements such as head banging and body rocking. These behaviors occur during the sleep–wake transition either at initial sleep onset or after arousal from sleep. These movements occur in normal infants and young children, typically beginning by 6 months of age and remitting by 5 years of age. Persistence into adolescence is unusual unless there are comorbid developmental disabilities such as mental retardation or autism. Reassurance and safety precautions (extra padding for head banging) are the treatments of choice.

Assessment

Initial workup for a sleep complaint in a child or adolescent should include a detailed history of sleep including sleep schedule and environment, unusual behaviors during sleep, and sleep-related breathing problems. The clinician must also assess daytime alertness by questioning the patient, parents, and possibly collateral sources such as teachers. Medical, developmental, and psychiatric histories are instrumental in considering differential diagnoses. Family sleep, medical, and psychiatric histories are important in assessing risk factors for certain conditions that run in families such as depression and RLS. The differential diagnosis of pediatric sleep disorders is listed in Table 15.4.

TABLE 15.4. ESSENTIALS OF DIFFERENTIAL DIAGNOSIS OF SLEEP DISORDERS

Medical	**Substances/Medications**
Allergies/eczema	Alcohol
Asthma	Antiepileptic drugs
Gastroesophageal reflux disease	Antidepressants
Migraine headaches	Antipsychotics
Neuromuscular disorders	Lithium
Arnold-Chiari malformation	Stimulants
Chronic renal failure	Opioids
Seizure disorders	Hypnotic agents
Ear infections	Corticosteroids
Diabetes mellitus	Caffeine
Pain syndromes	Nicotine
Iron deficiency anemia	Theophylline
Hyperthyroidism	
Hypothyroidism	**Psychosocial**
	Abuse
Psychiatric	Chaotic home life
Anxiety disorders	TV/computer in bedroom
Mood disorders	Parental sleep disorder
Disruptive behavior disorders	Inappropriate sleep-onset associations
Posttraumatic stress disorder	Marital conflict
Pervasive developmental disorder	New infant in home
Psychotic disorders	
Substance use disorders	
Reactive attachment disorder	
Obsessive compulsive disorder	

TABLE 15.5. ESSENTIALS OF EVALUATION FOR PEDIATRIC SLEEP DISORDERS

1. Must consider sleep disorders in the differential diagnosis when evaluating children and adolescents with cognitive, emotional, and behavioral problems.
2. Screen all children and adolescents for OSAS by asking parents about snoring, apnea, and labored breathing.
3. When assessing excessively sleepy youths, ask screening questions for narcolepsy (e.g., cataplexy, sleep paralysis, and hypnagogic hallucinations).
4. Carefully assess sleep schedules and sleep amounts on weekdays, weekends, and school holidays. Consider use of a sleep diary.
5. Remember that insufficient sleep is the most common cause of EDS.
6. Assess bedtime routines and sleep-onset associations, especially in younger children with behaviorally based sleep disorders.
7. Conduct a physical exam, particularly assessing risk factors for OSAS such as craniofacial anomalies, tonsillar size, and septal deviation of the nose.

OSAS, obstructive sleep apnea syndrome; EDS, excessive daytime sleepiness.

A tailored physical exam is also needed, especially in assessing risk factors for obstructive sleep apnea, such as micrognathia (small jaw), enlarged tonsils, and deviated nasal septum and abnormal palate and uvula. Weight and height measurements are important for assessing obesity, another risk factor for OSAS. Assessing mental status is important given the possibility of psychiatric conditions. Laboratory tests should be ordered on a case-by-case basis, depending on the condition suspected. Obstructive sleep apnea is common in hypothyroidism, so thyroid function testing may be indicated in patients with hypothyroid symptoms or signs. Drug screening should be considered in adolescents with EDS.

Questionnaires have a role in screening for specific sleep disorders. The Pediatric Sleep Questionnaire (PSQ) developed by Chervin for clinical research can be used to screen for pediatric sleep problems, particularly sleep-related breathing disorders, snoring, and sleepiness. It is a reliable measure validated by polysomnography. The Children's Sleep Habits Questionnaire (CSHQ) by Owens is a useful screening instrument for school-aged children. The CSHQ gives both a total score and eight subscale scores, reflecting the important sleep domains of the major behavioral and medical sleep disorders in this age group. There is also a role for scales that measure depression and anxiety (see Table 15.5).

A pediatric sleep specialist may use other assessment tools including an actigraph, which is worn on a patient's wrist for several weeks. The actigraph measures movement and correlates this with sleep/wake, allowing for objective assessment of sleep schedules over time. As mentioned previously, sleep studies are indicated for assessing medical causes of sleep disturbances such as OSAS, periodic limb movement disorder, and narcolepsy.

Referral to a pediatric sleep specialist is warranted when underlying sleep disrupters are suspected such as sleep apnea or periodic limb movements. Consultation is also indicated for the evaluation and management of EDS, RLS, or treatment-refractory parasomnias.

Treatment

Education of patient and family is the first step in treatment. In some cases, this may be the only treatment necessary, that is, when parents have inflated sleep expectations of children. Parents can be referred to various sources for education (see Suggested Readings). Improving sleep hygiene is important in almost every case and may be the only treatment needed in behavioral sleep disorders or insufficient sleep syndrome. Cognitive-behavioral interventions are invaluable in many pediatric sleep disorders. Deep breathing, guided imagery, and progressive muscle relaxation are specific techniques to be used, especially in psychophysiologic insomnia.

School interventions may be needed in certain situations. In correcting circadian rhythm disorders such as DSPS, it may be necessary to alter individual school start times at least temporarily. Excessive daytime sleepiness associated with narcolepsy can be treated with scheduled daytime naps at school.

Treatment of OSAS varies depending on etiology. In younger children, primarily ages 3 to 8, enlarged tonsils and adenoids are usually the culprits. Referral to a surgeon for adenotonsillectomy is the treatment of choice in this group of patients with OSAS. Older patients, especially those with comorbid obesity, are candidates for continuous positive airway pressure (CPAP), which uses a mask and positive air pressure to keep the airway open during sleep. Rare patients with craniofacial abnormalities and OSAS may need maxillofacial surgery.

Influencing circadian rhythms has a role in pediatric sleep medicine. Melatonin has been used in totally blind adults to entrain the free-running rhythm to the 24-hour environmental cycle, and research is underway to replicate this in children and adolescents. Melatonin also has been used successfully in treating irregular sleep–wake schedules in neurologically compromised patients. Melatonin appears to be generally well tolerated in this population although there are concerns for increasing seizure frequency in patients with epilepsy. DSPS can also be treated with melatonin dosed at bedtime. When recommending melatonin, one needs to keep in mind that it is not a Food and Drug Administration (FDA) approved drug but, instead, a nutritional supplement. There is a theoretical risk of exogenous melatonin affecting pubertal onset (postponing onset). Light therapy is also helpful in circadian rhythm disorders such as DSPS. The timing of light exposure is crucial. Light must be given in the morning after waking up in order to provide a corrective phase advance in DSPS. Depending on the season, natural light exposure can suffice, but often, especially in the winter at higher latitudes, artificial light is needed. Broad-spectrum light boxes, which provide 2,500 to 10,000 lux of nonultraviolet light, are preferred. Light exposure of 30 minutes is often enough in the morning.

There is minimal research on the pharmacologic treatment of pediatric sleep disturbances even though these problems are common and impairing. Despite the paucity of research, medications frequently are recommended and prescribed. Owens et al. report in a recent survey of primary care pediatricians that 75% of practitioners had recommended nonprescription medications and 50% had prescribed a sleep medication. These medications were prescribed most often for acute pain, travel, and children with special needs (autism, ADHD, and mental retardation). Antihistamines were the most commonly recommended nonprescription medications followed by melatonin. α-agonists such as clonidine were the most frequently prescribed medications. Other medications often prescribed include chloral hydrate, benzodiazepines, tricyclic antidepressants (TCAs), and trazodone. The non-benzodiazepine receptor agonists zolpidem and zaleplon, often considered first-line medicines to treat insomnia in adults, are occasionally used in pediatric insomnia, albeit without systematic research. Although not FDA approved for use in children, these hypnotics can be safely used off label with caution. Children and adolescents may be particularly at risk for hypnagogic hallucinations if these medicines are dosed too early prior to bedtime. Zolpidem and zaleplon have very short half-lives, making them much less likely to cause daytime sedation.

Diphenhydramine, which is available over the counter, is the most popular antihistamine used to facilitate sleep in children. Although this commonly used medicine will shorten sleep latency, it often causes significant side effects such as dry mouth and morning sedation. Chloral hydrate is frequently used to sedate young or disruptive children in

TABLE 15.6. ESSENTIALS OF TREATMENT FOR PEDIATRIC SLEEP DISORDERS

1. Refer suspected cases of OSAS and narcolepsy to a sleep center for further assessment with PSG and/or MSLT.
2. The treatment of choice for OSAS is adenotonsillectomy. CPAP can be used if surgery is not possible or if OSAS persists after adenotonsillectomy.
3. A follow-up polysomnogram should be done in any child continuing to have OSAS symptoms after adenotonsillectomy.
4. Initiation of pharmacologic treatment of narcolepsy is best left to a sleep specialist or neurologist with experience in managing narcolepsy patients. Alerting medications such as modafinil and stimulants are useful for EDS; TCAs and SSRIs are helpful for cataplexy.
5. DSPS is common and can be readily treated with chronotherapy, light therapy, and potentially melatonin as long as the patient is motivated.
6. Educate parents and the youth on sleep needs and hygiene and refer them to appropriate sources of information (see Suggested Readings).
7. Treat parasomnias with reassurance and safety measures, using benzodiazepines sparingly for severe, potentially dangerous cases.
8. Behavioral interventions are the treatment of choice for young children with bedtime struggles and frequent awakenings. Resist using medications unless the child is neurodevelopmentally compromised and unresponsive to behavioral treatments.

OSAS, obstructive sleep apnea syndrome; PSG, polysomnogram; MSLT, multiple sleep latency test; CPAP, continuous positive airway pressure; EDS, excessive daytime sleepiness; TCA, tricyclic antidepressant; SSRI, selective serotonin reuptake inhibitor; DSPS, delayed sleep phase syndrome.

order to perform selected examinations or to conduct mildly invasive procedures, but there are safety and tolerability concerns regarding long-term use. The active metabolite of choral hydrate, trichoroethanol, has a long half-life leading to next day sedation, especially in infants and young children.

Benzodiazepines have a role in treating severe parasomnias as they tend to decrease deep SWS. Clonazepam is most frequently used and can be effective in very small doses (0.25 to 0.5 mg at bedtime). TCAs and trazodone are often used for insomnia associated with psychiatric disturbances such as clinical depression and anxiety disorder. Trazodone, in particular, seems to be fairly well tolerated in the long term, at least anecdotally. Clonidine, an α-2-adrenergic receptor agonist, has been prescribed for sleep disturbances associated with ADHD and neurologic impairment. There is growing support in the literature for use of clonidine in these populations, although well-controlled studies are lacking.

There is more support for the use of medications to treat children and adolescents with narcolepsy. The treatment of narcolepsy is complicated and best left to a sleep specialist at least during the initiation phase. EDS can be treated with modafinil, a novel alerting agent, or stimulants such as methylphenidate. Cataplexy is treated with REM-suppressing medications such as protriptyline, fluoxetine, and venlafaxine. Sodium oxybate, also known as γ-hydroxybutyrate (GHB), is FDA approved for the treatment of cataplexy in adults, but due to its abuse potential, it should be judiciously used with close monitoring (see Table 15.6).

Conclusions

In conclusion, pediatric sleep disorders are common and disabling. The majority of pediatric sleep disorders are behavioral in origin, but medical conditions such as OSAS and RLS must be considered in the differential diagnosis. Clinicians should consider sleep disorders when assessing a child or adolescent with psychiatric complaints, as sleepiness often manifests as neurobehavioral problems. Consultation with a pediatric sleep specialist is indicated only for selected disorders, particularly those requiring sleep laboratory testing.

Case Vignette

Case vignette #1

Andrew presented to the sleep medicine clinic as a 6-year-old boy who had been disruptive and inattentive in his first-grade classroom. When assessed by his pediatrician, a history of nightly snoring was elicited and referral to the sleep medicine clinic was made. On further questioning, the parents confirmed habitual snoring and noisy breathing at night. A period of snoring would often end in a gasp or snort, and on occasion, they noted him to stop breathing for numerous seconds. He often awakened in the morning with a dry mouth and halitosis. Sleep was restless with frequent excessive sweating. During the day, he appeared to have "bags under his eyes" but did not complain of sleepiness. His first-grade teacher noted him to be distractible, hyperactive, and inattentive, leading to problems in relationships with peers and inability to complete work in class. Sleep attacks or napping were not reported in school. The teacher recommended that Andrew be assessed for ADHD. Past medical history was significant for frequent upper airway infections and otitis media. There was no history of ADHD or learning disabilities in the family.

The mother was particularly concerned that her son might have sleep apnea since her father and brother had been diagnosed with OSAS and benefited from CPAP treatment. The mother also had noted her husband to snore nightly with occasional cessation in breathing. Her concerns were confirmed when their pediatrician educated her about OSAS in children.

Physical examination revealed enlarged tonsils and edematous uvula. Micrognathia was noted as well. A 16-channel overnight PSG was performed with the mother present for the study. Objective evidence from this sleep study supported the diagnosis of OSAS. The child averaged three apneas and five hypopneas (partial airflow limitation) per hour of sleep. These events occurred primarily in REM sleep. Sleep efficiency was low for his age, and cyclic oxygen desaturations and arousals were noted in REM sleep.

On recommendation of the sleep specialist, the child was referred to a pediatric otolaryngologist who performed an adenotonsillectomy. The child recovered well from the procedure with resolution of snoring and witnessed apnea. Although inattention and hyperactivity in school did not fully resolve, it improved dramatically. Andrew was noted to "look more rested" with greater ability to engage and learn.

BIBLIOGRAPHY

Anders TF, Eiben LA. Pediatric sleep disorders: a review of the past 10 years. *J Am Acad Child Adolesc Psychiatry* 1997;36:9–20.

Carskadon MA. *Adolescent sleep patterns: biological, social, and psychological influences*. Cambridge, MA: Cambridge University Press, 2002.

Chervin RD, Hedger K, Dillon JE, et al. Pediatric Sleep Questionnaire (PSQ): validity and reliability of scales for sleep-disordered breathing, snoring, sleepiness, and behavioral problems. *Sleep Med* 2000;1:21–32.

Ferber R, Kryger M. *Principles and practice of sleep medicine in the child*. Philadelphia, PA: WB Saunders, 1995.

Garcia J, Rosen G, Mahowald M. Circadian rhythms and circadian rhythm disorders in children and adolescents. *Semin Pediatr Neurol* 2001;8:229–240.

Gaylor EE, Goodlin-Jones BL, Anders TF. Classification of young children's sleep problems: a pilot study. *J Am Acad Child Adolesc Psychiatry* 2001;40:61–67.

Guilleminault C, Pelayo R. Narcolepsy in children: a practical guide to its diagnosis, treatment and follow-up. *Pediatr Drugs* 2000;2:1–9.

Mindell JA, Owens JA. *A clinical guide to pediatric sleep: diagnosis and management of sleep problems.* Philadelphia, PA: Lippincott Williams & Wilkins, 2003.

O'Brien LM, Holbrook CR, Mervis CB, et al. Sleep and neurobehavioral characteristics of 5- to 7-year-old children with parentally reported symptoms of attention-deficit/hyperactivity disorder. *Pediatrics* 2003;111:554–563.

Osler W. *The principles and practice of medicine: designed for the use of practitioners and students of medicine,* 4th ed., New York: D. Appleton and Co, 1901.

Owens JA, Rosen CL, Mindell JA. Medication use in the treatment of pediatric insomnia: results of a survey of community-based pediatricians. *Pediatrics* 2003;111:e628–e635.

Owens JA, Spirito A, McGuinn M. The Children's Sleep Habits Questionnaire (CSHQ): psychometric properties of a survey instrument for school-aged children. *Sleep* 2000;23:1043–1051.

Picchietti DL, Walters AS. Moderate to severe periodic limb movement disorder in childhood and adolescence. *Sleep* 1999;22:297–300.

Reed MD, Findling RL. Overview of current management of sleep disturbances in children: pharmacotherapy. *Curr Ther Res Clin Exp* 2002;63:B18–B37.

Ross C, Davies P, Whitehouse W. Melatonin treatment for sleep disorders in children with neurodevelopmental disorders: an observational study. *Dev Med Child Neurol* 2002;44:339–344.

Sheldon SH, Spire J, Levy HB. *Pediatric sleep medicine.* Philadelphia, PA: WB Saunders, 1992.

Stores G. *A clinical guide to sleep disorders in children and adolescents.* Cambridge, MA: Cambridge University Press, 2001.

Stores G, Wiggs L. *Sleep disturbance in children and adolescents with disorders of development:its significance and management.* London: Mac Keith Press, 2001.

Wills L, Garcia J. Parasomnias: epidemiology and management. *CNS Drugs* 2002;16:803–810.

Wolfson AR, Carskadon MA. Sleep schedules and daytime functioning in adolescents. *Child Dev* 1998;69:875–887.

SUGGESTED READINGS

Ferber R. *Solve your child's sleep problems,* New York: Fireside, 1996.
(A classic book for parents who need help with their child's sleep problems.)

Loughlin G, Carroll J, Marcus C, eds. *Sleep and breathing in children: a developmental approach.* New York: Marcel Dekker Inc, 2000.
(A detailed comprehensive textbook of sleep disorders in children.)

Mindell J, Owens J. *A clinical guide to pediatric sleep: diagnosis and management of sleep problems.*

Philadelphia, PA: Lippincott Williams & Wilkins, 2003.
(Practical review of pediatric sleep disorders for clinicians. Includes a CD-ROM with excellent handouts and questionnaires.)

Sadeh A. *Sleeping like a baby: a sensitive and sensible approach to solving your child's sleep problems.* New Haven, CT: Yale University Press, 2001.
(Excellent review of infant and toddler sleep targeted for parents.)

CHAPTER 16

Learning Disorders

JENISE JENSEN
DAVID·BREIGER

Introduction

HISTORIC BACKGROUND

Reports of individuals who acquired a sudden inability to read, write, or perform mathematic calculations after some type of neurologic insult have been published since the 17th century. However, it was a description by Dr. W. Pringle Morgan in 1896 of a 14-year-old boy named Percy that led to the hypothesis that learning difficulties were due to a specific congenital or developmental disorder. Dr. Morgan's report of Percy's puzzling difficulty with learning to read, despite his overall bright cognitive abilities and intact visual and mental calculation skills, led another doctor, James Hinshelwood, M.D., to conclude that this difficulty was due to problems with the visual memory system for words. The term *congenital word blindness* was coined in the early 1900s to describe this condition and represents the beginning research into the field of learning disorders (LDs).

Later modifications to Hinshelwood's theory resulted in the hypothesis that the inability to learn to read was due to problems with left–right orientation and strephosymbolia, or twisted word imagery, that was caused by a lack of cerebral dominance. Therefore, it was reasoned that deficits in the visual system resulted in seeing letters backwards ("b" for "d") or transposing letters in words ("was" for "saw"). Until as recently as 20 years ago, this was one of the leading theories about the causes of developmental reading problems.

Another important point in the history of understanding childhood LDs was the 1918 flu pandemic. Many children who survived demonstrated attention, perceptual-motor, learning, and behavior problems despite having normal physical and neurologic examinations. Because these difficulties could not readily be attributed to mental retardation or other forms of social or emotional disturbance, the term *minimal brain damage* was used to indicate that these learning and attention problems were due to some congenital factor intrinsic to the child. Further research and debate resulted in the term *minimal brain dysfunction* to reflect that a specific brain insult was not required to cause these problems. Attempts to identify neurologic soft signs that might be diagnostic and predictive of which children would develop learning problems were also prominent throughout this period, to no avail.

It was not until the last 40 years that the official terms *learning disability* and *learning disorder* came into popular use. Dr. Samuel Kirk, a psychologist and special educator, first coined the term *specific learning disability* in 1963 to describe a group of children who had disorders of development in language, speech, reading, and associated communication skills that were not due to either sensory handicaps or mental retardation. This chapter summarizes the field's current understanding of LDs. The majority of this chapter will focus on reading disorders (RD) as they have been the most researched and, hence, the best understood of the LDs.

Clinical Definition

The term *learning disorders* is used in the *Diagnostic and Statistical Manual of Mental Disorders*, Fourth Edition, Text Revision (DSM-IV-TR) to refer to a group of disorders that are characterized by learning problems resulting in an individual's measured academic achievement falling substantially below the level expected given the person's chronologic age, educational level, and intellectual ability. As shown in Table 16.1, the three primary

TABLE 16.1. *DIAGNOSTIC AND STATISTICAL MANUAL OF MENTAL DISORDERS,* **FOURTH EDITION TEXT REVISION, DIAGNOSTIC CRITERIA FOR LEARNING DISORDERS**

I. **Reading disorder (315.00), mathematics disorder (315.1), and disorder of written expression (315.2)**

   A. Reading achievement, mathematical ability, or writing skills, as measured by individually administered standardized tests, are substantially lower given the person's chronologic age, measured intelligence, and age-appropriate education.

   B. The disturbance in criterion A significantly interferes with academic achievement or activities of daily living that require reading or mathematic skills or the composition of written texts (e.g., writing grammatically correct sentences and organized paragraphs).

   C. If a sensory deficit is present, the reading, mathematics, and writing difficulties are in excess of those usually associated with it.

Coding note: if a general medical (e.g., neurologic) condition or sensory deficit is present, code the condition on axis III.

II. **Learning disorder not otherwise specified (315.9)**

   A. Disorders in learning that do not meet criteria for any specific learning disorder outlined above.

   B. May include difficulties in all reading, mathematics, and written expression that together result in significant interference in academic achievement but do not individually meet criteria.

From American Psychiatric Association. *Diagnostic and statistical manual of mental disorders*, 4th ed, Text rev. Washington, DC: 2000, with permission.

LD diagnoses defined by the DSM-IV-TR are RD, mathematics disorder, and disorder of written language. The DSM-IV-TR also allows for the diagnosis of learning disorder not otherwise specified (LD-NOS) to account for learning problems that do not meet criteria for any specific LD.

The terms *learning disorder* and *learning disability* have largely been interchangeable in both the educational and psychiatric literature since the federal government officially adopted Kirk's term *specific learning disability* in 1975 with the passage of Public Law 94-142. This federal law mandated schools to provide publicly funded special education and related services to students whose disabilities adversely affected their educational performance. PL 94-142 is currently named the Individuals with Disabilities Education Act (IDEA) and defines the term *specific learning disability* as:

> A disorder in one or more of the basic psychological processes involved in understanding or in using language, spoken or written, that may manifest itself in an imperfect ability to listen, speak, read, write, spell, or to do mathematical calculations, including conditions such as perceptual disabilities, brain injury, minimal brain dysfunction, dyslexia, and developmental aphasia.

Although IDEA provides a federal definition of specific learning disabilities, states and local school districts have flexibility in how they identify which students meet criteria for special education services. The majority of school districts have traditionally used a discrepancy model to identify students with learning problems substantial enough to qualify for special education services under the classification of Specific Learning Disability. This formula requires a statistically significant difference of at least 1.5 to 2 standard deviations between assessed academic achievement and cognitive ability in order to qualify for special education. This type of identification system relies on categoric definitions of LD. However, there is also a debate that LDs, like many other medical and psychological disorders, may actually fall on a continuum and that a dimensional or spectrum model may be more appropriate. This type of identification system would allow children who would have otherwise been characterized as "poor readers," but not learning disabled, to receive needed services. For example, a student whose overall cognitive ability was measured in the "low average" range (standard score of 85) and single-word reading skills were in the "below average" range (standard score of 70) would not necessarily be identified as LD and receive services because the student's reading ability, while low, is interpreted as commensurate with his or her inherent ability using the discrepancy model.

Reading Disorder

CLINICAL FEATURES

RD, also known as dyslexia, is characterized by the presence of deficits in an individual's reading achievement despite having average intelligence and educational opportunities. Research in the past 20 years has demonstrated that dyslexia is related to deficits in processing the basic sounds that make up language, a skill that is referred to as phonological awareness. Specifically, these children demonstrate an isolated weakness with phonologic processing that results in difficulty with decoding or being able to "sound out" words, although higher order cognitive skills of thinking, reasoning, and understanding abstract concepts are intact, even advanced.

In order to become an effective reader, a child must first be able to hear and identify the individual sounds in a spoken word. These are called phonemes and are the basic building blocks of language. For example, the word "mat" is comprised of three phonemes:

"mmm," "aah," and "tuh." Phonologic processing allows one to identify, understand, store, and retrieve each of these sounds so that they can be put together to form a word or morpheme. This process occurs automatically in spoken language through a process called coarticulation, where individual phonemes are rapidly compressed or blended together to produce speech that is understandable and not taxing on the memory system. Hence, the spoken word "mat" is perceived as one single sound rather than the three separate phonemes that it actually contains.

In reading and writing, these individual phonemes are mapped onto letters that share the same structural sound properties. For example, the letter "B" makes the /b/ or "buh" sound. This process is termed the alphabetic principle. Reading requires that an individual be able to decode words by simultaneously segmenting each letter into its representative sound, retain these sounds in memory, and then blend them together to form a word. Effective reading also requires that an individual become fluent in this skill so that attentional and cognitive resources can be used for the purpose of recalling previous words and sentences in a paragraph in order to obtain meaning.

The core weakness of dyslexia lies in developing an awareness that spoken and written words are made up of phonemes. Hence, children with reading problems have difficulty recognizing that words are made up of much smaller segments representing individual sounds. These problems are then compounded further by the process of reading, which requires that a child learn that these sounds are tied to squiggly lines on paper called letters. Finally, a child must then understand that when these letters are put together to form words, they represent the same number and sequence of sounds that are heard in a spoken word. Children must first develop phonemic awareness in order to become effective readers and learn how to decode and decipher words into their representative phonemes.

Although children with dyslexia can be taught phonologic awareness skills, many continue to have difficulty with the automatization of this process that allows them to read fluently or in a quick, smooth, and accurate manner. Effective readers are able to identify individual words with little to no effort and, thus, are able to devote the majority of their cognitive resources to comprehension. Poor fluency can have an immense effect on comprehension when an individual is pressured by time or has a large volume of written material to understand and integrate. This is because so much energy must be dedicated to decoding text with few reserves left over for understanding critical pieces of information, recalling previously read material, and drawing inferences from prior knowledge. It is also important to note that because higher order cognitive skills are intact in dyslexic individuals, comprehension can be largely unaffected when they are allowed to read at their own pace or they are able to use visual cues to help them derive meaning from the text.

Although not directly related to the process of reading, many dyslexic individuals also have considerable difficulties with rote memorization and rapid word retrieval. This is often the most frustrating paradox of dyslexia since the inability to quickly find the correct word is often misinterpreted as the person being slow or dimwitted, when the converse is actually true. Individuals with dyslexia have been shown to have strong receptive vocabulary, syntactic, and grammar skills, but have difficulty retrieving words on demand due to the inability to use the phonemic properties of the word to assist with quick and easy access from long-term memory. In fact, sound-based slips of the tongue are often not indicative of poor understanding of the word's meaning but rather confusion regarding the words sounds (e.g., saying the word "intrepid" for "interrupted"). This is also one of the more persisting symptoms of dyslexia, as adults who have developed adequate reading skills will continue to demonstrate difficulties with rapid and fluent word retrieval and will have speech characterized by long pauses, fillers ("um"), and nonspecific language ("that thing").

CLINICAL COURSE

Previous theories about LDs posited that they represented a developmental lag that could be outgrown or effectively treated with a short-term "booster" of intervention that would allow a child to catch up. It is now understood that LDs can be persistent over time, although the manner in which the specific symptom is exhibited can vary. In fact, nearly 75% of children classified as RD in the third grade continue to demonstrate significant reading problems in the ninth grade. Specifically, adults who were identified as having an RD as children often continue to demonstrate difficulties with decoding unfamiliar words, spelling, and fluency. Reading can continue to be quite frustrating for these adolescents and adults whose comprehension often depends upon a laborious, time-consuming process of relatively slowed word retrieval. This is especially true for those bright individuals whose academic or vocational ambitions require a considerable amount of reading.

Many children with RD exhibit a reluctance to attend school, moodiness, self-derogatory comments about their ability, and disruptive behavior due to boredom, frustration, and/or shame. School dropout rates for youths with LD are estimated to be as high as 40%, resulting in major problems with employment as adults. Other lifelong correlates of dyslexia include self-perceptions of lower intellectual ability, more psychological distress, and less social mobility.

The term *Matthew effects* has been used to characterize the accumulated disadvantage of not being able to read fluently. Third grade has been identified as the turning point in school where instruction models switch from "learning to read" to "reading to learn." Unfortunately, if children have not learned adequate decoding and fluency skills by this age, the achievement gap between them and their peers in all academic areas begins to widen. Longitudinal studies of children who did not receive early and intense intervention have demonstrated that these students continue to lag behind their peers throughout high school in many academic areas, but especially in those areas that require a great deal of reading.

EPIDEMIOLOGY

RD is the most common form of LD, accounting for 50% to 80% of all diagnosed LDs. Prevalence in the DSM-IV-TR is estimated at 3% to 10% of the population with a male-to-female ratio of approximately 4:1. However, other studies suggest that the prevalence rate is closer to 17% to 20% with a more equal rate between boys and girls. The lower prevalence rates and bias toward boys cited in previous studies are likely due to these samples relying on children who were clinic referred or already qualified for special education services. Because boys are more likely to display disruptive behavior when confronted with academic challenges, whereas girls tend to display quietly inattentive behavior, boys are more often referred for evaluation. In fact, longitudinal studies with a representative sample of all young children entering school have found that the rate of RD is much higher than previously indicated, as well as more equal between girls and boys. It is also interesting that recent research has begun to question a previously held notion that dyslexia only occurs in individuals who speak alphabetic languages and not in individuals who speak logographic languages such as Chinese.

PATHOGENESIS

RD has been shown to be both familial and genetic with a nearly 80% concordance rate reported in monozygotic (MZ) twins in comparison to less than 50% concordance rate in dizygotic (DZ) twins and other siblings. Furthermore, if one family member is affected, the rates for other members are much higher than that in the general population. For example, the rates of reading problems in children of dyslexic parents have been found to be as high as 30% to 60%. Parents of children with RD are also more likely to have reading problems (25%–60%), with a higher risk for fathers (46%) compared to mothers (33%). Finally, linkage studies suggest a major role for chromosomes 6 and 15, with additional potential markers on chromosomes 1 and 2.

Structural and functional neuroimaging studies have demonstrated differences in brain structure and activation for children and adults with RD compared to matched normal controls. These results, while preliminary, are very promising. Structural studies have revealed possible differences in the left-hemispheric regions that support language in individuals with RD, most notably in the areas of the planum temporale, insular cortex, and corpus callosum. The most consistent findings have demonstrated that skilled readers generally demonstrate an asymmetry of the planum temporale favoring the left side, whereas individuals with dyslexia demonstrate a lack of, or reversed, asymmetry.

Functional neuroimaging studies have also supported left-hemispheric differences between individuals with and without RD, notably in the basal temporal, temporoparietal, and inferior frontal regions. Specifically, increased activation in the angular gyrus, Wernicke area, and basal temporal areas within the left temporoparietal region has been shown on word recognition tasks in skilled readers. In contrast, adults and children with RD exhibit increased activation in the anterior portions of the brain, as well as a reversed pattern of hemispheric activation in the right temporoparietal region, on these tasks.

Although there is strong evidence that RD is a genetic and neurobiologic disorder, the effect of the environment cannot be ignored. Parents who have reading problems often have fewer books in the home and are less likely to read to their children or to model reading as a rewarding activity. Furthermore, it is unclear what effect inadequate instruction has on brain development. Preliminary neuroimaging studies suggest that intense and early intervention that addresses the core phonologic deficit of RD produces changes in brain activation that resemble nondisabled readers. For these reasons, it is likely that neurobiologic and environmental factors interact to produce the phenotype currently defined as dyslexia.

DIFFERENTIAL DIAGNOSES AND COMMON COMORBIDITIES

The most common differential diagnoses for all LDs are summarized in Table 16.2. These include ruling out sensory problems related to vision or hearing difficulties and mental retardation. The DSM-IV-TR and special education definitions also specify that inadequate educational opportunities, poor motivation, and significant emotional problems must be ruled out as well. However, it is important to note that the mere presence of these factors does not rule out the diagnosis of LD. Instead, their presence can contribute to and interact with a comorbid learning disability, making a differential diagnosis quite difficult. Finally, methods of assessment and interpretation of testing results should be sensitive to an individual's ethnic or cultural background, as well as a child's current proficiency in developing a second language, to avoid possibly mislabeling a child as LD or mentally retarded.

LDs, including RD, frequently occur in association with several general medical conditions such as very low birth weight, prematurity, lead poisoning, fetal alcohol syndrome, and fragile X syndrome. However, the presence of these disorders does not necessarily indicate learning problems, and many individuals with LD do not have such a history.

TABLE 16.2. DIFFERENTIAL DIAGNOSES FOR ALL LEARNING DISORDERS

- Vision or hearing problems
- Mental retardation
- Psychological or mental health problems
- Environment
- Cultural factors

TABLE 16.3. COMMON COMORBIDITIES FOR ALL LEARNING DISORDERS

- Other learning disabilities
- Language disorders
- Disruptive behavior disorders
  - Attention deficit hyperactivity disorder (ADHD)
  - Oppositional defiant disorder (ODD)
  - Conduct disorder (CD)
- Mood disorders
- Anxiety disorders

The most common comorbidities with RD are primarily related to emotional and behavioral disturbances, as summarized in Table 16.3. Attention deficit hyperactivity disorder (ADHD) is the most frequently reported comorbidity with RD in both epidemiologic and clinical studies, regardless of whether individuals are selected for reading problems or for ADHD. Between 15% and 26% of individuals with dyslexia also meet criteria for ADHD, whereas 25% to 40% of individuals with ADHD have reading difficulties. Furthermore, the core deficits in language and phonologic processing specific to dyslexia have been shown to be independent of a comorbid diagnosis of ADHD.

RD can also take a high toll on children's psychological health. Emotional or physical symptoms (e.g., anxiety, depression, stomachaches, school refusal) are common in children with RD, with 14% to 32% experiencing depressive moods and feelings of lack of control and low self-efficacy. Twin studies have supported higher rates of all internalizing and externalizing disorders in individuals with RD. Gender differences have also been found with boys showing more externalizing symptoms and girls more internalizing symptoms.

ASSESSMENT

The essentials of assessment for RD are summarized in Table 16.4 and explicated here.

Children with normal reading processes spontaneously begin to identify and segment the sounds or phonemes in words around the ages of 4 to 6 years. For example, children at these ages are particularly attuned to and take pleasure in rhymes and can begin to group words by their initial and ending sounds. This has been shown to be a critically important skill for learning to read and, hence, difficulties in this area can be very predictive markers for reading problems. Early assessment of dyslexia usually focuses on three areas that are related to phonologic processing: (a) phonemic awareness or the ability to identify phonemes and manipulate words by removing and replacing sounds, (b) rapid automatic naming or the ability to quickly and efficiently retrieve phonologic information from long-term memory, and (c) phonologic working memory or the ability to temporarily store bits of verbal information.

The first area of assessment, phonemic awareness, can be measured in several ways, including sound comparison, segmentation, blending, and manipulation of phonemes in words. Sound comparison involves asking a child to decide which words are alike based on their initial, ending, or middle sounds. For example: "Which word begins with the same sound as pan: tub, pig, or can?" Segmentation can be measured by asking a child to either report how many sounds are in a word or to pronounce the sounds he or she hears. For example: "How many sounds are there in the word cat?" "Three" or "kuh" "aaa" "tuh." Alternatively, asking a child what sound "kuh" "aaa" and "tuh" requires him to blend these phonemes together to form a word. Finally, the most advanced phonemic awareness skill involves having a child add, move around, or delete sounds from one word in order to form another word. For example: "What word do you get if you take the /l/ sound away from the word *slide*?" It is important to note that most children have mastered the majority of these skills by the end of first grade.

TABLE 16.4. ASSESSMENT ESSENTIALS FOR READING DISORDER

Domain	Commonly Administered Measures (List Is Not Exhaustive)
Rule out sensory problems	Thorough screening of hearing and vision
Cognitive ability	
To obtain understanding of cognitive strengths and weaknesses and qualify for special education	Wechsler Intelligence Scale for Children (WISC)[a] Wechsler Adult Intelligence Scale (WAIS)[a] Stanford Binet[a]
Assessment of early language development	
Difficulties with rhyming	Developmental history
Poor articulation and pronunciation	Parent interview
Word finding problems	Observation
Poor knowledge of letter names and sounds	Ask child to name capital and lowercase letters and identify corresponding sounds
Areas of diagnostic assessment	
Family history	Parent interview
Phonemic awareness	Comprehensive Test of Phonologic Processing (CTOPP)[a]
Single-word decoding of real and nonsense words	Woodcock-Johnson Tests of Achievement[a] Letter-word Identification subtest Word Attack subtest
Reading fluency (oral and silent reading speed and accuracy)	Gray Oral Reading Test (GORT)[a] Rapid automatic naming
Reading comprehension	Woodcock-Johnson Tests of Achievement[a] Passage Comprehension subtest Wechsler Individual Achievement Test (WIAT)[a] Reading Comprehension subtest
Other assessment areas for differential diagnosis, comorbidity, and related problems	
Attention and concentration	Parent/teacher interview and rating scales Conners' Continuous Performance Test (CPT)[a]
Receptive and expressive vocabulary	Peabody Picture Vocabulary Test (PPVT)[a] Expressive One-word Vocabulary Test (EOWT)[a] WISC Vocabulary subtest[a]
Verbal fluency	NEPSY Verbal Fluency[a]
Listening comprehension	WIAT Listening Comprehension subtest[a]
Understanding of print conventions	Process Assessment of the Learner (PAL): test battery for reading and writing[a]
Problems with mood, anxiety, behavior problems, or self-esteem	Behavior Assessment Scale for Children (BASC)[a] Achenbach Child Behavior Checklist (CBCL)

[a]Indicates measure is standardized.

The second area, rapid automatic naming, is assessed by having a child name an array of stimuli arranged in rows on a card as quickly as he or she can. Because the purpose of the task is to assess how efficiently a child can retrieve information (rather than measure the child's vocabulary), the stimuli used are usually very familiar items such as letters, numbers, colors, or objects. Finally, phonologic working memory is a critical skill when learning to read as sounding out a word is a complex process that requires decoding letters into their sounds, storing these sounds in memory while decoding the remaining letters of a word, and then blending these sounds to form a word. Assessment of phonologic working memory usually involves having a child repeat strings of random numbers, letters, or words. Table 16.5 lists early warning signs in children who may exhibit RD.

Another important area of assessment in young children is knowledge of letter names and letter sounds. Developmentally, it is expected that children who are exposed to letter concepts will begin to show an interest in and be able to identify letters and their corresponding sounds by preschool with proficiency by early first grade. Difficulties with naming letters

TABLE 16.5. EARLY WARNING SIGNS OF READING DISORDER

- Early warning sign for children of reading disorder by end of kindergarten:
  - Delay in developing speech
  - Difficulties with articulation or pronunciation
  - Takes little enjoyment in hearing and repeating nursery rhymes
  - Difficulty with rhyming
  - Difficulty naming all upper- and lowercase letters
- Early warning signs for children of reading disorder by 1st grade:
  - Difficulty segmenting words and grouping them by their initial, ending, and middle phonemes
  - Difficulty naming letter sounds
  - Difficulty counting number of sounds in small words
- Expressive language seems to lag behind receptive language

and identifying their corresponding sounds by this age should warrant a referral for further evaluation. A commonly held notion that writing poorly formed or backwards letters represents a core symptom of dyslexia deserves comment. The base rate of this difficulty in young children is fairly high. Whereas children without dyslexia seem to outgrow this difficulty by second grade, many children with dyslexia continue to demonstrate such problems. Contrary to previous beliefs, the cause of this problem is not due to "seeing" letters backwards. Rather, these problems can again be attributed to poor phonologic processing skills that make it difficult and cumbersome for a child to tie letters with their corresponding sounds.

Three additional areas are generally targeted for assessment when evaluating for RD in school-aged children: (a) single-word reading, (b) reading fluency, and (c) reading comprehension. Assessment of single-word reading is fairly simple and involves having a child read aloud lists of real words, as well as phonetically regular nonsensical words. Nonsense words are a particularly important measure of phonologic decoding as many children with dyslexia initially try to learn to read by memorizing the letter groupings of real words. Reading fluency is a measure of an individual's speed and accuracy in reading. It is measured by timing how quickly and smoothly a child can read a list of single words, a group of sentences, or multiple paragraphs on a page without errors. Reading fluency is generally assessed through oral reading, although assessment of silent reading fluency can be important with older students or adults. Reading comprehension is measured by having an individual read a paragraph, story, or piece of text and then asking him or her questions about what was read. Although appearing to be a fairly straightforward concept, comprehension can be significantly affected by many task variables. These include differences in passage length and response format (free recall versus multiple choice), timed versus untimed reading of material, presence of other forms of contextual information (pictures, graphs, etc.), and an individual's previous knowledge of the material.

The role of assessing a child's cognitive or intellectual ability continues to this day to remain central in both educational and psychiatric diagnostic systems for learning disabilities. This harkens back to the originally proposed notion that problems with learning to read represent an *unexpected* difficulty that is not consistent with a child's innate cognitive ability. This hypothesis was based on research demonstrating a high correlation between cognitive ability and reading achievement in normal readers. However, current research on the role of phonologic processing with reading problems has demonstrated that overall cognitive ability and achievement are not highly correlated in individuals with dyslexia. In fact, intelligence quotient (IQ) tests are poor predictors of both later reading problems and response to treatment. Furthermore, the disturbing paradox with using IQ tests to diagnose or qualify a child with reading problems can be that many dyslexic children do not present with a significant enough discrepancy between their aptitude and achievement in the early grades and hence do not qualify for services. It is not until they have "failed" reading for several consecutive grades that their gap becomes wide enough to meet diagnostic or educational criteria, which can be too late to prevent subsequent academic and behavioral problems. For this reason, IQ tests are frequently not recommended in the assessment of early identification of reading problems, although understanding a child's overall cognitive ability can be useful in the development of other treatment goals. This difficulty further underscores the aforementioned controversy of using a discrepancy model rather than a continuum model in identifying children with RD or any LD.

TREATMENT

Early identification and intervention are essential for optimal prevention of further learning, emotional, and behavioral problems. Developing fluent reading skills requires the old adage of "practice, practice, practice." Hence, the older a child is before a diagnosis is made, the greater the gap between him or her and his or her peers. The essential pieces of an effective intervention include intense and high-quality instruction of sufficient duration. Specifically, it is recommended by Shaywitz that a child receive systematic and direct instruction in increasing phonemic awareness (noticing, identifying, and manipulating the sounds of language), as well as phonics (how written letters and letter groups represent the sounds of spoken language). Improving a child's ability to decode or sound out words; blend sounds together to form words; and recognize words by sight, spelling skills, and reading comprehension strategies is critical. Recent research has indicated that effective interventions for reading problems entail frequent instruction (between 30 and 60 minutes a day, 4 to 5 days a week) delivered in a one-to-one, or at most, a three-to-one setting. Other core elements to an effective reading program include an emphasis on letter identification, vocabulary development, the ability to recall and retell sentences and stories, and practice writing words and sentences with an emphasis on vocabulary development, planning, and organization of written material.

To facilitate reading fluency and comprehension, children with RD should be provided with materials that they are able to read easily, with an error rate of no more than 10%. It is further recommended that children receive practice in identifying key facts from written material to assist with developing an understanding of the structure of sentences, paragraphs, and stories and in being able to extract important concepts from reading material.

Several comprehensive reading programs are available that utilize a direct instruction approach with a systematic and integrated format that teaches phonetic skills in a structured and comprehensive manner. These include DISTAR, Reading Mastery, Open Court Reading, Success for All, and the REACH System to name a few. However, no single program is sufficient to meet all instructional reading needs, nor a panacea. Furthermore, the quality of instruction with teachers who are well trained in the technology of teaching reading is a critical part of any intervention.

Despite developing adequate decoding and reading skills, many older children and adolescents with dyslexia continue to demonstrate problems with fluency. These difficulties can represent a considerable impediment to their being able to access challenging learning opportunities and warrant academic accommodations. These may include providing extra time and/or alternate formats for tests (e.g., oral), a quiet environment for test taking, computer assistance, books on tape or CD-ROM, and recording lectures.

Three additional recommended interventions for a child with RD deserve mention. First, because of the impact reading problems can have on a child's self-confidence, it is critically important to focus on providing positive experiences that emphasize his or her strengths, provide him or her with enjoyment, and an opportunity to shine in his or her own way. Second, medications have not been beneficial for remediating reading or learning problems per se, but can be useful in addressing comorbid attention problems. Finally, several interventions that have not received empirical support for remediating reading problems, but nonetheless continue to be promoted, should be noted. These include treatment methods aimed at simultaneously stimulating several modes of sensory input to develop better "learning patterns," early motor training, improving eye–hand coordination, eye exercises, tinted lenses, biofeedback, and special diets.

Mathematics Disorder

Mathematic computation deficits have been less frequently reported historically but have been noted for as long as reading disabilities. Overall, educators, clinicians, and researchers have devoted less time to understanding mathematics disorders (MD) than RDs. This may be due to the central place that reading plays in academics and in vocational success.

Definitional issues in the area of arithmetic disabilities, like reading disabilities, are currently an area of considerable difficulty. Consistent standards or inclusion/exclusion rules to determine the presence of an LD in math do not exist, although several general terms are in common use, such as developmental arithmetic disorder, specific math disability, as well as dyscalculia. As in RD, the assumptions that underlie these terms are intact (normally developed) language, reading, and writing skills. Although deficits in math commonly occur with other LDs, it is possible for difficulties with math computation to occur in isolation. The relationship between language and reading problems on one hand with learning mathematic concepts on the other hand is unclear. However, difficulty with reading comprehension can interfere with a child's successful completion of arithmetic problems involving reading, for example, story problems. It can also interfere with being able to obtain information from textbooks.

CLINICAL FEATURES

Competence in the area of math involves mastering basic number skills, counting, and arithmetic. Basic number skills involve learning the English number words and the correct sequence of numbers, for example, 1, 2, 3. The quantities associated with the number words and number digits must be learned, for example, two and 2 are symbols that indicate a group of any two things. In addition, children must learn to translate numbers from one form to another, for example, "twenty-two" into "22." Several other skills must be mastered including an understanding that numbers can be decomposed into smaller numbers or combined to make larger numbers. The most challenging feature of the number system is that it is based upon a base-10 structure, and it is necessary to understand this in order to master other domains in arithmetic. Generally, youths with MD do not have a basic inability in understanding or learning basic number skills.

Learning to count in order, for example, "one, two, three," is mastered by most children. Learning the concepts and rules that allow for effective and accurate counting are critical skills to develop. These basic rules include one-to-one correspondence, stable order, cardinality, abstraction, and order irrelevance, that is, items do not have to be adjacent to be counted. Research indicates that children with math disabilities in first and second grade understand the concepts of one-to-one correspondence, stable order, and cardinality as well as children without MD. However, many children with MD experience difficulty on tasks that require an understanding of the order-irrelevance principle, that is, items do not have to be adjacent to be counted.

Many children with math disabilities recall fewer basic arithmetic facts, such as $5 + 5 = 10$, and are slower retrieving the facts they do know. This pattern appears to be chronic and not one that is "outgrown." Children with MD use immature problem-solving procedures or strategies that are more commonly used by younger, typically learning

TABLE 16.6. FREQUENTLY EXHIBITED PROBLEMS IN CHILDREN WITH MATHEMATICS DISORDER

- Concentration
  - Difficulty maintaining attention to steps required for problem solving
  - Difficulty sustaining attention/concentration to instruction
- Memory/retrieval
  - Inability to retain mathematic facts
  - Difficulty counting from within a sequence
  - Forgetting steps in algorithm
  - Performing poorly on review lessons
  - Difficulty telling time
  - Difficulty solving multistep word problems
- Visual-perceptual/visual-motor
  - Losing place on page
  - Difficulty keeping numbers aligned, writing straight across page
  - Difficulty with directional aspects, e.g., up-down, left-right
  - Difficulty using number line

children. For example, when solving the problem 5 + 4, the immature approach would be to hold up nine fingers and begin counting from one. The more mature approach would be to begin with five and then add on the smaller number, for example, six, seven, eight, nine. Although a sizable number of children with MD catch up to their peers by the middle of elementary school, a subset demonstrates persisting difficulties in counting procedures throughout elementary school and sometimes later. A list of problems frequently exhibited by children with arithmetic disabilities can be found in Table 16.6.

CORE PROCESSES

Recent research has identified two problem areas in children with arithmetic disabilities: basic math processes and procedural difficulties. The problem of basic math processes affects a child's ability to learn mathematic concepts, representing concepts, and retrieving math facts. Difficulties with these processes will be expressed as slow computational speed, as well as inaccurate or inconsistent computations. Some children will use counting because they are unable to retrieve a math fact with minimal effort. The problem with mastering the procedural aspects of math will appear as difficulties with counting. The underlying processes for both of these problem areas seem to be related to working memory and executive function skills. Poor working memory skills are defined as difficulties with temporarily storing and manipulating information in order to solve a cognitive task. Executive function skills utilized in math include strategy knowledge and the ability to use working memory efficiently. Both of these have been found to be related to math disabilities.

Children with both RD and MD are more impaired on language-related tasks than are children with only single-word decoding deficits. These children have difficulty with all aspects of math, for example, learning math facts, retaining, and easily retrieving math facts. Neuropsychological studies have attempted to subtype LDs based on different patterns of performance related to patterns of academic achievement. For example, groups of children with low achievement in arithmetic relative to reading and spelling demonstrate low scores on visual-perceptual and visual-spatial measures. In contrast, their performance on measures of auditory-verbal measures are higher relative to children with low achievement in reading and spelling.

EPIDEMIOLOGY

The prevalence of MDs has been estimated to be 5% to 6% of school-aged children. No consistent evidence of gender differences in math achievement has been found and little is known of the developmental course. It does appear that a significant number of children with MDs identified in elementary school will continue to meet the diagnostic criteria several years later. Like RD, MDs appear to be chronic and persist through school. Little is known about the development and course of children with deficits only in math and not reading.

ETIOLOGY AND PATHOGENESIS

MDs have been found to be more common in some families. One study found concordance between parents and siblings to be between 40% and 66%. Other studies have also found substantial shared variance between RD and MD. It is important to note that approximately 40% to 60% of individuals with a disability in one area such as math will also have a disability in another such as reading.

Studies of either brain structure or brain function have not been carried out on children with MD. Research in adults has suggested that calculation involves the inferior prefrontal cortex in the left hemisphere as well as the angular gyrus. These areas are also involved in language.

DIFFERENTIAL DIAGNOSES AND COMORBIDITY

RD is very common in children with math disabilities. Specifically, 50% or more of children with MD will also experience difficulty learning to read. Please refer to Table 16.2 for additional common differential diagnoses. Furthermore, it is not uncommon that children with MD have difficulties on tasks requiring visual-perceptual and visual-motor integration.

TREATMENT

Much less is known about effective remediation approaches to MD as compared to RD. In large part this is because little is known about the nature and course of MD. The DISTAR Arithmetic Program has been shown to increase computational and math problem-solving skills using such approaches as teacher modeling, strategy training, direct instruction, and cooperative learning groups. A number of other techniques have also been validated for children with MD including: (a) providing demonstration, modeling, and feedback; (b) increasing fluency; (c) using concrete/abstract teaching sequence; (d) setting goals; (e) combining demonstration with permanent model; (f) using verbalization while solving problems; (g) teaching strategies for computation and problem solving; and (h) using computerized instruction.

Disorder of Written Language

No current definition of disorder of written language or disorder of written expression clearly articulates the variety of component processes necessary for adequate writing skills. Written expression is linked and likely dependent upon oral expression skills. In addition, written expression performance will not exceed reading competence in most children. However, written expression is also related to basic skills such as handwriting and spelling, as well as executive functions such as planning, self-monitoring, organizing, and perspective taking. In general, selective difficulties with psychomotor skills or spelling are not considered to be disorders of written expression.

CORE PROCESSES

Written expression is a complex activity that involves a host of cognitive and executive functions, as well as the automatization of lower level skills. Cognitive and executive functions needed include expressive vocabulary skills, general world knowledge, and planning/organizational skills. Lower level skills include the production of letters and spelling, as well as understanding rules of grammar. Additionally, other factors that can affect writing skills include motivation, speed of processing, sustained attention, and interest in and knowledge of a topic. In summary, it appears that difficulties with writing can include problems with handwriting, spelling, or the ability to express ideas through text, all of which have different underlying subcomponents. Spelling is related to phonologic analysis, knowledge of letter-sound correspondence, and single-word reading. Handwriting is related to fine motor skills, motor planning, and rapid retrieval of symbols. Finally, written expression is related to executive functioning, including working memory and language skills.

EPIDEMIOLOGY

Most children with LDs have difficulty with at least one aspect of writing, for example, handwriting, spelling, content, or form. Epidemiologic data are lacking regarding the prevalence of disorders of written language. However, given the rate of developmental language disorders and RD, deficits in written language likely affect 15% to 25% of school-aged children.

PATHOGENESIS

The number of skills necessary for the development of writing makes it likely that a large number of etiologies are possible and interact with each other. These include biologic causes, genetic, psychosocial, and environmental (including instructional variables). Difficulties with language-related skills (e.g., phonologic analysis, rapid retrieval), executive functioning (e.g., working memory), visual-spatial skills, and motor systems could each impede the development of writing skills. Component skills related to writing such as spelling and reading have been found to have significant heritability although their specificity with regards to writing is unclear.

There is limited information regarding the causes, course, prognosis, and treatment of disorders of written language. The distinction between children who demonstrate differences with motor versus idea generation may be an important clinical and research goal. Specifically, children with expressive writing difficulties that are not primarily due to language-based disorders may have different etiologic causes compared to children with language problems.

DIFFERENTIAL DIAGNOSES AND COMORBIDITY

Children with RD will invariably have difficulty with written expression as well. Common problems may involve any aspect of writing, including spelling, sentence structure, grammar, fluency, and clarity of ideas. Please see Table 16.2 for a list of common differential diagnoses for disorders of written expression. Furthermore, it is important to evaluate for the presence of visual-motor and language disorders.

TREATMENT

There are a number of intervention components that have been shown to improve the writing of children with learning disabilities. These include: (a) consistently using a basic framework of planning, writing, and revision; (b) direct instruction of the critical steps in the writing process; (c) providing consistent feedback regarding the child's writing; and (d) providing early intervention. When planning what to write, it is helpful if teachers use such techniques as semantic maps to help a child respond to questions such as "Who am I writing for?", "Why am I writing?", "What do I know?", "How do I group my ideas?", and "How will I organize my ideas?" Providing feedback of already written material is often directed at such aspects of writing as organization, punctuation, and interpretation.

Case Vignette

Case vignette #1

Tim is a 9-year-old who is in the third grade. He is brought to the pediatrician's office by his parents due to concerns regarding his behavior at home and school. Specifically, Tim has demonstrated increased difficulty with homework completion, incomplete assignments, and below average reading scores on school tests. His teacher reports that he is often off task and fails to complete assignments on time.

Tim's developmental history is unremarkable. The family history is notable for difficulty in learning to read by Tim's father, who reports he is a poor speller and does not read book-length material for pleasure, although he did graduate from college. His parents report that Tim was not interested in Dr. Seuss type books as a preschooler, did not seem to enjoy word play or rhyming, and did not learn the letters of the alphabet until the summer after kindergarten. They remarked that this was different from his older sister who was a good student. Tim's parents became concerned with his reading development in kindergarten. They reported that he was given some extra reading time at the end of first grade, which continued through second grade. His current third grade teacher has raised concerns regarding Tim's attention and activity level, as well as poor performance on reading tasks.

The pediatrician referred them for a neuropsychological evaluation. The results indicated that Tim had average cognitive skills, but that his single-word reading was slow and his accuracy was below average. Reading comprehension and written math calculations were average. Spelling and writing skills were low to below average. Tim performed below average across a number of tasks that assess skills shown to be important in the development of reading. In particular, he exhibited deficits in the area of phonemic awareness, phonemic analysis (e.g., the ability to deal explicitly and segmentally with sound units smaller than the syllable), and rapid naming. He did not demonstrate a pattern of difficulty on tasks involving speed of processing, sustained effort, inhibition, or planning. Behavioral questionnaires completed by parents and teachers highlighted concerns with learning, homework completion, and completing academic work involving reading and writing.

DISCUSSION OF VIGNETTE

Tim demonstrated several disruptive behaviors that could be suggestive of an attentional or behavioral disturbance, including clowning around when called on to read aloud, off task or inattentive behaviors, poor sustained effort with school assignments and homework, non-compliance, and anger directed at his parents regarding his school performance. Although ADHD, emotional disturbance, or parent–child problems are appropriate differential diagnoses in this case, further evaluation revealed that Tim's difficulties with reading were the cause of these other problems. Specifically, his early history of difficulty with precursors to phonologic analysis (e.g., rhyming), and the father's history of early reading and spelling problems are very important. Results from his neuropsychological testing indicated that Tim had difficulty with reading single words and decoding nonsense and unfamiliar words, as well as poor fluency and spelling. His reading comprehension, in contrast, was superior to his decoding skills when there were no time limits. Moreover, the use of standardized behavior questionnaires did not reveal a pattern of significant or pervasive inattention, impulsivity, or overactivity. Taken together, these do not support a diagnosis of ADHD.

The recommendations from the evaluation included reading interventions that are empirically validated and would include sustained and systematic instruction with an emphasis on: (a) phonemic analysis—detection of sounds that comprise words; (b) synthetic phonics—production of sounds that comprise letters and practice in blending; and (c) reading fluency—additional practice in reading.

BIBLIOGRAPHY

Aylward EH, Richards TL, Berninger VW, et al. Instructional treatment associated with changes in brain activation in children with dyslexia. *Neurology* 2003;61:212–219.

Beitchman JH, Young AR. Learning disorders with a special emphasis on reading disorders: a review of the past ten years. *J Am Acad Child Adolesc Psychiatry* 1997;36:1020–1032.

Boetsch EA, Green PA, Pennington BF. Psychosocial correlates of dyslexia across the life span. *Dev Psychopathol* 1996;8:539–562.

Denckla MB, Cutting LE. History and significance of rapid automatized naming. *Ann Dyslexia* 1999; 49:29–42.

Gertsten R, Baker S. *Teaching expressive writing to students with learning disabilities: a meta-analysis.* Eugene, OR: University of Oregon, 1999.

Grigorenko EL. Developmental dyslexia: an update on genes, brains, and environments. *J Child Psychol Psychiatry* 2001;42:91–125.

Hinshelwood J. Congential word-blindness. London: H.K. Lewis & Co. Ltd, 1917.

Kirk SA. Behavioral diagnosis and remediation of learning disabilities. In: *Proceedings of the conference on exploration into problems of the perceptually handicapped child.* Chicago: Perceptually Handicapped Children, 1963.

Kronenberg WG, Dunn DW. Learning disorders. *Neurol Clin North Am* 2003;21:941–952.

Lyon GR, Fletcher JM, Barnes MC. Learning disabilities. In: Mash EJ, Barkley RA, eds. *Child psychopathology*, 2nd ed. New York: Guilford Press, 2003:520–586.

Lyon GR, Shaywitz SE, Shaywitz BE. Specific reading disability (dyslexia). In: Behrman RE, Kliegman RM, Jenson HB, eds. *Nelson textbook of pediatrics*, 17th ed. Philadelphia, PA: WB Saunders, 2004: 110–112.

Morgan WP. A case of congential word blindness. *Brit Med J* 1896; 2:1378.

Pennington BF. Toward an integrated understanding of dyslexia: genetic, neurological, and cognitive mechanisms. *Dev Psychopathol* 1999;11:629–654.

Semrud-Clikeman M, Biederman MD, Sprich-Buckminster S, et al. Comorbidity between ADHD and LD: a review and report in a clinically referred sample. *J Am Acad Child Adolesc Psychiatry* 1992;31:439–448.

Shaywitz SE. Dyslexia. *Sci Am* 1996;275:98–104.

Shaywitz BA, Fletcher JM, Shaywitz SE. Defining and classifying learning disabilities and Attention-Deficit/Hyperactivity Disorder. *J Child Neurol* 1995;10:S50–S57.

Snowling M. Dyslexia as a phonological deficit: evidence and implications. *Child Psychol Psychiatry Rev* 1998;3:4–11.

Stuebing KK, Fletcher JM, LeDoux JM, et al. Validity of IQ-discrepancy classification of reading disabilities: a meta-analysis. *Am Educ Res J* 2002;39:465–518.

Temple E, Deutsch GK, Poldrack RA, et al. Neural deficits in children with dyslexia ameliorated by behavioral remediation: evidence from functional MRI. *Proc Natl Acad Sci USA* 2003;100:2860–2865.

Whitmore K, Hart H, Willems G, eds. *A neurodevelopmental approach to specific learning disorders.* London: Mac Keith Press, 1999.

Willcutt EG, Pennington BF. Comorbidity of reading disability and attention-deficit/hyperactivity disorder: differences by gender and subtype. *J Learn Disabil* 2000a;33:179–191.

Willcutt EG, Pennington BF. Psychiatric comorbidity in children and adolescents with reading disability. *J Child Psychol Psychiatry* 2000b;41:1039–1048.

Yin WG, Weekes BS. Dyslexia in Chinese: clues from cognitive neuropsychology. *Ann Dyslexia* 2003;53: 255–279.

SUGGESTED READINGS

Pennington BF. *Diagnosing learning disorders: a neuropsychological framework.* New York: Guilford Press, 1991.

Rayner K, Foorman, Perfetti CA, et al. How psychological science informs the teaching of reading. *Psychol Sci Pub Interest* 2001;2:31–74.

Shaywitz SE. *Overcoming dyslexia: a new and complete science-based program for reading problems at any level.* New York: Knopf, 2003.

Special Issues

CHAPTER 17

Suicidality and Youth: Identification, Treatment, and Prevention

BRENT COLLETT
KATHLEEN M. MYERS

Introduction

Few presenting complaints concern clinicians more than child and adolescent suicidality. Whether encountered in the emergency room (ER) after an attempt or in the primary care physician's office as depressed mood with passive suicidal ideation, the suffering of these youths is palpable. Clinicians are faced with difficult decisions regarding the management of these patients, such as when to recommend hospitalization, how to facilitate outpatient treatment, dealing with recurrent suicide attempts, and ameliorating the social chaos that often surrounds these youths. These decisions are taxing for even experienced physicians. All too often, they have either limited training in mental health, such as the primary care physician, or limited experience with youths, such as general psychiatrists.

In a broader sense, suicide represents a major public health concern. During the 1980s and 1990s increasing rates of suicide by youths led the Public Health Service to issue a "call to action" for suicide awareness and prevention. In addition to the loss of life, the premorbid distress experienced by suicidal youths and the costs associated with caring for those with recurrent suicidality call out for public attention.

Some authors draw parallels between suicide and self-injury enacted without intent to die, referring to these nonlethal behaviors as "parasuicide" or "suicidal gestures." Understanding these phenomena is important, as a subset of youths use self-injury to manage negative affect and/or communicate their distress to significant others. However, for the purposes of this chapter, we consider suicidality to include *preoccupations and overt behaviors enacted with intent to cause one's own death*. Although intent to die is an essential element of this definition, it is important to note that children need not have a mature concept of the finality of death or an accurate assessment of the lethality of their behavior. If youths expect that their behavior will bring about death, then that behavior should be considered a suicidal act. This conceptualization is of relevance for younger and developmentally delayed children who do not fully understand death and may engage in low lethal behaviors in a genuine attempt to kill themselves.

In this chapter, we review the salient features of child and adolescent suicidality with an emphasis on primary care physicians and general psychiatrists who often first encounter youths at risk. We delineate an approach for the assessment of suicidality and disposition of suicidal youths from the primary care or general psychiatrist's office to other services. We then review the literature on the management and treatment of suicidal ideation and attempts and the prevention of completed suicide.

Clinical Presentation and Course

Suicidality can be thought of as a continuum ranging from nonspecific or passive ideation (e.g., "Life is not worth living," "I wish I were dead"), to ideation with specific intent and/or a suicide plan, to actual suicidal behavior. Support for this view comes from research showing that most individuals who attempt suicide have had previous suicidal ideation; that it is difficult to discern patients with specific intent from those who actually attempt suicide; and that youths who are psychiatrically hospitalized for severe suicide attempts closely resemble those who complete suicide. Although this approach has been questioned, and there is some evidence that individuals who attempt suicide are distinct from those who merely think about and plan suicide, it is helpful to consider where a youth falls in this spectrum from passive suicidality to active plan or attempts when evaluating risk and determining the most appropriate interventions.

The majority (over 90%) of adolescents who commit suicide were suffering from a psychiatric disorder, usually for over 2 years. Similarly, most youths with suicidal ideation and attempts suffer from an underlying disorder, usually a mood disorder, yet most will not be referred because of their mood-related symptoms. More common scenarios involve youths presenting with changes in behavior or suicide threats that bring them to the attention of parents, teachers, peers, or the juvenile justice system. The mood disorder becomes evident upon clinical interview. Both major depression and bipolar disorder confer risk for suicide. Bipolar disorder has the highest risk for completed suicide of all psychiatric disorders due in part to the poor judgment of the manic phase as well as the despair of the depressed phase of illness. Other psychopathology that frequently co-occurs with mood disorders and seriously heightens the risk for suicide includes conduct disorders, substance use disorders, and thought disturbances or affective dysregulation due to other disturbances such as personality disorders. Overall, youths presenting with suicidality and a mood disturbance in combination with any factor that lowers the threshold for violence should be considered very high risk.

Many youths do not demonstrate clear symptoms of suicidality or even of a mood disorder, and it is only in retrospect that the cardinal symptoms were evident. Parents often describe such youths as more "moody," "closed up," not communicating, and spending long periods of time in their rooms. They may listen to suicidal and nihilistic lyrics in music. Alternatively, their school essays might demonstrate themes of death, the meaninglessness of life, despair, and feeling unconnected to others and life. Of course, many parents state that most teenagers show these symptoms and behaviors at times of stress and change. Thus, it is most important to note these problems if other aspects of the youth's life are also compromised, such as deteriorating grades or lack of peer contact.

Once the youth's underlying psychopathology has been clarified, the clinician can focus on "why now?" By the time youths come to clinical attention, they have generally been distressed for some time. Therefore, asking what brings the family to clinical attention will help to determine the potentiating risks, to identify targets for intervention, and prioritize the level of care needed. Acute precipitants include difficulties in important interpersonal relationships, real or perceived losses, legal involvement, or other disciplinary crises. Of course, youths with preexisting long-standing depression, conduct disturbances, and substance use are prone to create such crises. These crises, in turn, dangerously raise the ante for acting on suicidal impulses or for precipitating new suicidal tendencies. Therefore, such stressors should be considered in the context of a youth's psychopathology, as well as in the context of a youth's personal attributes. For example, falling out with a close friend may be less threatening for a youth who is socially skilled than for a youth who has difficulty forming and maintaining friendships. A disciplinary crisis at school may be less distressing for a youth who has a supportive family than for a youth with a blaming and conflictual family.

The course of suicidal behavior is episodic, and, thus, recurrent suicidality is common, especially when youths express such feelings so early in life. Furthermore, the best predictor of future suicidality is past suicidality. Thus, the assessment of prior suicidal ideation and attempts is critical to the determination of present risk and the needed restrictiveness of intervention. For youths who are hospitalized, it is important to ensure that adequate safety measures are taken in the period immediately following hospitalization, and again after hospital discharge, as these are times of heightened risk. Special vigilance is needed with the reemergence of new depressive symptoms.

Epidemiology

COMPLETED SUICIDE

Rates and methods

In the United States, approximately 2,000 adolescents commit suicide each year. The Centers for Disease Control (CDC) report that between 1999 and 2001, suicide was the twelfth leading cause of death (0.46 per 100,000) among children aged 13 and younger and the third leading cause of death (8 per 100,000) for those aged 14 to 18. The rate of suicide among 15- to 24-year-olds more than tripled between 1950 and 1990, but has stabilized and fallen somewhat in recent years. To put these numbers into perspective, more adolescents die of suicide than cancer, stroke, heart disease, acquired immunodeficiency syndrome (AIDS), birth defects, chronic lung disease, pneumonia, and influenza combined.

In the United States, firearms are the most common method of suicide for both sexes followed by hanging, jumping, carbon monoxide poisoning, and self-poisoning. Firearms are more often used in rural areas where guns are readily available for a variety of purposes; jumping is more prevalent in urban areas; and asphyxiation by carbon monoxide is most common in suburban areas where teens have access to a car and garage. Firearms are by far the most lethal method of suicide attempt, being 200 times more likely than drug overdose to end in death. Firearms have been found in the homes of suicide completers more often than in the homes of comparison groups, including suicide attempters. The rate of suicide by firearms has increased much faster than the suicide rate by other methods (2.5-fold versus 1.7-fold) among minors, particularly boys. Only 2% of adolescent and young male suicides are committed by ingestion. However, it is not known whether firearm ownership is an independent risk or whether it is associated with other risks for suicide. At the time that suicide by firearms among men increased dramatically in the United States, suicide also increased markedly in Europe, Australia, and New Zealand where suicide by firearms is rare. Therefore, it has been hypothesized that some other factor is operative worldwide to increase male suicides.

The proportion of suicide victims who have detectable blood alcohol levels has also risen dramatically. Youths who use firearms to kill themselves are more likely to have been drinking than those who choose other methods. Thus, the use of alcohol combined with access to firearms has emerged as the major factor differentiating completed suicides from attempts that are serious enough to warrant hospitalization.

Demographic aspects

Juvenile suicide rates increase with age, with older victims tending to show greater suicidal intent. The lower rate of completed suicide among prepubertal children has been attributed to children's "protection" against suicide by their cognitive immaturity, which may prevent them from planning and executing a lethal suicidal attempt, despite suicidal impulses. Another explanation relates to increasing risk factors, such as psychiatric and substance use disorders, in adolescence which independently increase the risk of suicide.

Suicide attempts by boys are over 100 times more likely to end in death than are attempts by girls. Thus, boys commit suicide 5 times more often that do girls. In fact, the increased rate of adolescent suicides from the 1950s to 1990s predominantly reflected suicide by boys. These data represent the greater number of nonlethal attempts by girls as well as boys' choice of more lethal and irreversible means of suicide. As boys are likely to have a disruptive behavior disorder and to be intoxicated at the time of their suicide, their impulsivity and impaired judgment may lead to the choice of more lethal methods. A prior suicide attempt is predictive of later completed suicide for both genders, but is the most potent predictor of eventual suicide by boys, followed by depression, substance abuse, and disruptive behavior. For girls, the most potent risk factor is depression, followed by a prior suicide attempt.

Culture is important. The suicide rate is higher among white versus African-American youths. However, in the 1980s and early 1990s, the rate among African-American boys rose dramatically, nearly eliminating the racial differential. African-American suicide victims tend to be from upper socioeconomic families. Thus, it has been hypothesized that greater educational and employment achievement have led to closer identification with the majority white culture, along with the erosion of some traditional protective values. Since 1994, suicide rates have been declining for both races.

Young Native American boys have an especially high suicide rate, reportedly among the highest in the world. For those ages 15 to 24, suicide rates are 2 to 3 times higher than the national average, up to 62 per 100,000. There is great variability among Native American and Alaska Native tribes. Rates appear highest within tribes that have experienced erosion of traditional culture and that have high rates of delinquency, alcoholism, and family disorganization. Data on suicide among Asian-American and Pacific Islander youths are limited, but the risk appears comparable to or lower than that of white youths. Although suicide attempts appear to be more common among Hispanic-American youths, data are equivocal with regard to the rate of suicide completions. Similarly, the rate of completed suicide for gay, lesbian, and bisexual youths is unclear.

Religion may offer protection against suicidality due to religious proscriptions, community involvement, and other beneficial effects of spirituality. However, the protective role of religion is often confounded with reductions in other risk factors, such as substance abuse and parental divorce, precluding firm conclusions.

Psychosocial factors

Psychosocial factors promoting suicide are many but rarely comprise a sufficient cause for suicide. These factors are discussed below under nonlethal suicidal behaviors.

NONLETHAL SUICIDAL BEHAVIORS

Rates and methods

It is more difficult to determine rates of nonlethal suicidal behaviors, both because suicidality is not consistently defined across studies and because there is no standardized method for collecting such information across the states. Nevertheless, some data are available from epidemiologic and clinical studies and from the state of Oregon, which nationally has the highest rate of suicide and which monitors suicide attempts.

Suicidal ideation and nonlethal suicide attempts are common and a major concern for youths at all ages. Overall, it has been estimated that each year in the United States two million adolescents attempt suicide, but only 25% ever come to medical attention, suggesting that many of these youths are missed by current systems of care. In epidemiologic samples, approximately 3% of adolescents report current suicidal ideation and 19% report a lifetime history of suicidal ideation, with up to 3 times more girls than boys reporting such ideation. In the Methods for the Epidemiology of Child and Adolescent Mental Disorders (MECA) study of 9 to 17 year olds, 5.2% of youths reported suicidal ideation and 3.3% reported having attempted suicide. Across studies, rates of suicide attempts within the prior year have ranged from 1.7% to 8.3%, and rates of suicide attempt over the lifetime have ranged from 7% to 9%.

Data for adolescents who have been hospitalized for suicidality indicate reattempt rates of roughly 6% to 15% per year with the highest risk shortly after discharge. Similarly, in community samples of youths with prior suicide attempts, 25% will reattempt suicide within 3 months after an initial attempt. Finally, postmortem data suggest that between 10% and 46% of youths who eventually complete suicide had prior suicidal behaviors. Overall, these findings indicate that suicidality is a recurrent phenomenon and increases in severity over time and with age.

Suicidal ideation is also common among prepubertal youths. In community and school samples, up to 14% of children have endorsed suicidal thoughts or acts, up to 7% have endorsed recurrent thoughts of hurting themselves and/or committing suicide, and 2% have endorsed thinking a lot about killing themselves. Approximately 1% of children report having made a suicide attempt in the past year. Furthermore, children who report suicidal ideation or make a suicide attempt are at greatly increased risk to attempt suicide during adolescence. Again, these findings suggest the importance of talking with all youths about previous suicidality. Of greater concern, such a history may not be known to caregivers who tend to be unaware of their children's subjective distress.

Self-poisoning, or overdose, is by far the most common method of nonfatal suicide attempt, followed by cutting and piercing injuries (mostly lacerations of the wrists). The method chosen varies by sex, age, and opportunity. Girls favor ingestions while boys and older attempters choose suffocation/hanging, cutting/piercing, and firearms, that is, in general more lethal methods. It should be noted that suicide attempt by unusual methods and medically serious attempts are predictive of further suicide attempts, as well as of eventual completed suicide.

Demographic aspects

There appears to be an interaction of age and gender in determining risk for attempted suicide. Nationally, girls attempt suicide 2 to 4 times more often than boys and the rate of attempted suicide increases with age. However, suicide attempts tend to peak at age 15 for girls but continue to increase with age for boys.

Etiology and Risk Factors

Although the exact etiology of suicide is unknown, multiple risk factors have been identified, as summarized in Table 17.1.

TABLE 17.1. ESSENTIAL RISK FACTORS FOR SUICIDALITY

- History of suicidality (past attempts predict future suicidality)
- Lethality of suicide attempt/medical compromise (intent)
- Psychiatric disorders (fuels suicidality)
  - Major depression
  - Bipolar disorder, depressed, or manic phase
  - Psychosis
  - Substance abuse, especially alcohol
  - Conduct disorder, especially impulsive/aggressive
- Personality traits (act on suicidal thoughts)
  - Impulsivity
  - Aggressiveness
  - Inflexibility
  - Perfectionism
  - Hopelessness
- Family factors (modeling, alienation, reduced supervision)
  - Parental suicidality
  - Parental mood disorders
  - Parental substance abuse
  - Family conflict and communication
- Acute stressors (why now?)
  - Disciplinary crises
  - Legal involvement
  - Incarceration
  - Loss events: parents, peers, romantic, prestige
  - School failure
- Access to means (decreased time to consider options)
  - Firearms, especially in rural areas
  - Other highly lethal means
  - Inadequate supervision

Note: Risk factors are cumulative in predicting suicide. Severity of risk factors is important in predicting suicide, especially severe acute stressors.

NEUROBIOLOGIC MECHANISMS

Although most research on neurobiologic mechanisms has been conducted with adults, this has relevance for youths. Neurobiologic risk factors are especially intriguing as the development of biologic markers may hone the identification of at-risk youths and lead to earlier intervention with more specific treatments.

In particular, there is great interest in markers of serotonergic function, such as the 5-HT transporter gene; the 5-HT_{1A}, 5-HT_{2A}, and 5-HT_{1B} receptors and genes; and the tryptophan hydroxylase gene. Monoamine oxidase A and its gene are also of interest. Most research supports a role for central serotonergic functioning. Less clear is whether serotonergic functioning influences suicidality directly or, alternatively, indirectly by mediating other systems such as impulsivity or mood, which also place youths at risk. Indeed, there is some evidence to suggest a common link between suicidality and the transmission of impulsive aggression. On the other hand, the clinical "activation" associated with serotonergic medications suggests a primary role for serotonin.

PSYCHOPATHOLOGY RISKS

As noted previously, most suicidal youths have a major psychiatric disorder regardless of the severity of suicidality. A psychiatric disorder increases the risk for suicide 35-fold. Most of these youths suffer from major depression, suggesting that suicidality may represent a severe variant of depression rather than a separate construct. Among adults, bipolar disorder has consistently been found to present a very high risk for suicidality, but this association has yet to be clarified for youths.

Conduct disorder also places youths at risk, in part due to the impulsivity, low threshold for violent behavior, and poor judgment observed in this population. It might also reflect these youths' recurrent disciplinary crises, peer difficulties, and social alienation. One might also speculate that these youths are more likely to have access to lethal weapons. Substance abuse, major depression, psychosis, or any interference in self-regulation, judgment, and perception confer risk for suicide. Such disturbances in the absence of clear psychiatric disorder may be observed in emerging personality disorders, particularly traits of borderline personality disorder.

INDIVIDUAL RISKS

Individual factors, such as attributional style, hopelessness, interpersonal problem solving, anger/hostility, and sexual orientation have all been found related to suicidality to varying degrees. Attributional style refers to individuals' approach to explaining negative events as due to oneself but positive events as random occurrences, and it has been associated with juvenile depression as well as suicidality. Hopelessness has been considered a risk for adult suicide. However, it is also a type of attributional style. In youths, it is unclear whether hopelessness provides a unique role in predicting suicide after accounting for its association with major depression. Poor interpersonal problem solving is also commonly observed among suicidal youths who appear to generate fewer approaches to problems than do other youths. These deficits in problem solving have been found to discriminate suicidal youths from nonsuicidal peers even after controlling for depression. It seems likely that such deficits serve to alienate these youths from their peers and prevent them from accessing social supports during times of stress. Although they do not appear to be at increased risk for suicide completion, there are some data to suggest that homosexual and bisexual youths are at increased risk for suicide attempts. It appears that this risk is mediated by other risk factors that are commonly observed in this population, such as depression, substance abuse, family history, and history of abuse. Finally, research suggests that suicidal youths have elevated levels of chronic anger and hostility, supporting the role of abnormal serotonergic function. These individual risks can be considered liabilities which are expressed during times of stress when a youth's coping resources are tested, rather than considered the primary force driving suicidality.

PSYCHOSOCIAL RISKS

Debate continues over the relative importance of psychosocial stressors in explaining suicidal behavior. Overall, there appears to be a unique role for selective life stressors, such as interpersonal losses, school problems, poor parent–child communication, and legal or disciplinary crises, in accounting for suicidal behavior. The relative contribution of these stressors may even be comparable to that of primary psychopathology. In particular, stressors such as legal and disciplinary crises provide additional "predictive value" in the assessment of suicide risk after controlling for the presence of psychiatric disorders.

Child and adolescent maltreatment of all types is associated with the development of depression and suicidality. Sexual abuse is especially prevalent among suicide attempters and increases the risk of repeated suicide attempts up to eightfold, independently of associated factors such as depression or the contextual factors under which the abuse occurred. Physical abuse also contributes to repeated suicide attempts during adolescence. A recent 18-year longitudinal study has indicated that maladaptive parenting and early maltreatment lead to profound interpersonal difficulties in middle adolescence. In turn, these interpersonal difficulties mediate the association between maladaptive parenting/abuse and suicide attempts during later adolescence and young adulthood. Children with such adverse early experiences may have difficulties in developing skills that are essential for the maintenance of healthy relationships with both adults and peers. Without these skills, youths may become interpersonally isolated, leading to suicidality when under stress. Perhaps such early adverse life experiences also account for the tendency of suicidal youths to engage in other risky behaviors.

Even in the absence of overt maltreatment, family dysfunction has consistently been identified as a salient factor in the lives of young suicide victims and attempters. Risks include lack of an intact family, depressed mothers, fathers with police or legal difficulties, and a family history of suicidal behavior. The families of suicidal youths have also been characterized as less supportive, more conflicted, and more hostile, with poor communication. Such families may also provide less supervision of their children. Family problems appear to be the major risk for prepubertal youths who attempt suicide. Suicidal adolescents have described their families as experiencing difficulties in adapting to change, problem solving, and prone to crisis, with insufficient, ineffective, or confusing communication. They also report power struggles and ineffective methods of control. Family members have been perceived as either emotionally disengaged or enmeshed, that is, lacking appropriate emotional attachment.

Another family issue relates to the increased risk conferred by a family history of suicidality, although the relative contribution of genetic mechanisms on the one hand and of social learning on the other remains unclear. Both mechanisms are almost certainly operative to some extent. Additionally, with either mechanism, part of the risk is mediated by the environmental concomitants of having a psychiatrically ill parent.

Interpersonal problems with peers have long been identified as precipitants to suicidal behaviors. In particular, conflicts with and separations from a romantic relationship play an important role as precipitants to both attempted and completed suicide. The risk may be especially poignant for boys. "Breaking up" may leave a boy with little social support, as intimacy for boys may be more restricted to a single relationship with the opposite sex, whereas girls may establish intimate and confiding relationships with same sex and opposite sex peers. More generalized social alienation also appears to pose substantial risk. Such youngsters may give the impression of "drifting" without affiliation with a school, community, or work institution.

Comment is needed regarding ecologic precipitants to suicidality. Studies of suicide "contagion" among high school students suggest that students with current major depression and those with past depression and suicidality may be the most likely to become suicidal subsequent to a peer's suicide. Furthermore, prior and current psychopathology appears to predict suicidality to a greater degree than does closeness of the relationship to the suicide victim. However, students who are close friends of a suicide victim may become suicidal at a lower threshold of psychopathology than exposed students who were not as close to a victim.

Finally, the directionality of psychosocial risks and suicidality is not always clear. The stressors leading to suicidality may be normative outcomes of uncontrollable events, such as a death in the family; alternatively, such stressors may ensue from the underlying mental disorder, for example, legal crises for conduct-disordered youths. The important issue is that the youth with a mental disorder may be faced with greater numbers of stressful events or such a youth may perceive events as more stressful.

Differential Diagnosis

Suicidality is not a disorder in its own right. Thus, a "differential diagnosis" focuses on discerning self-injurious behavior and high-risk behaviors without intent to die. Although these are clinically important differentials, such nonlethal behaviors are a concern in that they do have an association with suicidality.

As noted earlier, youths with emerging personality disturbance, highly dysregulated affect, and dissociative features often engage in self-injurious behaviors, such as cutting or burning, in an effort to manage negative affect and/or communicate distress to others but without an intent to die. They may report a sense of relief upon such injury or may acknowledge that they wanted to "get back at" a significant other for a perceived transgression. Self-injurious behaviors without suicidal intent are more likely to be highly repetitive with multiple injuries over relatively short periods of time.

High-risk behaviors such as reckless driving, frequent accidents, and running in front of vehicles must be differentiated from suicide attempts. There is some suggestion that suicidal individuals engage in endangering behavior, even at a very young age. Youths with disruptive behavior disorders put themselves in harm's way, either without consideration of the consequences or with the assumption that nothing bad will happen to them, such as driving fast, provoking police, or binging on drugs or alcohol. Open-ended questioning about such youths' assumptions regarding their intent and the expected outcome of their behavior helps to differentiate suicide from self-injurious behavior.

Assessment

The importance of the primary care physician, general psychiatrist, or other front-line clinician in assessing and preventing suicide is suggested by three factors. First, only a minority of these youths will access mental health treatment and, of those who are referred for such care, many will not receive the most effective treatments and/or will "drop out" of treatment prematurely only to resurface during crises. Second, many suicidal youths seek medical attention for factors unrelated to their suicidality in the months prior to an attempt. Third, physicians will often have contact with a child and another family member over a prolonged period of time and can, therefore, monitor behavioral and environmental changes that may suggest that a youth is at risk. Having an awareness of the factors that place youths at risk and developing a systematic approach for assessing suicidality can help to identify these patients early and prevent tragic outcomes.

METHODS OF ASSESSMENT

The basic assessment constitutes an interview with the youth and a parent. It is important to obtain information from relevant adults, not just the youth. Both sources of information are important as parents are often unaware of their child's suicidality, even previous suicide attempts. Parents may not even be aware that their child has been depressed, although they will be more aware of their children's disruptive behaviors. Youths may reveal stressors that their parents would be reluctant to share such as abuse, domestic violence, or parental psychopathology including substance abuse. Thus, it is critical to conduct an interview with the youth alone. In conducting these interviews, it is most effective to begin with broad, open-ended questions (e.g., "It sounds like you have been feeling really sad lately, how bad has it gotten?") and follow-up probes to assess specific risk factors (e.g., "Have you had any thoughts about hurting yourself?"). Questions should be posed in a developmentally appropriate manner, with attention given to the specificity, lethality, and anticipated outcomes that the youth associates with a suicide attempt. Clinicians may be reticent to ask specific questions about suicide out of fear that they will "plant ideas." However, there is no evidence that inquiring about suicidal thoughts in a clinical situation will initiate, encourage, or exacerbate suicidal behavior. Rather, such inquiry lets the youth know that he or she can safely discuss it and obtain help. Thus, simple inquiry may instill some hope. Promises of confidentiality should be avoided because the care provider may need to break such confidence in order to provide appropriate interventions. Inquiry about a youth's reasons for *not* committing suicide will reveal potential protective factors that the clinician can draw upon and will help to establish the severity of risk. Such inquiry may also steer the youth's attention to reasons for living. For some, these reasons may include religious or cultural proscriptions against suicide, fear of physical pain, knowledge of the emotional pain inflicted on loved ones, or even awareness of missing some pleasurable event in later life. These steps may also provide a brief therapeutic intervention by making suicide seem a less viable "solution" to life's problems and by instilling hope. Overall, the clinician should ascertain the type and degree of suicidality, including whether and how often the youth thinks about suicide and whether the youth ever attempted such. If suicidal ideation or recent suicidal behavior is expressed by a depressed teen, that youth should continue to be monitored while other evaluation and triage are undertaken.

Parents are better reporters of their child's "acting out" behaviors and can therefore clarify the youth's impulsivity and judgment. Young children, in particular, often have difficulty reporting the course of their symptoms over time and may struggle to identify the relationship between precipitants and the onset of their suicidality. Even though they may not be aware of the degree of their child's distress, parents can often provide insight into environmental stressors. An interview with parents also serves a preventive role as clinicians can provide information regarding risks for parents to monitor and review proactive steps such as limiting a youth's access to potential means for suicide and providing appropriate supervision. Interviewing other relevant adults, such as teachers and counselors, can also elucidate precipitants as well as sources of monitoring.

APPROACH TO TRIAGE

Despite the accumulating data regarding the risk factors for suicidality in youths, suicide prediction remains elusive. No single risk factor is pathognomic for suicide; rather, it is the interplay between the various risk and protective factors that offers the best prediction of outcomes. We propose a four-dimensional model for assessment and triage of suicidal youths. These dimensions include: (a) underlying psychopathology, (b) environmental catalysts, (c) personal skills and/or deficits, and (d) access to means. Factors relevant to these four dimensions are summarized in Table 17.2.

Psychopathology that has long gone undetected by parents and other relevant adults is present in most suicidal youths. Thus, clinicians should routinely screen for mental health problems and substance use. In particular, impulsiveness, rapid mood shifts, or thought disturbances, regardless of actual diagnosis, decrease opportunities to delay suicidal impulses and to generate options. Clinicians can then provide appropriate referral for further assessment. Follow-up is advised to ensure that patients actually access and utilize recommended mental health care.

Environmental catalysts are often given undue weight as "the reason" for a youth's suicide. Nonetheless, being aware of the effects of environmental stressors may lead to further assessment. In particular, youths with a history of maltreatment should be carefully assessed as new crises may ignite self-reproach and suicidality as fear of parental discipline recapitulates the maltreatment of earlier life. Similarly, youths in the juvenile justice system may fear rejection by their families or prolonged incarceration leading to suicide as a quick "solution" to escape their psychological distress.

Personal skills and/or deficits may attenuate or exacerbate a youth's risk and should be considered in conjunction with a youth's underlying psychopathology and environmental stressors. For example, a youth with strong religious beliefs or a close family might better

---

TABLE 17.2. ESSENTIAL ASSESSMENT OF SUICIDALITY

Underlying psychopathology
- Determining a youth's psychopathology and its severity is critical; especially look for disturbances in mood, thinking, or impulsivity, *regardless of specific diagnosis.*
- The clinical interview of the youth is the critical element in determining suicidality. The *youth should be interviewed separately from the parents* with developmentally appropriate questions, particularly to determine internalizing pathology, substance abuse, physical or sexual abuse, and self-injurious behavior.

Environmental catalysts
- Are there recent stressors at home, in school, in the community, or with peers that are beyond the youth's ability to tolerate?
- *Parents should be interviewed separately from the youth* to clarify issues at home, particularly domestic violence, parental problems, and communication.
- How aberrant are the communications between youth and parent?

Personal skills
- Can youth form an alliance to report suicidal impulses or contract for safety?
- Youth's personal attributes such as commitment to others, investment in activities, and past resilience in adversity help to determine severity of risk, as well as disposition to *less restrictive* intervention.
- Youth's personal deficits such as self-reproach, perfectionism, hopelessness, inflexibility, perceived lack of options, and social alienation help to determine disposition to *more restrictive* interventions.

Access to means
- *Both the youth and parents* should be queried about access to lethal means of harm in the home, especially firearms and their proximity to ammunition.
- The parents should be queried about access to alcohol in the home.
- Parent's ability to supervise youth physically and emotionally should be ascertained if youth is to be sent home.

survive personal loss. However, a youth who lacks the interpersonal skills needed to access social support during times of distress would be considered at greater risk than a youth who has such skills. A depressed youth with perfectionistic traits might suffer the loss of prestige poorly. A youth who is feeling hopeless may drop out of treatment. The depressed youth who turns to alcohol in times of rejection and/or discipline will likely not survive.

Access to means for suicide is becoming more important, especially for youths with decreased judgment such as those who are intoxicated or impulsive or younger children who may lack problem-solving strategies. Both children and their parents should be queried about access to firearms, knives, means for hanging, and medications or other toxic substances that may be ingested. Firearms should be explicitly addressed. Parents may assume that routine safety measures, such as locking firearms or storing ammunition and guns in separate places, will ensure safety. This is not the case. Youths frequently have greater awareness of how to access these weapons than their parents realize. Strongly encouraging other options, such as storing guns elsewhere, should be included as part of the assessment and prevention effort. However, many families living in rural communities own many firearms and use them in daily life. When the parent who owns the guns (usually the father) is not present for such discussion, it is unlikely that the firearms will be removed. Thus, other protective options within the home should also be discussed, including increased supervision.

When a youth endorses suicidal thinking or a past attempt, many clinicians obtain a "no-suicide agreement" or "no harm contract," in which the patient promises to (a) refrain from hurting him- or herself and (b) to notify a therapist, parent, or other appropriate adult if he or she feels suicidal again. A contract is useful to help identify potential future precipitants and a clear sequence of alternative behaviors that the youth can employ for future crises. It is also helpful in the assessment process to start turning the interview away from dying and toward living. The very process of defining the terms of the "no harm contract" helps the clinician to better understand the youth's desire to live or die, his or her strengths and weaknesses, and whether returning home is a reasonable disposition. It may also offer some face-saving after discharge from the office. Such "no harm contracts" comprise a community standard of care making them an appropriate intervention. Also, if the youth refuses to contract, the next step is clearly laid out, that is, hospitalization. However, such "no harm contracts" have never been subjected to scientific scrutiny and their role in actually preventing suicide is not known. The youth might not be in a mental state to accept or understand the contract, and both family and clinician must know not to relax their vigilance just because a contract has been signed. Also, the "no harm contract" is mostly used in ERs with a clinician whom the youth will never see again and with whom such a therapeutic relationship is tenuous at best. If the relationship with one's own family and friends would not deter a youth from suicide, why would a brief encounter with a clinician in the ER? Overall, the "no harm contract" seems a more therapeutic tool with a clinician who is known to and trusted by the youth, such as a front-line provider. However, it is not often used in those settings. Finally, the "no harm contract" provides no legal protection. Thus, no clinical or legal refuge can be found in negotiating a "no harm contract." Careful clinical assessment and disposition are the cornerstones to preventing suicide.

Rating scales are an efficient method for collecting information, particularly for following a youth's progress during treatment, although their relevance to non–mental health settings is unclear. Some youths are more forthcoming in revealing their level of suicidality on a rating scale than in a personal interview. Several useful scales are summarized in Table 17.3 and are more thoroughly discussed in Chapter 2. Scales assessing depression might also be helpful, and several readily available scales are presented in Chapter 10.

TABLE 17.3. RATING SCALES FOR ASSESSING SUICIDALITY

Youth Self-report Scale	Author	Ages	Purpose	Length/items
Hopelessness scale for children (HSC)	Kazdin et al., 1986	Children and adolescents	Assesses hopelessness	17 true/false items
Beck hopelessness scale (BHS)	Beck, 1993	Adults and adolescents	Assesses hopelessness	20 true/false items
The Columbia suicide screen (CSS)	Shaffer et al., 2004	Adolescents	Screens for suicidal behavior, ideation, mood, substance abuse, and risk factors	11 items
Suicidal ideation questionnaire (SIQ) and (SIQ-JR)	Reynolds, 1987	Adolescents (SIQ) and children Suicide ideation questionnaire-Jr (SIQ-JR)	Measures frequency and severity of suicidal ideation	30-item (high school) or 15-item (junior high)
Suicidal probability scale (SPS)	Cull and Gill, 1993	14 yr old and over	Clinical index of suicide risk	1 page
Reasons for living inventory for adolescents (RFL-A)	Gutierrez et al., 2000	Adolescents [adaption of Linehan's reasons for living inventory (RFL)]	Measures life-affirming, adaptive beliefs, which may distinguish suicidal from nonsuicidal youths	14 items
Child and adolescent suicide potential index	Pfeffer et al., 2000	Children and adolescents	Assesses potential for any suicidality	36 true/false items
Clinician-administered Scales	**Author**	**Ages**	**Purpose**	**Length/items**
Child suicide potential scale	Pfeffer et al., 1979	6 to 12 yr old	Assesses suicidal behaviors and risk factors	17 pages (battery of 8 scales, but first scale often used alone to assess severity)
Suicide behavior interview (SBI)	Reynolds, 1987	11 to 18 yr old	Evaluates suicide risk	4 pages, 22 items
Scale for suicide ideation (self-report version available)	Beck et al., 1979 Beck et al., 1988	Adolescents	Measures frequency, intensity, and duration of suicidal ideation	4 pages, 19 items

DISPOSITION (PSYCHIATRIC HOSPITALIZATION VERSUS OUTPATIENT TREATMENT)

Most clinicians overpredict suicide, resulting in many "false positives." This is a reasonable approach given the severe consequences of failing to identify a youth at risk. Nonetheless, this leaves critical decisions regarding the most appropriate disposition in the face of limited resources available to a family or community.

In some cases, the most appropriate disposition for a suicidal youth will be clear, and the only questions will relate to how to access resources. The depressed and/or substance abusing youth with a recent suicide attempt will require hospitalization. When a youth of the age of consent refuses hospitalization, involuntary commitment may be needed. On the other end of the spectrum, when a youth who is in mental health treatment expresses suicidal

TABLE 17.4.   TRIAGE OF SUICIDAL YOUTHS IN OUTPATIENT SETTINGS

- **Suicide attempt**
  - Hospitalize
  - Emergency room, or other emergent evaluation, if psychiatric bed not readily available or if patient does not agree to hospitalization

- **Suicidal ideation with plan or suicidal ideation with highly lethal thoughts**
  - Urgent outpatient psychiatric assessment if interim safety can be ensured
  - Parents must agree to supervise adequately and to secure lethal means of self-harm in home while awaiting urgent outpatient assessment
  - Emergent evaluation if interim safety cannot be ensured

- **Suicidal ideation without plan**
  - Routine psychiatric assessment if within reasonable time, if parental supervision is adequate, and if removal of means of self-harm ensured
  - Urgent psychiatric assessment if due to exacerbated psychiatric disorder, if routine appointment not readily available, or if parent cannot adequately supervise or secure means of self-harm

Note: "emergent" is defined as that day, as soon as possible; "urgent" evaluation is defined variably as within 48–72 h; "reasonable time" and "routine" refer to within 3 wk but also according to family's ability to safely supervise in interim.

ideation, referral back to the treating clinician may be the appropriate step; a depressed teen with mild suicidal ideation without plan or intent may be pharmacologically treated by the primary care provider. In between these extremes are multiple scenarios for which the next step is not so clear. Relevant information to gather in making a disposition includes assessment of risk factors, the severity of depression and/or a disruptive behavior or substance use, whether an attempt has been made in the past, the seriousness of past and current suicidal intent including a plan, access to means, and the physical and emotional availability of relevant adults to provide ongoing supervision. A minimal algorithm for assistance in determining disposition from the outpatient office is provided in Table 17.4.

Many clinicians will need to send the youth home while awaiting appropriate outpatient services. Discharge can be considered if the clinician is satisfied that adequate supervision and support will be available while awaiting formal outpatient treatment and that the supervising adults have rid the home of potentially lethal means.

Treatment/Interventions

Before considering specific treatments or the contexts of treatment for suicidal youths, the clinician encountering the youth in the outpatient setting should have a "game plan" or some general principles to establish a helping relationship and begin the therapeutic process. Most suicide attempters and their families benefit from straightforward interventions determined by the youth's mental status and family circumstances. Some such interventions that are easily implemented in the clinician's office are summarized in Table 17.5. Note that these in-office interventions are educational, directive, and almost prescriptive in nature, recognizing the family's need for a professional to assure them that something can be done and to jump start the process.

There have been few empiric studies of treatments for suicidal youths. In general, treatment focuses on addressing known risk factors on the aforementioned four levels: treating underlying psychiatric illnesses, family psychoeducation and conflict resolution to address environmental catalysts, ameliorating social and problem-solving deficits, and decreased access to lethal means. Also, because of the need to respond to a suicidal crisis, treatment should ideally be provided within a continuum of care that includes resources for inpatient, short- and long-term outpatient, and emergency interventions, as well as respite care and/or in-home stabilization when possible. These treatment essentials are summarized in Table 17.6.

TABLE 17.5. ESSENTIAL IN-OFFICE INTERVENTIONS

- Be aware of own ability and limitations in predicting youth's behavior, forming a therapeutic bond, and eliciting family's compliance with recommendations.
- Be aware that suicidality tends to be recurrent; therefore, establish rapport for longer term and plan for future triage and/or other referrals or interventions; have an "emergency" plan established.
- Be prepared for the tendency of suicidal youths and their families to "split" care providers and/or to present predominantly during crises.
- Considering the risk for suicide completion, educate youth and parents about the nature of suicidality in young people, particularly its relationship to psychiatric disturbance and the need for treatment of such.
- Considering the response of suicidal youths to parental difficulties and family dysfunction, educate parents about the need for minimizing harmful family environments; encourage parents to get help for themselves, if indicated.
- Obtain commitment from youth to not hurt self while awaiting further care; identify community supports such as a special peer, adult, or organization.
- Offer hope and encouragement through relationship with youth; note youth's success with past distress.
- Educate youth and parents about the disinhibiting effects of alcohol and drugs, particularly on judgment. Actively advise against the use of such substances.
- Obtain parental commitment to secure firearms and other means of harm.
- Obtain parental commitment to provide appropriate supervision.
- Obtain parental commitment to obtain mental health care for youth.
- Determine that appointment for mental health care has been made *and kept.*
- Consider pharmacotherapy, especially if ongoing mental health care is delayed; especially relevant for rapid mood swings or psychosis.

TREATMENT OF UNDERLYING PSYCHIATRIC ILLNESS

Treatment of underlying psychopathology is the most obvious locus for intervention. The reader is directed to the relevant chapters throughout this text for detailed information regarding the treatment for child and adolescent psychiatric disorders, particularly depressive disorders (see Chapter 10), substance use disorders (see Chapter 6), and conduct disorder (see Chapter 5). As most recommended treatments increasingly include both pharmacologic and psychotherapeutic components, this often means that suicidal youths are treated by a team of clinicians, due to the dearth of child and adolescent psychiatrists. Primary care physicians will frequently find themselves addressing pharmacologic needs, while mental health clinicians provide psychotherapy. There are many advantages to such an interdisciplinary approach as these youths can be taxing for caregivers. However, ongoing communication among providers is vital to ensure that all team members are aware of the treatment plan and able to reinforce one another's efforts. Special care must be taken to avoid "splitting" by suicidal youths and their families. "Splitting" is a maladaptive defense

TABLE 17.6. TREATMENT ESSENTIALS FOR SUICIDAL YOUTHS

- Identification and development of a continuum of interventions including use of emergency room, crisis services, inpatient unit, outpatient services, "wrap around" services, and respite care
- Development of a treatment team that includes various providers: primary care provider, primary mental health clinician, child and adolescent psychiatrist, school counselor, and other clinicians as needed and available
- Active diagnosis and aggressive treatment of psychiatric illness
- Individual therapies emphasizing the development of problem-solving skills and impulse control, cognitive-behavioral therapies, and dialectical behavior therapy
- Development of family and community resources; emphasize community supports for youths with psychiatrically compromised parents or from unsupportive homes
- Family interventions emphasizing the development of nonviolent conflict resolution skills
- "Harm reduction" through modifications of stressful life obligations such as school schedule

in which the individual, and/or family, perceives one provider as "all good" and the other as "all bad." At such times, patients and families place blame on one clinician and then another creating turmoil as the patient and family feel abandoned, poorly treated, or otherwise distressed. It is important to not be drawn into this dynamic, but rather to pull together to alter the treatment plan so as to provide optimal care.

Psychotherapeutic treatments vary depending on the underlying psychopathology, and they are discussed in more detail in other relevant chapters. For depressive disorders this generally includes some form of cognitive-behavioral therapy (CBT) or interpersonal therapy (IPT) augmented by family therapy and pharmacotherapy as needed. For substance use disorders, enrollment in outpatient substance use programs is the recommended approach, although sometimes inpatient stabilization is needed first. For conduct disorders, a behavioral and/or community approach is advocated, such as multisystemic therapy (MST). Psychotic disorders, as occur with schizophrenia and sometimes bipolar disorder, are generally only amenable to supportive interventions until the core symptoms are contained with medications.

A few comments are warranted regarding pharmacologic treatment of depressive disorders, particularly with selective serotonin reuptake inhibitors (SSRIs). This issue is reviewed in Chapter 22 and will be briefly addressed here with focus on the SSRIs' alleged ability to precipitate suicidal impulses. The Food and Drug Administration (FDA) recently mandated labeling on antidepressants regarding the risks of suicidal impulses associated with these medications. However, this issue is complex. It appears that approximately 3% of youths treated with SSRIs compared with 1% of placebo-treated youths develop new onset suicidal thinking. However, other work has recently shown that about 12% of medication-naive youths treated with psychotherapy alone also develop new onset suicidal thinking, attributed to the "activation" due to recovery from the depression. Thus, suicidal thinking and impulses are often part of the depressed state and/or can be precipitated as youths pull out of their depression, whether "activated" by spontaneous resolution of the depression, psychotherapy, or medication. Thus, it is not yet clear whether the suicidality associated with the use of SSRIs during juvenile depression is directly due to these medications.

On the other hand, one needs to consider that the SSRIs have shown only modest effectiveness in treating depression, better with adolescents than with children. Furthermore, even for those youths who do respond, only partial resolution of symptoms has been reported and placebo-response rates are very high. Furthermore, most of the published studies enrolled youths with mild-to-moderate depression, the severity range most likely to show placebo response. Thus, although published studies do suggest effectiveness of SSRIs over placebo, the benefits are not robust. Thus, the SSRIs' modest benefits together with their potential to precipitate active suicidal thinking may pose a high cost/benefit ratio, at least for mild-to-moderate depression. For youths with serious depressions, and especially those who have not responded adequately to psychotherapy, less is known and the cost/benefit ratio may be more favorable.

Thus, in clinical practice most youths should be enrolled in psychotherapy first, with medication reserved for those youths who do not respond well to psychotherapy. However, for youths who are seriously depressed, combined treatment still appears most appropriate. Interestingly, more severely depressed youths are also more likely to benefit from antidepressant treatment. In cases for which antidepressant treatment is elected, especially with the SSRIs, careful consent with the youth and parent should be obtained, regular monitoring should be instituted, and vigilance for suicidality explicitly addressed, as it is likely that serotonergic "activation" of the SSRIs can place some youths at risk.

The situation differs for youths with bipolar disorder or psychotic disorders. Even in the absence of clear treatment algorithms, pharmacotherapy will be essential for most such youths to control lethal impulsivity, rapid mood shifts, and idiosyncratic thinking. Such youths are more likely to need hospitalization and subsequent intensive monitoring.

FAMILY PSYCHOEDUCATION AND CONFLICT RESOLUTION

Adolescent suicide attempts occur most frequently during the late afternoon/evening between school and bedtime, a time that may be unstructured and/or unsupervised. When social support is increased, suicide-risk behaviors and even depression decrease. Focused awareness and supervision are especially important after precipitants such as family fights and increased parent–child discord as these are common precipitants for suicide and suicidal behaviors, especially among girls. Increased supervision is an easy intervention to recommend in any clinician's office, particularly for at-risk youth for whom parents are motivated to make changes at home.

Similarly, this is a good time to recommend lowering openly expressed conflict at home. The concept of "high expressed emotion" is likely applicable for suicidal youths, as it is for depressed and psychotic youths. Families that express high rates of negative emotion, blaming others, and discounting one another greatly impact already depressed youths, resulting in higher levels of needed care, often due to intensification of suicidal impulses. Thus, another psychoeducational recommendation that can easily be made in the office is for families to better contain their conflict. While psychotherapy may be advisable, many of these families will not pursue such services. However, they might be willing to make other changes when the home is linked to the youth's welfare.

Remediation of social and problem-solving deficits

Suicidal youths tend to have difficulty in problem solving, especially generating alternatives to suicide as a means to solve their life problems. Thus, many research endeavors and evidence-based programs focus on practical skills such as improving problem solving and teaching social skills, especially for youths who are at risk for dropping out of school. Core components of such programs include regular monitoring of mood, school behaviors, and drug use, as well as skills training in four areas: self-esteem enhancement, decision making, personal control (anger, depression, stress management), and interpersonal communication. Other programs include key elements of peer group and teacher support, monitoring, and skills training, generally over short-term group or individual sessions. Some programs also involve family interventions (family support, family goals met, and family distress/conflict). Such programs have found success in decreasing suicide-risk behaviors and emotional distress with the most efficacious components appearing to be reinforcing personal skills such as increased personal control and problem-solving coping.

There is one psychotherapy that has been developed specifically to help suicidal and self-harming patients improve their skills at self-management. Marsha Linehan at the University of Washington has developed dialectical behavior therapy (DBT), which addresses the core deficits in suicidal patients, such as underlying psychiatric illness, psychoeducation, and conflict resolution to contain potential environmental catalysts, amelioration of social and problem-solving deficits, and decreased access to means of suicide. DBT was originally developed for suicidal adults, although child and adolescent mental health professionals are increasingly adapting the model with youths. In brief, DBT is a structured psychotherapy that incorporates features of CBT with philosophies and strategies related to Eastern practices, such as acceptance and mindfulness. The basic hypothesis underlying this approach is that suicidal patients show a core deficit in emotion regulation. Interventions are utilized to address a hierarchy of therapeutic needs including reduction of suicidal and self-injurious behaviors, reduction of behaviors that interfere with therapy, enhancement of quality of life and reasons for living, and building interpersonal skills. DBT is an intensive, multimodal, team-based approach, which includes individual therapy and group therapy to facilitate skills training. There is also recognition of the high demand that these patients place on clinicians, and consultation groups are used to reduce therapist burnout. There is a solid research base supporting DBT with adults, and an evidence base with adolescents is forthcoming. Some other therapies have adapted components of DBT into their curricula.

Means restriction

Restricting access to easy means of suicide is an ecologic intervention that may be the most economic and most effective means of suicide prevention. As noted previously, the most common means of suicide among young people is firearms, particularly among impulsive youths or those abusing alcohol or drugs. There has been increasing effort to educate the public in general, and parents of at risk youths in particular, about the danger of having firearms at home. The American Academy of Pediatrics has sponsored a campaign to educate pediatricians of the need to ask about firearms at home and to educate families about firearm safety as part of routine pediatric practice. At a minimum, routine safety measures and appropriate storage of firearms should be recommended, that is, suggesting locking firearms, storing weapons unloaded, and keeping guns and ammunition in separate locations. For acutely suicidal youths, recommending storage of weapons outside of the home is warranted. However, families show low compliance with such a recommendation, even when they are compliant with other safety recommendations. Education should include a variety of firearm storage options that are directed specifically at the parent who is the primary gun owner, usually the father. Other recommendations might focus on removing potentially toxic substances and knives and other potential instruments for cutting and piercing. Removal of alcohol may also decrease risk. Given that it is unlikely that families will be able to remove all potentially dangerous means for suicide, perhaps the most important recommendation is to increase parental supervision.

Suicide Prevention

As part of the United States Healthy People 2000 and 2010 campaigns, former Surgeon General, David Satcher, M.D., called for a public health approach to reducing suicide. In response, multiple grassroots movements have developed on both the state and local levels. Programs such as the Suicide Prevention Advocacy Network have brought relatives of suicide victims together with academic and governmental institutions to educate policy makers of the need for a national suicide prevention initiative. Many communities have initiated educational activities to increase awareness of suicide and its prevention. As these public health and community movements indicate, the prevention of suicide incorporates a continuum of approaches which can be classified as *universal programs* that benefit the general population, *selective programs* that target at risk populations, and *indicated programs* that focus on high-risk individuals.

The Centers for Disease Control and Prevention (CDC) has responded to the increasing suicide rate and communities' concerns by identifying a series of prevention strategies with the assumption that effective prevention will need to incorporate several different strategies simultaneously. These strategies fall into two conceptual categories: (a) those designed to increase recognition of youths at risk and facilitate referral to mental health services, and (b) those designed to address risk factors. The major strategies outlined by the CDC (discussed below) include educational, screening, and peer support programs;

school and community gatekeeper training; crisis services/hotlines; and interventions after a suicide to prevent "contagion."

EDUCATIONAL, SCREENING, AND PEER SUPPORT PROGRAMS

Many supportive strategies have focused on increasing knowledge about suicide warning signs and mental health referral sources, as well as participation in programs that educate youths about helpful and harmful ways of coping with stress and/or suicidal ideation. Such programs tend to conceptualize suicidality as a normative response to stress. However, the proportion of youths who would ask a teacher, counselor, or parent about how to contact a mental health professional outside of school and the proportion of youths who indicate they know how to get help outside of school does not seem affected by such programs. Nonetheless, there is some suggestion that such programs do help youths to decrease reliance on social withdrawal as a response to stress and thus engage in less wishful thinking, less blaming others, and decreased hopelessness.

More recent efforts at educational programs have emphasized the need to link suicide with mental health problems rather than presenting suicide as a normative response to stress. When this link is made, more young people appear willing to seek help from an adult if a peer was thinking about suicide, to seek help from a friend if they had thoughts of self-harm, or to seek help from a mental health professional. Also, more youths endorse understanding the association between suicide and mental health concerns. The downside is that youths who are at greatest risk, that is, those who view suicide as a solution to problems, may not change their view after these universal school-based interventions. The overall impression is that such programs need to state clearly that suicidal behavior is a symptom of mental health problems that can be effectively treated.

SCHOOL AND COMMUNITY GATEKEEPER TRAINING

Several programs over the last decade have focused on increased gatekeeper training efforts, typically in conjunction with other prevention strategies. Several types of gatekeeping have been explored. Many programs have focused on training students in the schools on the premise that youths who are suicidal are more likely to talk to a peer than to a parent or other adult. These programs also have the intuitive and nonstigmatizing appeal of conceptualizing suicide as a response to stress, rather than focusing on suicide as a sign of mental illness. Thus, these programs aim to increase awareness of suicide as a problem and to teach students, teachers, and parents how to recognize youths who might be at risk and refer them to appropriate resources. However, more recent investigators have questioned the efficacy and cost-effectiveness of these brief, universal, school-based, general education programs, particularly those that present suicide as a response to normal adolescent stressors rather than as an indication of serious emotional distress. Instead, they argue for a case-finding approach that would identify youths with emotional problems and facilitate their referral to mental health services. This approach has also emphasized the importance of focusing prevention efforts on very high-risk adolescent boys who have made a previous suicide attempt or who are depressed.

Overall, school-based suicide prevention programs continue to be controversial. This is because many still follow a stress-related model, assume a universal rather that an indicated prevention approach, and assess changes in attitudes rather than actual suicide-related behaviors. Other approaches have been explored.

More comprehensive gatekeeper training programs have been developed as part of comprehensive suicide prevention initiatives in the United States, Canada, and Australia.

These programs generally consist of several stages with public education, gatekeeper training for adult educators and/or caregivers, and enhancements to existing crisis services. Generally, gatekeeper training of both youths and adults is highly effective in increasing public awareness about suicide prevention, gatekeepers' knowledge of suicide warning signs and competencies in assessing suicide risk, and their ability and readiness to initiate prevention steps. Furthermore, such increased knowledge and capability by the gatekeepers appear to be sustained over several months. However, other aspects of training gatekeepers are more challenging. For example, facilitating access to youth-friendly crisis services has proven difficult due to limited funding and high utilization of existing services. There may also be difficulties related to families following through with recommended services.

SUICIDALITY IN THE EMERGENCY ROOM

ER staff may also be considered gatekeepers as they provide an important role in case finding, risk assessment, and disposition. ER staff also provide clinical interventions geared to de-escalating the crisis, making safety plans, and/or referring for acute services. Surprisingly, despite the frequent presentation of youths to the ER for acute care following suicide attempts, and their risk for repeated attempts and completed suicide, prevention efforts in the ER have not been well examined. This is a particularly difficult population to study as they frequently fail to keep appointments scheduled at the time of the suicide gesture.

One intervention termed "Successful Negotiation Acting Positively" (SNAP) has shown preliminary success in engaging families in follow-up treatment and in decreasing their distress. Success appears related to engaging the families when they present to the ER. This first stage of the two-part intervention includes training ER staff and having parents and teens view an educational video aimed at increasing their understanding about youth suicide, the need for treatment, and what to expect from treatment. Additionally, an on-call therapist works with the family while in the ER and helps with their transition to outpatient treatment. This ER intervention has shown effectiveness in decreasing youths' depression and suicidal ideation, improving families' participation in follow-up treatment, and fostering in mothers a positive attitude regarding treatment.

The second component is a six-session CBT for working with suicidal youths and their families. It is designed to increase positive feelings and problem-solving skills among family members while also demonstrating that therapy can be helpful so that these families will seek help again when problems arise. Both suicidal teens and their mothers have reported lower levels of depression and decreased distress 18 months after participation in SNAP. However, the SNAP program has not yet been fully evaluated, and more information is needed regarding such early interventions in the ER when youths are most symptomatic and motivated for care.

Conclusions

Suicide among young people is a serious psychiatric problem of growing concern for both children and adolescents. Even suicidal behaviors without completion confer great morbidity and interfere with the quality of young people's lives. Suicidality is a complex, multifaceted, and multidetermined problem with roots at the neurobiologic, psychodynamic, family, and societal level. While these multiple sources of difficulty may seem overwhelming, they also provide multiple points for intervention. The outpatient clinician may provide the first intervention point by identifying suicidality, appropriately triaging the youth to services, by participating in the youth's care as part of a treatment team, and by providing a safe haven when things go awry.

Treatment is multifaceted, often with a team of clinicians. Overall, it is important to minimize the family's "splitting" of the treatment team by these challenging families so that team members can work together effectively and not "burn out." Treatment may evolve through different stages depending on the acuity and recurrence of suicidality, moving from more restrictive and intensive interventions to customary outpatient care as safety allows. Treatment generally combines psychotherapy and pharmacotherapy geared to the under-lying psychopathology, remediating problem-solving deficits, building interpersonal skills, and containing family dysfunction. Until more evidence-based interventions are available, community standards of care are utilized.

AVAILABILITY OF SCALES ASSESSING SUICIDALITY

Beck A. *Beck Hopelessness Scale (BHS) manual*, Psychological Corporation, 555. San Antonio, TX: Academic Court, 1993:78204–72498; 1-800-211-8378; www.psychcorp.com; or available through The Beck Institute at beckinst@gim.net.

Beck AT, Kovacs M, Weissman A. Assessment of suicidal intention: The Scale for Suicide Ideation. *J Consult Clin Psychol* 1979;47:343–352; Available through The Beck Institute at beckinst@gim.net.

Beck AT, Steer RA, Ranieri WF. Scale for suicide ideation: psychometric properties of a self-report version. *J Clin Psychol* 1988;44:499–505; Available through The Beck Institute at beckinst@gim.net.

Cull JG, Gill WW. *Suicide Probability Scale (SPS) manual*. Los Angeles, CA: Western Psychological Services, 1993; 12031 Wilshire Blvd. Los Angeles, CA 90025-1251. (800) 648–8857; www.wpspublish.com.

Gutierrez PM, Osman A, Kopper BA, et al. Why young people do not kill themselves: the reasons for living inventory for adolescents. *J Clin Child Psychol* 2000;29:177–187; The RFL-A is available through Augustine Osman PhD, Department of Psychology, University of Northern Iowa, 334 Baker Hall, Cedar Falls, IA 50614-0505; augustine.osman@uni.edu.

Kazdin AE, Rodgers A, Colbus D. The Hopelessness Scale for Children: psychometric characteristics and concurrent validity. *J Consult Clin Psychol* 1986;54:241–245; The HSC is available through Alan E. Kazdin, Ph.D., Child Study Center, Yale University School of Medicine, 230 S. Frontage Road, New Haven, CT 06520-7900; Phone (203) 785-5759; Fax (203) 785-7402; alan.kazdin@yale.edu.

Pfeffer CR, Conte HR, Plutchik R, et al. Suicidal behavior in latency age children: an empirical study. *J Am Acad Child Psychiatry* 1979;18:679–692; The *Child Suicide Potential Scale (CSPS)* are available through Cynthia R Pfeffer MD, Department of Psychiatry, Weill Medical College of Cornell University, New York Presbyterian Hospital, 21 Bloomingdale Road, White Plains, NY 10605; cpfeffer@med.cornell.edu.

Pfeffer CR, Jiang H, Kakuma T. Child-Adolescent Suicidal Potential Index (CASPI): a screen for risk for early onset suicidal behavior. *Psychol Assess* 2000;12:304–318; The *CASPI* is available through Cynthia R Pfeffer MD, Department of Psychiatry, Weill Medical College of Cornell University, New York Presbyterian Hospital, 21 Bloomingdale Road, White Plains, NY 10605; cpfeffer@med.cornell.edu.

Reynolds WM. *Suicidal Ideation Questionnaire (SIQ): professional manual*. Odessa, FL: Psychological Assessment Resources, Inc 1987, 16204 N. Florida Avenue, Lutz, FL 33549, 1-813-968-3003; www.parinc.com; *the Suicide Behavior Interview* is available through William Reynolds PhD at Humboldt State University; wr9@humboldt.edu.

Shaffer D, Scott M, Wilcox H, et al. The Columbia Suicide Screen: validity and reliability of a screen for youth suicide and depression. *J Am Acad Child Adolesc Psychiatry* 2004;43:71–79; The CSS is a available through David Shaffer MD, Department of Child Psychiatry, New York State Psychiatric Institute, Columbia University, 1051 Riverside Drive, Unit 78, New York, NY 10032; shafferd@childpsych.columbia.edu.

BIBLIOGRAPHY

Brent DA. Risk factors for adolescent suicide and suicidal behavior: mental and substance abuse disorders, family environmental factors, and life stress. *Suicide Life Threat Behav* 1995;25:52–63.

Brent D, Baugher M, Birmaher B, et al. Compliance with recommendations to remove firearms in families participating in a clinical trial for adolescent depression. *J Am Acad Child Adolesc Psychiatry* 2000;39:1220–1225.

Brent D, Bridge J, Johnson B, et al. Suicidal behavior runs in families. A controlled family study of adolescent suicide victims. *Arch Gen Psychiatry* 1996;53:1145–1152.

Brent DA, Perper JA, Goldstein CE, et al. Risk factors for adolescent suicide. A comparison of adolescent suicide victims with suicidal inpatients. *Arch Gen Psychiatry* 1988;45:581–588.

Brent DA, Perper JA, Moritz G, et al. Firearms and adolescent suicide. A community case-control study. *Am J Dis Child* 1993;147:1066–1071.

Brown J, Cohen P, Johnson JG, et al. Childhood abuse and neglect: specificity of effects on adolescent and young adult depression and suicidality. *J Am Acad Child Adolesc Psychiatry* 1999;38:1490–1496.

Centers for Disease Control. Suicide among black youths, United States youth suicide fact sheet. *MMWR Morb Mortal Wkly Rep* 1998;47:193–196.

Gould MS, Greenberg T, Velting DM, et al. Youth suicide risk and preventive interventions: a review of the past 10 years. *J Am Acad Child Adolesc Psychiatry* 2003;42:386–405.

Johnson JG, Cohen P, Gould MS, et al. Childhood adversities, interpersonal difficulties, and risk for suicide attempts during late adolescence and early adulthood. *Arch Gen Psychiatry* 2002;59:741–749.

King CA, Segal H, Kaminski K, et al. A prospective study of adolescent suicidal behavior following hospitalization. *Suicide Life Threat Behav* 1995;25:327–338.

King RA, Schwab-Stone M, Flisher AJ, et al. Psychosocial and risk behavior correlates of youth suicide attempts and suicidal ideation. *J Am Acad Child Adolesc Psychiatry* 2001;40:837–846.

Lewinsohn PM, Rohde P, Seeley JR. Psychosocial risk factors for future adolescent suicide attempts. *J Consult Clin Psychol* 1994;62:297–305.

Lewinsohn PM, Rohde P, Seeley JR. Adolescent suicidal ideation and attempts: prevalence, risk factors, and clinical implications. *Clin Psychol Sci Pract* 1996;3:25–46.

Lieb K, Zanarini MC, Schmahl C, et al. Borderline personality disorder. *Lancet* 2004;364:453–461.

Linehan MM. *Cognitive-behavioral treatment of borderline personality disorder.* New York: Guildford Press, 1993.

Mann J, Brent DA, Arango V. The neurobiology and genetics of suicide and attempted suicide: a focus on the serotonergic system. *Neuropsychopharmacol* 2001;24:467–477.

Office of Disease Prevention and Health Promotion. *Healthy People 2000: National health promotion and disease prevention objectives.* Rockville MD: Department of Health and Human Services, 1992: 634–666. www.healthypeople.gov/Publications/

Office of Disease Prevention and Health Promotion. *Healthy People 2010: Mental health and mental disorders. Objectives for improving health. Part B: Focus Area 18.* Rockville MD: Department of Health and Human Services, 2003: 3–33. www.healthypeople.gov/Publications/

Olfson M, Shaffer D, Marcus SC, et al. Relationship between antidepressant medication treatment and suicide in adolescents. *Arch Gen Psychiatry* 2003; 60:978–982.

Pfeffer CR, Klerman GL, Hurt SW, et al. Suicidal children grow up: rates and psychosocial risk factors for suicide attempts during follow-up. *J Am Acad Child Adolesc Psychiatry* 1993;32:106–113.

Rotheram-Borus MJ, Piacentini J, Cantwell C, et al. The 18-month impact of an emergency room intervention for adolescent female suicide attempters. *J Consult Clin Psychol* 2000;68: 1081–1093.

Shaffer D, Craft L. Methods of adolescent suicide prevention. *J Clin Psychiatry* 1999;60:70–74.

Shaffer D, Gould M, Hicks RC. Worsening suicide rate in Black teenagers. *Am J Psychiatry* 1994;151: 1810–1812.

Sorenson SB, Shen H. Youth suicide trends in California: an examination of immigrant and ethnic group risk. *Suicide Life Threat Behav* 1996;26: 143–154.

Thompson EA, Eggert LL, Randell BP, et al. Evaluation of indicated suicide risk prevention approaches for potential high school dropouts. *Am J Public Health* 2001;91:742–752.

Trautman PD, Stewart N, Morishima A. Are adolescent suicide attempters noncompliant with outpatient care? *J Am Acad Child Adolesc Psychiatry* 1993;32:89–94.

Velez CN, Cohen P. Suicidal behavior and ideation in a community sample of children: maternal and youth reports. *J Am Acad Child Adolesc Psychiatry* 1988;27:349–356.

Verona E, Sachs-Ericsson N, Joiner TE Jr. Suicide attempts associated with externalizing psychopathology in an epidemiological sample. *Am J Psychiatry* 2004;161:444–451.

Wallace L, Calhoun A, Powell K, et al., Homicide and suicide among native americans, 1979–1992. *Centers for disease control and prevention, national center for injury prevention and control: violence surveillance summary series, No. 2.* Atlanta GA: CDCP, 1996. ohcinfo@cdc.gov

CHAPTER 18

Violence by Children and Adolescents

KAY M. REICHLIN

Introduction Violent behavior in children and adolescents is not a diagnosis but rather a behavior with multiple determinants. It has become much more common in the last century in the United States. Some aggressive behaviors, such as temper tantrums, playground scuffles, and shoving matches, are minor or self-limited and often do not require attention outside the family. However, if such behaviors are frequent and lasting, families may seek help from pediatricians, family practitioners, counselors, and mental health professionals. The continuum of care includes outpatient treatment, foster placement, residential treatment, and hospitalization. Severe violence is a much more rare event but one that must be studied in order to prevent it as much as possible. The most severe forms of violence are addressed through court proceedings and possibly incarceration. Thus, violence may bring great suffering and financial cost to individuals, families, and society.

HISTORIC NOTES

Violent behavior by children and adolescents has been a significant concern for some time. The first juvenile court in the United States was started in Chicago in 1899. The child guidance clinic movement began in the 1920s with a model of collaboration by psychologists, psychiatrists, and social workers. Specialized child psychiatry training began in the 1940s. Aggressive behavior has been one of the most frequent reasons for seeking psychiatric care as it can result from a number of disorders and conditions. Violent behavior often falls on the cusp between mental health treatment and legal consequences.

Juvenile detention centers and correctional facilities have grown in most states in recent years due to a prevailing attitude in legislatures and among voters to hold individuals of younger ages more accountable for criminal behavior. These facilities, which had a focus on child welfare and rehabilitation in past decades, have moved in the direction of jails. In the past, juveniles were handled in juvenile court unless they were mature enough and the crime serious enough that they were remanded to adult court. By the mid 1990s, over half the states had passed laws that automatically remanded juveniles to adult court for certain serious crimes. According to the United States Bureau of Justice statistics, by 1997 the courts had sentenced 7,400 juveniles to adult prisons and 2% to 3% of death sentences were given to juveniles. Although the frequency of violent juvenile crime has been falling since that time, the more punitive trend may result in hardening of the youthful offender rather than rehabilitation as it may repeat the very experiences that contributed to his or her violence in the first place: abuse, coercive discipline, and lack of appropriate nurturing or positive socialization. In time, the pendulum may again swing toward a more rehabilitative model of justice. Prevention strategies, requiring early intervention to help children at risk for developing a long-standing problem with violence, should be tried.

Clinical Presentation and Clinical Course

The clinical course of aggressive behavior in the child or adolescent depends in large part on its root causes. Aggressive or violent behavior can be a symptom of mental disorder such as mood disorder, psychotic disorder, intermittent explosive disorder, attention deficit hyperactivity disorder (ADHD), or posttraumatic stress disorder (PTSD). In mood disorders, general impulsiveness and irritability can erupt into violence. In psychotic disorders, violence may result from paranoia, delusions, disorganization of thought process, or misperceptions. ADHD, intermittent explosive disorder, and pervasive developmental disorder involve impulsiveness and poor frustration tolerance, often resulting in aggression. PTSD can cause irritability, misperceptions, and flashbacks that can cause the individual to strike out. Anything that alters thought processes or normal functioning can result in violence. Such alterations occur most notably with intoxication with substances and in medical illnesses that can cause delirium or psychosis. Methamphetamine and phencyclidine (PCP), in particular, have been associated with severe aggressive behavior. Intoxicants such as alcohol, cocaine, and marijuana seriously affect judgment and impulse control. Medical conditions which affect frontal lobe functioning, whether traumatic, infectious, or metabolic, result in decreased impulse control and/or judgment and can contribute to aggressive behavior. Static organic impairments, such as low intellectual functioning and, more rarely, seizure disorders and interictal states, can contribute to violent episodes.

Violence can also occur without concomitant mental disorders in retaliation, in self-defense, or in pursuit of a particular goal or outcome, for example, attacking someone in order to steal a purse. Gang violence is sometimes of this type when directed outside the gang.

There is also intra-gang violence in which physical aggression is used to initiate gang members and to enforce gang hierarchy and cooperation. Youths who are attracted to gangs tend to be disaffected from society, to be from dysfunctional or abusive backgrounds, and to do poorly in school. Membership in a gang may then provide a sense of belonging and structure so as to make school and personal failures seem irrelevant.

Adult antisocial behavior has usually been established as a pattern by late adolescence, but not all antisocial children become antisocial adults. Factors that mitigate continuance into adulthood are good parental and school involvement and a positive peer group. In *Deviant Children Grown Up; A Sociological and Psychiatric Study of Sociopathic Personality*, Lee Robins described a very long-term follow-up study of 524 juveniles referred to a St. Louis clinic and 100 age-, sex-, and demographically matched controls regarding antisocial behavior, mental illness, and adjustment in adulthood. The referrals occurred in the late 1920s, and the follow-up was completed from 1955 to 1966. Twenty-eight percent of the juveniles referred for antisocial behavior were diagnosed as having sociopathic personality in adulthood. By comparison, if the referrals had been for any other reason, the follow-up rate of sociopathy was 4%. Rate of sociopathy was higher in those who had police contact in childhood than in those who did not. Follow-up found that 16% of the children with antisocial behavior had no disorder in adulthood, but 11% had psychoses, 14% neuroses, and 23% had some undiagnosed (presumably mental) illness. In contrast to sociopathy, rates for mental disorders in adulthood were not appreciably different between the clinic population and control group. Sociopathy tended to decrease after a median age of 35.

With respect to mortality in 2000, the United States Bureau of Justice statistics reported a juvenile homicide rate of 9.3 per 100,000 population in the 14- to 17-year-old group and 27.3 per 100,000 population in the 18- to 24-year-old group. In the same year, homicide was the second highest cause of death in the 10- to 19-year-old group. Property crimes and other violent crimes involving juveniles as either offender or victim continued a decreasing trend through 2002. Between 1993 and 1999, about 7% to 8% of high school students were victims of violent crimes at school. In 1999, 7% of students surveyed reported carrying a weapon on school property in the preceding month. Since then, "zero tolerance" policies of schools may have decreased the frequency of carrying weapons. Students who use drugs are more likely to be involved in crimes as both victim and offender.

Epidemiology

The United States has a higher prevalence of violent crime than other countries. The rate of violent crime among juveniles increased rapidly from 1987 to 1994 and has been decreasing since then. Despite the overall decrease in the past 10 years, multiple victim school shootings not associated with gang violence have increased. These events, such as the Thurston High School shootings in May 1998 and the Columbine High School shootings in April 1999 and their media coverage have shocked and frightened parents, teachers, and students alike.

In most species including humans, males are the perpetrators of aggression most of the time. In the aforementioned 524 referrals to the St. Louis clinic in the 1920s, just over three fourths of both sexes had demonstrated antisocial behavior, but boys were referred for antisocial behavior about 2.5 times as often as girls. For this reason, several recent studies have included only boys. However, if the type of aggression is considered, that is, overt versus covert aggression, referrals are similar for boys and girls until about age 7. Bullying and manipulation are covert forms of aggression which are used by either sex, but tend to be used more often by girls. After age 7, boys begin to show more overt aggression and girls more covert aggression. Girls do become overtly violent, though at a much lower frequency than boys. In several of the school shootings, the young perpetrators complained of feeling alienated from their peers and of having been bullied. A review of adult studies showed more violence by men in the community but more equal violence among male and female psychiatric populations.

Nonwhites are overrepresented in population statistic data regarding violent crime. Rates of homicide and use of a firearm are significantly higher for African-Americans than for whites, and arrest rates follow a similar pattern. On the other hand, self-report surveys show more comparable rates of aggression in these racial groups. The meaning of racial differences in violence and arrest rates is unclear. There is speculation as to whether the statistics suggest differential arrest and prosecution or reflect adverse environmental experiences of a larger percentage of racial minorities.

Socioeconomic factors are very important in the distribution of violent behavior. Although violence is becoming more common in suburban and rural areas and other socioeconomic groups, violent crime is most common in poor inner-city areas which are plagued by gang activity and substance abuse. Adults who do poorly in society, engage in illegal behavior, fail to hold a job, and use drugs or alcohol, tend to drift to lower socioeconomic areas. They may neglect or abuse their children who are also surrounded by adults with problems. The children accumulate multiple risk factors for continued aggression including genetic, constitutional, and environmental causes. Their brains may also have been affected by poor nutrition, psychosocial deprivation, abuse, illness, accidents, or substances.

Aggressive behavior can be normal during the preschool years but is sometimes severe enough to result in clinical referral. Aggressive behavior is only part of the problematic behavior subsumed under conduct disorder, but two patterns have been identified and incorporated into the *Diagnostic and Statistical Manual of Mental Disorders*, Fourth Edition (DSM-IV) criteria for conduct disorder. These are childhood onset, beginning prior to age 10, and adolescent onset. According to Moffitt, the childhood-onset pattern is a "life-course-persistent" variety, whereas adolescent-onset, called "adolescent-limited" by Moffitt, antisocial behavior is more likely to resolve by the third decade of life. During adolescence, there is no difference in the seriousness of the antisocial behavior between these two groups. Robins gives the median age of onset of antisocial behavior in boys at 7 years and in girls at 13 years. While overt aggressive behavior declines through the elementary school years, more covert behaviors can persist and then become more overt again in adolescence. The severity and dangerousness of aggressive behavior, if it persists, increases with age, size, and access to weapons into the teen years.

Etiology and Pathogenesis

As noted above, violent behavior is not itself a disorder but is associated with several different diagnoses. It can also occur outside the context of mental illness, either in a moment of high stress or emotionality or as a planned event. Studies relating to causation are varied in approach and in theory. One set of theories described by Patterson, Moffitt, and others differentiates early-onset aggression (childhood) from late-onset aggression (adolescent). Vitiello describes the model derived from animal studies and divides aggression into "an impulsive-reactive-hostile-affective subtype and a controlled-proactive-instrumental-predatory subtype."

Genetic investigations of aggressive and violent behavior have not yielded clear-cut results thus far. However, many studies indicate that children of antisocial fathers are more prone to be antisocial themselves whether or not they are raised by their fathers, suggesting that genetic factors may outweigh environmental factors in antisocial behavior. While violence can be a component of antisocial behavior, it is not always present. Environmental factors such as severe deprivation and abuse are also associated with the development of violence.

Genes affect neurotransmitter manufacture and metabolism. Research on possible biochemical determinants of aggression has focused on the neurotransmitters serotonin, norepinephrine, and dopamine in animals and to a lesser extent in humans. Decreased brain serotonin and increased norepinephrine and dopamine have been associated with aggression, but the significance of these findings remains unclear.

Clinical and sociologic studies have also addressed the frequency and apparent determinants of aggressive behavior. As described by Perry in Schetky and Benedek's *The Principles and Practice of Child and Adolescent Forensic Psychiatry,* violence in childhood can affect brain development and neurophysiology. The cortical modulation of behavior can be damaged either by regression of established structures and processes or by failure of adequate development. Causes of regression include effects of illness and trauma. The author reviews work suggesting that normal brain development can be adversely affected by the experience of violence in childhood, resulting in a persistent state of fear, increased tendency to dissociate, increased startle response, and hypervigilance, which can be symptoms of PTSD. This predisposing violence experience may include enduring abuse personally, as well as witnessing violence to others, and, in vulnerable individuals, viewing media violence.

Patterson and others in the Oregon Youth Study devised a behavioral theory through their longitudinal study of antisocial boys. The boys' own antisocial behavior causes peer problems and school-behavioral problems that then result in the parents responding in a "coercive" fashion, that is, responding with "thoughtless, angry reflexes rather than responses that will help socialize their children." This study describes the "early starters," who may be symptomatic by age 3 or 4 and are at the greatest risk of arrests at an early age, and the "late starters," who begin antisocial behavior in midadolescence and have had the opportunity to develop some appropriate social skills. Patterson's group theorizes that among late starters, family stressors are a strong influence.

From a sociologic perspective, poverty, abuse, and weakened family and neighborhood structure appear closely related to violence in young people. Many more children live in poverty in the United States than in European countries, which have lower rates of juvenile violence. Many youths are severely abused or neglected, and the most severe abuse correlates with the most violent behavior.

Psychopathology

Diagnoses that are frequently associated with aggressive behavior are ADHD, conduct disorder, mood disorders, psychoses, PTSD, and mental retardation. Epidemiologic studies with adults have shown that an increased occurrence of aggressive behavior occurs with schizophrenia, affective disorder, posttraumatic stress disorder, and personality disorders, and the same is likely true for adolescents with these disorders. Personality disorders, especially with narcissistic, paranoid, or passive-aggressive traits, are associated with violence in adolescence. Often, children who resort to aggression are impulsive and inflexible, tolerating little frustration and requiring that their environment meet their needs in very exacting ways. These characteristics are often found in children and adolescents with pervasive developmental disorder, Asperger disorder, ADHD, and obsessive-compulsive disorder.

Repeated serious violence is associated with a history of severe abuse in childhood. Dorothy Otnow Lewis and Bruce Perry have written extensively of the association of central nervous system impairments with aggressive behavior. These impairments themselves may result from severe abuse. Otnow Lewis et al. found that serious violence is an infrequent event that is most often associated with a history of brutal abuse; paranoia, which may not be of a delusional level; and brain damage, which may be subtle, undiagnosed, and related to prenatal or very early insults to the infant.

Concomitant substance abuse, including alcohol, increases the risk of violence in major mental disorders. Intoxication with hallucinogens, PCP, methamphetamine, and cocaine can result in violence. Unusual causes of violence are seizure disorders and prodromal confusion associated with migraine headaches.

ASSOCIATED FAMILY DYNAMICS

Farrington et al. found that broken homes, large family size, and gang membership are associated with violent behavior. These homes may be characterized by chaos, lack of respect, inappropriate boundaries, and lack of routines that promote security in normal homes. Some homes include adults or teens who may openly use substances. Violent children and adolescents have often been abused severely and/or chronically in their homes. The child's or adolescent's temperament may not mesh well with that of one or both parents, and this may lead to conflict. Parents may be struggling with environmental stresses such as poverty or joblessness and are overwhelmed by their children's problems and do not know what to do. Some may try to ignore the child and the problems. Others may try to gratify the child's demands in an effort to postpone or divert the anticipated tantrum or aggression. Still others will try spanking, possibly verging on abuse, other severe punitive discipline such as long periods of grounding or time out, or removal of items to which the child is attached. Verbal abuse such as berating, name calling, and threats of withdrawal of affection may occur. Patterson refers to this pattern of harsh discipline as "coercive."

ASSOCIATED ENVIRONMENTAL FACTORS

Violent children and adolescents have often experienced violence by being abused in their homes or witnessing domestic violence. They often spend time with delinquent or substance-abusing friends. They tend to be truant from school and to have little or no supervision after school. Thus, they have much free time in which to get into trouble. An increased risk of juvenile violence exists in a few of the largest cities in the United States. These large cities contain areas characterized by severe poverty, unemployment, single parent homes, and gang activity. Being part of a deviant peer group, such as a gang, encourages violent behavior that may have started even prior to association with these peers. Many adolescents have access to guns or regularly carry guns or other weapons. The presence of guns in the home increases the risk of homicide to members of the household.

MEDIA VIOLENCE

Many studies have suggested that media violence increases aggressive behavior in children. Work by Huesmann et al. has shown that viewing violent tapes increases arousal, aggressive thinking, and aggressive acts. Longitudinal studies by the same author in other countries demonstrated a correlation between the hours of television viewed and subsequent child aggression. Recent years have seen a tremendous increase in exposure to violence through television, movies, the Internet, music videos, and video games. If the viewing child or adolescent also experiences violence in the neighborhood and at home, violence is reinforced as a real option. While ratings of violence in music, videos, and computer games are meant to help with parental supervision, parents do not always use these tools and/or may not have control of what is provided by older siblings or friends. Movies can be viewed repeatedly on VCRs or DVD players that are widely available. Many writers

TABLE 18.1. ESSENTIALS OF MANAGING MEDIA VIOLENCE

- Limit the time that children spend alone with TV, video, and video games.
- Watch and discuss television, movies, etc. with children.
- Make it clear that violence is not acceptable, even if it is acted out by the hero/heroine.
- Take note of parental advisory rating on movies, video games, and CDs.
- Ensure that children have adequate after-school adult supervision.
- Limit the amount of time that children spend using the Internet, especially chat rooms.

From Al-Mateen CS. Effects of witnessing violence on children and adolescents. In: Schetky DH, Benedek EP, eds. *Principles and practice of child and adolescent forensic psychiatry.* Washington, DC: American Psychiatric Publishing, 2002:213–224, with permission.

have noted that the realism inherent in newer video games and cartoons may enhance the realism of the violence. Parental involvement in media decisions tends to decrease the level of violence exposure for their children, as summarized in Table 18.1.

Assessment

A full assessment is recommended when a child or adolescent presents with a complaint involving violence or aggression. Assessment includes an interview that covers chief complaint; present illness; psychiatric, psychosocial, educational, and family history; neurologic and medical history; and mental status examination. It may include physical and neurologic examination, laboratory work, electroencephalogram (EEG), and imaging studies. In addition, any special tests that may be indicated by the history, physical examination, or mental status examination, such as human immunodeficiency virus (HIV) antibody test, Wilson disease, porphyria, or other potential medical causes of aggression, should be done. A careful review of medical records may contribute important clues to contributing medical conditions.

The clinician must approach the patient in a polite, friendly, and calm manner, and one which respects the patient's boundaries. Once comfortable, most children and teenagers will talk about their experiences. The goal is to complete an interview, physical and neurologic examination, and obtain cooperation for any indicated laboratory or other studies. If the child or adolescent makes the clinician feel unsafe, having another person in the room will be helpful. This could be a family member of the patient or a member of the clinic staff. In high acuity settings such as emergency rooms, or if weapons and overt hostility are a concern, it may mean alerting security staff to stand by. The individual should be asked about weapons, and, if present, they should be removed. If they are not surrendered, the interview should be suspended until police or security staff can ensure safety.

The interviewer should ask about the patient's understanding about why the interview is occurring. Recent stresses or changes may be important. Neutral topics such as his or her interests and leisure activities can be interspersed with more probing questions regarding past history of violence or aggression, school history, legal history, and substance abuse. Important areas are violence in the home, past abuse, and substance abuse by the patient and family. Ask directly about suicidal and homicidal ideation and include whether there is active planning or an available method; a feasible plan makes an immediate intervention necessary, as does an assessment that the individual is psychotic or delirious and, therefore, unpredictable. The presence of hallucinations, gross disorganization of thought process, or a conviction that he or she is being forced to behave in uncharacteristic or dangerous ways suggest psychosis. If violent themes spontaneously arise in the patient's conversation, this could be a clue to dangerousness and could indicate a risk of violence during the interview. The essential aspects of history taking are summarized in Table 18.2.

The formal mental status examination includes orientation to person, date and place, memory test, serial subtractions or spelling a word forward and backward, and testing for

TABLE 18.2. ESSENTIALS OF TAKING A HISTORY OF VIOLENCE

- Recent stresses
- Aggressive and delinquent behavior, including legal history and gang involvement
- Relationships with peers, fights with peers, and being picked on
- School history (suspensions or expulsion) and performance
- Substance abuse
- Depression, suicidality, and self-abuse
- History of head or other injuries, periods of dizziness, headaches, or blackouts
- Birth and pregnancy history
- History of verbal, physical or sexual abuse, or witnessing violence or sexual abuse
- Family history of violence, mental disorder, incarceration, substance abuse
- Familiarity with weapons, especially guns, and access to weapons
- If a violent episode has already occurred, ask about it in detail to determine the course of events, reasoning about it, and memory of it

From Dubovsky SL, Weissberg MP. *Clinical psychiatry in primary care,* 2nd ed. Baltimore: Lippincott Williams & Wilkins, c1982:257–263, and Schetky DH. Risk assessment of violence in youths. In: Schetky DH, Benedek EP, eds. *Principles and practice of child and adolescent forensic psychiatry*. Washington, DC: American Psychiatric Publishing, 2002:231–246, with permission.

abstract thinking using similarities or proverbs. Without specifically asking these questions, the clinician could miss a delirium and a potentially treatable medical illness. Table 18.3 summarizes steps in the mental status examination.

PHYSICAL ASSESSMENT

Assessment of health status should include a medical history, including information from parents or other informants, and physical examination. Pertinent information includes headaches, dizzy spells, blackouts, appetite, and sleeping patterns. As always, serious medical conditions that could underlie the psychiatric presentation should be ruled out. For patients presenting in a confused state, a medical and laboratory evaluation is crucial to rule out substance use, infectious and medical causes of delirium, or head injury that the individual is not reporting. Components of the physical examination are presented in Table 18.4.

RATING INSTRUMENTS AND PSYCHOLOGICAL TESTING

These tools are not generally applicable in an emergency but may be helpful or required to clarify diagnosis or to follow treatment response at other times. Standardized instruments

TABLE 18.3. ESSENTIALS OF THE MENTAL STATUS EXAMINATION FOR EVALUATING VIOLENCE

- A connection with the interviewer through words, eye contact, body language; remoteness or lack of connection is worrisome
- Paranoia, delusions, or hallucinations; does the patient feel threatened by someone in particular or that he or she is the victim of a plot?
- Thoughts of injuring or killing someone, especially someone in particular, who may need a warning
- Serious depression with suicidal ideation or a recent suicide attempt
- Hostile or threatening manner, or statements
- Orientation to person, place, and date
- Confusion, distractibility
- Depression with ideas or plans of suicide or self-abuse
- Preoccupation with violent ideas or violent movies

From Dubovsky SL, Weissberg MP. *Clinical psychiatry in primary care,* 2nd ed. Baltimore: Lippincott Williams & Wilkins, c1982:257–263, and Schetky DH. Risk assessment of violence in youths. In: Schetky DH, Benedek EP, eds. *Principles and practice of child and adolescent forensic psychiatry*. Washington, DC: American Psychiatric Publishing, 2002:231–246, with permission.

TABLE 18.4. ADJUNCTIVE DIAGNOSTIC TOOLS FOR ASSESSING VIOLENCE

- Vital signs; fever could suggest infection and/or delirium
- Physical and neurologic examination
- Urine drug screen to check for substances, legal and illicit, that may increase aggression
- WBC if elevated could suggest infection
- Chemistry screen and TSH to check for thyroid abnormalities or other metabolic abnormalities that could result in delirium
- EEG and MRI or CT scan of the head to look for electrical or structural abnormalities that may be associated with aggression or poor impulse control
- Neurologic consultation for tremors, abnormal movements, seizure or absence spells, abnormal EEG or neuroimaging.

WBC, white blood cell; TSH, thyroid-stimulating hormone; EEG, electroencephalogram; MRI, magnetic resonance imaging; CT, computed tomography.

From Tardiff K. Evaluation and treatment of violent patients. In: Stoff DM et al., eds. *Handbook of antisocial behavior*; New York: John Wiley and Sons, 1997:445–495, Lewis DO, Yeager CA, eds. Juvenile violence. *Child Psychiatric Clin North Am* 2000;9:733–891, and Pincus J. Neurologic evaluation of violent juveniles. *Child Adolesc Psychiatric Clin N Am* 2000;9:777–792, with permission.

may provide more reliable and objective information than the interview. Many of these instruments are not geared to aggression but provide other helpful information regarding a youth's intellect, attitudes, personality, or other factors. Consultation with a child psychologist for formal testing may also be helpful. Some popular tests used with aggressive youths are presented in Table 18.5.

TABLE 18.5. HELPFUL PSYCHOLOGICAL TOOLS FOR ASSESSING VIOLENCE

Rating Instruments and Tests	Focus or Use
Child behavior checklist (CBCL) and Teacher's Report Form (TRF; Achenbach TM)	Widely used, but the aggression subscale addresses mainly disruptive and oppositional behaviors
Conners' rating scales	For diagnosing and monitoring treatment of ADHD
Wechsler intelligence scale for children, 3rd Edition (WISC-III), Brief intelligence test for children (K-BIT), or Stanford-Binet scales of intelligence	Intellectual tests to be used when cognitive ability or executive thinking skills are an issue
Minnesota multiphasic personality inventory— adolescent version (MMPI-A), millon adolescent personality inventory (MAPI)	Self-report questionnaires for adolescents that can yield personality information; contain validity indices to detect deception or overreporting
Overt aggression scale (OAS; Yudofsky, 1986), Modified OAS (MOAS; Kay, 1988)	Developed for adults and useful for adolescent inpatients to track progress in treatment; MOAS tracks behaviors over a week, particularly in the outpatient setting
Children's aggression scale, parent and teacher versions (CAS-P and CAS-T; Halperin, 2003)	A newer scale covering ages 7–11 for outpatient settings and modeled on the Overt aggression scale
Neuropsychological assessment	If deficits are suspected; consists of a number of different individualized tests addressing specific constructs of functional abilities, such as logical sequencing, perceptual-motor integration, planning, impulsivity, explicit memory, and implicit memory

ADHD, attention deficit hyperactivity disorder.

From Collett B, Ohan J, Myers K. Ten-year review of rating scales. VI: scales assessing externalizing behaviors. *J Am Acad Child Adolesc Psychiatry* 2003;42:10–29, Halperin JE, McKay KE, Newcorn JH. Development, reliability, and validity of the children's aggression scale-parent version. *J Am Acad Child Adolesc Psychiatry* 2002;41:245–252, Lewis DO. Development of the symptom of violence. In: Lewis M, ed. *Child and adolescent psychiatry; a comprehensive textbook*, 3rd ed. Philadelphia, PA: Lippincott Williams & Wilkins, 2002:387–399, Pincus J. Neurologic evaluation of violent juveniles. *Child Adolesc Psychiatric Clin N Am* 2000;9:777–792, and Yudofsky SC, Silver JM, Jackson W, et al. The overt aggression scale for the objective rating of verbal and physical aggression. *Am J Psychiatry* 1986;143:35–39, with permission.

Collateral information

With children and adolescents, more often than adults, the evaluator can access collateral sources of information, such as the parents, caretakers, and teachers. Records of previous evaluations and periods of treatment should be obtained. Friends and recent contacts may be able to shed light on precipitants of the current problem. Except in severe emergencies, a proper release of information should be obtained before contacting others. A summary of the clinical evaluation for violent youths is provided in Table 18.6.

Treatment

If violence has occurred or seems imminent without intervention, parents must be involved, weapons removed, and, if necessary, the individual placed in a setting such as a hospital that can prevent the possible dangerous action. It may be necessary to consider whether identified potential victims should be warned as mandated by the Tarasoff decision or related laws in some states. Rapid psychiatric consultation is advisable. If the violence is less serious and more chronic, an outpatient evaluation may be undertaken. The evaluator can sometimes organize the caretakers to be more vigilant and helpful to the child during an assessment if there is not an imminent risk of harm to self or others.

The practitioner must determine whether an emergency exists and whether an underlying condition treatable by a particular type of medication is present. An emergency in which violence may be imminent or the patient is already combative requires sedation and hospitalization and, perhaps, seclusion or seclusion and restraint. The patient in need of immediate intervention is overtly threatening with a feasible plan and access to the means to put the plan into action. Severe disorganization, agitation, paranoia, or psychosis also are more safely evaluated and treated in a hospital.

Patients whose threats are more vague and/or whose symptoms are less acute and who are likely to cooperate with responsible caretakers can be evaluated in the home as outpatients. A treatment plan should be formulated to include medication and referrals to

---

TABLE 18.6. ESSENTIAL CLINICAL EVALUATION FOR VIOLENCE

- Begin the interview with a calm voice and respectful manner, being aware of a quick way to leave the interview room if necessary. Avoid challenging or arguing with the patient.
- Evaluator should be aware of whether the youth engenders a feeling of uneasiness in him or her, as this is clue to dangerousness.
- Inquire as to what is bothering the youth and listen carefully.
- Appearance of intoxication should increase the level of concern.
- Assessment of dangerousness includes discussion of the violent ideation or behavior, victims or intended victims, methods, and availability of weapons.
- Suicidal feelings can accompany violence and should be assessed.
- Support system should be explored. Is there a place or persons that would allow the youth to feel safe and secure without the need to act violently?
- Mental status examination and careful observation of physical status may suggest the need for neurologic and physical examination, EEG, imaging, or laboratory work.
- Continued outpatient assessment can be used if the patient has the ability to make a safety commitment, has no access to weapons, and has a safe and well-supervised setting in which to stay. This may be possible with a patient who responded to emergency medication and is willing to continue to take the medication.
- Assessment, clinical reasoning, and plan should be carefully documented.

EEG, electroencephalogram.

From Dubovsky SL, Weissberg MP. *Clinical psychiatry in primary care,* 2nd ed. Baltimore: Lippincott Williams & Wilkins, c1982:257–263, and Schetky DH. Risk assessment of violence in youths. In: Schetky DH, Benedek EP, eds. *Principles and practice of child and adolescent forensic psychiatry.* Washington, DC: American Psychiatric Publishing, 2002:231–246, with permission.

mental health professionals. In difficult or complex cases, child psychiatric consultation should be obtained early, perhaps at the first presentation.

When concomitant mental disorders exist, treatment of the primary mental disorder with a combination of medication and psychosocial interventions should result in improvement of the violent or aggressive behavior or ideation. In the case of predatory, or proactive, aggression, which is carried out without significant arousal and for a specific antisocial reason, behavioral interventions may be more effective. Medication use in these cases is less specific to the cause of the behavior.

In the Robins study described above, psychotherapy appeared helpful, but less so for both the most severe and least severe cases. Psychotherapy is likely helpful in many cases, but outcome studies are available only with more structured psychotherapy techniques. Outcome studies show good results with parent management training, cognitive problem-solving skills training, and multisystemic therapy. Many patients who were deemed to need treatment in the Robins study did not get it for various reasons. Premature termination of treatment poses a significant problem with aggressive children and adolescents.

PHARMACOTHERAPY

There is no single reliable medication for aggressive behavior or conduct disorder. Moreover, no medication has been approved by the Food and Drug Administration (FDA) for violence, although chlorpromazine and haloperidol have indications for severe behavioral problems. While many psychotropic medications have limitations on age or indication by the FDA, many are supported in the literature for use with children and adolescents, sometimes for a number of indications. Few have been tested in randomized double-blinded studies.

If the presumed cause of the violence or threatened violence is a disorder usually treatable by medication, for example, psychosis, bipolar disorder, major depression, ADHD, or others, then medications specific for those disorders should be tried first. Please refer to the corresponding chapters in this text for treatment guidelines. For explosive aggressive behavior occurring in the absence of other mental disorders, recommendations were recently formulated by Schur, Pappadopoulos, and others. These recommendations emphasize the use of psychosocial interventions first, if possible. When medication is used, monotherapy is encouraged; and when an antipsychotic is used, an atypical rather than typical antipsychotic is strongly encouraged.

Emergency situations

If there is threatening, severe agitation, or striking out, the child or adolescent may require emergency medication for the safety of all. Reassurance, crisis management, and listening techniques should be tried first. An atypical antipsychotic, such as risperidone or olanzapine, may be given orally to calm with minimum side effects. Zydis, a rapidly dissolving oral form of olanzapine, can be given without liquid if "cheeking" is likely. Zydis has the same pharmacodynamics as olanzapine tablets. Intramuscular olanzapine has recently become available. Intramuscular ziprasidone is available but can cause lengthening of the QTc interval on electrocardiogram (ECG). If an intramuscular medication is required, olanzapine or haloperidol can be used. To minimize the needed dose of haloperidol, it may be combined with lorazepam. Since haloperidol can cause acute dystonic reactions or extrapyramidal (parkinsonian) side effects, diphenhydramine or antiparkinsonian agents such as benztropine may also be given, either orally or intramuscularly, especially in young men who are at greatest risk of dystonic reactions. Both lorazepam and diphenhydramine occasionally cause increased behavioral problems due to either disinhibition or central anticholinergic effects, but diphenhydramine generally is safe in younger children. Once the child or adolescent is calm, the evaluation can proceed.

Nonemergency use

Typical antipsychotics historically have been most commonly prescribed for nonemergency use. Concerns about cognitive effects, sedation, and tardive dyskinesia have led to use of newer antipsychotic medications and other classes of psychotropic medications with less risk of serious side effects. Atypical antipsychotics are preferred over typical antipsychotics and are becoming first-line medications for aggressive behavior by younger patients. Psychostimulants, especially methylphenidate, have been shown to decrease the aggressive behavior with conduct disorder, both with and without concomitant ADHD. Lithium and antipsychotic medications have been shown to be helpful in aggressive children and adolescents. Anticonvulsant mood stabilizers, α-agonists, and β-blockers are also used to dampen aggressive behavior. These are briefly outlined below, and the reader is referred to Chapter 22.

Monotherapy is recommended. However, those patients with the most treatment-resistant aggression may eventually be treated with more than one medication in an attempt to prevent danger to others. Partially effective antipsychotics or antidepressants are often paired with a mood stabilizer. The clinician should be vigilant about side effects and/or lack of effectiveness. It is important to discontinue any medication that is not effective, but this should be done in a gradual and deliberate manner. Polypharmacy is more frequent in treatment-resistant patients, as well as in disorders such as fetal alcohol effects, low intellectual level, and PTSD. Table 18.7 reviews medications commonly used to treat violent youths.

Atypical antipsychotics

Atypical antipsychotics (risperidone, olanzapine, quetiapine, ziprasidone, aripiprazole, clozapine) are presumed less likely to cause tardive dyskinesia than typical antipsychotics but can occasionally cause extrapyramidal side effects. In general, they are better tolerated than typical antipsychotics, and this leads to better medication compliance. Many cause

TABLE 18.7. ESSENTIAL PSYCHOPHARMACOLOGY FOR VIOLENT YOUTHS

Target Symptom	Medication
Impulsivity	Psychostimulants: methylphenidate, amphetamines; atomoxetine
Poor frustration tolerance, explosiveness, high arousal	α-2 agonists: clonidine, guanfacine; β-blockers: propranolol; atypical antipsychotics: risperidone, olanzapine, quetiapine, ziprasidone, aripiprazole
Anxiety, obsessions, compulsions, depression	SSRIs: fluoxetine, sertraline, citalopram, escitalopram, fluvoxamine (paroxetine currently contraindicated); tricyclics: clomipramine; buspirone; α-2 agonists
Mania	Mood stabilizers: lithium, valproate, carbamazepine, topiramate, lamotrigine, oxcarbazepine; antipsychotics: atypicals, typicals; benzodiazepines: lorazepam, clonazepam, diazepam, alprazolam
Paranoia or psychosis	Antipsychotics: atypicals, typicals
Aggression (reactive, hostile, affective)	Atypical antipsychotics; lithium; anticonvulsants/mood stabilizers; typical antipsychotics; α-2 agonists
Aggression (predatory or proactive)	Behavioral methods should be tried first except in emergencies; psychostimulants, antipsychotics, or lithium may be considered

SSRIs, selective serotonin reuptake inhibitors.

From Green WH. *Child and adolescent clinical psychopharmacology*, 3rd ed. Philadelphia, PA: Lippincott Williams & Wilkins, 2001, with permission.

significant weight gain and sometimes elevated cholesterol, triglycerides, and/or glucose, which should be monitored. This has led to interest in the newer ziprasidone and aripiprazole, which are supposed to be less hyperphagic and thus weight neutral. Some studies of these medications in children and adolescents are available, but data are preliminary and no definitive conclusions can be drawn.

Typical antipsychotics

Typical antipsychotics, a few of which are FDA approved for behavioral disorders and use in younger children, carry a risk of parkinsonian side effects and of tardive dyskinesia as well as weight gain, subjective dysphoria, and cognitive dulling. Thioridazine was once approved for treating severe behavioral disorders in children but is no longer approved due to "black box" warning for cardiac arrhythmia. It is approved only for schizophrenic patients who do not respond to other antipsychotic medications. Haloperidol is a frequent choice among the typical antipsychotics for emergency situations, in part due to availability of an intramuscular preparation. Fluphenazine or trifluoperazine can also be used.

Mood stabilizers

The use of lithium has been studied for children and adolescents with bipolar disorder, severe aggression, and conduct disorder with encouraging results. Valproic acid has been studied for adolescent mania, for children and adolescents with mental retardation and mood disorders, and for adolescents with explosive mood disorders. Carbamazepine shows mixed results in studies on the treatment of aggression, and it can occasionally worsen symptoms.

α-agonists and β-blockers

Clonidine, guanfacine, and propranolol have been used with aggressive youths. Clonidine and guanfacine are frequently used in PTSD as they decrease arousal states. They can cause hypotension and postural hypotension when given with atypical antipsychotics. Propranolol has been used for aggressive behavior in head trauma, autism, and schizophrenia. It may be an effective adjunct but also can exacerbate hypotension with atypical antipsychotics. These classes of medication are also used in cases of poor frustration tolerance or explosiveness.

Antidepressants

There are few reports of reduction of impulsive aggression with antidepressants in the class of selective serotonin reuptake inhibitors (SSRIs). However, if the aggression is associated with significant depression or suicidality, treatment with an SSRI would be appropriate. Please refer to the Chapters 10 and 22 for details on using SSRIs with youths. Antidepressants generally need several weeks of administration to become effective. Trazodone causes some immediate sedation and has been used down to age 6 for aggression. Concerns are drowsiness, dizziness, dry mouth, and priapism. The latter should result in immediate discontinuation and, if it persists, medical consultation. With all antidepressants, there is a risk of activation or precipitation of a manic episode.

PSYCHOSOCIAL INTERVENTIONS

In emergency situations, crisis management techniques such as listening, problem solving, and offering medication or a quiet place to calm, or using a diversionary activity can be helpful. In the most severe situations, seclusion or restraint may be needed. In chronic situations or longer term treatment, anger management skills, conflict resolution, stress management classes, and behavioral programs designed to reinforce prosocial behaviors are helpful. If stresses in the home environment are aggravating the youth's difficulties, a structured setting, such as a residential program or hospital, often helps the child or adolescent gain control of his or her impulses even without medication. Parents often feel blamed for their child's problems and will be relieved if they receive empathy about the difficulty of the situation. The clinician should make it clear that interventions are to help the whole family to get along better.

Parent management training

Parent management training is a behavioral technique that is well investigated with conduct disorders. It is especially effective with preadolescent patients but has been studied with adolescents as well. This method focuses on adjusting the ways in which parents interact with their troubled children. The theory is that parents inadvertently reinforce problem behaviors and can be taught to modulate their own responses and reinforce the desired prosocial behaviors. As reviewed by Kazdin, outcome studies support the effectiveness of these techniques. Manuals, such as McMahon and Forehand's *Helping the Noncompliant Child* and Patterson's *A Social Interactional Approach,* are available.

Problem-solving skills training

Problem-solving skills training is a model of cognitive intervention in which children or adolescents are taught in stepwise fashion to first solve hypothetical problem situations and then gradually more real-life situations. Many anger management classes are of this type. This technique is more useful at age 10 and above due to level of cognitive development.

Multisystemic therapy

This treatment, based on systems theory and social ecology, is highly individualized to the patient and situations being addressed and uses parts of other techniques and interventions. It has been most studied and used with delinquent older adolescents. The patient is conceptualized as a part of many systems, for example, family, school, peer group, neighborhood, and so on and may need specific interventions to help with each system with which he or she is involved. Kazdin describes this technique as particularly useful for those youths whose aggression has been resistant to less elaborate interventions. Multisystemic therapy is intensive and requires wraparound services to be available and coordinated. *Multisystemic Treatment of Antisocial Behavior in Children and Adolescents* by Henggeler et al. is a detailed manual for this model of treatment.

Family interventions

Parenting classes and/or family therapy may help the parents respond to a particular child in a more effective way in order to improve the aggressive behavior. Family therapy is often conducted in a family systems model or a psychodynamic model for which there is limited research, though it is likely helpful to many families.

Group therapies

Group therapies can be helpful with aggressive and conduct-disordered youths, but they appear to be more effective if the groups are heterogeneous. Groups with mostly conduct-disordered members tend to reinforce the negative values in each other.

CONTINUUM OF CARE NEEDS

Younger children can more often be treated while remaining in their home settings unless the family is too dysfunctional or the child too dangerous. For the more dangerous behaviors that could be harmful to members of the family or community, hospital care or residential care combined with an assessment of future treatment needs may be necessary. Day treatment or partial hospitalization may prevent the need for 24-hour hospital care or facilitate successful transition back home. Longer term residential or foster care is important for some young people to stabilize and, if possible, transition back to their homes. Several professional disciplines may be needed to complete an adequate treatment or evaluation. Social service agencies, local mental health agencies, child psychiatrists, and child psychologists may be able to assist in assessment or provide referral sources for various levels of care.

OTHER INTERVENTIONS

Occupational therapy for sensorimotor treatment can be helpful to children or adolescents who have processing difficulties or pervasive developmental disorders and who may disorganize in stressful situations. Patients learn how to use movement or soothing sensations to calm themselves. An occupational therapy assessment can determine whether this would be helpful. Speech and language therapy can also be helpful if the child's or adolescent's ability to communicate his or her needs and feelings is compromised. Subtle language deficits can be difficult to diagnose without a complete speech/language evaluation. Deafness or primary languages other than English may necessitate using interpretive services to assess properly and to treat the patient.

If the youth has become involved in the legal system and is on probation or parole, participating in treatment and/or taking medication can sometimes be made a condition of probation or parole. This can ensure better cooperation in treatment and prevent premature termination of treatment. The essential aspects of treatment are summarized in Table 18.8.

TABLE 18.8. ESSENTIALS FOR THE TREATMENT OF VIOLENT YOUTHS

- For emergency sedation, consider atypical antipsychotic. A typical antipsychotic, either orally or intramuscularly, with a benzodiazepine or diphenhydramine may be used.
- Use the proper medication for the presumed diagnosis if possible.
- Ensure removal of weapons accessible to the individual.
- Consider whether a potential victim needs to be warned (Tarasoff).
- Decide whether hospitalization is needed and, if so, arrange it.
- Hospitalize if there is overt threat or aggression, especially with access to weapons, active psychosis, or suicidal ideation with urge to act on it. Decompensated mental illness or intoxication can increase risk and also may require hospitalization.
- If members of the support system are frightened or overwhelmed, but the patient does not have the above indicators, use crisis residence or foster home. The child welfare agency, child protective services, police, or a social worker in the emergency room may be able to assist with access.
- For those not in need of immediate hospitalization, follow-up care should be arranged and risk should be reassessed at each meeting.
- Underlying conditions leading to violence or potential violence should be vigorously treated.
- Plan for appropriate psychosocial interventions.

From Dubovsky SL, Weissberg MP. *Clinical psychiatry in primary care,* 2nd ed. Baltimore: Lippincot Williams & Wilkins, c1982:257–263, and Schetky DH. Risk assessment of violence in youths. In: Schetky DH, Benedek EP, eds. *Principles and practice of child and adolescent forensic psychiatry*. Washington, DC: American Psychiatric Publishing, 2002:231–246, with permission.

Case Vignettes

Case vignette #1

GT, a 10-year-old white boy, was referred to a child psychiatric inpatient unit for evaluation of aggressive, assaultive, oppositional behavior. He had broken windows at school and had threatened to kill his younger sister. His problems had worsened throughout the school year, and he was failing all subjects. He did not get along with his family, and his mother felt she had to watch him constantly. He had seldom seen his father since a divorce 3 years before, but his father was reported to have hit him in anger. GT had talked of killing himself and was isolated from peers, having no friends. There had been some minor sexual acting out and vandalism. GT had temporal lobe epilepsy due to an illness in infancy. He was being treated with diphenylhydantoin and primidone at the time of admission and had been seizure free for some time.

On mental status examination, GT had no abnormal movements and was well nourished and well developed. He had a hard time sitting still and seemed to expect criticism. He was excessively upset when he thought he gave a wrong answer. Overall, knowledge was limited for age. He made eye contact but frequently hid his face. He reported worries about being disciplined if the doctor did not like him and cried easily. He also exaggerated his abilities in sports.

Physical examination was normal except for gingival hyperplasia and some difficulty with fine motor movements. In the hospital, GT had an abnormal EEG with right temporal spikes. IQ testing showed a low normal verbal IQ with a borderline performance IQ. On projective testing he disorganized under stress but showed no overt psychosis. Speech-language evaluation showed weak auditory memory and impaired expressive language.

GT's behavioral difficulties were thought to be due in part to his treatment with primidone, which can cause irritability and emotional disturbance. With pediatric neurology consultation, it was slowly tapered while carbamazepine was added with the ultimate goal of being able to discontinue both primidone and diphenylhydantoin. He did not require the addition of any other psychotropic medication. The carbamazepine may well have been beneficial for the aggressive behavior. He also received group, individual, and speech/language therapy. Behaviorally, he improved in the hospital but did strike out at peers occasionally. He had difficulty sharing attention with others and tolerating limits.

After some weeks of hospitalization, GT continued to need treatment and was transferred to residential treatment. A few months after his discharge, he was doing well. He was no longer fighting and was performing well in school. He continued to take carbamazepine with good seizure control and decreased irritability.

In summary, GT was not manageable in his home. The etiology of his aggressive behavior was multifactorial, including his difficult relationship with his mother and relative loss of his abusive father, brain dysfunction due to infantile illness with subsequent seizure disorder, and behavioral side effects of his anticonvulsant medication. In addition, his behavior had led to alienation from peers and family, and he expected only criticism and harsh discipline, which made him anxious and sad.

Case vignette #2

LP was a 14-year-old mixed-race boy who was admitted to an acute care psychiatric hospital in a manic state, showing pressured speech, flight of ideas, elevated mood, and decreased sleep. He was extremely irritable and easily erupted into aggressive behavior toward others. After attacking others, he would say they deserved it. He stated he had been "beaten" into a gang and acted tough. He had frequently run away from home, and he sometimes lived on the street and sometimes with older gang-involved individuals, where he also engaged in promiscuous sexual behavior. He admitted frequent use of alcohol and marijuana and sometimes bragged about how much he had used.

LP was born of a normal pregnancy and had normal developmental milestones. During his early years, his parents fought and were involved in alcohol and methamphetamine use. Older siblings also had substance abuse and legal problems. After his parents separated when LP was 5 or 6 years old, a stepfather with whom LP had conflicts entered the home. LP was identified as having ADHD in first grade and required an individual education plan and psychostimulant medication throughout elementary school. Nevertheless, there were many suspensions for aggressive and disruptive behavior. At home, LP was destructive of property, unable to share, oppositional to limits, and threatening to family members. Mother and stepfather fought about how to discipline him, and some corporal punishment was used.

LP was not stabilized in acute care but was medicated with divalproex sodium and risperidone and moved to residential care. There his aggressiveness and efforts to stir his peers into open revolt resulted in his being hospitalized at a longer term facility. LP was no longer manic but remained inflexible, irritable, and prone to physical attack on others for any perceived disrespect or frustration of his wishes. LP was aggressive toward both peers and nursing staff. After aggressive episodes, he sometimes was angry at himself and made impulsive self-abusive acts or suicidal statements. Intellectual testing showed low average IQ, but LP seemed to function below this level.

After several medication trials including psychostimulants, mood stabilizers, atypical and typical antipsychotics, and α-2 blockers, LP stabilized on bupropion, clonazepam, dextroamphetamine, lithium, olanzapine, and small divided doses of trazodone. Improvement also required extensive work with 1:1 staffing and occupational therapy services to increase frustration tolerance. The psychologist provided a behavioral plan to reward nonaggressive behavior, which was very helpful. LP was eventually able to share a room with two peers successfully. His family was very involved and spent much time visiting at the hospital and then providing passes of slowly increasing length.

LP was discharged back home with a day treatment program that included special education; group, individual, and family therapy; and psychiatric follow up. Occupational therapy services were also planned. If aggressive behavior occurred, it was to be handled with either brief hospitalization or brief stays in detention.

BIBLIOGRAPHY

Bloomquist ML, Schnell SV. *Helping children with aggression and conduct problems; best practices for intervention.* New York: Guilford Press, 2002.

Collett B, Ohan J, Myers K. Ten-year review of rating scales. VI: Scales assessing externalizing behaviors. *J Am Acad Child Adolesc Psychiatry* 2003;42:10–29.

Dishion TJ, McCord J, Poulin F. When interventions harm; peer groups and problem behavior. *Am Psychol* 1999;54:755–764.

Dubovsky SL, Weissberg MP. *Clinical psychiatry in primary care,* 2nd ed. Baltimore: Lippincott Williams & Wilkins, c1982:257–263;

Farrington DP, Loeber R. Epidemiology of juvenille violence. Child Adolesc Psychiatric *Clin N Am* 2000;9:733–748.

Green WH. *Child and adolescent clinical psychopharmacology,* 3rd eds. Philadelphia, PA: Lippincott Williams & Wilkins, 2001.

Halperin JE, McKay KE, Newcorn JH. Development, reliability, and validity of the children's aggression scale-parent version. *J Am Acad Child Adolesc Psychiatry* 2002;41:245–252.

Huesmann LR, Moise JF, Podolski CL, et al. The effects of media violence on the development of antisocial behavior. In: Stoff DM, Breiling J, Maser JD, et al., eds. *Handbook of antisocial behavior.* New York: John Wiley and Sons, 1997:181–193.

Johnson JG. Adolescent personality disorders associated with violence and criminal behavior during adolescence and early adulthood. *Am J Psychiatry* 2000;157:1406–1412.

Kay SR, Wolkenfeld F, Murrill LM. Profiles of aggression among psychiatric patients. I. Nature and prevalence. *J Nerv Ment Dis* 1988;176:539–546.

Kazdin AE. Parent management training: evidence, outcomes, and issues. *J Am Acad Child Adolesc Psychiatry* 1997;36:1349–1356.

Kellerman AL, Rivara FP, Rushforth NB, et al. Gun ownership as a risk factor for homicide in the home. *N Engl J Med* 1993;329:1084–1091.

Klassen D, O'Connor WA. Demographic and case history variables in risk assessment in violence and mental disorder. In: Monahan J, Steadman JH, eds. *Violence and mental disorder; developments in risk assessment.* Chicago, IL: University of Chicago Press, 1994:227–257.

Klein RG, Abikoff H, Klass E, et al. Clinical efficacy of methylphenidate in conduct disorder with and without attention deficit hyperactivity disorder. *Arch Gen Psychiatry* 1997;54:1073–1080.

Lewis DO. Development of the symptom of violence. In: Lewis M, ed. *Child and adolescent psychiatry; a comprehensive textbook,* 3rd ed. Philadelphia, PA: Lippincott Williams & Wilkins, 2002:387–399.

Lewis DO, Shanok SS, Pincus JH, et al. Violent juvenile delinquents: psychiatric, neurological, psychological and abuse factors. *J Am Acad Child Adolesc Psychiatry* 1979;18:307–319.

Lewis DO, Yeager CA, eds. Juvenile violence. *Child Psychiatric Clin North Am* 2000;9:733–891.

Mandoki MW, Sumner GS, Matthews-Ferrari K. Evaluation and treatment of rage in children and adolescents. *Child Psychiat and Human Devel* 1992;22:227–235.

Moffitt TE. Adolescence-limited and life-course-persistent antisocial behavior: a developmental taxonomy. *Psychol Rev* 1993;100:674–701.

Nestor PG. Mental disorder and violence: personality dimensions and clinical features. *Am J Psychiatry* 2002;159:1973–1978.

Pappadopulos E, MacIntyre JC II, Crismon ML, Findling PS, et al. Treatment recommendations for the use of antipsychotics for aggressive youth (TRAAY), Part II. *J Am Acad Child Adolesc Psychiatry* 2003;42:145–161.

Patterson GR. *Antisocial Boys,* A Social Interactional Approach. Vol. 4. Eugene, OR: Castalia, 1992.

Pincus J. Neurologic evaluation of violent juvenniles. *Child Adolesc Psychiatric Clin Am* 2000;9:777–792.

Robins LN. *Deviant children grown up; a sociological and psychiatric study of sociopathic personality.* Baltimore, MD: Williams & Wilkins, 1966.

Schetky DH, Benedek EP, eds. *Principles and practice of child and adolescent forensic psychiatry.* Washington, DC: American Psychiatric Publishing, 2002:191–203, 213–224, 231–246.

Schur SB, Sikich L, Findling RL, et al. Treatment recommendations for the use of antipsychotics for aggressive youth (TRAAY). Part I: a review. *J Am Acad Child Adolesc Psychiatry* 2003;42:132–144.

Stoff DM, Breiling J, Maser JD, eds. *Handbook of antisocial behavior.* New York: John Wiley and Sons, 1997:181–193, 445–453, 474–495.

Vitiello B, Stoff DM. Subtypes of aggression and their relevance to child psychiatry. *J Am Acad Child Psychiatry* 1997;36:307–315.

Yudofsky SC, Silver JM, Jackson W, et al. The overt aggression scale for the objective rating of verbal and physical aggression. *Am J Psychiatry* 1986;143:35–39.

SUGGESTED READINGS

Garbarino J. *Lost boys: why our sons turn violent and how we can save them.* New York: Anchor Books, 1999.
  (*A thoughtful review of the development of violence in youths, written for families and interested lay persons.*)

Garbarino J, Bedard C, *Parents under siege: why you are the solution, not the problem, in your child's life.* New York: Free Press, 2001.
  (*This readable book is written particularly for the parents of difficult children.*)

Greenspan S, Salmon J. *The challenging child; understanding, raising, and enjoying the five "Difficult" types of children.* Reading, MA: Addison Wesley, 1995.
(*Especially chapters 5 and 7. A readable book for parents of younger children, emphasizing understanding and firmness, with many vignettes and example interactions.*)

Henggeler SW, Borduin CM, Schoenwald SK, et al. *Multisystemic treatment of antisocial behavior in children and adolescents.* New York: Guilford Press, 1998.
(*This is a detailed manual for this model of treatment.*)

Lewis DO, Yeager CA, eds. Juvenile violence. *Child Adolesc Psychiatr Clin North Am* 2000;9(4), 733–891.
(*An excellent general review for clinicians.*)

McMahon RJ, Forehand RL. *Helping the noncompliant child: family-based treatment for oppositional behavior,* 2nd ed. New York: Guilford Press, 2003.
(*A treatment manual for practitioners for teaching parents how to deal with their noncompliant 3–8 year olds. Based on behavioral principles and very detailed.*)

CHAPTER 19

Diagnosis and Treatment of Trauma in Children

ROY LUBIT

Introduction   Freud initially believed that trauma played a major role in the development of psychopathology in children. Freud and Breuer argued that the symptoms of hysteria are due to the repressed memories of traumatic events. In time, however, Freud came to believe that conflict over fantasies and wishes, rather than an actual history of trauma, was pathogenic. In recent decades, there has been a slow but steady realization that Freud's initial assessment was correct and that trauma is indeed at the root of much childhood psychopathology.

Serious emotional trauma is a common occurrence. Millions of children worldwide experience physical and sexual abuse, natural or technologic disasters, collapse of buildings or other structures, transportation accidents, invasive medical procedures, community violence, domestic violence, assault, bullying, terrorism, or war. The emotional impact of direct or vicarious exposure to violence often goes unappreciated and untreated. Even when children exhibit symptoms that adversely affect their ability to learn academic and social skills and to enjoy life, caregivers and others miss the connection between trauma and emotional consequences.

There are several key elements to the definition of trauma that may not be immediately apparent. First, trauma is not simply any stress, but a serious threat or assault on bodily integrity, one that can involve the risk of death. However, sexual assaults without perceived risk of death are sufficient to cause emotional trauma. The threat of injury or violation of bodily integrity can be to someone close to the child, such as a parent or sibling. Witnessing or learning about the injury, near injury, or sexual violation of a loved one can be traumatic. How an individual interprets a situation affects the degree to which it is traumatic.

This chapter begins with a discussion of the epidemiology and process of trauma, then reviews the impact of trauma on children, including both diagnosable and nondiagnosable sequelae. This chapter also discusses the intergenerational transmission of trauma and why it is often difficult to recognize which children have been traumatized and need help. It closes with a discussion of treatment and prevention issues.

Epidemiology of Trauma

Trauma is a common occurrence in our communities. Each year hundreds of thousands of children are in serious car accidents or have serious accidents at home or play. The National Center on Child Abuse and Neglect in 1997 reported that three million children a year are referred to child protective services for abuse or serious neglect. One-third of these cases are substantiated and half of these (0.5 million) are so severe that the children are removed from their homes. Estimates of the number of children who witness domestic violence run from 3 to 10 million. According to the Bureau of Justice statistics, 44% of rape victims are under the age of 18 and 15% are under age 12. The Commonwealth Fund Survey found that in grades 9 to 12, 12% of girls and 5% of boys reported being sexually abused. There are approximately 249,000 rapes, attempted rapes, and sexual assaults each year, not including the roughly 1 in 6 that occurred to children 12 years and under according to the 2000 National Trauma Victimization Survey.

Community violence is a very serious issue in inner cities. Fitzpatrick and Boldizar, studying low-income African American youths aged 7 to 18 attending a federally funded summer camp program, found that more than 70% of the children and adolescents reported being victims of at least one violent act, close to 85% reported having witnessed at least one violent act, and 43% reported having witnessed a murder. Jenkins and Bell studied teenagers in a public high school on Chicago's South Side and found that almost two-thirds had seen a shooting and almost one half had been shot at themselves. Forty-five percent reported that they had seen someone killed. Among sixth, eighth, and tenth graders in New Haven, Connecticut, Schwab-Stone et al. found that 40% of the youths reported exposure to a shooting or stabbing in the past year. Before September 11, Hoven found that 64% of New York City public school children in grades 4 to 12 had been exposed to a traumatic event. Trauma exposure for these children will continue to increase as they grow older.

The Impact of Trauma

There are many theories about what happens to individuals who are traumatized. Freud defined trauma as the experience of having the ego rendered helpless by overstimulation. He noted that psychic trauma led to two types of symptoms: (a) fixation to the trauma with subsequent repetition compulsion and (b) defensive reactions of avoidance, inhibition, and phobia. Janet described the intense emotional reactions and progressive weakening which follow traumatic events. Horowitz argued that posttraumatic stress disorder (PTSD) arises from an overwhelming and negative experience that is incongruent with existing schema. Kardiner believed that trauma could lead to a "physioneurosis" in which there is biologic dysregulation and enduring hypervigilance to threat. Like Janet, Kardiner believed that crucial to the outcome of a trauma was the meaning of the trauma, the interplay of the event with the individual's coping mechanisms, and the resulting alteration of the victim's adaptive processes. Rado postulates that a traumatic experience may lead to traumatophobia, that is, the anxious child feels continually on the verge of experiencing another trauma. Van der Kolk et al. proposed that PTSD involves a combination of a conditioned fear response to trauma-related stimuli, altered cognitive schemata and social apprehension, and altered neurobiologic processes leading to increased arousal and unusual handling of memory. These theories provide important insights into the many effects of traumatic experiences.

CONDITIONED FEAR RESPONSE

Following a traumatic event, one develops a conditioned fear response to the situation and to stimuli that remind one of the incident. Stimuli that remind a person of the dangerous situation can cause considerable anxiety and physiologic arousal. With time, the conditioned fear response usually weakens. For some, however, it can remain strong and expand to include increasing numbers of traumatic reminders. Encountering these traumatic triggers causes intense emotional discomfort. Complicating the conditioned fear response is the brain's uncharacteristic handling of memory in traumatic situations. Traumatic memories are stored largely in the amygdala rather than in the hippocampus. Individual experiences and memories of the traumatic incident may feel as if they are still taking place or had just happened, rather than occurring in the past. Intrusive recollections of the event may arise either from a conditioned fear response and attempts to be alert to a recurrence, or an attempt to integrate the experience and to accommodate existing cognitive schema to the new information. Numbing and withdrawal are attempts to cope with the pain of the memories. Victims sometimes engage in increased risk-taking behavior and substance abuse, either to deal with the feelings of withdrawal or to block out the painful intrusive memories.

ALTERED COGNITIONS

Traumatic experience changes one's perceptions of self and the world. After a traumatic experience, self-confidence often declines while the world seems increasingly dangerous. People frequently develop an increased sense of vulnerability and guilt or shame. Changes in threat perception, a tendency to interpret other people's behavior as aggressive, and a predisposition to choose aggressive ways of dealing with conflict impair social relationships and can lead to social isolation. Trauma can catastrophically destroy a child's illusion of omnipotence and belief in his or her parents' protection. Identification with the aggressor can occur in an attempt to gain power, control, and escape the horrifying world of the victim. Another altered cognition is a foreshortened image of the future. This can have a tremendous impact. It can lead to dropping out of school, having children prematurely, and engaging in risk-taking behavior.

AUTONOMIC DYSFUNCTION AND NEURODEVELOPMENTAL IMPACT

The hyperarousal that results from trauma (hypervigilance, increased startle, irritability, and difficulty sleeping) arises from a combination of neurobiologic changes and new cognitive schema depicting the world as a dangerous place. In children, the neurobiologic changes may lead to long-term impact on the development of the brain.

According to the cascade model, early trauma not only activates the stress response system, but leads to changes in brain development that affect later responses to stress. Stress hormones have a profound effect on the brain development of a child and affect patterns of myelination, neurogenesis, synaptogenesis, and neural morphobiology. Enduring neurophysiologic effects include size reduction in the midportion of the corpus callosum, decreased right/left hemispheric integration, electrical irritability of limbic circuits, decreased functional activity of the cerebellar vermis (and therefore decreased ability to inhibit limbic irritability), and attenuated left hemisphere development. Studies show mixed effects of stress on the size of the hippocampus. Teicher et al. hypothesize that these changes increase risks for PTSD, depression, dissociation, substance abuse, and borderline personality disorder. Animal research has shown that early stress interferes with the development of benzodiazepine and γ-aminobutyric acid (GABA) receptors, which inhibit the amygdala. In addition, prolonged stress or maternal inattention interferes with the glucocorticoid receptors in the hippocampus that provide negative feedback to cortisol release, leading to augmented release of stress response hormones. Several studies have shown that early stress also results in decreased levels of oxytocin mRNA in the hypothalamus. Oxytocin is a key factor in affiliative love, maintenance of monogamous relationships, and normal nonsexual interactions.

INCREASED VULNERABILITY TO TRAUMA

Sensitization and kindling make the traumatized person more vulnerable to further trauma in the future. "Kindling" processes have been described as subclinical abnormal electroencephalogram (EEG) activity. While "temporal lobe kindling" has been associated with epilepsy, kindling in the amygdala has been associated with anxiety in animal models. Learned helplessness makes individuals less able to protect themselves in potentially dangerous situations. Research has shown that people who dissociate after a trauma have decreased blood flow to the frontal lobes when dissociating. Hence, a trauma victim's cognitive capabilities, and ability to get out of a dangerous situation, are impaired in future dangerous situations.

Traumatic experiences change our perception of the risk and dangers of the world. Some people face high levels of anxiety and become inhibited in a wide variety of situations. Others, in order to deal with the anxiety, use denial. In order to avoid facing the high levels of anxiety after a trauma, they deny the risks involved in these situations. While denial is less painful in the short run than experiencing anxiety, it permits individuals to engage in some important developmental experiences. It can also place them in harm's way. This is another reason some traumatized individuals become risk prone.

Children who have been abused or exposed to domestic violence are at increased risk for becoming involved in abusive relationships or abusing their own children. The early abuse provides them with a model of the world in which violence is used in intimate relationships. This leaves them at greater risk for becoming perpetrators or tolerating being abused.

In addition, the fear and anger that result from the early trauma are likely to be played out in adult relationships.

SYMPTOMS AND DIAGNOSABLE DISORDERS

Exposure to violence has multiple effects on children, each of which should be addressed. Exposure to trauma can cause psychopathology and neurophysiologic changes. It may also impair ability to control affect and result in inappropriate responses to social situations, in addition to distorting a child's emotional development, core identity, and view of the world. The central issue in assessing the impact of trauma, and deciding if a child needs treatment, is the degree of impairment in social skills, academic functioning, and self-care.

According to the *Diagnostic and Statistical Manual of Mental Disorders,* Fourth Edition,Text Revision (DSM-IV-TR), PTSD trauma begins with the experience of intense fear, helplessness, horror, or disorganized and agitated behavior in response to exposure to an event that caused or threatened serious injury or violation of body integrity.

The likelihood that a traumatic situation will result in PTSD is based on a variety of factors. The intensity of trauma exposure is a key element in the development of PTSD. For example, close proximity to a traumatic event is more likely to result in PTSD then vicarious witnessing. Similarly, high media exposure of the traumatic event may repeat the emotional insult and increase the intensity of the trauma exposure. A history of previous trauma, abandonment, or insecure attachment also predisposes a child to developing PTSD. A prior history of anxiety and depressive symptoms, low resilience, and high reactivity to stimuli also increases vulnerability. Parents' level of stress and ability to respond to their children's needs and maintain normal routines and rules are also significant risk factors. How quickly and fully children are brought to a safe and comfortable place, the unexpectedness and duration of a disaster, whether the disaster was an act of nature or of human cause, and whether the child feels guilty over acts of omission or commission associated with trauma are also influential factors affecting prognosis. Other signs that indicate PTSD is likely to develop include dissociation at the time of the trauma, having a prolonged startle reaction, and having negative thoughts about oneself and others after the trauma.

After a trauma most people have significant symptoms, but, after time, recover. Therefore, chronic PTSD may be conceptualized as a disorder of recovery. Two factors that contribute to the ability of people to recover include the presence of supports and minimization of secondary stresses. For children, the presence of parents and their calm support is vital (see Table 19.1).

PTSD is only one of several diagnosable disorders that can arise from trauma. Depression, anxiety disorders, substance abuse, and subsyndromal PTSD are all common responses to trauma and can be very debilitating. Hoven found in NYC following the September 11 disaster that 26.5% of NYC public school children living in Manhattan below 110th Street appeared to meet criteria for a psychiatric disorder. The rate was more than double the estimated baseline rate.

PTSD symptoms overlap with those of other disorders, so clinicians may focus on symptoms but miss the underlying trauma syndrome. Depression and generalized anxiety disorder are particularly common responses to traumatic events. Weinstein et al. note that the hyperactivity, distractibility, impulsivity, and interpersonal problems that often come from trauma can lead to a diagnosis of attention deficit hyperactivity disorder (ADHD) instead of PTSD. Pelcovitz and Steiner describe how the trauma symptoms, such as loss of impulse control and aggression, can lead to diagnoses of oppositional defiant disorder (ODD) and conduct disorder (CD). Children with ODD have very high rates of traumatic victimization, but not of accidents or nonvictimization traumas.

TABLE 19.1. SALIENT CRITERIA FOR POSTTRAUMATIC STRESS DISORDER PER *DIAGNOSTIC AND STATISTICAL MANUAL OF MENTAL DISORDERS,* FOURTH EDITION, TEXT REVISION

Category	Criteria
Trauma exposure	• The child has been exposed to a traumatic event(s) directly in person or as a witness and is confronted with actual or threatened death or serious injury, or a threat to the physical integrity of self or others. • The child's response to the trauma may be expressed by disorganized or agitated behavior instead of the intense fear, helplessness, or horror seen in adults.
Trauma reexperience	• In young children, repetitive play may occur in which themes or aspects of the trauma may be expressed. In older children, the adult symptoms of recurrent intrusive distressing recollections of the event, including images and thoughts, may be evident. • Recurrent distressing dreams of the event. In children, there may be frightening dreams without recognizable content. • Acting or feeling like the traumatic event was recurring, e.g., experiencing flashbacks. In young children, trauma-specific reenactment may occur. • Intense psychological distress at exposure to internal or external cues that symbolize or resemble an aspect of the traumatic event. • Physiologic reactivity on exposure to internal or external cues that symbolize or resemble an aspect of the traumatic event.
Trauma avoidance	• Persistent avoidance to avoid activities, places, and individuals that arouse recollections of the traumatic event. • Persistent efforts to avoid thoughts, feelings, or conversation of the trauma. • Inability to recall important aspects of the event. • Markedly diminished interest in significant activities of daily living. • Feeling detached or estranged from others. • Restricted range of affect. • Sense of foreshortened future.

From American Psychiatric Association. *Diagnostic and statistical manual of mental disorders*, 4th ed. Text rev. Washington, DC: American Psychiatric Association, 2000, with permission.

In teenagers, it can be difficult to distinguish between PTSD and borderline personality. Herman reports that 60% to 80% of women with a diagnosis of borderline personality disorder report a history of childhood sexual abuse. Van der Kolk and Herman posit that borderline personality disorder may be a severe, chronic manifestation of PTSD-related character pathology. Substance abuse is a common comorbidity that may represent a failed effort to relieve distress through self-medication. Postconcussive syndrome (headaches, anxiety, emotional lability, concentration impairment, memory problems) and head injuries without loss of consciousness can be confused with PTSD. The aggression, difficulty concentrating, sleep problems, labile mood, and risk taking of PTSD can lead a clinician to diagnose bipolar disorder. The loss of interest in previously enjoyed activities, withdrawal from family and peers, and sleep problems may result in the diagnosis of major depression. Schwarz and Perry found that somatization is a prominent symptom in traumatized children and can lead to a focus on finding a medical problem. Therefore it is important to evaluate for the presence of PTSD in children with multiple somatic complaints.

DEVELOPMENTAL DISTURBANCE

Trauma can have a profound effect on a child's ability to mature, including the development of affect and behavior regulation, core identity, and social skills. This impact, however, is not captured by any of the DSM-IV-TR diagnoses. Traditional trauma treatment plans tend to overlook these sequelae and focus on symptoms such as intrusive recollections and sleep disturbance. As a result, the child is less likely to fully recover and reach his or her previctim potential.

Regulation of affect and behavior

Pynoos et al. observe that the intense negative affective states that arise after disasters can interfere with a child's developing ability to regulate, identify, and express emotions. The intense emotional experience caused by traumatic reminders interferes with the child's ability to reflect, examine, label, express, and control affect. As a result, traumatized children often are unable to develop adequate control of their affective experiences and responses to stressful situations.

Intensified startle reactions, hypervigilance, numbing, and withdrawal can interrupt the acquisition of affect control. These symptoms interfere with attempts to reflect, express, and manage emotions. Pollak et al. postulate that traumatic victimization often leads to distrust and intolerance of one's emotions and interferes with the development of self-control skills. It is difficult to engage successfully in social and work activities when contending with hypervigilance, startle reflexes, numbness, and withdrawal. Without normal developmental experiences, opportunities to habituate to stressful situations and to develop effective coping skills will be lost. Hypervigilance can also lead to exaggerated perceptions of danger. Pynoos et al. note that these distortions of the intentions of others can markedly impair social relationships.

The child's ability to inhibit aggressive impulses can deteriorate after experiencing a trauma. Watching violence may interfere with the development of appropriate impulse control. Moreover, revenge and retaliation fantasies often follow, which may foster identification with the aggressor and the self-righteous belief that one is entitled to behave violently. Even vicarious experiences of violence can lead to preoccupation with aggression, rumination on violent images, and a tendency to watch or engage in aggression. For some children the fear of aggression may promote inhibitions that can interfere with the appropriate use of assertiveness. The resulting inability to be assertive can fuel an image of oneself as a victim and lead to more intense anger as the individual fails to cope with competitive situations. In time, there may be compensatory outbursts of aggression. Children and adolescents may also turn to substance abuse in order to manage the painful emotions created by the trauma of a disaster. Both van der Kolk et al. and Pynoos et al. hypothesize that revenge fantasies, narcissistic rage, adolescent omnipotence, and access to drugs and weapons may result in an explosive combination that can lead the child to engage in violent behavior, radical ideologies, and hate groups.

Core identity

Trauma markedly affects a child's core identity. The sense of powerlessness in being a victim damages the sense of self-efficacy. The tendency of children to blame themselves for problems, along with magical thinking, can promote a deep sense of guilt or shame. Moreover, the belief that one did not perform well during a crisis, either due to a harsh superego, objective failure, or someone's unfortunate comment, can lead to further damage to self-esteem. This shameful or guilt-ridden self-image can become embedded into the core of the personality and have a negative effect on personality development. Children may become chronically dysthymic, socially isolated, or risk-prone as a way to disprove the tarnished self-image. Shame, self-blame, and seeing oneself as ineffective can also interfere with adaptive and social functioning. Ultimately, these problems can interfere with the development of empathy and prosocial behavior.

Trauma can also distort representations of the self, others, and the world, and can activate conflicts from earlier developmental periods. In young children, trauma can derail central organizing fantasies around which the sense of self is established, leading to developmental arrest. The traumatic disruption of early narcissistic fantasies can leave archaic grandiose fantasies unresolved and lead to a perpetual search to merge with powerful figures. Disaster can also interfere with consolidation of identity or even to the formation of a negative identity.

The experience of disaster may destroy the child's glorified images of parents and self. In normal development, children slowly come to terms with the limited abilities of their parents. Premature and sudden collapse of these images may lead to a variety of problems. A child's attachment to his parents may be weakened, and the child may search for other parental figures with whom to identify. The child may become anxious and withdraw from social and school activities essential to social development. The child can also develop a pervasive sense of defectiveness that constitutes a risk for narcissistic psychopathology, including vulnerability to grandiosity and narcissistic rage.

Traumatic anxiety can interfere with the development of prosocial, moral behavior. Children must overcome anxiety to counter the wishes of delinquent peers to maintain morally appropriate behaviors in peer group situations. Anxiety can also block a child's engagement in the social relationships and experiences needed for moral development.

Efforts to master the fear and sense of vulnerability elicited by exposure to a disaster may foster enduring identifications. Pynoos et al. describe one possible identification with rescuers leading to a long-term preoccupation with saving people. Another possibility is preoccupation with revenge fantasies arising from identification with the aggressor. Revenge fantasies can also foster a combined identification with both aggressor and victim that can be disorganizing or dangerous. Recent mass shootings by teenagers at Columbine and Thurston High Schools demonstrate this dynamic.

Social skills

Perhaps the two most destructive aspects of PTSD are the damage to the child's ability to engage in normal developmental experiences and the markedly increased vulnerability to trauma in the future. Trauma-induced anxiety may cause withdrawal, regression, and interfere with participation in normal developmental activities, such as socializing with other children and participating in school activities. The impact of this can be greater than the direct impact of the symptoms of PTSD.

Traumatic victimization fosters oppositional defiant behavior. The oppositional defiant behavior, in turn, can increase the risk of further victimization and lead to a cascade of problems including depression, engagement with a deviant peer group, substance abuse, truancy, petty criminal activity, and even aggressive delinquency. Victimization predisposes children to see benign actions as hostile and to select aggressive responses, seeing them either as a good choice or the only choice possible. These children demonstrate a resentful and resigned coping style.

Types of Trauma and Sequelae

Although there is significant overlap of symptoms in response to different types of trauma, there are also differences. According to Terr, one of the most important differences is whether the trauma was a single or multiple event. Having addressed some of the underlying psychological and neurophysiologic processes that are activated in trauma, the following sections discuss the findings of symptoms in children traumatized in different ways.

SINGLE EVENT TRAUMA SYMPTOMS

Following a disaster, accident, or assault, most children will develop significant psychiatric symptoms, and many will have a diagnosable disorder. The most common symptoms are fear, anhedonia, and attention and learning problems. New onset reactivation or intensification of specific fears, along with dependent and regressed behavior, is also common. A trauma can cause a wide range of depression and anxiety-like symptoms. These include dissociation, sleep dysregulation, nightmares, trauma-related fears, repetitive trauma-related play, regression, clinginess, separation anxiety, intrusive recollections, numbing and withdrawal, hyperarousal, problems with concentration, irritability, dysphoria, and somatic complaints. Substance abuse, personality disorders, and decreased ability to protect oneself from dangerous situations leading to revictimization may also occur. Belief that omens predicted the disaster, along with subsequent attention to possible warning signs and sense of a foreshortened future, are also prominent at times. While PTSD symptoms have a tendency to progressively lessen over time, anxiety, depressive symptoms, and behavior problems may be greater during the latter months than in the initial weeks after trauma. Moreover, the onset of PTSD may be delayed.

Children's symptoms vary as a function of age and developmental phase (see Table 19.2). Young children are likely to have the new onset of aggression or a fear not directly related to the trauma, such as separation anxiety or fear of the dark. Numbing and withdrawal may appear as regression and loss of previously acquired skills. Intrusive memories in young children are likely to take the form of repetitive, joyless play with traumatic themes. Repetitively drawing pictures of the trauma or acting out the trauma in play occurs frequently. Generalized anxiety, along with heightened arousal and exaggerated startle reactions, are common. Many children have sleep problems, nightmares without clear content, and somatic complaints. Regression, including loss of skills and increased attachment behavior, is particularly common in young children. Young children develop renewed separation anxiety and new fears, avoid new activities, become aggressive, lose verbal skills and sphincter control, wish to sleep in their parents' bed, whine and have temper tantrums, and develop stage-four sleep disorders.

School-aged children may become obsessed with the details of the disaster in an attempt to cope or enter a state of constant anxiety and arousal to prepare for future dangers. Some children withdraw into their own quiet world while others engage in increased aggressive behavior. Concentration problems, distractibility, poor sleep, and nightmares are common in this age group, along with preoccupation with danger and reminders. Somatic symptoms continue to be a common expression of distress at this age. School-aged children may become inconsistent in their behavior, vacillating between being cooperative and argumentative, or from exuberant to inhibited. To avoid painful feelings associated with the disaster, children may avoid social activities and school and may instead focus their energies on repetitive retelling of the event and traumatic play. School-aged children can engage other children in playing out games recreating the trauma. Their play and comments may show misunderstandings about what occurred. School-aged children can have an inappropriate sense of responsibility for the disaster, reinforced by a tendency toward magical thinking. A tendency to "time skewing" results in a child erroneously sequencing events when retelling what happened in a traumatic event.

As children move into adolescence, their trauma reactions become similar to those of adults. They are likely to have symptoms of numbing and withdrawal, as well as hyperarousal and intrusive memories. To manage their painful feelings they may retreat from others or throw themselves into various activities. They may become unusually aggressive and oppositional. Adolescents develop a foreshortened view of the future and may precipitously enter into adult activities, like leaving school to find a job or marry. They may engage in

TABLE 19.2. TRAUMA RESPONSE AND DEVELOPMENTAL AGE

Developmental Age	Trauma Response
Preschoolers	• Likely to not report symptoms of numbing and withdrawal, but are likely to have the new onset of aggression or a fear not directly related to the trauma, such as separation anxiety or fear of the dark. • Intrusive memories are likely to take the form of repetitive, joyless play with traumatic themes, or repetitively drawing pictures of the trauma or acting it out. • Regression; lose verbal skills and sphincter control. • Renewed separation anxiety and new fears and avoidance of new activities. • Become aggressive, whine, and have temper tantrums. • Develop stage-four sleep disorders; wish to sleep in their parents' bed.
School age	• Become obsessed with the details of the disaster in an attempt to cope, or enter a state of constant anxiety and arousal to prepare for future dangers. • Withdraw into their own quiet world while others engage in increased aggressive behavior. • Concentration problems, distractibility. • Poor sleep and nightmares, along with preoccupation with danger and reminders. • Somatic symptoms are a common expression of distress at this age. • Become inconsistent in their behavior, vacillating between being cooperative and argumentative, or from exuberant to inhibited. • Can engage other children in playing out games recreating the trauma. • Play and comments may show misunderstandings about what occurred. • Inappropriate sense of responsibility for the disaster, reinforced by a tendency toward magical thinking.
Adolescents	• Reactions become similar to those of traumatized adults. • Likely to have several symptoms of numbing and withdrawal, as well as hyperarousal and actual intrusive memories. • To manage their painful feelings, they may retreat from others or throw themselves into various activities. • May become unusually aggressive and oppositional. • Develop a foreshortened view of the future and may precipitously enter into adult activities, leave school to find a job, or marry. • May engage in high-risk behavior including life-threatening reenactments of the trauma situation, substance abuse, and unsafe sexual behavior to counter the pain of the trauma. • May harbor revenge wishes. • May become depressed and withdraw, with sudden shifts in relationships. • Eating disturbances, sleep problems, and nightmares are common. • Combination of concentration problems, hyperarousal, dysphoria, and irritability can simulate ADHD, oppositional defiant disorder, conduct disorder, and even bipolar disorder.

ADHD, attention deficit hyperactivity disorder.

high-risk behavior including life-threatening reenactments of the trauma event, substance abuse, and unsafe sexual behavior. They may harbor revenge wishes. Some become depressed and withdraw, and there may be sudden shifts in relationships. Eating disturbances, sleep problems, and nightmares are common. The combination of concentration problems, hyperarousal, dysphoria, and irritability can simulate ADHD, ODD, CD, and even bipolar disorder.

Single incident trauma can have a profound and long-lasting effect. Two years after the Buffalo Creek Dam collapse, 37% of children evaluated met some DSM-III-R PTSD criterion, and 17 years after the collapse 7% still met the minimum number of criteria for having the disorder. All of the children in the Chowchilla bus hijacking had posttraumatic symptoms 4 years later. Another study showed that 7 years after a bus/train accident, those having relatively high levels of exposure had relatively high levels of somatization, depression, phobic anxiety, psychoticism, and PTSD symptoms. Half of victims generally recover within 3 months, but many remain ill for a year or more. Symptoms may reemerge following a subsequent trauma, life stresses, or reminders of the original trauma.

COMPLEX TRAUMA

Complex trauma consists of multiple exposures to stressful events over time. Complex trauma, such as repeated episodes of physical abuse, is known to cause PTSD. In a study of children abused by their parents, 40% met criteria for PTSD upon removal from their parents' homes and 33% still met criteria 2 years later. Widom found a 37.5% lifetime prevalence for PTSD in victims of substantiated childhood abuse and neglect. The primary symptoms in chronic trauma are impairment of affect regulation, chronic destructive behavior (self-mutilation, eating disorders, drug abuse, oppositional behavior, violence to others, risk taking, suicidality), dissociation, and problems with attention, somatization, problematic relationships, altered threat perception, and shame. These problems resulting from trauma have been referred to as disorders of extreme stress not otherwise specified (DESNOS).

Complex trauma can lead to perceptual disturbances, possibly due to limbic system malfunction. Teicher et al. found that adult outpatients with childhood histories of physical and sexual abuse had significantly increased rates of limbic system symptoms commonly seen in temporal lobe seizures, including dissociative phenomena, perceptual distortions, and brief hallucinatory events.

Complex trauma may result in affective instability and impaired concentration abilities. Physically abused infants demonstrate high levels of negative affect and limited positive affect. Emotionally neglected infants tend to have blunted affect. Maltreated toddlers are found to be angrier, more frustrated, and more noncompliant during an experimental task than nonmaltreated comparison children. During the preschool years, these children were rated as more hyperactive, distractible, lacking in self-control, and evidencing a high level of negative affect. In kindergarten, maltreated children are rated more inattentive, aggressive, and overactive by teachers. As maltreated children reach adulthood, they show increased rates of depression and domestic violence. It may take years for symptoms and behavioral deficits to manifest in youths exposed to complex trauma. Many children exposed to extreme violence under the Pol Pot Regime in Cambodia, which killed 10% of the country's population, did not reveal emotional problems until years later.

Maltreated infants and toddlers also show a preponderance of atypical attachment patterns. Cicchetti and Toth note that "internal representational models of these insecure and often atypical attachments, with their complementary models of self and other, may generalize to new relationships, leading to negative expectations of how others will behave and how successful the self will be in relation to others."

Physically abused children have heightened levels of physical and verbal aggression in peer interactions, and they may respond with anger and aggression to friendly overtures or signs of distress in other children. Maltreated toddlers have been shown to react to peer distress with anger, fear, and aggression, rather than empathy and concern. Maltreated children are often avoidant of peer interactions. In a new peer group, maltreated children show less social competence than controls, fewer positive emotions, direct less behavior toward peers, initiate fewer interactions, and engage in less complex play. Maltreated children are more attentive to and distracted by aggressive stimuli than controls. Peers see maltreated children as evidencing more aggressiveness and disruptive behavior and less leadership and sharing. A 16-year longitudinal study of maltreated preschool children showed that adolescent assaultive behavior is related to severe physical discipline, being sexually abused, and experiencing negative mother-child interactions. Abused preschoolers also have a tendency toward aggression and lack of empathy to others, withdrawal in interactions with adults, and distortions in information processing. Abused children tend to see their nonabusing mothers as unavailable, untrustworthy, unloving, and unreliable, and they may develop an oppositional defiant stance as a defense against betrayal or vulnerability to any emotion.

SEXUAL ABUSE

Sexual abuse is traumatic in several ways. Sexually abused children often feel like victims of physical aggression. Sexual abuse may also involve betrayal of a child's trust with subsequent depression and difficulty trusting. Sexually abused children often feel weak and vulnerable. The associated shame, low self-esteem, and self-destructive behavior may perpetuate a trauma cycle.

Sexualized behavior from abused children is common and is manifested as sexual play with dolls, excessive or public masturbation, seductive behavior, requests for sexual stimulation from adults or children, and age-inappropriate sexual knowledge. Preschoolers tend to suffer from anxiety, nightmares, disruptive behavior, and inappropriate sexual behavior. School-aged children tend to show fear, aggression, nightmares, school problems, hyperactivity, and regressive behaviors. Adolescents show depression, withdrawal, suicidality, self-injury, somatic complaints, delinquency, running away behavior, and substance abuse. Survivors of sexual abuse often have poor social adjustment, fewer and less close friends, and see themselves as unworthy of healthy relationships. Avoidance and tension-reducing symptoms include dissociation, substance abuse, promiscuity, eating disorders, and self-mutilation.

DOMESTIC VIOLENCE

Witnessing domestic violence is a serious trauma for a child. Several studies have reported that children exposed to domestic violence exhibit more aggressive and antisocial behaviors (often called "externalized" behaviors) as well as fearful and inhibited behaviors ("internalized" behaviors) when compared to nonexposed children. Children exposed to domestic violence show responses similar to children who have been directly physically or sexually abused. These children show lower social competence than children not exposed to domestic violence and are found to show higher levels of anxiety, depression, trauma symptoms, aggression with peers, negative affect, and inappropriate responses to social situations than children who are not exposed to violence at home. These children tend to feel worthless, mistrust intimate relationships, are aggressive, and have delayed intellectual development. Very young children often identify with the aggressor and may lose respect for victimized peers. Older children often feel guilty. Girls tend to become anxious, passive, and withdrawn, while boys demonstrate aggressive and disruptive behavior. Compared to children who received corporal punishment, children who witnessed interparental aggression are more likely to be convicted of an index crime such as larceny, auto theft, burglary, assault, attempted rape, rape, kidnapping, attempted murder, or murder. Spaccarelli et al. found that among a sample of 213 adolescent boys incarcerated for violent crimes, those who had been exposed to family violence believed more than others that "acting aggressively enhances one's reputation or self-image" and holding this belief significantly predicted violent offending. The Silvern et al. study of 550 undergraduate students found that exposure to violence as a child is associated with adult reports of depression, trauma-related symptoms and low self-esteem among women and only trauma-related symptoms among men.

COMMUNITY VIOLENCE

Community violence is an endemic problem in many cities in the United States. High levels of community violence exposure predict peer-rated aggression, alcohol and drug use, carrying knives and guns, defensive and offensive fighting, and trouble in school, as well as fear and anxiety, depression, helplessness and hopelessness, emotional withdrawal, somatic symptoms, impaired social relationships, and increased general activity and restlessness. The experience of chronic danger has a marked effect on a child's ability to explore his or her environment and develop social skills. Desensitization, resignation, and addiction are frequent results of experiencing community violence. Perceptions of others and interpreting social interactions are also affected.

In 1992, Garbarino et al. noted that preschool children exposed to community violence tend to have passive reactions and regressive symptoms in response. School-aged children tend to have aggression, inhibition, somatic complaints, and learning difficulties. Adolescents tend to enter into adulthood prematurely, use substances, and display aggression, promiscuity, and increased risk taking.

BULLYING

Bullying is the abuse or harassment of weaker individuals. It differs from typical age-related quarreling or teasing by being prolonged, one sided, and malicious. It may consist of physical aggression (hitting, kicking, robbing, pushing, unwanted sexual touching), be verbal in nature (insulting, threatening, taunting), or include psychological cruelty (extortion, intimidation, spreading rumors, excluding). Bullying is a serious problem for children and hurts both perpetrators and victims. Studies have shown that up to 17% of school-aged children are bullied at school and 19% had bullied others. Six percent of students are frequently both bullied and bully others. Finally, it is estimated that 1.6 million children in grades 6 through 10 alone are bullied on a weekly basis in the United States.

Perpetrators frequently fail to learn appropriate inhibitions against hurting others and instead receive gratification for being abusive. Victims experience the typical range of trauma-related symptoms, including academic impairment, depression, isolation, fear and anxiety, humiliation, and poor self-esteem. Victims may also later develop substance abuse, criminal behavior, and PTSD. Students who are both bullied and bully others tend to have particularly poor outcomes. Those who witness bullying probably suffer some negative effects, too.

Whether emotional abuse and trauma fit the DSM-IV-TR criteria for trauma is debatable. Being unable to go anywhere else and being dependent on parents for basic needs places children in marked states of vulnerability so that neglect can be as threatening as assault. Children's emotional dependence on adults leaves them vulnerable to emotional abuse in ways adults are not. Assaults on the sense of self can be as damaging and invasive as a sexual assault is on bodily integrity. Whether or not one sees emotional abuse and neglect as types of trauma, it is clear that they have devastating effects on children.

DEATH OF A LOVED ONE

Bereavement and complex bereavement are very common problems. Bereavement affects 6 million Americans a year. Of those, 20% have complex bereavement. Complex or traumatic bereavement is a combination of a trauma reaction and bereavement. In classic bereavement, the cardinal symptoms include sadness or other dysphoria, social withdrawal, loss of interest or pleasure in daily activities, and somatic symptoms. In complex bereavement, however, a persistent intense grief reaction, unusual difficulty separating, and a trauma reaction are present. Certain beliefs are common in complex grief: sense of guilt and hopelessness, the feeling that one will not be able to cope, an abiding sense of the world as dangerous and unjust, and believing that the intensity and continuance of one's grief is a measure of love for the deceased and, thus, ceasing to grieve would constitute betrayal.

Adults often miss the fact that children are grieving because their reactions are different from those of adults. Children may be preoccupied with who will take care of them. They lack a mature understanding of death and may nearly simultaneously note that the loved one is lost and then ask if they will be back for the upcoming holiday.

Complex grief is particularly likely under certain situations such as witnessing an unexpected or violent death by the bereaved. Other situations that increase the risk of complex grief include ambivalent feelings about the deceased, death related to negligence by the bereaved, and guilt related to feelings of betrayal or permanent loss.

The process of grieving a loved one entails remembering the good and bad times, coming to a well-rounded picture of the relationship, and changing the relationship from one in real life to a relationship in memory. When one has a trauma reaction, and one's thoughts of the person are preoccupied with violent images of how he or she died, it is not possible to go through the normal grieving process.

INVASIVE MEDICAL PROCEDURES

Invasive medical procedures and serious illness can also cause posttraumatic stress disorder. Children with cancer, burns, and those undergoing transplantation of bone marrow or livers are all at considerable risk for PTSD. The repetitive nature of certain medical treatments results in complex trauma. Children receiving chemotherapy, in particular, may experience their multiple treatments as complex trauma. The initial pain associated with intravenous line placements is followed by the terrible side effects of nausea, vomiting, malaise, and, in some cases, disfigurement from alopecia or cachexia. Children with most types of cancer need multiple chemotherapy treatments and must endure these experiences numerous times during the course of their illness. For children with burns, sometimes the repeated debridements and skin-grafting procedures are more painful then the initial burns. Despite the trauma caused by medical treatments and procedures, treatment of PTSD in these children can significantly improve medical compliance and outcomes.

INTERGENERATIONAL TRANSMISSION OF TRAUMA

The intergenerational transmission of trauma is a particularly serious problem in our society. Trauma has become an endemic problem as a result of intergenerational transmission phenomenon. Children who are abused are far more likely to abuse their own children than are nonabused children. Boys who witness domestic violence are more likely to abuse romantic partners, and girls who witness domestic violence have an increased rate of being abused themselves. In fact, the best predictor of whether an individual will be abusive is whether he or she had been abused as a child.

Several mechanisms are notable. As described earlier, experiencing trauma increases an individual's predisposition to behaving aggressively by creating narcissistic injuries and predisposing the individual to feel threatened and violated by interactions with people. Trauma also interferes with affective development and control. Second, abuse interferes with the development of normal attachment. Insecure attachments are a prelude to subsequent adult emotional problems. Third is the internalization of parental models of violence. Related to this, social learning theory argues that much of human behavior is learned by observing others. Children try out behaviors they have seen others model and then refine their own behavior based on the feedback they receive. Internalization of observed behavior is particularly likely if the model has high status and if the observer has low self-esteem. Behavior is also influenced by the inner standards one develops about appropriate behavior. These inner standards arise from the experience of having limits prescribed during childhood and by seeing how peers and adults modulate or do not modulate their own actions.

Identifying and Treating Trauma Victims

Identifying the children who are having emotional problems because of exposure to trauma is a difficult and fundamental problem for all childcare workers. The ability of children to shift from painful affective states to play often leads parents incorrectly to assume that the child has recovered. Studies indicate that counselors and teachers identify fewer than 50% of adolescents with significant, treatable emotional problems. Pediatricians do even more poorly, probably due to their more limited time for interaction, and identify only 25% of those with diagnosable mental disorders. While the literature on treating emotional trauma in children is somewhat limited, teachers, pediatricians, and other child healthcare professionals need to receive more training in recognizing children who have been traumatized and in referring them for treatment (see Table 19.3).

ASSESSMENT

Children may avoid telling their parents about difficult feelings because it is painful to talk about them and because they do not want to worry their parents. Parents, meanwhile, are often stressed themselves after a disaster or car accident and are not at their best as observers of their children. Changes in children's behavior are often seen as moodiness or a phase rather than a reaction to a traumatic incident. Teachers are often better at picking up the signs of a traumatized child since they see the child interacting with others and attempting to concentrate over a period of several hours every day. Teachers, however, are mainly responsible for teaching their lessons and maintaining order in their classes. This leads them to pay more attention to the disruptive child and to overlook the child who is quietly in pain.

TABLE 19.3. ESSENTIALS FOR ASSESSMENT OF TRAUMA IN CHILDREN

- Very young children are less likely to have any of the traditional signs of trauma, and, the younger the traumatized children the less likely they are going to talk about their trauma. Assessing clinicians should be aware of the developmental variations of presentation.
- Assessing clinicians should always ask direct questions about the trauma of the traumatized children; however, they may need several sessions to elicit trauma history in severely anxious traumatized children.
- Clinicians trying to obtain history from traumatized children should not expect them to talk directly about their traumatic experiences. The use of projective techniques such as storytelling, play, and expressions through artwork may be the only avenue to the inner life of the traumatized child.
- While data from a structured rating instrument is a valuable part of a comprehensive evaluation of traumatized children, no rating scale can be used as a substitute for clinical interviews in making a trauma-related diagnosis.
- Parental history is often limited since they are often stressed themselves after a disaster or traumatic event and are not at their best as observers of their traumatized children. Thus, the diagnosis of trauma psychopathology should not rely entirely on the parental history.
- The over diagnosis of trauma psychopathology is due to a lack of awareness of the specific diagnostic criteria required and the notion that the presence of trauma history and anxiety or affective dysregulation following exposure to an extreme stressor are all that are needed to make these diagnoses.
- The underdiagnosis of trauma psychopathology is most often due to assessing clinicians not asking direct questions about the trauma and the reexperience of trauma.

Assessment for trauma should include the basic components of a psychiatric assessment. Trauma history needs to be taken in context of developmental and social domains. As noted earlier, trauma symptoms vary with chronologic age. History should be gathered from multiple sources including parents, teachers, therapists, child welfare case-workers, and child protective service providers. Externalizing symptoms are more readily reported by parents, teachers, and other adults than the affected child. Internalizing symptoms, however, are more likely to be elicited from the traumatized child than from parents and other adults. Because the signs and symptoms of trauma greatly overlap with most of the psychiatric disorders found in children, special attention should be given in discerning the difference between externalizing and internalizing symptoms due to nontrauma childhood psychopathology and those secondary to trauma. When interviewing the child, the examiner should attempt to ask direct questions about the traumatic event. Often, children will reveal details of the event, despite the discomfort in the recounting of the trauma. If a child declines to share during the initial evaluation, pressure to self-disclose should be minimized. The child should be reassured that questions about the trauma can come later when he or she is feeling less overwhelmed.

As noted earlier, preschool-aged children will often demonstrate violent themes in their play during the mental status exam. While school-aged children are often uncomfortable talking about their traumatic experiences, when requested they usually will draw pictures of the traumatic event. Asking the child to tell the story behind the picture often provides a window into the child's experience of the trauma. Adolescents are able to respond like adults during the mental status exam and are able to answer questions about their mood and thought content. Obsessive thoughts about the trauma are common. Flashbacks may be reported as hallucinations. These experiences may be distinguished from psychotic pathology if they are only associated with trauma triggers. Queries about suicidal and homicidal ideations should be made in traumatized teens as they frequently suffer from comorbid depression and anxiety or revenge fantasies in cases of abuse or being bullied. Concentration and focus are often impaired in traumatized youths. The negative affect usually associated with trauma differentiate these children from those with ADHD.

A number of rating scales maybe helpful in assessing trauma. Two examples of commonly used assessment tools that are used specifically for measuring trauma include the Trauma Symptom Checklist for Children (TSCC) and the Child Posttraumatic Stress-Reaction Index (CPTS-RI). These instruments are meant to be used as part of a comprehensive evaluation. They are not intended to be used individually to make the diagnosis of trauma-related psychopathology.

TREATMENT

Cognitive-behavioral therapy

Optimal treatment of trauma using cognitive-behavioral therapy (CBT) techniques integrates the following five components. The first is a combination of psychoeducation, stress inoculation, and relaxation training. In addition, some children will need help in learning to put feelings into words. Second is the creation of a narrative of what occurred. This will help to desensitize the child to painful memories and traumatic reminders and decrease the child's withdrawal and avoidance. Depending upon the child's age, one may talk directly about what occurred, or create a book or a make-believe radio show about the events. The third component is exploring the way in which the child has been affected by the trauma and replacing unhelpful thoughts with more helpful ones. The fourth component is working on social skills so that the child's relationships improve. The final component is safety planning: what active steps can the child take to deal with dangerous situations in the future? Whenever possible, parents should receive guidance in parallel with the child's therapy.

Therapy begins by providing an orientation to CBT and stress inoculation. Stress inoculation typically consists of education and training of coping skills, including deep muscle relaxation training, breathing control, assertiveness, role playing, modeling, thought stopping, positive thinking, and self-talk. The indications for therapy are discussed. If the child has a limited understanding, the clinician can acknowledge that the child has been through a traumatic experience, and, that when terrible things happen, people have strong feelings and often do not want to talk about them. When children are able to talk about the event it helps them to feel better. Feelings identification, relaxation training (deep breathing and muscle relaxation), thought stopping, and cognitive coping are all important techniques to consider teaching the child depending upon his or her specific symptoms. For children having nightmares, dream control techniques in which the child thinks about a more benign end to the nightmares can be helpful. Relationship and trust building are essential elements of the first part of therapy. The most important factor in healing is the development of a trusting relationship in which patients feel that their therapist truly understands and is concerned about them.

These techniques help a child to begin feeling better and generally make it possible to begin talking about what occurred and the impact of the event on the child's feelings about the world and him- or herself. Central to treatment is the examination of the impact of the event on the child's images of self and the world. To begin this process, instruction is given about the difference between thoughts and feelings, and about how thoughts about events affect feelings and behavior. The tendency to automate thoughts and the possibility of replacing them with thoughts that are more helpful need to be practiced. Critical areas to examine include self-image, ability to trust others, sense of safety, and images of and plans for the future. Adolescents will generally be able to relate what occurred. Younger children may do better by creating a storybook of the event. The child's thoughts and feelings during the trauma should be noted. Therapists should ask about the worst moment. Distortions about what happened should be corrected as they arise in the storytelling. Relaxation techniques and distraction are important tools to modulate the child's affect. Having the child write a corrective story or doing corrective drawings can often help. Whether using drawings or storytelling, the therapist must never leave the child focused on the images of pain, fear, and loss. Instead, move on to how the child wants to rebuild things, what he or she has learned, and how he or she wants the future to be (see Table 19.4).

TABLE 19.4. ESSENTIALS FOR TREATMENT OF TRAUMATIZED CHILDREN

- Psychoeducation and parental guidance and counseling should be provided in parallel with individual treatment of the child.
- Coercing or forcing a child to talk about or recall trauma can make symptoms more intense and overwhelming.
- Creation of a narrative of the traumatic event is useful to help desensitize traumatized children.
- Safety planning with the traumatized child is particularly important in situations involving domestic and community violence.
- The treatment of traumatized children will often be unsuccessful if their traumatized parents are not treated concomitantly.
- Parents should be coached to avoid contaminating the child with their own feelings and verbalizing that their child may be damaged from the traumatic event.
- To prevent future symptoms and psychopathology, children with complex trauma should receive treatment even if they do not manifest any overt signs and symptoms.
- Care should be given to treating any secondary psychopathology and behavioral problems such as depression, phobias, aggression, or school avoidance.
- Despite the paucity of research showing the efficacy of psychotropic agents for the treatment of trauma, empiric treatment with psychotropic medications should be used as adjunctive treatment for clearly defined target symptoms.

Other psychotherapeutic aspects of treatment

It is destructive for children to suffer a significant period of poor psychosocial functioning. Poor social or academic functioning lasting a few months can cause a child to fall significantly behind peers. Once symptoms resolve it can still be difficult for them to catch up, particularly for those who sustain psychiatric sequelae from the trauma. Therefore, it is important for therapists to help their patients complete basic developmental tasks. Moreover, therapists should encourage parents to arrange for assistance in keeping their child from becoming developmentally derailed to prevent falling behind peers. Assistance may include social skills building and behavioral interventions that can disrupt the maladaptive coping patterns resulting from trauma.

Creating a safety plan and helping children to deal with dangerous situations is also a fundamental part of treatment. Without this, it will be difficult for traumatized children to feel safe enough in their environment to learn, socialize, and grow. In addition, the child may need a safety plan for use in ongoing dangerous situations. Children from homes of domestic violence, in particular, are in need of specific responses to risk situations. Coaching the child and appropriate family members in how to use the plan is part of the safety planning process. Role-playing may be needed to induce behaviorally inhibited children to practice safety plans so they will actually use them when necessary.

It is important to work with the parents and to treat the parents for their own trauma if necessary. Multiple studies have shown that parents' reactions are the most influential factors affecting a child's outcome. If the parents' stress, depression, or anxiety is untreated, significant therapy for the child will be of limited help.

It can be very helpful to have a joint session with the parent and child in which the child can "teach" the parent about PTSD and relaxation techniques, cognitive processing (how our thoughts affect our feelings), and the impact the trauma has had. The child can share the narrative/storybook of the trauma. All of this needs to be reviewed by the therapist and parents prior to the joint session. The joint session facilitates the ability of the child and parent to talk about what happened and to continue to work together to counter problematic cognitions and trauma symptoms.

All children with complex trauma should receive an assessment even if they do not manifest any symptoms. Adults often do not see children's internalizing symptoms because children deny that they are feeling bad. Hidden effects on the child's sense of self and views of the world may have a profound effect on development, but preventive work can help the child avoid serious problems in the future.

Complex bereavement also requires special techniques. Before helping the individual with grief, one treats the trauma reaction. In addition, the child needs help in working through ambivalent feelings about the lost person, guilt over unpleasant words or actions during the relationship, saying goodbye to the relationship, and reconnecting to life. Letters written to and imagined discussions with the deceased can be very helpful.

Many trauma researchers note the value of using creative ways to help children tell the story of their traumatic event. One of the most innovative researchers is van der Kolk. He suggests the use of dance, song, and theater to help children express themselves, rather than sitting and talking. He also argues for the critical role of helping children develop a sense of competence and achievement as they work in nontraditional creative ways on ameliorating the effect of their trauma.

Pharmacotherapy

There is a dearth of scientific evidence for using psychotropic medications in the treatment of childhood trauma-related psychopathology and PTSD. At this time, there are only two Food and Drug Administration (FDA)-approved psychotropic medications for the treatment of

PTSD in adults, but no approved medications for the treatment of pediatric PTSD. Despite the lack of data for practicing evidence-based psychotropic treatment, the majority of medical practitioners use pharmacologic interventions. The goal of pharmacologic interventions is to decrease or eliminate the major symptoms of trauma and treat secondary disorders. Hyperarousal, insomnia, anxiety, and agitation are the common target symptoms for trauma victims. A review of the meager research literature reveals that clonidine, propranolol, imipramine, citalopram, nefazodone, and carbamazepine have been in studies of the treatment of PTSD in children and adolescents. These studies had small sample sizes and all reported some improvement for some of their subjects. Despite these published studies, selective serotonin reuptake inhibitors (SSRIs) seem to be the most popular treatments for pediatric PTSD. Sertraline and paroxetine are FDA approved for the treatment of PTSD in adults but not in children. Both fluoxetine and sertraline, however, are FDA approved for use with children for other psychiatric disorders. Hence, sertraline and fluoxetine are commonly used in the treatment of PTSD in youths. The clinical experience of using SSRIs in children seems to parallel the positive outcomes found in adults. The citalopram study of eight adolescents in 2001 reported that all PTSD symptom clusters showed response to treatment. However, it is interesting to note that self-report depression scores did not improve. By reputation, these medications are thought to have a very favorable side-effect profile, though the recent FDA advisory on the use of all the SSRIs in children calls this into question (see Chapter 22 for details). Some clinicians also consider the α-2a agonists, clonidine and guanfacine, first-line treatments for PTSD. They seem particularly effective in decreasing the associated symptoms of insomnia, nightmares, hyperarousal, and agitation. Antipsychotic medications should be reserved for traumatized children who have associated psychotic symptoms, extreme aggression, or serious self-injurious behaviors. Domon and Andersen report that nefazodone is effective in treating the insomnia and hyperarousal found in youths with PTSD. The recent FDA warning for nefazodone-induced liver failure, however, makes its use in children very unappealing. For data about other medications in the treatment of PTSD, see Table 19.5.

Prevention

Prevention of trauma is preferable to having to treat trauma sequelae. There is a strong tendency to rescue a particular individual with a name and face who has suffered a tragedy rather than taking actions to decrease trauma risk. Calabresi notes this is neither cost-effective nor optimal for the well being of children.

Society can do far more to address child abuse. One approach is to encourage adolescent boys and girls to mentor young children. By learning about childhood development and becoming used to the normal behavior of young children, those adolescents will develop invaluable patience and understanding before becoming parents themselves.

Antibullying programs are effective and should be in every school. In these programs, students and teachers are taught about the destructive effects of bullying. Students are also taught about respect, kindness, compassion, and to include rather than exclude others. Students learn to negotiate conflict among peers and to intervene safely in bullying situations. They are taught that reporting on bullying is not tattling but protecting the rights of others. Effective programs often involve surveys to assess the extent of the problem, role-playing of difficult situations, individual work with bullies and the bullied, parental involvement, and increased supervision of areas and times in which bullying frequently occurs. Because bullying peaks between the fourth and seventh grade, efforts to prevent it should begin in the second and third grade.

Programs in social and emotional intelligence, such as those offered by the Center for Social and Emotional Education, may decrease the development of chronic PTSD and other emotional problems in traumatized children. Youths who can deal constructively with trauma, build relationships, access support, express feelings, and develop friendships

TABLE 19.5. MEDICATIONS USED IN THE TREATMENT OF POSTTRAUMATIC STRESS DISORDER

Medication Category	Examples Commonly Used in Pediatric Populations	Target Symptoms/Comments
Serotonerigc agents	Fluoxetine, sertraline, citalopram, nefazodone	Reported to be effective in treating hyperarousal, agitation, and insomnia; considered a first-line treatment for PTSD.
α-2a agonists	Clonidine, guanfacine	Also reported to be effective in treating hyperarousal, agitation, insomnia, and nightmares; also considered a first-line treatment for PTSD.
β-blocker	Propranolol	Shown effective for treating target symptoms of hyperarousal and agitation; considered second line because of problems with side effects and dizziness.
Tricyclic antidepressants	Imipramine, desipramine	Good for sleep dysregulation and associated enuresis; considered second line because of the cardiotoxicity side-effect profile.
Benzodiazepines	Lorazepam, diazepam, clonazepam	Brief use for insomnia; probably underutilized in children because of worries of abuse or dependence (short-term use would minimize this risk); look out for disinhibition; considered second line by many.
Mood stabilizers	Valproate, carbamazepine, oxcarbazepine	Carbamazepine is shown to be effective in decreasing flashbacks, nightmares, intrusive memories, and sleep dysregulation in children and adults; considered second line by some because of side-effect profile and the need for blood testing.
Antipsychotics	Risperidone, olanzapine, quetiapine, aripiperazole, ziprasidone, haloperidol	Should be reserved for youths with associated psychotic symptoms or extreme aggression or self-injurious behaviors.

PTSD, posttraumatic stress disorder.

with those who have experienced trauma will be better able to minimize the harmful impact of the trauma. Social and emotional intelligence programs could address the most serious problem in helping traumatized children by giving them the skills to request help. The programs in social and emotional intelligence shown to be effective are those that take a holistic approach. In addition to teaching children in workshops and giving them opportunities to role-play, teachers and parents are taught to create a more supportive and caring environment, and issues around conflict resolution and understanding the feelings of others are brought into the social studies and language arts curricula.

Community support networks provide adults with the support they need, which can decrease their frustration, substance abuse, and related abuse of children. A study of two impoverished communities in Chicago showed considerably less child maltreatment in the community after social networks were fostered.

Electronic entertainment is also a serious source of violence exposure for our children. Television shows disasters repeatedly, and commercials for computer games, movies, and TV shows are full of violent images. This is not helpful to children, particularly those who have been traumatized. Care should be taken in supervising and limiting electronic entertainment media choices.

Conclusion

The impact of trauma on children is far greater than generally appreciated. Many traumatized children are never recognized or treated. When they do receive treatment, the traumatic origin of their symptoms is often missed. Moreover, many of the effects of trauma on development and personality are overlooked when a child has been clearly traumatized and brought to treatment. Recent years have seen rapid increase in trauma treatment protocols. These protocols, however, are underutilized and need to be more widely adopted by treating clinicians. Meanwhile, far more needs to be done to prevent traumatic events and foster resiliency so that traumatized youths will not develop chronic sequelae.

BIBLIOGRAPHY

American Academy of Child and Adolescent Psychiatry. Practice parameters for the assessment and treatment of children and adolescents with posttraumatic stress disorder. *J Am Acad Child Adolesc Psychiatry* 1998;37(Suppl. 10):4S–26S.

Briere J, Johnson K, Bissada A, et al. The Trauma Symptom Checklist for Young Children: reliability and association with abuse exposure in a multisite study. *Child Abuse Negl* 2001;25:1001–1014.

Calabresi G, Bobbitt P. Tragic Choices. New York: Norton, W.W. & Company Inc., 1990.

Cicchetti D, Toth SL. A developmental psychopathology perspective on child abuse and neglect. *J Am Acad Child Adolesc Psychiatry* 1995;34:541–565.

Cloitre M, Scarvalone P, Difede J. Posttraumatic stress disorder, self-and interpersonal dysfunction among sexually retraumatized women. *J Trauma Stress* 1997;10:437–452.

Cohen J. Practice parameters for the assessment and treatment of children and adolescents with posttraumatic stress disorder. *J Am Acad Child Adoles Psychiatry* 1998;37(Suppl. 10):4S–26S.

Costello EJ, Costello AJ, Edelbrock C. Psychiatric disorders in pediatric primary care: prevalence and risk factors. *Arch Gen Psych* 1988;45:1107–1116.

Deblinger E, Lippman J, Steer R. Sexually abused children suffering posttraumatic stress symptoms: initial treatment outcome findings. *Child Maltreat* 1996;1:310–321.

Deykin EY, Buka SL. Prevalence and risk factors for posttraumatic stress disorder among chemically dependent adolescents. *Am J Psychiatry* 1997; 154:752–757.

Dodge K, Lochman J, Harnish J, et al. Reactive and proactive aggression in school children and psychiatrically impaired chronically assaultive youth. *J Abnorm psychol* 1997;106:37–51.

Domon SE, Andersen MS. Nefazodone for PTSD. *J Am Acad Child Adolesc Psychiatry* 2000;39:942–943.

Fitzpatrick KM, Boldizar JP. The prevalence and consequences of exposure to violence among African-American youth. *J Am Acad Child Adolesc Psychiatry* 1993;32:424–430.

Ford JD, Racusin R, Ellis C, et al. Child maltreatment, and other trauma exposure, and posttraumatic symptomatology among children with oppositional defiant and attention deficit hyperactivity disorders. *Child Maltreat* 2000;5:205–217.

Freud A, Burlingham D. *War and children*. New York: Ernest Willard, 1943.

Garbarino J, Dubrow N, Kostelny K, et al. *Children in danger: coping with the consequences of community violence*. San Francisco: Jossey-Bass, 1992.

Herman JL, Perry JC, van der Kolk BA. Childhood trauma in borderline personality disorder. *Am J Psychiatry* 1989;14:490–495.

Horowitz M. Stress response syndromes. New York: Jason Aronson, 1976.

Hoven C. *Effects of the world trade center attack on NYC public school children*, Senatorial Field Hearing Chair, Hillary Rodham Clinton, New York State Senator. New York: Senate Health, Education, Labor and Pensions (HELP) Committee, June 10, 2002.

Janet P. Du rôle de l'émotion dans la genèse des accidents névropathiques et psychopathiques. *Revue Neurologique* 1909;17(II):1551–1687.

Jenkins EJ, Bell CC. Exposure to violence, psychological distress, and risk behaviors in a sample of inner city high school students. In: Friedman S, ed. *Anxiety disorders in African Americans*. New York: Springer Publishing Co, 1994:76–88.

Kardiner A. The traumatic neuroses of war. New York: Hoeber, 1941.

Langan PA, Harlow CW. Bureau of Justice Statistics, Child Rape Victims 1992, 1994. Available at: http://www.ojp.usdoj.gov/bjs/pub/ascii/chilrape.txt. Accessed October 1, 2004.

Laor N, Wolmer L, Mayes LC, et al. Israeli preschool children under scuds: a 30-month follow-up. *J Am Acad Child Adolesc Psychiatry* 1997;36:349–356.

Marans S, Cohen D. Children and inner-city violence. In: Leavitt L, Fox N, eds. *The psychological effects of war and violence on children*. Hillsdale NJ: Lawrence Erlbaum, 1993:281–301.

McCord J. A forty year perspective on effects of child abuse and neglect. *Child Abuse Negl* 1983;7: 265–270.

National Center for Victims of Crime. *Trauma of victimization, FYI*. Arlington, VA: National Center for Victims of Crime, 1997.

Pelcovitz D, Kaplan S, Goldenberg B. Post-traumatic stress disorder in physically abused adolescents. *J Am Acad Child Adolesc Psychiatry* 1994;33: 305–312.

Pollak S, Cicchetti D, Klorman R. Stress, memory and emotion: developmental considerations from the study of child maltreatment. *Dev Psychopathol* 1998;10:811–828.

Pynoos RS, Steinberg AM, Wraith R. A developmental model of childhood traumatic stress. In: Cicchetti D, Cohen DJ, eds. *Developmental psychopathology: risk, disorder, and adaptation*. New York: Wiley, 1995:72–95.

Rado S. Pathodynamics and treatment of traumatic war neurosis (traumatophobia). *Psychosom Med* 1942;4:362–368.

Schwab-Stone ME, Ayers TS, Kasprow W. No safe haven: a study of violence exposure in an urban community. *J Am Acad Child Adolesc Psychiatry* 1995;34:1451–1459.

Schwarz ED, Perry B. The post-traumatic response in children and adolescents. *Psychiatr Clin N Am* 1994;17:311–326.

Seedat S, Stein DJ, Ziervogel C, et al. Comparison of response to a selective serotonin reuptake inhibitor in children, adolescents, and adults with posttraumatic stress disorder. *J Child Adolesc Psychopharmacol* 2002;12:37–46.

Silvern L, Karyl J, Waelde L, et al. Retrospective reports of parental partner abuse: relationships to depression, trauma symptoms and self-esteem among college students. *J Fam Violence* 1995;10:177–202.

Spaccarelli S, Coatsworth JD, Bowden BS. Exposure to serious family violence among incarcerated boys: its association with violent offending and potential mediating variables. *Violence Vict* 1995;10:163–182.

Steinberg AM, Brymer MJ, Decker KB, et al. The University of Los Angeles post-traumatic stress disorder reaction index. *Curr Psychiatry Rep* 2004;6: 96–100.

Teicher MH, Glod CA, Surrey J, et al. Early childhood abuse and limbic system ratings in adult psychiatric outpatients. *J Neruopsychiatry Clin Neurosci* 1993;5:301–306.

Terr L. Children of Chowchilla: a study of psychic trauma. *Psychoanal Study Child* 1979;34:547–623.

The Commonwealth Fund. The commonwealth fund survey of parents with young children, 1996. Available at: http://www.cmwf.org/surveys/surveys_show.htm?docZ_id=240205. Accessed October 18, 2004.

Twemlow SW, Fonagy P, Sacco F. An innovative psychodynamically influenced approach to school violence. *J Am Acad Child Adolesc Psychiatry* 2001;40:377–379.

United States Department of Health and Human Services, National Center on Child Abuse and Neglect. *Child Maltreatment 1997: Reports from the states to the national child abuse and neglect data system*. Washington, DC: GPO, 1999.

Van der Kolk BA, Hostetler A, Herron N, et al. Trauma and the development of borderline personality disorder. *Psychiatric Clin N Am* 1994;17: 715–730.

Van der Kolk BA, Perry C, Herman JL. Childhood origins of self-destructive behavior. *Am J Psychiatry* 1991;148:1665–1671.

Weinstein D, Staffelbach D, Biaggio M. Attention-deficit hyperactivity disorder and posttraumatic stress disorder: differential diagnosis in childhood sexual abuse. *Clin Psychol Rev* 2000;20:359–378.

Weston D, Ludolph P, Misile B, et al. Physical and sexual abuse in adolescent girls with borderline personality disorder. *Am J Orthopsychiatry* 1990;60:55–66.

Widom CS. Posttraumatic stress disorder in abused and neglected children grown up. *Am J Psychiatry* 1999;156:1223–1229.

Yehuda R, Spertus I, Golier J. Relationship between childhood traumatic experiences and PTSD in adults. In: Eth S, ed. *PTSD in children and adolescents*. Washington, DC: American Psychiatric Publishing, 2001:117–146.

SUGGESTED READINGS

Center for Social and Emotional Education Website. http://www.csee.net, 2005.
(*A website to refer parents, educators and counselors for information and strategies on promoting social and emotional growth and preventing childhood trauma*).

National Children's Traumatic Stress Network Website. http://www.nctsn.org, 2005.
(*Contains a wealth of information for both families and clinicians, highly recommended*).

Pfeffer C, ed. *Severe stress and mental disturbance in children*. Washington, DC: American Psychiatric Press, 1996.

(*For Clinicians interested in overview of childhood trauma and its sequelae.*)

Terr L. *Too scared to cry: psychic trauma in childhood*, New York: Basic Books, 1992.
(*A classic read for all interested in the effects of trauma on children; special emphasis on Chowchilla bus victims.*)

Yehuda R, ed. *Treating trauma survivors with PTSD*. Washington, DC: American Psychiatric Press, 2002.
(*A good overview of trauma interventions with a good chapter on childhood treatment.*)

CHAPTER 20

Child Maltreatment

ANN M. CHILDERS

Introduction

When the United States was in its infancy, child maltreatment was not recognized as such. Society considered family members the property of the male head of the household, and domestic events were sacrosanct. As in Great Britain, protection of children followed that of animals. Both countries enacted laws to protect the helpless, particularly children, the mentally ill and incompetent, and domestic animals from willful and malicious acts of cruelty. However, until the British Parliament passed the Martin Act for animal protection in 1822, cruelty to animals was criminal only when severe enough to constitute a public nuisance. Two years later Richard Martin formed the Society for the Prevention of Cruelty to Animals. The Cruelty to Animals Acts of 1849 and 1854 protected animals, but it was not until 1884 that the first British law was passed to protect children from cruelty as well.

The movement to protect dependent individuals and animals spread throughout Europe and to the United States, and in 1866 the American Society for the Prevention of Cruelty to Animals (ASPCA) was established in New York City. Children came under the umbrella of this organization's charter in 1877, when the ASPCA became the American Humane Association. In all states, state and local laws mandate that parents guilty of bodily cruelty to, or moral corruption of, their children can be punished, and the children may be removed from them to become wards of the state. In the United States, child maltreatment continues to be a prominent public health concern. Statistics suggest that during the 1990s the United States led other industrialized nations in child maltreatment deaths by a significant margin and also leads in child poverty, teen birth rates, and one-person households.

Definitions

The Child Abuse Prevention and Treatment Act (CAPTA) was enacted in 1974 and reauthorized in 1996. This Act provides federal funding to states to prevent, identify, and treat child abuse and neglect. It created the National Center on Child Abuse and Neglect, developed standards for receiving and responding to reports of child maltreatment, and established a clearinghouse on the prevention and treatment of abuse and neglect. Changes in 1996 established Community-based Family Resource and Support Grants, which are used to fund state programs.

The CAPTA also features the Federal definitions of child abuse and neglect and is the standard each state and U.S. territory must incorporate into their child abuse and neglect legislation. The CAPTA allows each state and territory to provide its own statutory definitions, which must meet or exceed CAPTA guidelines.

Four major types of maltreatment are identified by the CAPTA: physical abuse, child neglect, sexual abuse, and emotional abuse. CAPTA's operational definitions can be found in Table 20.1.

On the basis of CAPTA guidelines, state and territory legal definitions describe the acts and conditions that determine the grounds for state intervention in the protection of a child's well being. Standards for what constitutes abuse varies from state to state and often include the words "threatened harm" as well as "harm" to a child's well being. Some states use the terms "serious harm or threat of serious harm." While meeting the CAPTA guidelines, states and territories may be purposefully broad in their definitions. Broader definitions provide local Department of Human Services (DHS) agencies with greater discretion in determining what constitutes child maltreatment. Most specify exceptions to their definitions, the most common being a religious exemption for parents who choose not to seek medical care for their children due to religious beliefs. Other common exceptions include corporal punishment, cultural practices, and poverty (vs. "neglect"). In recognition of

TABLE 20.1. CHILD ABUSE PREVENTION AND TREATMENT ACT: OPERATIONAL DEFINITIONS OF CHILD MALTREATMENT

- Physical abuse: infliction of physical injury as the result of punching, beating, kicking, biting, burning, shaking, or otherwise intentionally harming a child
- Sexual abuse: fondling a child's genitals, intercourse, rape, sodomy, exhibitionism, and commercial exploitation through prostitution or the production of pornographic materials
- Neglect: failure to provide for a child's basic needs; four major subcategories under the umbrella of neglect: (1) physical neglect, (2) educational neglect, (3) emotional neglect, and (4) medical neglect
- Emotional abuse (psychological/verbal abuse, mental injury): acts, or failures to act, by parents or other caregivers that have caused or could cause serious behavioral, cognitive, emotional, or mental disorders

"throwaway" children (children whose parents or guardians will not permit them to live at home), many states and territories now include abandonment in their definition of neglect.

Epidemiology

Other than the fact that child maltreatment crosses gender, cultures, and socioeconomic classes, its true nature and prevalence remains an area of social data collection riddled with methodologic problems. Among the myriad factors that make accurate estimates difficult are the absence of universal definitions for child maltreatment and the variety of ways in which existing definitions are interpreted.

Currently, the primary sources of national statistics on child abuse and neglect are two studies sponsored by the U.S. Department of Health and Human Services: the National Incidence Study (NIS), and Child Maltreatment: Reports from the States to the National Child Abuse and Neglect Data System (NCANDS). NIS is designed to estimate the *actual number* of abused and neglected children, including cases reported and cases not reported to child protective services (CPS). The most recent NIS survey (NIS-3) examines data from 1993, while the previous survey was conducted in 1986. Estimates generated by the NIS are based on a nationally representative sample of professionals and agencies using only two sets of standardized definitions of abuse and neglect. The NCANDS is the national database that combines and analyzes data from all child protective agencies in the United States. Statistics generated by the NCANDS rely on ways in which child maltreatment is substantiated, which varies from state to state due to variables like agency reporting and investigation practices, and legal definitions adopted by individual states.

The most recent NIS is based on data generated after 1986 and before 1993. Published in 1996, the Executive Summary of the Third National Incidence Study of Child Abuse and Neglect was released. This report presents the results of the congressionally mandated Third National Incidence Study of Child Abuse and Neglect (NIS-3). NIS-3 findings are based on a nationally representative sample of over 5,600 professionals in 842 agencies serving 42 counties, using two sets of standardized definitions of abuse and neglect: the Harm Standard and the Endangerment Standard. The NIS-3 provides insights about the incidence and distribution of child abuse and neglect and changes in incidence since the previous studies.

The most recent published report, the NIS-3, indicates the number of abused and neglected children doubled between 1986 and 1993, from 1.4 million to more than 2.8 million. The study estimated that the number of children who were seriously injured during that period quadrupled from approximately 143,000 to nearly 570,000. The researchers explain that only a portion of these increases in child abuse and neglect can be attributed to increased public awareness and recognition of the problem, as well as real increases in the scope of the problem. Highlights from the NIS-3 include:

- Substantial and significant increases in the incidence of child abuse and neglect since the previous NIS, conducted in 1986.
- Under the Harm Standard definitions, the total number of abused and neglected children was two-thirds higher in the NIS-3 than in the NIS-2, suggesting that a child's risk of experiencing harm-causing abuse or neglect in 1993 was 1.5 times the child's risk in 1986.
- Under the Endangerment Standard, the number of abused and neglected children nearly doubled from 1986 to 1993. Physical abuse nearly doubled, sexual abuse more than doubled, and emotional abuse, physical neglect, and emotional neglect were all more than 2.5 times their NIS-2 levels.
- The total number of children seriously injured and the total number endangered both quadrupled during this time.

The most current report for the NCANDS at this writing, entitled *Child Maltreatment 2002,* was released in April of 2004. This NCANDS indicates nearly 900,000 reports of child maltreatment were substantiated by child protection agencies in 2002. Highlights from the 2002 NCANDS include:

- 896,000 reports of child maltreatment were substantiated in 2002
- substantiated reports of maltreatment comprised 30% of all reports
- 60% of substantiated reports involved child neglect
- 20% of substantiated reports involved child physical abuse
- 10% of substantiated reports involved child sexual abuse
- 7% of substantiated reports involved emotional maltreatment
- nearly 30% of substantiated reports involved multiple maltreatment types
- an estimated 1,400 children died of maltreatment in 2002
- one third of the 1,400 children died of neglect
- three fourths of the 1,400 children were younger than 4 years old
- infant boys had the highest rate of fatalities, at nearly 19 deaths per 100,000 boys of the same age in the national population
- 80% of perpetrators were parents
- women accounted for 58% of perpetrators and were younger overall than their male counterparts
- men accounted for 42% of perpetrators
- less than 3% of all parent perpetrators were associated with sexual abuse
- nearly 29% of sexual perpetrators were other relatives
- nearly 25% of sexual perpetrators were in nonrelative or non–child caring roles.

Special mention is made here regarding head injuries and neglect. A history of head injury is common to maltreated children, regardless of abuse type. Nonaccidental head injury is the leading cause of head-injury related deaths in children less than 2 years of age and the leading cause of death among maltreated infants of this age. Nonaccidental head injury occurs most often at a stage of infant development particularly vulnerable to lifelong neurologic disability and death from brain injury, and it is considered the leading cause of permanent disability among all maltreated children.

Child neglect presents with a myriad of manifestations and sequelae, including but not limited to: social and emotional handicaps, medical and dental conditions, accidents, sexual abuse and exploitation, physical abuse, exposure to harsh environmental elements, and malnutrition. Significant neglect, particularly at early developmental stages, exerts a lasting impact on child health and development. Malnourishment in infants ages 0 to 3 years, for example, is a well-recognized contributor to mental retardation, as is mental understimulation (e.g., institutionalization).

Clinical Features

In terms of maltreatment, children are variable reporters. Children who do not feel threatened, whose accounts have not been contaminated by suggestions by others, and who clearly recall events as they occurred generally make good witnesses. But perpetrators frequently coerce or extort silence from their victims. They may contaminate a victim's accounts via term substitutions (e.g., "worm" for "penis") and rehearsed false information. Physically (e.g., head injury) and emotionally traumatized children often fail to recall their traumatic experiences clearly enough to describe them. Victims too young to describe what happened, and those whose disabilities interfere with communication and recall, are particularly handicapped in their abilities to convey their experiences to adults. Nonoffending adults who are shocked by the story or aligned with the offender may rebuff children who give accurate accounts. Children with poor social skills and those with a history of telling untruths are at special risk for disbelief from adults. Clinical signs and symptoms may be all the evidence a healthcare provider has to establish a suspicion of child maltreatment.

A number of signs and symptoms should alert providers to the possibility of child maltreatment. Histories from witnesses and caregivers comprise a key feature. When descriptions of a victim's behaviors leading up to a traumatic event make no practical or developmental sense, when stories change between witnesses, or when stories from the same witness alter significantly from one report to the next, child maltreatment becomes part of the differential diagnosis.

A common feature of physical abuse is the history that does not match the injury. In the case of significant nonaccidental head injuries in children <2 years of age, studies report nontraumatic histories were most often given to healthcare providers by children's caretakers. Here, the fall height described aids the clinician in raising or lowering his or her index of suspicion. Studies of accidents witnessed and reported by persons other than the caretakers responsible, and studies of falls from beds and examining tables in hospitals, demonstrate that falls of <10 ft (3 m) onto a hard surface did not cause serious, let alone life-threatening, head injuries. Where extenuating circumstances such as a recent traumatic brain injury or surgery are absent, significant head injuries from falls described as <4 ft are considered suspicious for maltreatment.

Signs of physical abuse are seldom specific to maltreatment, but certain patterns of injury raise the index of suspicion. In general, physically abused children sustain more injuries to the chest and abdomen, areas where children are not normally injured. Burn injuries without splash on infants, especially burn areas that are limited and circumscribed, suggest dunking into very hot or scalding water by a larger person; injuries with outlines that suggest implements of abuse, such as hand-shaped bruising, are suspect. Multiple doctor visits, emergency room visits, scars, bruises, and old (healed and healing) fractures suggest maltreatment, particularly when the caretaker's story does not match the injury (for example, a caretaker who attributes wounds and scars on a coordinated child to "clumsiness").

The child's behaviors provide additional clues to maltreatment. A child's response to a dangerous event differs from that of adults, expressed as disorganized or agitated behavior rather than intense fear, helplessness, or horror. Children are less likely to complain of intrusive thoughts and flashbacks and more likely to demonstrate distress and recall aspects of the event through repetitive play. In the absence of reasonable alternative explanations, a sudden change in behaviors, such as tantrums, poor appetite, disinterest in play, avoidance of specific people and/or places, nightmares, developmentally inappropriate sexual behaviors, difficulty concentrating, and the sudden appearance of enuresis and/or encopresis raises suspicions for trauma. Children subject to painful physical attacks may become aggressive, especially boys. In the office setting, caregivers may emphasize the child's sleep dysregulation and physical aggression, as these are most likely to interfere with function and the child's acceptance at home, school, and community.

Frequent office visits to a primary healthcare provider can signal family distress, such as domestic violence, mental illness in a caregiver, and a caregiver's despair over the child's disruptive behaviors. Repeat episodes of a mysterious illness in a young child may be the product of Munchausen syndrome by proxy, an uncommon disorder in which a parent seeks attention from physicians and the community by making the child ill. Neglect is suspect in children who are soiled and unkempt, wear the same clothes each day, have poor dentition, hoard and steal food at school, take things from others, do not receive routine vaccinations and well child visits, and have extensive school absences.

Physical and historic evidence specific to sexual maltreatment is elusive. Tissues of the rectum and genitalia heal quickly, and events other than molestation can inflict lesions in these areas. A strong and reportable indicator is the presence of a sexually transmitted disease, particularly gonorrhea. In its 1998 policy statement entitled *Gonorrhea in Prepubertal Children*, the American Academy of Pediatrics states, "The presence of *N. gonorrhea* infection in a child is diagnostic of abuse with very rare exception. By law, all known cases of gonorrhea in children must be reported to the local health department. A report also should be made to a child protective services agency. An investigation should be conducted to determine whether other children in the same environment who may be victims of sexual abuse are also infected." Regression in toileting and avoidance of adults of the same gender as the abuser are common. Children may wet the bed at night out of regression or to deter nighttime visits by the abuser. They may develop urinary tract infections. They may become constipated and encopretic, particularly when rectal penetration is involved. Other reported manifestations include sexual play, sexual precocity, sexual aggression, and public masturbation.

Maltreatment without acute adverse effects seldom attract the attention of healthcare providers, yet effects over time can result in long-term health impairments, etiologies of which are not immediately apparent. One example is "social medication." The "old wives'" practice of soaking a washcloth in liquor to stop a teething baby from crying is one example. Another is the administration of over-the-counter medications (OTCs) to children. In a 2004 study, Allotey reported Australian parents of children less than 5 years of age administered OTC medications for behavioral control. These "social medications" were perceived by parents as controlling behaviors they perceived as fractious and irritating. By controlling their children, parents reported OTCs assisted them with time management. Of note, acetaminophen was perceived by many Australian parents to have "almost miraculous properties in calming, sedating, and lifting the mood of children." In the United States, Kogan et al. published a paper in 1994 based on interviews of parents of more than 8,000 children less than 3 years of age and discovered more than two-thirds had administered acetaminophen to their child in the preceding 30-day period.

A number of legal documents and reports describe use by caregivers of physical methods perceived as effective and nonlethal to calm children. The reputation of the "sleeper hold" (also known as a "carotid restraint," or "choke hold"), made popular by its use in law enforcement, martial arts, and professional wrestling, is that it subdues opponents quickly and effectively without producing marks or injuries. Legal documents describe emulation of this technique by adult caregivers to subdue infants, children, and adolescents with lethal results.

Maltreatment can interfere with neurodevelopment, damaging a child's personality, social capacity, and ability to attach to other human beings. Physical damage to specific areas of the brain, such as the prefrontal cortex, can exert profound effects on attention, mood, and personality. A 1998 article by Andrews compared 27 children with traumatic brain injury to 27 control subjects. The traumatically brain-injured children had significantly lower levels of self-esteem and adaptive behavior, as well as higher levels of loneliness, maladaptive, aggressive, and antisocial behavior than children not known to have brain damage.

Social maltreatment or neglect can have similar outcomes. The importance of caregiver-child attunement to the mental and physical health of developing human beings cannot be overemphasized. In the first 3 to 4 years of life, anatomic brain structures that govern personality traits, learning processes, and coping with stress and emotions are established and made permanent. Insufficient interpersonal attunement between a child and his or her caregivers contributes to poor ego development, a diminished capacity to develop empathy, and an impaired ability to develop and sustain healthy relationships. When neglect is severe and the infant is isolated, these effects are compounded. Studies of children adopted from institutionalized settings demonstrate profound adverse effects on communication, attachment, sensory organization, and empathy. Reactive attachment disorder of infancy and early childhood and conduct disorder are among the psychiatric disorders of children featuring impaired relational abilities. Infants with global developmental delays who do not exhibit separation anxiety between 6 and 9 months of age and children who seem uninterested in people or demonstrate indiscriminate attachments to strangers and children who lack remorse may be victims of maltreatment.

For reasons not fully understood, the quality of a child's relationship with his or her caretaker exerts an independent influence on physical development. Statures of children with *psychosocial short stature* (PSS) remain at less than the 5th percentile for age and inheritance, despite adequate nutrition. Sometimes referred to as "psychosocial dwarfism," PSS is a disorder of short stature or growth failure and/or delayed puberty in development, with sustained disturbances of growth hormone, somatomedin, and thyroid functions. As with reactive attachment disorder of infancy and early childhood, criteria for PSS include a pathologically disturbed relationship between child and caregiver. Manifestations of PSS depend on the stage of development at which maltreatment occurs. Children with PSS present with abnormal and bizarre behaviors including, but not limited to, hoarding food, drinking water from toilets, polydypsia and polyphagia despite adequate food and water, self-injurious behaviors, apathy, developmental delays and disabilities, sleep disturbance, and pain agnosia. Diagnosis of PSS is confirmed by the removal of the child from the unsafe or nonnurturing environment and observation of the catch-up growth, behavioral improvement, and normalization of hormonal disturbances over time.

A remarkable plasticity of mind and behavior allows human beings to survive extremes of environment. Posttraumatic stress disorder (PTSD), an anxiety disorder common to maltreated children, is considered by some to be adaptive, a "normal" response to abnormal conditions. Hypervigilance, chronic physiologic hyperarousal, and avoidance of situations reminiscent of the traumatic event are protective in times of crisis; but when the threat is long absent, this chronic state of alertness interferes with activities of daily living, making this once-protective condition maladaptive. Insomnia, a common comorbidity, further impairs daytime function.

In cases of child maltreatment, symptoms of PTSD may not be as elusive as a history for the precipitating event, which can evade the best examination. Establishing a timeline for the child's behavior changes and exploring family, home, social, and school environments in the interview provides a good (albeit imperfect) chance of uncovering the event or events responsible for the child's symptoms. Because unhealthy family relationships are common precipitants of trauma, the clinician may glean more accurate and pertinent information by interviewing parents and other family members individually. The child's diagnostic comorbidity pattern may also provide clues (for example, social phobia that is comorbid with a number of specific phobias is a pattern commonly seen in cases of maltreatment). Also, behaviors speak volume (for example, a child who suddenly avoids adults of one gender may be generalizing the dangerousness of the abuser to adults of the same gender; a child who suddenly develops enuresis and/or encopresis may have been abused in a bathroom or rectally sodomized; a child who refuses to play in the backyard may have been whipped by a switch cut from a tree growing there).

In susceptible individuals and/or when trauma is chronic and severe, children and adolescents may protect themselves through *dissociation*, a process whereby the mind "wanders" away from traumatic events. Dissociation can be involuntary or voluntary (e.g., self-hypnosis). In Landesman's 2004 New York Times report, a child prostitute describes teaching other child captives "how to float away so things didn't hurt."

Dissociation interferes with memory for events, even when victims are presented with convincing evidence the events occurred. When trauma is chronic and severe, victims may develop a dissociative disorder, a pattern of dissociation that robs them of conscious awareness of periods of stress that interferes with routine function, even under safe conditions. Individuals with a dissociative disorder perceive losses of time and continuity. A child may describe daily headaches, "popping" into conversations he or she is not prepared to engage in, and periods of time for which he or she cannot account. By interfering with the daily activities and function of children, dissociative episodes puzzle and aggravate caregivers and children alike. These persistent maladaptive patterns share a number of features in common with some neurologic disorders and can be mistaken for epilepsy.

Significant head injuries occur in every category of maltreatment, are far more common than realized, and frequently go undetected. Children less than 2 years of age are particularly vulnerable to inflicted head trauma; more than 80% of lethal head injuries in this population result from maltreatment. The presence of a cranial injury is deceptive, frequently coexisting with other signs and symptoms of maltreatment in the absence of head injury-related symptoms. A study of medical records submitted to the National Pediatric Trauma Registry by U.S. hospitals over a 10-year period found abused children were nearly 3 times more likely to sustain injuries to the skull than children with accidental injuries. A retrospective review of medical records of children admitted to a metropolitan children's hospital also found a major difference in injuries between children with accidental injuries and those whose injuries were nonaccidental. In the accident group, subdural hematoma was diagnosed in 10% and subarachnoid hemorrhage was found in 8%. Significant brain injuries in the nonaccidental group were far higher, with 46% sustaining a subdural hematoma and 31% found to have subarachnoid hemorrhage.

Risk Factors

A multitude of factors place children at risk for maltreatment. In published reports, no single factor or finding has been found to predict a particular type of abuse. The purpose of this chapter is to acquaint the reader with ways in which risk factors may arise and interact. For further information, tables are provided at the end of this chapter.

Current theories of child maltreatment integrate risk factors into four primary systems: (a) the child (see Table 20.2), (b) the family (see Table 20.3), (c) the community (see Table 20.4), and (d) the society (Table 20.4). Although no child deserves maltreatment, a child's characteristics may significantly elevate the likelihood of maltreatment. Such characteristics include, but are not limited to, low birth weight, physical disabilities, and developmental disabilities, such as autistic spectrum disorders, mental retardation, attention deficit hyperactivity disorder, and being the infant child of a single mother. The needs of children with these characteristics can overwhelm the coping skills of parents who lack the personal and community resources and support required to care for them. Limitations in mobility and communication render children with cognitive and physical disabilities

---

TABLE 20.2.   CHILD RISK FACTORS FOR MALTREATMENT

- Premature birth, birth anomalies, low birth weight, exposure to toxins *in utero*
- Temperament: difficult or slow to warm up
- Physical/cognitive/emotional disability, chronic or serious illness
- Childhood trauma
- Antisocial peer group
- Age
- Child aggression, behavior problems, attention deficits

TABLE 20.3. PARENT AND FAMILY RISK FACTORS FOR MALTREATMENT

- Personality factors
- External locus of control
- Poor impulse control
- Depression/anxiety
- Low tolerance for frustration
- Feelings of insecurity
- Lack of trust
- Insecure/conflicted attachment with own parents
- Childhood history of abuse
- High parental conflict, domestic violence
- Family structure: single parent with lack of support, high number of children in household
- Social isolation, lack of support
- Parental psychopathology
- Substance abuse
- Separation/divorce, especially high conflict divorce
- Age
- High general stress level
- Poor parent–child interaction, negative attitudes, and attributions about child's behavior
- Inaccurate knowledge and expectations about child development
- Unskilled/low employability
- Disability

more vulnerable to sexual exploitation. Being a girl, especially an adolescent girl, places children at higher risk for sexual abuse, whereas serious physical abuse is inflicted most often on boys. In the vicious cycle of maltreatment, a child's reaction to victimization increases the likelihood of future maltreatment. Examples include physically abused boys, whose disruptive behaviors attract negative attention from caregivers, and sexually abused girls, who exhibit inappropriate sexuality and whose views of love, privacy, sex, and personal rights in their relationships with adults have been distorted.

Substance abuse in families places children at risk. In 2001, the Child Welfare League of America reported substance abuse to be present in 40% to 80% of families in which children are victimized. Substance use disorders may occur in response to, create, and/or exacerbate a number of psychiatric conditions. Disruptive behavior disorders, such as attention deficit hyperactivity disorder, major depressive disorder, bipolar affective disorder, and psychosis, occur more frequently in families engaged in substance abuse and domestic violence. Poor parenting skills, communication skills, and parent misconceptions about the developmental capabilities of children also heighten the risk of child maltreatment. Domestic violence between adults is a risk factor for child maltreatment, as is having a parent who is a victim of domestic violence. The impairment of empathy in

TABLE 20.4. SOCIAL AND ENVIRONMENTAL RISK FACTORS FOR MALTREATMENT

- Low socioeconomic status
- Stressful life events
- Lack of access to medical care, health insurance, adequate child care, and social services
- Parental unemployment, homelessness
- Social isolation/lack of social support
- Exposure to racism/discrimination
- Poor schools
- Exposure to environmental toxins
- Dangerous/violent neighborhood
- Community violence

Note: Factors are associations and do not imply causality.

caregivers with borderline, narcissistic, or antisocial personality disorders may place children at particular risk due to the impairment of empathy inherent in these disorders.

A key community risk factor, poverty, exerts a powerful influence on family function, affecting parents and children. Poverty is positively associated with substantiation of child maltreatment and strongly associated with neglect. Supporting data from the NIS-3 is noteworthy. The authors estimate that between 1986 and 1993, 27 of every 1,000 children were neglected in families with incomes of $15,000 or less. For families with incomes of $30,000 per year, the incidence of neglect fell 96%, to less than 1 in 1,000 children. Costello published a study in 2003 of 1,420 children on an Indian reservation, of which 68% lived below the federally defined poverty line. On average, the impoverished children exhibited more behaviors consistent with psychiatric disorders, including stubbornness, temper tantrums, stealing, bullying, and vandalism. Subsequently, the reservation opened a casino which raised families' average income levels. Four years later, youths' disruptive behaviors decreased to the level observed for children who had never lived in poverty.

High among societal risk factors for child maltreatment are teen pregnancy rates and children born to single mothers. In 2001, 34% of infants were born to unmarried mothers, including 4 out of 10 firstborns. In the United States, an estimated 4 of every 10 teenagers becomes pregnant. Year 2002 statistics estimated about one-fifth (23%) of children lived with only their mothers, 5% lived with only their fathers, and 4% lived with neither of their parents. Teen pregnancies are higher risk for pregnancy and birth complications; children of unmarried mothers are more likely to have low birth weight and to live in poverty.

Approximately half of persons living in poverty today are children of unmarried mothers (see Table 20.5). The lack of education and marketable skills in young parents, especially young single mothers, prevents upward mobility. A full-time job does not guarantee escape from poverty; families where the head of the household works full time for minimal wage remain below the poverty line. Food insecurity and diminished parenting resources, household goods, and services negatively influence the entire family, and sibling relationships are no exception. Sibling competition for these resources elevates the risk of "sibling rivalry" (sibling relational problem) and, for some sibling sets, intersibling maltreatment. Conflicts can escalate to the point of dangerousness, and it is estimated that 3 of every 100 children are at risk for serious physical abuse by a sibling. Sibling sexual maltreatment is thought to be vastly underreported. Current information suggests that siblings whose parents do not meet their emotional needs and who experience their home lives as unhappy may look to one another for emotional support and, in some cases, engage one another sexually.

TABLE 20.5. MALTREATMENT RISKS FOR CHILDREN IN SINGLE PARENT HOMES VERSUS TWO PARENT HOMES

- 77% greater risk of being harmed by physical abuse and a 63% greater risk of experiencing any countable physical abuse
- 87% greater risk of being harmed by physical neglect and a 165% greater risk of experiencing any countable physical neglect
- 74% greater risk of being harmed by emotional neglect and a 64% greater risk of experiencing any countable emotional neglect
- 3 times greater risk of being educationally neglected
- 80% greater risk of suffering serious injury or harm from abuse or neglect
- 90% greater risk of receiving moderate injury or harm as a result of child maltreatment
- Two times greater risk of being endangered by some type of child abuse or neglect.

From Sedlak, AJ, Broadhurst DD. *Executive summary of the third national incidence study of child abuse and neglect.* U.S. Department of Health and Human Services, Administration for Children and Families Administration on Children, Youth and Families, and National Center on Child Abuse and Neglect, 1996, with permission.

Protective Factors

Increasingly, factors that prevent maltreatment, cultivate family stability, and foster resilience in maltreated children attract attention from researchers, policy makers, and practitioners. As with risk factors, protective factors cover a spectrum ranging from child to family to society. In 1987, Mrazek and Mrazek described three case studies of children in high-risk environments. They identified key characteristics contributing to the resilience of the children, including the ability to recognize danger and adapt, distance oneself from intense feelings, create relationships that are crucial for support, and project oneself into a time and place in the future in which the perpetrator is no longer present.

A number of other factors have been identified since. Child factors with potential to protect children include good health, an above-average intelligence, hobbies or interests, good peer relationships, an easy temperament, a positive disposition, an active coping style, positive self-esteem, good social skills, an internal locus of control, and a balance between seeking help and autonomy.

Parent and family protective factors that may protect children have also been identified and include secure attachment with children, parental reconciliation with their own childhood history of abuse, supportive family environment, household rules and monitoring of the children, extended family support, stable relationship with parents, family expectations of prosocial behavior, and high parental education.

A middle-to-high socioeconomic status is among social and environmental risk factors protective to children. Family Support Network 2002 cites additional factors, which include adequate access to health care and social services, sufficient housing, steady parental employment, participation by family in a religious faith, good schools, and adults outside the family who serve as supportive role models or mentors. Marriage protects women and children from poverty. Referencing data from the 1998 U.S. Census Bureau's Survey of Income and Program Participation, Lerman, in 2002, reported pregnant women who did not marry encountered a poverty rate of 47%, whereas the population who married sometime between pregnancy and childbirth experienced a 20% poverty rate, less than half that of unmarried mothers. Families with two married parents enjoy more stable home environments, fewer years in poverty, and less material hardship.

Clinical Course

Clinical course over the long term depends largely on the nature of maltreatment, combined with the absence and presence of risk and protective factors in children, families, and their communities. The likelihood of permanent brain compromise results from child maltreatment is high, but establishing cause and effect is difficult to impossible in the majority of cases. A lack of prenatal care, low birth weight, and compromised early nutrition, even in the absence of traumatic head injury, places young brains at risk.

Child maltreatment exacts a price from society in terms of morbidity, mortality, unemployment, and social services that too often extends from generation to generation. Studies link child maltreatment with an increased risk of low academic achievement, substance use disorders, teen pregnancy, juvenile delinquency, and adult criminality.

Teen pregnancy is both a risk factor for, and potential outcome of, adolescent pregnancy. Currently, 4 of 10 adolescents become pregnant before of age 20 years, resulting in approximately 900,000 teen pregnancies each year. A 2004 article by Hillis et al. defines adverse childhood experiences (ACEs) as "emotional, physical, or sexual abuse; exposure to domestic violence, substance abusing, mentally ill, or criminal household member; or separated/divorced parent," and reports strong associations between ACEs and adolescent pregnancy, long-term psychosocial consequences, and fetal death.

Maltreatment increases demands for mental health and substance abuse treatment programs, police, courts and correctional facilities, welfare, Medicaid, and many other public assistance programs. With losses in productivity and the increase in human suffering added in, the cost to victims and society is significant.

Assessment

Before undertaking any mental health examination, a mental healthcare provider should clearly define his or her role in the process and in the system. The provider's role can be obscured in a number of ways. One way a potential interviewer may unearth conflicting interests and roles is by asking questions such as "Whose mental health provider am I?", "Who pays for my services?", and "Do personal, financial, political, or other constraints exist that could adversely influence my clinical performance in this case?" Conflicts should be resolved before proceeding with an interview, with consideration for the safety of children and families and medical ethics prevailing.

How patients and families process language used in the assessment largely depends upon the cognitive, emotional, and developmental status of participants. Abstractions will likely be lost on children and adolescents who think concretely, and children with language disorders may incorrectly process what is said. Information is best understood when provided in a language and conceptual framework that corresponds with the recipient's cognitive abilities and stage of development.

To begin the assessment, the mental health professional shares his or her role and potential conflicts of interest with parents, guardians, and patients. Statements should describe the types of disclosures shared with outside parties and which parties disclosures may reach. Basic disclosures by minors, which must be shared with other parties, include child maltreatment toward the patient and related minors, recent suicide and homicide attempts and ideations, and patient threats of serious harm to self and others. The minor's stage of development determines how these rules are interpreted and presented. Young children should know issues caretakers could help with. Sibling problems, fears, and sadness may be shared with guardians. Teens should be informed that hazardous behaviors such as intravenous drug abuse and needle sharing may be shared with parents and/or agencies as appropriate.

Open-ended questions regarding bullying, neglect, and physical, sexual, and emotional abuse, as well as violence at home and the child's treatment of other children should be part of the formal mental status examination. When allegations of abuse arise *de novo* during routine interviews, questions surrounding the disclosure should remain open. Questions such as "Do you know who did it?" are less likely to contaminate a child's account to authorities than direct questions like "Did your uncle molest you?"

When maltreatment is suspected, the local CPS agency should be contacted as soon as possible, preferably before the child and accompanying adult(s) leave the healthcare setting. CPS can ensure the safety of children. In emergencies, CPS can assume the protective custody of minors and provide consents required for hospitalization and medical treatment.

Most communities have protocols in place by which forensic data can be gathered from minors in an unbiased fashion. This process is usually initiated by CPS and related agencies. At the point an evaluator decides to file a report of suspected maltreatment to CPS, he or she may elect to steer the interview away from continued disclosure to avoid complicating and contaminating future forensic interviews. If the child is stable and the situation permits, it may be useful to gather information related to the child's physical and mental health instead.

For various reasons, some reports of suspected child maltreatment may not result in substantiation of maltreatment or even initiate an investigation. It is important that such failures not deter providers from continuing the practice of reporting. Of all reports received by CPS, those submitted by healthcare providers see the highest rate of substantiations. CPS and other agencies recognize the value of reports from the healthcare community, which support case documentation over the long run, whether or not investigations and substantiations result.

Children frequently undergo more thorough mental health assessments after investigations of child maltreatment reports have concluded. Most community agencies that recognize unsubstantiated reports do not guarantee the absence of maltreatment and may continue to offer assistance to children and families involved.

All children suspected of being maltreated should undergo complete medical and dental examinations. Examinations should include a survey of skin and scalp. Bruises and their approximate stage of healing should be documented, along with scars, dents in bone, and other findings. Dental findings should be documented with like care, as abused children frequently suffer dental and facial injuries. Objective documentation in keeping with the forensic nature of the examination is invaluable.

Mental health evaluations are geared to the developmental stage of the child. Chronologic age is frequently inconsistent with the maltreated child's mental age and stage of development. Even under the best of circumstances, children with developmental disabilities may exhibit emotional immaturity, and those receiving pathologic care can present as episodically or chronically regressed. Children with higher intellectual functioning may process well intellectually, yet regress emotionally to far younger emotional ages in the presence of their abuser and other emotionally charged situations.

As previously described, children's risk factors for maltreatment range widely across physical, biologic, psychological, and social realms. The assessment of maltreated children and adolescents should generate a picture of functioning across environments and key relationships. A formal psychiatric examination by itself is useful; when part of a multidisciplinary evaluation spanning key biopsychosocial aspects, the value of the psychiatric assessment is magnified (see Tables 20.6 and 20.7).

TABLE 20.6.   SIGNS AND BEHAVIORS SUGGESTIVE OF SEXUAL ABUSE

Physical signs that suggest sexual abuse:
- Difficulty in walking or sitting
- Bladder or urinary tract infections
- Pain, swelling, and redness or itching in the genital area
- Bruises, contusions, bite marks, or bleeding in perineum or hymenal disruption
- Presence of suspicious stains, blood, or semen on child's body, underwear, or clothing
- Presence of sexually transmitted diseases
- Painful bowel movements or retention of feces
- Early, unexplained pregnancy in a nonsexually active child

Behaviors that suggest sexual abuse:
- Unwilling to participate in certain physical activities; wears extra layers of clothing
- Engages in delinquent acts or runaway behavior
- Has poor peer relationships, low self-esteem, social isolation, is secretive
- Displays bizarre, sophisticated, or unusual sexual knowledge or behavior
- Fear of the dark and recurrent nightmares, sleep disturbances
- Changes in eating behaviors
- Regressive behavior
- Hostile, aggressive, acting-out behaviors and play
- Decline or change in academic performance, school avoidance
- Excessive, inappropriate fears
- Hiding clothing

TABLE 20.7. EVALUATION ITEMS THAT SUGGEST PHYSICAL ABUSE

History
- Failure to thrive
- Delay in obtaining care
- Multiple previous injuries
- Absent or uninterested caregiver
- Fluctuating or conflicting histories
- History not consistent with injury, developmental level of victim, or alleged child perpetrator

Cranial/HEENT examination
- Shaken baby syndrome: child <2 yr old, without external trauma, and with retinal and subarachnoid hemorrhages on funduscopic examination (usually dilated)
- Ear cupping and/or ear asymmetry (size/induration may be L > R if ear pulled by right- handed individual)
- Tin ear syndrome: unilateral ear bruising, ipsilateral cerebral edema, and retinal hemorrhages
- Hemorrhaging that suggests violent shaking, hitting, or throwing of the child
- Retinal hemorrhages
- Concomitant head injury common with any nonaccidental skeletal fracture

Abdominal examination
- Swelling of the abdomen
- Localized tenderness or complaints of pain in the abdominal area
- Chronic emesis

Chest
- Rib fractures: multiple, bilateral, posterior, different ages
- Trunk encirclement bruises

Integument and mucosa
- Bruises in various stages of healing
- Abrasions on the back or arms, legs, or torso.
- Any lacerations or abrasions to external genitalia
- Absence of hair or hemorrhaging beneath the scalp due to hair pulling
- Bruises found on any of the following: face, lips, mouth, genitalia, ear lobes, torso, back, buttocks, thighs
- Clustered bruises—suggests repeated contact with the hand or instrument
- Bruises in unusual patterns that reflect the implement used to inflict the injury such as:
  - Bite marks (adult mouth intercanine distance >3 cm)
  - Pinch marks: paired ovals
  - Slap marks: parallel stripes, hand mark
  - Cord or belt marks: loops, stripes
  - Rope marks

Burns
- Rope burns on the arms, legs, neck, or torso
- "Wet burns" that suggest dunking in a hot liquid
- Cigar or cigarette burns: round, 4–8-mm diameter, especially on the soles of the feet, palms of the hand, the back, or buttocks
- Patterned or dry burns, indicative of being forced to sit on a hot surface or hot implement applied to skin
- Cuts or tears or scratches on an infant's face, such as tears to the gums
- Circumferential, uniform depth, multiple, no splash
- Buttock, perineum, back, dorsal hand, stocking glove

Skeletal extremities
- Metaphyseal "chip" or "bucket handle"
- Diaphyseal spiral (<9 mo of age)
- Transverse midshaft long bone
- Femur fracture (<2 yr of age)
- Acromion process of scapula
- Proximal humerus

Skull
- Multiple or bilateral skull fractures
- Skull fracture in falls <4 ft.

HEENT, Head, Eyes, Ears, Neck, Throat; L, left; R, right.

Differential Diagnosis and Common Comorbidities

It is said that children are "not little adults," and no one knows this better than those who provide services to this population. Development, the dynamic process at the core of pediatric medical care, can respond to and/or change a child's internal milieu. It both impacts and responds to his or her environment and influences the developing patient's mental health status, which is in a constant state of flux. What looks like bipolar disorder today may turn out to be a language disorder and attention deficit disorder tomorrow; the same hyperactive child who runs around the classroom and climbs excessively at age 6 years sits in his chair and bounces his knee at age 14. Development sets child mental health evaluations into a state of constant evolution. Seasoned pediatric mental health professionals familiar with this pattern accept conflicting and changing diagnoses as part of the process.

Known biopsychosocial risk factors for child maltreatment contribute to a particularly broad diagnostic differential. To illustrate, comorbidities and differentials generated by a suspicion of nonaccidental head injury alone may include breathing-related and other sleep disorders, epilepsy, learning disabilities, attention deficit hyperactivity disorder, chronic headaches, language disorders, intermittent explosive disorder, mood disorders, and developmental coordination disorder. Common comorbidities and differential diagnoses are provided in Table 20.8.

Treatment

No matter how much data is gathered, mental health professionals working with maltreated minors can never be entirely certain of the nature and duration of maltreatment their patients experienced. From a broad standpoint, psychiatric treatment addresses symptoms that cause suffering, interfere with daily functioning, and engender developmental derailment. It is useful to generate diagnoses and conditions via a thorough evaluation, and organize them according to the *Diagnostic and Statistical Manual of Mental Disorders*, Fourth Edition (DSM-IV) Axes I through V. The ability to guide the course of treatment is inherent in this system, and it provides a framework with which to describe patients to other providers. Axes should be updated periodically, preferably at every visit, to track the evolution of symptoms and the impact of treatment.

In concert with the mental health assessment, treatment should involve biologic, psychological, and social approaches. The term *child maltreatment* is not a diagnosis but a description. Therapies for maltreated children are individualized, based on diagnoses generated from a complete developmental psychiatric or multidisciplinary evaluation that incorporates a developmental psychiatric component.

The first and most important intervention is to separate the child from danger. Children who endure ongoing threats to physical and psychological integrity cannot be expected to

---

TABLE 20.8. COMORBIDITY IN CHILDHOOD POSTTRAUMATIC STRESS DISORDER

- Major depressive disorder
- Dysthymia
- Substance use disorders and addictions
- Other anxiety disorders
- Attention deficit hyperactivity disorder
- Conduct disorder
- Oppositional defiant disorder
- Enuresis/encopresis

---

improve, medications and other interventions notwithstanding. Healthcare providers can assist children for whom maltreatment is unsubstantiated but suspected by assisting them in developing emergency plans, such as escaping to the home of a trusted neighbor and calling 9-1-1 when endangered.

PTSD is commonly diagnosed in maltreated children. Although a variety of pharmacotherapies have been investigated for their application in childhood PTSD, no double blind placebo-controlled studies have been published. A list of agents commonly used to treat symptoms of trauma is outlined in Chapters 19 and 22. Weller also provides a review of medications used in the treatment of traumatized children including clonidine, propranolol, carbamazepine, serotonin reuptake inhibitors, and other antidepressants.

Cognitive-behavioral therapy may be considered first-line therapy for PTSD. Therapeutic interventions should maximize the child's abilities and cultivate his or her strengths, especially those that contribute to resilience, while addressing problems and conflicts that affect the child's current functioning and may impair functioning in the future. If the child will live in the family home, the same approach applies to his or her family. A balanced approach that is strength based while addressing difficulties instills hope and strengthens capabilities.

Family dynamics leading to maltreatment must be addressed, including emotional, educational, and financial aspects. Interventions to promote healthy changes to the child's environment and relationships begin with the family and extend to schools. In addition to protecting young victims, CPS provides access to child and family mental health treatment and medical care for children and their families. Caseworkers are assigned to families in crisis to coordinate services, such as basic care, transportation, or meals. Under the provisions of a public law entitled the Individuals with Disabilities Education Act (IDEA), infants, children, and adolescents with special physical, cognitive, and emotional needs and their families may qualify to receive mental health and other services through their schools as well.

Conclusions

Child and adolescent maltreatment is common and increasing. Significant contributors include poverty, young parenthood, single parenthood, mental disorders, parental substance abuse and addictions, infant prematurity, and child disabilities. Child victims of all types of maltreatment are at significant risk for head injury, which is the leading cause of morbidity and mortality in child abuse and which often goes undetected. Infants and young children are at greatest risk for mortality. More than 80% of lethal head injuries in children less than 2 years of age are inflicted intentionally. Maltreatment establishes a vicious cycle: by increasing child dysfunction, maltreatment increases child risk factors for maltreatment. This epidemic presents an opportunity for clinicians to assist at local and community levels. Clinicians who harbor a high index of suspicion for abuse in young patients and report to CPS as indicated increase the likelihood that medical treatment rendered will be effective, and patients and families will receive the community assistance they require to break the cycle of maltreatment.

BIBLIOGRAPHY

Allotey P, Reidpath DD, Elisha D. "Social medication" and the control of children: a qualitative study of over-the-counter medication among Australian children. *Pediatrics* 2004;114:e378–e383.

American Academy of Pediatrics, Committee on Child Abuse and Neglect. Gonorrhea in prepubertal children. *Pediatrics* 1998;101: 134–135.

American Academy of Pediatrics, Committee on Child Abuse and Neglect. Guidelines for the evaluation of sexual abuse of children. *Pediatrics* 1991;87:254–260.

Andrews TK, Rose FD, Johnson DA. Social and behavioural effects of traumatic brain injury in children. *Brain Inj* 1998;12:133–138.

Association National Clearinghouse on Child Abuse and Neglect Information Web Site. Child maltreatment, 2002. Available at: http://nccanch.acf.hhs.gov/pubs/factsheets/canstats.cfm. Accessed November 9, 2004.

Costello EJ, Compton SN, Keeler G, et al. Relationships between poverty and psychopathology: a natural experiment. *JAMA* 2003; 290: 2023–2029.

Federal Interagency Forum on Child and Family Statistics. *America's children: key national indicators of well-being 2003 federal interagency forum on child and family statistics.* Washington, DC: Government Printing Office, 2003.

Hillis SD, Anda RF, Dube SR, et al. The association between adverse childhood experiences and adolescent pregnancy, long-term psychosocial consequences, and fetal death. *Pediatrics* 2004;113:320–327.

Jenny C, Hymel K, Ritzen A, et al. Analysis of missed cases of abusive head trauma. *JAMA* 1999;281:621–626.

Kirby D. *Emerging answers: research findings on programs to reduce teen pregnancy.* Washington, DC: National Campaign to Prevent Teen Pregnancy, 2001.

Kogan MD, Pappas G, Yu SM, et al. Over-the-counter medication use among US preschool-age children. *JAMA* 1994;272:1025–1030.

Landesman P. The girls next door. New York Times January 25, 2004, Sunday Late Edition - Final, Section 6, Column 1, 2004:30.

Lerman R. *Married and unmarried parenthood and the economic well-being of families: a dynamic analysis of a recent cohort.* Washington, DC: The Urban Institute, 2002.

Madigan A, Dowell K. *Emerging practices in the prevention of child abuse and neglect.* Washington, DC: Department of Health and Human Services, 2003.

Mrazek PJ, Mrazek DA. Resilience in child maltreatment victims: a conceptual exploration. *Child Abuse Negl* 1987;11:357–366.

Reece RM, Sege R. Childhood head injuries: accidental or inflicted? *Arch Pediatr Adolesc Med* 2000; 154:11–15.

Rose E. *A mother's job: the history of day care, 1890-1960.* New York: Oxford University Press, 1999.

Sjoberg RF, Lindblad F. Limited disclosure of sexual abuse in children whose experiences were documented by videotape. *Am J Psychiatry* 2002;159: 312–314.

Weller E, Shlewiet B, Weller R. Traumatized children: why victims of violence live out their nightmares [Current Psychiatry Online Web Site], 2003. Available at http://www.currentpsychiatry.com/2003_01/0103_ptsd.asp. Accessed November 9, 2004.

Zitelli B, Davis H. *Atlas of pediatric physical diagnosis,* 4th ed. Saint Louis, MO: Mosby, 2002.

INTERNET RESOURCES

ChildStats (http://www.childstats.gov)

International Society for Traumatic Stress Studies (www.istss.org)

National Center for Children Exposed to Violence (http://www.nccev.org)

National Center for PTSD (http://www.ncptsd.org) '

National Childrens Trauma Stress Network (http://www.nctsn.org)

Parents Anonymous Inc. (http://parentsanonymous.org)

The PTSD Alliance (http://www.ptsdalliance.org)

CHAPTER 21

Child Custody Evaluations

ROY LUBIT

Introduction

Each year, approximately one million families with children divorce. By the age of 18, 40% of children have experienced divorce. In 10% of divorces, litigation arises over issues of custody and visitation.

Over the years, there have been major changes in how parents obtain custody of their children. Before the 20th century, society considered children the property of their fathers, and so fathers usually were granted custody after a divorce. If the mother obtained custody, the father had no monetary obligations for the support of the child. For most of the 20th century the "tender years doctrine," under which young children were believed to always be better off with the mother, dominated court rulings. In the 1960s and 1970s, fathers received greater equality. Two books by Goldstein et al., *Beyond the Best Interest of the Child* and *Before the Best Interest of the Child*, along with the Uniform Marriage and Divorce Act, helped to change the basis of custody decisions to the "best interests of the child." Today, in all states, the best interest of the child, and not the interests of the parents, is the standard upon which courts make custody decisions. Nevertheless, for many judges, there is at least tacit belief in the "tender years doctrine" that small children (younger than 7 years of age) should be with their mother.

Solnit et al. argued for a child to have the stability of having a single custodian. In recent years, however, joint custody has become common. The hope is that this arrangement keeps both parents actively involved in the child's life.

The role of the psychiatrist in a forensic psychiatric evaluation relating to a custody dispute is different from the typical clinical role. The evaluator's role is not to be a therapist but to render expert opinions to the court. Although it is not a therapeutic intervention, care should be taken to do no harm, including damaging the ability of any of the family members to trust and work with mental health professionals in the future. Unlike therapeutic interventions, a custody evaluation is not confidential since the evaluator will inform the court of the results of the assessment. The evaluating clinician or psychiatrist must clarify the terms of the evaluation, including the lack of confidentiality with the client. However, information should only be released with the client's permission or as required by law. Finally, the clinician should provide only the information required for the particular decision under consideration by the court.

> *Treating clinicians are advocates or agents for children and ideally are partners with parents or guardians in the therapeutic alliance. In contrast, the forensic evaluator, while guided by the child's best interest, has no duty to the child or his parents. The forensic evaluator reports to the court or attorney involved rather than to the parties being evaluated. Thus, the aim of the forensic evaluation is not to relieve suffering or treat, but provide objective information and informed opinions to help the court render custody decisions.*—Practice Parameters for Child Custody Decisions, AACAP 1997.

Forensic evaluators should be experienced in working with both children and adults. They should be familiar with child development and the research on the effect of various custody arrangements. The evaluator should know the basic family law and legal procedures in the state. The therapist can be a fact witness but not an expert witness in the case, since expressing a preference for either parent could impair or destroy the relationship between the therapist and the other parent. This could impede cooperation with that parent and lead to conflicts in continuing therapy relationships.

In an ideal world, all parties in a custody case would focus on the best interests of the child. Instead, lawyers work for their clients' interests, and the judge applies the existing law to the case at hand. Theoretically, law guardians are focused on the child's best interest. However, their ability to do this is often weakened by a lack of knowledge of child development or a willingness to fight for whatever the child wants, particularly if the child is a teenager.

It is the psychiatrist's responsibility to gather all relevant data, to make a sound recommendation, and to educate the court concerning why this recommendation is best. Although some judges and law guardians have a deep understanding of child development and children's needs, this is not universally the case. In providing testimony, child psychiatrists must base their opinions not on pet theories or the wishes of the party that hired them, but on scientific evidence. In 1993 the U.S. Supreme Court ruled in *Daubert versus Merrill Dow* that scientific evidence, and not simply generally accepted practice, was the rule for expert testimony in federal courts.

The evaluator comments on two issues: legal custody and physical placement. The person with legal custody has control of issues such as medical treatment, schooling, religious choices, and early entrance into the military or marriage. Physical placement issues focus on where and with whom the child will live and what visitation arrangement is best.

Impact of Divorce

Conflict between parents may be the most critical factor in adjustment for children in divorcing families. In fact, on average, children in divorced families with low levels of conflict are better adjusted than children in intact families that have high levels of conflict. Children are particularly prone to developing emotional problems when they feel caught between their parents. Many children have significant emotional and behavioral problems during the first year or two after a divorce, including sleep problems, sadness, anger, worry about themselves and their family, and aggressive behavior. These problems tend to abate after 2 years.

After separation, children are stressed by the collapse of their nuclear family and home situation, change in routines and decreased access to friends, the need to transition between two houses, loss of family income, and their parents' stress. Family dynamics are compromised when angry, clingy, and possibly oppositional children are combined with parents whose emotional resources are stretched past the breaking point. Children caught in the battles between their parents are likely to blame themselves for the collapse of the marriage. Those who do so are at higher risk to develop emotional problems.

Young children are egocentric and engage in magical thinking. They tend to see themselves as the cause of things that happen for other reasons. Hence, they can blame themselves for the divorce and for how their parents are coping afterward. The forensic evaluator needs to be aware of these issues since they may color the child's statements.

Another important issue is that after a divorce many children are parentified and become emotional supports for their parents, listening to their problems, giving them advice, and perhaps even acting as an intermediary between them. This is generally very destructive to the child's development and can interfere with the individual being able to forge and maintain appropriate adult relationships in the future.

Children often fear abandonment by their parents. Children of divorced parents are, on average, more aggressive, inattentive, and socially unpopular. They tend to have earlier sexual experiences and use more alcohol and drugs.

Perhaps the biggest effect of divorce occurs when children grow up and seek their own relationships. They lack an inner model for lasting adult relationships and tend to see family and marital relationships as fragile. Wallerstein observes they can impulsively jump into relationships with people they do not know well or have difficulty committing themselves.

Essential Aspects of Child Development

An understanding of child development is essential to designing placement and visitation arrangements that appropriately meet children's needs after a divorce. First, the young child's experience of time is different from that of an adult. Time seems to pass much more slowly for children. They cannot look back on having had many hundreds of weeks and dozens of holidays during their lifetime. Not only is their life span shorter, but they also cannot remember their preverbal experiences. Young children have a limited sense of object constancy and object permanence, so separations are much more stressful. A child's experience of time needs to be a central factor in designing visitation schedules, particularly overnight visits and vacations.

While the preschooler's life centers on the home, as the child moves into school age and adolescence, ties to the community and friends become increasingly important. The child's living arrangement must allow for the normal developmental experiences of childhood in order for the child to develop skills and interests. For example, spending every weekend with the visitation parent in a neighborhood without friends is acceptable for a 3-year-old, but not for a school-aged child or adolescent. It would be unusual for any adolescent to spend every weekend solely with a parent rather than seeing friends.

The internalization of morals and development of a coherent identity are two critical developmental tasks of childhood and adolescence. That work requires a child to have positive images of his or her parents to internalize. If one parent is engaging in undesirable behaviors, the key issue should be whether the child is affected. For example, if a parent has multiple sexual partners but behaves discreetly, it does not necessarily hurt the child. However, a parent filled with anger and negative statements about the other parent can cause lasting damage to his or her child.

Amidst the turbulence of the divorce, sources of security and stability outside of the relationship with the parents take on added importance in the child's life. These include religion, ties to friends, adults in the community, and sibling relationships. Maintaining these ties should be part of the custody decision.

Crucial questions include: Which parent can best support the child's development? Which parent best provides support and encourages the child to learn new skills? Which parent can best help the child deal with anxiety-provoking situations and to provide the child with the emotional sustenance, support, and encouragement to engage in them and develop new skills? Which parent is best able to help the children learn to think about new situations, develop trust in themselves and validate their feelings? Does one of the parents fail to protect the child adequately from dangers in the community or from their own mistakes? Which parent provides more assistance and encouragement with school work and learning opportunities outside of school? Which parent can better guide the child to learn social skills? Which parent more accurately observes and reasonably responds to the child's feelings? Does one of the parents invalidate the child's emotional experience? Which parent is better able to assess a child's abilities and emotional needs accurately and adjust their parenting style to fit the developmental needs of the child? Children's fantasies are a large part of growing up. How each parent is able to help the child with fantasies is an important part of parenting and something to be assessed in the custody evaluation. Which parent can best support the child's fantasy attachment or admiration to a powerful, admirable figure and which responds with jealousy or belittling of the child's attachment to an outside hero?

There are many child-rearing approaches in our country because of our diverse population. While it is important for evaluators not to allow biases and cultural background to affect decisions on optimal parenting, it is also important to not abandon any attempts to assess what is appropriate out of respect for cultural pluralism. Severe corporal punishment or isolating a child from interactions with others is inappropriate, even if they are part of a child's cultural heritage. Research has shown that children's school performance tends to be better when children and parents share work and play. Authoritative parents who emphasize encouragement, who provide support for efforts initiated by the child, and who provide clear communication and a focus on the child's needs are preferable to authoritarian ones. Research has also shown that child-centered discipline, in which general acceptance of the child is communicated and disciplinary measures are modified based on the child's response, is best at leading to the development of internal controls and values. Inconsistent and harsh parenting can lead to oppositional behavior. Antisocial behavior can also arise from ineffective monitoring.

Decisions about the best parenting situation should not be based on stereotypes of parental roles and gender-based traits or on general statements about good parenting styles. Rather, the clinician needs to evaluate the ability of parents to relate to the child's specific needs and temperament. Good parenting for a child with one temperament and set of needs is not optimal for a child with a different temperament and set of emotional needs.

Mrazek identified five "key dimensions of parenting." They are emotional availability (warmth), type of control (flexibility and permission), psychiatric health versus disturbance (including personality disorders), knowledge base (understanding of parenting role and how it changes over the course of development), and commitment. As they grow, children need to be involved in making decisions about their lives and not simply subject to parental dictates if they are to develop their own good judgment, self-control, and confidence. Invasive parents who make all decisions, particularly during adolescence, interfere with the child's ability to become an independent adult. At the same time, the parent needs to protect the child from disastrous decisions. Some parents are not able to distinguish between situations that have dangerous or long-term serious destructive impact from ones with limited risk and cost. Parents also need to be able to maintain a warm supportive stance with children who are rebelling against them. Parents need an understanding of the different phases of development and the emotional health and flexibility to be able to modify their behavior to meet their child's changing needs.

Visitation Schedules

The underlying principle to be followed is that a child needs to have a secure base and the developmental supports and experiences needed to grow. Being constantly in transition between homes is stressful, but visits that are too far apart or too short in duration can turn the visiting parent into a visitor rather than a parent with destructive effects on the child. Regularity of visits is particularly important. Children need as much contact as possible with each parent and with other important relatives such as grandparents. Time with friends is also important.

One common plan is the alternate weekend plan. Another is that one parent has primary placement when school is in session (10 of 14 days) and the other parent has the child during most vacation time (9 of 14 days, alternating 3- and 1-night weekends). It is best if children can see both parents on a holiday rather than alternating holidays.

Infants need very frequent visits, every day or every other day, but should not stay overnight. Visits should last a couple of hours and should allow the noncustodial parent to engage in various aspects of caretaking. Some feel that between 18 months and 3 years, an occasional overnight with a noncustodial parent to whom the child is well bonded is acceptable, but that the very young child should not go longer than this without contact with the primary caretaker. Moreover, the child should have phone calls, photographs of each parent, and transitional objects available when needed. Between 2 and 7 years, overnights can gradually increase to a point of *de facto* joint custody.

For adolescents who are generally separating from their parents and highly invested in peer relationships, maintaining their ability to see friends is important. Weekend visits should not involve pulling them away from normal activities. If a child is spending the summer with the noncustodial parent, there should be daily phone calls and visitation if possible.

It is important for siblings to stay together. Siblings provide each other with a sense of continuity, security, and a continuing relationship. To rob them of this support at any time, but particularly in the midst of the parents splitting up, is destructive. Separating children also denies them the opportunity to learn socialization and sharing skills. However, siblings' visitation schedules do not need to be simultaneous. Children benefit from one-on-one time with parents.

Visitation with a parent who is inappropriate, mentally ill, or abusive should be supervised. If the behavior continues even under supervision, then visitation may be suspended until the adult's destructive behaviors resolve.

Custody

When both parents are equally fit, there is a tendency to award custody to the parent who has been the primary caretaker in 10 specific areas: preparation and planning of meals; bathing, grooming, and dressing; buying, cleaning, and caring for the child's clothes; medical care; arranging social activities; arranging child care; putting the child to bed and waking them; discipline; religious, cultural, and social education; and teaching basic skills. Evaluators should not give too much weight to this practice if the other parent is equally capable of taking care of these functions but has not done so because of a division of chores. Although mothers generally perform these roles, there is some evidence that boys do better when in their father's custody.

When parents can work together, joint custody has the significant advantage of keeping both parents actively involved in the child's life. For joint custody to work, however, the parents need to be able to communicate and cooperate. Geographic proximity is also important. Judges tend to opt for sole custody if the parents cannot work together, there was domestic violence, or if one of the parents is a substance abuser, has serious emotional problems, or abused the child.

Special Situations: Allegations of Domestic Violence, Physical Abuse, Sexual Abuse

At times, sexual abuse, physical abuse, and domestic violence are issues in a custody war. The presence of any of these generally means that the nonoffending parent will obtain custody, but the next step is to determine how much visitation the offending parent will have and whether visits will be supervised or unsupervised. People who abuse their spouses frequently abuse their children as well. One parent's tendency toward violent behavior, even if originally limited to the spouse, can include the children in the future. Therefore, an absence of direct physical abuse to a child, in the presence of domestic violence, does not mean that the child can see the offending parent without supervision.

Clinicians making custody decisions need to closely examine their negative stereotypes about the victims of domestic violence. People often look very negatively on the victim, as well as the perpetrator, of domestic violence. Victims stay in an abusive relationship for a number of reasons. They often blame themselves for the abuse due to low self-esteem or violence they experienced as a child. They believe the spouse's promises that the abuse will stop. Abusive relationships often involve financial dependence. A real and realistic fear of many victims is that the abuser will track down and harm them or their children. Experiencing domestic violence can result in "Stockholm syndrome," in which the victim becomes protective of the abuser, since this is less painful than realizing the degree to which one is vulnerable and a victim.

The perpetrator of violence is likely to deny that it occurred, to declare that he or she was actually victimized himself or herself, and that his or her ex-spouse has psychological problems. Assessing the propensity of each parent for violence and other inappropriate behavior in such situations is both very difficult yet critical to the assessment. False allegations of abuse can arise from a histrionic, narcissistic, or antisocial spouse. At times, people create false abuse allegations to keep their children to themselves and prevent their former spouse from having custody or visitation. At the same time, many psychological problems presented by parents can come from the experience of being victimized. Victimization can lead to depression, self-destructive behavior, anxiety and traumatic stress, feelings of isolation, poor self-esteem, a tendency towards revictimization, substance abuse, difficulty trusting others, and sexual maladjustment.

It is important to remember that men are sometimes the victims of domestic violence. Societal beliefs and male egos, however, make it very difficult for men to complain.

When Children Do Not Want Contact with a Parent

When a child does not want to see a parent and alleges mistreatment by that parent, the parent is likely to allege that the child has been turned against them by the other parent. In these situations, many evaluators, law guardians and judges almost automatically disbelieve allegations of mistreatment of a child that occur within the context of custody battles, stating that it is simply a matter of what Richard Gardner called "parental alienation syndrome" (Rand 1997 a, b; Warshak 2001). There certainly are many children who are placed under great pressure by a parent to reject the other parent and, as a result, become fearful of the second parent and object to visitation. However, the concept has been misunderstood and overused. Research has failed to support the common practice of ignoring abuse allegations made within the context of a custody dispute. Accusations of abuse must always be taken seriously (Thoennes 1990; Everson 1989; Association of Family and Conciliation Courts Research Unit 1988).

Unfortunately, parents who allege abuse can be seen as manipulative and psychologically unstable. Those who have not done extensive work with domestic violence, abuse, and trauma do not realize that the anxiety and pressured responses of these individuals are normal responses to being victimized or facing the possibility of leaving the child in an abusive situation. Parents often find themselves in the painful position of being threatened with losing custody to an abusive parent if they do not force their frightened children to comply with court-mandated visitation. These situations need extensive evaluation by people trained in evaluating abuse. Moreover, the forensic examiner needs to understand these issues in depth and be able to explain them to the court.

There are a variety of factors that can help evaluators distinguish between cases of abuse and PAS. If the alleged abuser has a history of impulsive and aggressive behavior and does not cooperate with the evaluation, while the accusing parent supports evaluation and the maintenance of contact with the alleged abuser under safe circumstances, it is more likely that the abuse allegations are true. On the other hand, if the abuse is alleged to have suddenly begun after separation, the accusing parent avoids evaluation, and the accused parent has no history of impulsivity or aggression, then parental attempts to turn the child against the other parent seem more likely. In addition, the child might appear coached or rehearsed, and the child might need reminders from the accusing parent in order to tell the story of the bad things. A truly abused child will require few reminders.

What to Evaluate in Custody Disputes

Central issues in deciding the capability of each parent include:

- Better role model
- Placing the child's needs over one's own needs
- Preparing the child for the future
- Loving the child as a person and not for his or her accomplishments
- Fostering the child's curiosity
- Validating the child's feelings and experiences
- Listening to the child
- Treating the other parent well and fostering continued contact between the child and the other parent
- Fit between child's temperament and needs, and parent's parenting style and personality
- Able and willing to spend time with the child
- Interacts appropriately with the child in all areas
- Bond between parent and child
- Parents' flexibility and openness to professional advice

According to the Uniform Marriage and Divorce Act, the evaluating psychiatrist should assess:

- The wishes of the parents regarding custody
- The wishes of the children
- Interaction and relationships of the child, parents, siblings and others who affect the child's well-being.
- The mental and physical health of the people involved
- Other pertinent factors to the specific case

There is no set amount of time needed to assess the important factors in a case. Some cases are much more complex than others, either because information is highly contested or neither parent is clearly superior to the other. In addition, there may be limitations on how many hours you are allocated to work on a case. In general, however, one should generally spend two or more hours with each child and four hours with each parent. Moreover, one should spend a couple of hours with each parent in combination with the child. Optimally this would include a home visit. Other good evaluation locations are a toy store, the park, or a restaurant. Seeing the parent and child in a community setting provides a better sense of how the parent is able to set limits, play with the child, and support the child. The evaluator should also speak with others who may have pertinent information, including the child's pediatrician, babysitters, teachers, activity or club leaders, grandparents, and other key relatives.

Evaluators need to be careful in how they ask questions and interpret the answers. If one parent says many negative things about the other, it could be an indication of the objective problems of the second parent or the out-of-control anger and tendency to splitting and externalization by the first parent. Children's statements also require interpretation. Evaluators should discern if a desire to live with one parent over the other is arising from a deeper connection to that parent, from an emotional need to take care of this parent who is not functioning well on his or her own, or from transient anger with the other parent who is better able to set appropriate limits. Some children will turn against one of their parents. While this could result from the abuse, emotional abandonment, or chronic disconnection from one parent, it could also arise from fear of losing the other parent's love or from actions and statements of the other parent that encourage the hatred. A child's alienation from a parent necessitates very close evaluation. The evaluator needs to address the following items:

Which parent has been the primary caretaker?

- Buying clothing and dressing
- Washing
- Taking to the doctor
- Helping with homework
- Taking to school and after school activities

Which parent is best able to help the child with their particular needs?

- Usual emotional and developmental needs
- Child's specific emotional needs and issues
- Emotional and behavior problems resulting from the divorce
- Medical needs
- Educational needs
- Sensitivity to the child's role model needs

Factors that may affect a parent's ability to take care of a child's needs include:

- Parents' emotional health
- Parents' physical health
- Parents' time availability, work schedule, child-care plans
- Stresses the parent is under that may impede caring for the child
- Unhealthy parental habits
- Good fit between parenting style and child's needs including style of discipline and ability to be flexible
- Attachment to the parent
- Willingness to support contact with the other parent
- Larger family and community support system each parent would provide
- Problematic value systems and ethics

KEY ITEMS FOR THE EVALUATION

Parental assessment

Parents should be informed that the interviews are not privileged and that a written report will be submitted to the court. This is a forensic evaluation and not therapy. The parents' discussion of the history of their relationship, the child's development, and of the deterioration of their marriage reveals a great deal about their psychological functioning, flexibility, and capacity to relate to others. The parent should be questioned about the child in detail. This provides the evaluator with an understanding of the parent's ability to understand the child and the child's needs, and his or her ability to appropriately respond to those needs. Topics to be covered include the following list:

- Strengths of the child
- What the child likes and wants for the future; parent's attitude toward those wishes
- Needs of the child
- Frequency, intensity, duration of problematic behaviors, and the way the parent deals with the behavior
- Traumas and stresses the child has had

- Child's developmental history
- Who has taken care of which needs of the child in the past: buying clothing, going to school, cooking, play dates, going to the pediatrician, helping with homework, bathing, talking to teachers
- Concerns about the other parent's relationship with and caretaking of the child
- Response to allegations by the other parent

Parents should be asked for specific plans for taking care of their child. The list below is a sample of commonly asked items. Information regarding these items will help supply the evaluator with information about which parent will provide the child with the best developmental experiences:

- Contact with the other parent
- Schooling
- Contact with relatives
- Recreational activities
- Socialization with other children
- Religious activities
- Special needs
- Emotional stress around the divorce

Parent's history and functioning

In determining which parent is more stable and has the better emotional balance and intellectual ability to provide the child with the structure, emotional support, and role model needed to grow into a capable adult, the following items should be examined in the parent history:

- Parent's family of origin, education, work history, history of relationships, current relationship, cultural/religious ties, family ties
- Prior marriages, if any, and history
- Children from prior marriages, those custody relationships and why, how those relationships will affect children from the current marriage
- History of psychological/substance abuse problems and treatment, medical history, legal history
- Use of alcohol and other drugs
- Parent's beliefs about discipline and how to support the child
- Parent's understanding of the child's needs
- Feelings about the child having contact with the other parent
- Extended family with whom they want the child to have contact
- Family psychiatric and medical problems
- Does the child remind the parent of someone?
- Does the parent identify with the child?

Child custody evaluators should also gather information about parental thoughts on the current family situation. Topics for exploration include the following items:

- History of the relationship, including reason for the divorce
- Current living situation
- Current visitation arrangements and problems with the arrangement
- Why the parent feels he or she would be the better custodial parent
- Concerns about the other parent having custody
- Beliefs about the other parent's concerns about them
- Ability to identify and acknowledge one's own weaknesses and shortcomings
- Ability to appreciate mental or physical health problems the child has or might develop and willingness to cooperate with physicians or clinicians in evaluation and treatment

Attention should be paid to whether parents are able to focus on the child's needs or are preoccupied with their own needs or anger at their spouse. In addition, evaluators should interview stepparents to assess their ability to relate appropriately to the child and meet the child's needs.

Child assessment

The parents should be instructed to tell their children that an evaluator will be meeting with the family to make recommendations on how they can best take care of the children now that they are living apart. When assessing a young child, begin by seeing the parent and child together and then transition to having the parent leave the room. How they separate and how they react when reunited can be very informative. Explain to the child that the evaluator's job is to help the judge to decide where it is best for the child to live. The interview of the child should include the following topics:

- Child's likes
- Child's dislikes
- Daily activities
- Relationships with friends, family members, and teachers
- Child's view of the problem
- History of sexual or physical abuse
- Worst thing that ever happened to the child
- What the child's understanding of the family's situation is and what the child expects to happen
- What it would be like to live with each parent and why
- Does the child have a preference on where to live?
- Does the child appear to have been coached? One can ask the child if anyone told him or her to say something in particular.

A custody evaluation of the child should include a discussion of feelings toward parents. It would also include feelings about the divorce situation. The following questions about the divorce situation and parents should be broached in the assessment of the child:

- What is your understanding of the breakup of the family?
- What do you do with each parent: homework, play, talking?
- Who can you talk to about how you feel?
- Who do you go to for help with different things?
- What makes each parent upset and how do the parent reacts when upset?
- What does each parent do for the household and for the child?
- What were/are the household rules?
- When you are bad how does each parent punish you?
- Did either parent ever hurt you?
- Did either parent ever hurt the other?
- What did your mother (father) tell you to be sure to tell me?
- When your mother (father) talks to you about your father (mother), what does he or she say?
- What would be best about living with each parent?
- What would not be so good about living with each parent?
- How would you feel if the judge said you should live with your father and why?
- How would you feel if the judge said you should live with your mother and why?
- Do you want more or less time than you now have with your mother and your father and why?

Projective questions are often illuminating. The following questions are commonly used in a child custody evaluation:

- What would you do if you had a million dollars?
- What would you ask for if you had three wishes?
- What type of animal would you like to be and why?
- What type of animal would you not like to be and why?
- If you had two houses, who would live in each?
- If you were going to be stranded on a desert island, and there was only room on the island to have one person with you, who would you want to be there?
- A baby bird and his or her parents were caught in a storm. They were blown in different directions by the wind. The baby bird could only fly a little bit. The wind decreases. What happens next?
- If a martian came to visit, how would you describe your parents to him or her?
- What is the best age to be and why?

Drawings can often provide valuable information, particularly in younger children or those who are not inclined to talk. Pictures of the following are part of a standard child custody evaluation:

- Free drawing
- House
- Tree
- Person
- Person of the opposite sex
- Family

OBSERVATION OF CHILD AND PARENT

A fundamental part of the child custody evaluation is to observe the child's interaction with each parent in play and nonplay situations. An evaluator should watch how the parent relates to the child. Observing a parent and child over lunch, in a park, and in a toy store can reveal important evaluation data. An evaluator should ask the parent and child to perform a task together. Specific interaction items to observe include the parent's ability to focus on the child's needs, to relate appropriately, to encourage the child, to provide support, to talk with the child, to have fun with the child, and to set limits. The following questions should be considered when observing a child with a parent:

- Which parent can best support the child's development?
- Which parent best provides support and encourages the development of new skills?
- Which parent can best help the child deal with anxiety-provoking situations and provide the child with the emotional sustenance, support, and encouragement to engage in these challenging circumstances, and develop new skills?
- Which parent is best able to help the child learn to think about new situations, develop trust in the child, and validate the child's feelings?
- Does one of the parents fail to protect the child adequately from dangers in the community or from their own mistakes?
- Which parent provides more assistance and encouragement with schoolwork and learning opportunities outside of school?
- Which parent can better guide the child to learn social skills? Which parent more accurately observes and reasonably responds to the child's feelings?
- Does one of the parents invalidate the child's emotional experience?
- Which parent is better able to accurately assess a child's abilities and emotional needs and adjust their parenting style to fit the developmental needs of the child?

Other information that is pertinent to a child custody evaluation may come from contact with medical and mental health providers the parents and children have used. It is also important to obtain school information and reports from teachers. Consideration should be given to a home visit and interviewing extended family members, neighbors, friends, alternative caregivers (babysitters), and new partners of the parents.

The child custody evaluation should be made available to the court in an organized format. Table 21.1 is an example of a written child custody evaluation report.

Pitfalls

There are a number of common pitfalls in doing custody evaluations. The evaluator needs to create a comfortable atmosphere in which the child can feel free to speak. One must be careful not to lead the child into saying things. Children try to tell interviewers what they think the interviewer wants to hear. It is important to evaluate if coaching occurred. Use developmentally appropriate language and clarify any possibly ambiguous statements. Ignoring signs of important issues and reading interview or situational stress as a sign of psychopathology are other common errors.

TABLE 21.1. OUTLINE OF CHILD CUSTODY EVALUATION REPORT

Child:	name, age, DOB
Mother:	name, age, DOB
Father:	name, age, DOB

Identifying Information

Confidentiality Statement
Father and mother were advised that the normal confidentiality of a psychiatric interview did not apply and that Dr. X would be writing a report to the court based on the interviews that occurred and the review of records seen. They were told that this evaluation was not therapy.

Sources of Information
Clinical interviews
- Interview with father X hours (date)
- Interview with mother X hours (date)
- Interview with child 1 X hours (date)
Documents reviewed
Phone contacts

History by Source of Information
History as per father
Mental status examination of father
History as per mother
Mental status examination of mother
Interview with child
Observation of mother and child
Observation of father and child

Conclusions
Strengths of father
Weaknesses of father
Strengths of mother
Weaknesses of mother
(No DSM-IV-TR diagnosis is necessary.)

Recommendations
Custody
Timeshare
Therapy recommended

DOB, date of birth; DSM- IV-TR, *Diagnostic and Statistical Manual of Mental Disorders*, Fourth Edition, Text Revision.

TABLE 21.2. ESSENTIALS OF CHILD CUSTODY EVALUATION

- The main goal of a child custody evaluation is to provide clinically informed information and recommendations to the court, not to provide assistance or counseling to the involved parties.
- Child custody evaluations are not confidential. Parents and children should be informed of this lack of confidentiality at the beginning of the assessment process.
- The custody evaluation should include individual interviews with all the involved parties and clinical observations of parent–child interactions.
- The "best interests of the child" should be the guiding principle in developing recommendations for custody.
- Recommendations should be supported with explanations based on objective clinical observations and scientific evidence, not on clinical intuition or personal theories.
- Recommendations regarding the primary custody should be primarily based on an assessment of the ability of a parent to understand and be able to provide for the child's specific needs and temperament.
- In performing a child custody evaluation, care should be taken to avoid damaging the ability of any of the family members examined to trust and work with mental health professionals in the future.

A common misconception is that a parent who is calm and personable is credible, and an agitated parent is not. The truth is that an agitated parent may be psychologically unstable or traumatized, while a personable, calm parent may be a stable healthy individual or a well-defended abuser. While psychologists tend to rely on psychological testing, psychiatrists generally do not use them, with the possible exception of the Minnesota Multiphasic Personality Inventory (MMPI) II. The MMPI II can provide information on whether each parent is providing accurate information, their abilities to be empathic with the child, and the presence of psychopathology.

Another pitfall concerns every clinician's own blind spots, pet theories, and biases. Projecting one's own beliefs about family is likely to have a silent and powerful effect. As much as possible, the evaluator should focus on data and discuss it with colleagues to see if they would have similar reactions (see Table 21.2).

Conclusions

Approximately 50% of American children come from homes of divorce. As high as 1 in 10 of these divorces result in custody litigation. The role of the psychiatrist in a custody dispute is different from the characteristic clinical role. The child custody evaluation is a type of forensic assessment. Hence, a clinician's role in this situation is not to be a therapist, but to render expert opinions to the court. The custody evaluation is not protected by patient confidentiality. While clinicians are usually advocates for children and their parents or guardians, the forensic evaluator is not primarily concerned with ameliorating suffering or caring for the child and family. Providing objective information and clinically informed opinions to the court are the principal goals of a custody evaluation.

BIBLIOGRAPHY

Allison P, Furstenberg R. How marital dissolution affects children: variation by age and sex. *Dev Psychol* 1989;25:540–549.

Amato P. Children's adjustment to divorce: theories, hypotheses, and empirical support. *J Marriage Fam* 1993;55:23–38.

Amato P. Life-span adjustment of children to their parent's divorce. *Child Divorce* 1994;4:143–164.

American Academy of Child and Adolescent Psychiatry. Practice parameters for child custody evaluation. *J Am Acad Child Adolesc Psychiatry* 1997; 36(Suppl. 10):57s–68s.

American Psychological Association. *Report of the APA presidential task force on violence and the family.* Washington, DC: American Psychological Association, 1996.

Association of the Family and Conciliation Courts Research Unit. *The sexual abuse allegations project, final report*. Denver, CO: Association of the Family and Conciliation Courts Research Unit, 1988.

Bryant B. The neighborhood walk: sources of support in middle childhood. *Monogr Soc Res child Dev* 1985;50:1–122.

Buchanan C, Maccoby E, Dornbusch S. Caught between parents: adolescents' experience in divorced homes. *Child Divorce* 1991;62:1008–1029.

Clarke-Stewart K, Hayward C. Advantages of father custody and contact for the psychological well-being of school-age children. *J Appl Dev Psychol* 1996;17:239–270.

Collins W, Harris M, Sussman A. Parenting during middle childhood. In: Bornstein M, ed. *Handbook of parenting*, Vol. 1. Mahwah, NJ: Lawrence Erlbaum Associates, 1995.

Dunn J, Hedrick M. The parental alienation syndrome: an analysis of sixteen selected cases. *J Divorce Remarriage* 1994;21:21–38.

Everson MD, Boat BW. False allegations of sexual abuse by children and adolescents. *J Am Acad Child Adolesc Psychiatry* 1989;28:230–235.

Faller K. The parental alienation syndrome: what is it and what data support it? *Child Maltreat* 1998;3:100–115.

Galatzer-Levy, Cohler B. *The essential other: a developmental psychology of the self*. New York: Basic Books, 1993.

Gardner RA. Differentiating between parental alienation syndrome and bona fide abuse-neglect. *Am J Fam Ther* 1999;27:97–107.

Healy J, Steward A, Copeland A. The role of self-blame in children's adjustment to parental separation. *Person Soc Psychol Bull* 1993;19:279–289.

Herman S Child custody evaluations. In: Schetky D, Benedek E, eds. *Principles and practice of child and adolescent forensic psychiatry*. Washington, DC: American Psychiatric Publishing Inc, 2001.

Hetherington EM. An overview of the Virginia longitudinal study of divorce and remarriage with a focus on early adolescence. *J Fam Psychol* 1993;7:39–56.

Hetherington E, Cox M, Cox R. Effects of divorce on parents and children. In: Lamb M, ed. *Nontraditional families*. Hillsdale, NJ: Lawrence Erlbaum Associates, 1982:233–288.

Issacs M. The visitation schedule and child adjustment: a three-year study. *Fam Proc* 1988;2:251–256.

Lamborn S, Mounts N, Steinberg L, et al. Patterns of competence and adjustment among adolescents from authoritative, authoritarian, indulgent and neglectful families. *Child Dev* 1991;62:1049–1065.

Lubit R, Billick S. Adolescent moral development. In: Rosner R, ed. *Textbook of adolescent psychiatry*. London: Arnold Press, 2003a.

Lubit R, Billick S. Juvenile delinquency. In: Rosner R, ed. *Principles and practice of forensic psychiatry*, 2nd ed. London: Arnold Press, 2003b.

Maccoby E. Middle childhood in the context of the family. In: Collins W, ed. *Development during middle childhood: the years from six to twelve*. Washington, DC: National Academy of Sciences Press, 1984:217–234.

Mrazek D, Mrazek P, Klinnert M. Clinical assessment of parenting. *J Am Acad Child Adolesc Psychiatry* 1995;34(3):272–282.

Pruett M, Pruett K. Fathers, divorce, and their children. *Child Adolesc Psychiatric Clin North Am* 1998;7:389–407.

Rand DC. The spectrum of parental alienation syndrome (part 1 & 2). *Am J Forensic Psychol* 1997;15:23-52–39-92.

Smith R, Coukos P. Fairness and accuracy in evaluations of domestic violence and child abuse in custody determinations. *Judges J* 1997;Fall 36:38–56.

Thoennes N, Tjaden PG. The extent, nature, and validity of sexual abuse allegations in custody/visitation disputes. *Child Abuse Neglect* 1990;14:151–163.

Tolan P, Loeber R. Antisocial behavior. In: Tolan P, Cohler B, eds. *Handbook of clinical research and practice with adolescents*. New York: Wiley-Liss, 1993:307–331.

Veltkamp L, Miller T. Clinical strategies in recognizing spouse abuse. *Psychiatr Quar* 1990;61:179–187.

Warshak R. Current controversies regarding parental alienation syndrome. *Am J Forensic Psychol* 2001;19:29–59.

Wood C. The parental alienation syndrome: a dangerous aura of reliability. *Loyola LA Law Rev* 1994;7: 1367–1368.

SUGGESTED READINGS

Ackerman M. *Clinicians guide to child custody evaluations*. New York: John Wiley and Sons, 2001.
(A comprehensive review for serious clinicians who perform child custody evaluations.)

Galatzer-Levy R, Kraus L. *The scientific basis of child custody decisions*. New York: John Wiley and Sons, 1999.
(For clinicians who conduct custody evaluations, an objective and comprehensive overview of research pertinent to child custody process.)

Goldstein J, Freud A, Solnit A. *Before the best interest of the child*. New York: Free Press, 1979.
(This is a classic volume for clinicians, judges, and lawyers who are involved in child custody cases.)

Nurcombe B, Partlett D. *Child mental health and the law*. New York: Free Press, 1994.
(This is a comprehensive review of the legal issues regarding divorce and other mental health laws pertaining to children.)

Wallerstein J, Blakeslee S, Lewis J. *The unexpected legacy of divorce: the 25 year landmark study*. New York: Hyperion, 2001.
(An elegant review of the research on children of divorce for clinicians and parents.)

Treatment

CHAPTER 22

Psychopharmacology

ANN M. HAMER

Introduction

Pediatric psychopharmacology is an ever-expanding area of study. It is thought that the first reports of psychotropic drug use in adolescents occurred in the 1930s with the publication of *The Behavior of Children Receiving Benzedrine* by Charles Bradley. Since that time, many therapeutic agents have been marketed for a variety of psychiatric disorders. But, until recently, very few clinical studies have been conducted to support the use of these agents in young patients. In fact, the majority of indications for the use of psychotropic agents in children are considered "off-label" and are not supported by the Food and Drug Administration (FDA). Despite this lack of information, the prevalence of psychotropic drug use in children has steadily increased and is at an all-time high.

In an attempt to increase available information regarding medications for children, the United States passed the Food and Drug Administration Modernization Act (FDAMA 1997). This act encourages pharmaceutic companies to conduct pediatric studies of drugs by allowing these companies an additional 6-month market exclusivity for new and already marketed drugs. The Secretary of Health and Human Services makes a written request for such studies. A year later, the FDA also passed regulations that require drug manufacturers to evaluate the safety and effectiveness of new drugs and biologic products in pediatric patients if the drugs are likely to be applicable to children. With the institution of these new regulations, consumers and medical providers have been assured a larger database of scientific evidence for the use of psychotropic medications in young patients.

This chapter presents general principles for the use of psychopharmacology as well as describes the major groups of psychotropic medications used to treat mental disorders in children.

General Principles and Clinical Considerations

Psychotropic medications are often poorly understood, and, as stated previously, there exists a paucity of evidence recommending their use in children. The decision to use pharmacotherapy in children should thoughtfully include the general principles and clinical considerations that are listed in Tables 22.1 and 22.2.

A comprehensive psychiatric evaluation should precede the prescription of psychotropic medications. In addition to the patient interview, information should also be gathered from the child's parents or caretakers and, if possible, teacher. A further discussion of the psychiatric assessment of children with mental disorders is available in other chapters of this book.

Prior to the start of any psychotropic medication, a physical examination should be completed. The rationale for a physical exam is threefold. First, it is important to rule out the contribution of underlying medical illnesses in the diagnosis of psychiatric symptoms. Second, it is important to identify all medical illnesses that may be exacerbated or further complicated by the introduction of psychotropic medications. Finally, certain medications will require the routine assessment of physical parameters [e.g., electrocardiogram (ECG)] and laboratory values [e.g., complete blood count (CBC), electrolytes, glucose, calcium, thyroid-stimulating hormone, liver function tests, and renal tests]. Baseline information is needed for later comparison.

Pharmacotherapy for the treatment of mental disorders should not be used as a substitute for other interventions such as behavior therapy, family therapy, or individual psychotherapy. In order for the patient to benefit from the use of psychotropic medications, there must be clear target symptoms that are pharmacologically sensitive. While certain chemical entities are capable of altering the dynamics of neurotransmitters, no chemical will change a poor living situation or erase the memories of abuse.

TABLE 22.1. EVALUATION ESSENTIALS FOR THE USE OF PSYCHOPHARMACOTHERAPY

1. Conduct a comprehensive psychiatric evaluation of the child or adolescent.
2. Interview the patient and caregiver regarding the youth's psychiatric symptoms.
3. Perform a physical examination.
4. Collect baseline laboratory and physical assessment data where warranted.
5. Determine the indicated nonpharmacologic interventions for the diagnosed disorder.
6. Consider the risks and benefits of pharmacotherapy as opposed to other interventions.
7. Consider the risks and benefits of specific medications relevant to the disorder.
8. Conduct a formal consent procedure with the parent and youth.

TABLE 22.2. ESSENTIALS OF PHARMCOTHERAPY

1. Review patient's medication history, drug allergies, and past drug reactions.
2. Identify treatable symptoms and establish treatment goals.
3. Initiate drugs at low doses and evaluate need for multiple daily doses based on patient's metabolism.
4. Monitor therapy regularly:
   - Ask patient about the presence of side effects.
   - Ask parents about the presence of adverse reactions.
   - Perform routine physical assessment.
   - Use rating scales to assess side effects as available.
5. Limit and manage side effects:
   - Start medications at low doses and titrate slowly.
   - Avoid adding medications that may cause drug interactions.
   - Identify need for medications that treat side effects (e.g., benztropine, diphenhydramine).
6. Treatment duration:
   - Evaluate effectiveness of current dose after 2–6 wk.
   - Duration of therapy will depend upon the diagnosis, however, need for ongoing treatment should be evaluated every 6 mo.
7. Minimize duplicate therapy and polypharmacy:
   - Monotherapy is preferred when possible.
   - Consider potential drug–drug interactions when combining medications.
8. Coordination of care should exist with the patient, caretakers, and all health care providers, including the family's pharmacist.

Prior to instituting any medication trial, formal consent to medication treatment should be obtained. The consent process includes documentation stating that discussion of possible adverse reactions has occurred. Some county health agencies also prefer that the consent language include a risk-benefit ratio statement that the risks of not treating the patient's symptoms with a particular medication outweigh the possible risks of developing adverse reactions.

Once treatable symptoms are identified, drug selection should incorporate rational and realistic expectations for drug therapy outcomes. Many psychotropic medications are not immediately effective and, in fact, may require daily treatment for up to 2 months before optimal effects are seen. Thus, prescribers should not escalate the dose unnecessarily. Elevated doses are often not more effective but may be more harmful and more costly. Thorough knowledge of drug products underlies rational prescribing.

Benign psychotropic medications do not exist. On the basis of therapeutic expectations, the benefits of drug treatment should outweigh the risks from adverse effects. Patients and caretakers should be made aware of both short- and long-term adverse effects associated with the use of the prescribed medication. Adverse outcomes from drug treatment range from sedation, fatigue, and insomnia to psychosis, delirium, obesity, and lipid abnormalities. A formal understanding of potential harm is an important part of the decision-making process.

The best way to minimize medication adverse effects is to utilize the lowest effective dose possible. All psychotropic medications, particularly in children, should be initiated as a low dose and titrated slowly over time. Slowly increasing the dose will ensure that the prescriber has identified the lowest dose at which the patient will maximize benefit and minimize risk. It should also be recognized that some adverse effects may be unavoidable.

Drug pharmacokinetics in young children can present as a challenge to clinicians, particularly as it applies to medication dosing. By age 2, many of the systems responsible for drug disposition, metabolism, and elimination function at adult levels. Paradoxically, between 2 and 12 years of age, drug clearance greatly increases and often exceeds adult levels. Half-lives are shorter and dosing requirements are frequently greater than for adults. It is not uncommon to see once-daily medications dosed twice a day in adolescents, elementary, and middle school-aged children.

Ongoing assessment of the patient's response (positive and/or negative) to pharmacotherapy is important. The therapeutic evaluation of drug therapy should include the amelioration of target symptoms, the occurrence of side effects, and the need for continuing therapy. Sufficient treatment durations vary by diagnosis. On an average, the need for ongoing treatment with a psychotherapeutic agent should be evaluated every 6 months.

Patient care extends beyond the office of the prescriber into the patient's home, school, other health care providers' offices, and the family pharmacy. Information gathered from each participant can enable the provider to maximize therapy and minimize drug interactions and therapeutic duplication. The inclusion of each variable will ensure a well-coordinated and thoughtful approach to psychopharmacology for the pediatric patient.

Stimulant Medications

Stimulants are sympathomimetic drugs that are structurally similar to the endogenous catecholamines. They act both centrally and peripherally by enhancing both dopaminergic and noradrenergic transmission, although their mechanisms differ to some degree. They improve both cognitive and behavioral functioning.

Stimulants are the most prescribed psychotropic agent for children in the United States and are considered first-line medications in the treatment of attention deficit hyperactivity disorder (ADHD). Traditional stimulant medications include methylphenidate, dextroamphetamine, mixed salts of amphetamine (75% dextroamphetamine and 25% levoamphetamine), and pemoline. Zito et al. have described the pharmacoepidemiology of stimulant use in the United States during the 1990s. From 1987 to 1996 there was a marked increase in stimulant prescriptions ranging from three- to sixfold. The change was most notable in children over the age of 15 and in children of preschool age (ages 3–4). Current evidence suggests that as many as 30 per 1,000 (3%) children or adolescents are prescribed stimulant medications.

The popularity of stimulant medications is partially due to their high rate of effectiveness. At least 70% of children with ADHD will have a positive response to a stimulant during the first trial. Target symptoms shown to improve with therapeutic doses of stimulants include easy distractibility; difficulty in sustaining attention; problems with on-task functioning; excessive nonpurposeful motor activity; disorganization; and associated functional impairment in classroom, peer, and family functioning. Response to stimulants is highly variable and patient dependent; not all patients and not all symptoms will respond. Predictors of response to methylphenidate, for example, include a high IQ, considerable inattentiveness, young age, low severity of disorder, and low rates of anxiety.

All stimulant medications are equally efficacious in group studies, although individual youths may respond to one stimulant and not to another. Many studies have been conducted comparing methylphenidate to other traditional stimulant medications. In randomized, double-blind studies comparing Adderall to methylphenidate, the two medications appear to be equally efficacious if given at equivalent doses. A review of 22 different studies showed no differences between methylphenidate and dextroamphetamine nor among the different forms of these stimulants.

Selection of stimulant medication in clinical practice is not based on differences in effectiveness. Factors to take into consideration include dosing frequency, compliance, feasibility of medication administration during the school day, behavior that requires treatment in the late afternoon, side-effect profiles, and cost.

Methylphenidate and dextroamphetamine products are available in both immediate- and sustained-release formulations. Immediate-release products have a quick onset of action, however, the duration of action for these products is typically short (2 hours), necessitating multiple daily doses. Longer-acting, sustained-release preparations, while eliminating the need for medication administration during the school day, can be limited by duration of action (up to 8 hours), a slower onset of action, and decreased effectiveness compared to immediate-release dosage forms. A combination of immediate-release and sustained-release methylphenidate is commonly used to overcome the limitations of both products and is a very useful combination in the treatment of ADHD.

Pemoline (Cylert) is a nonamphetamine stimulant medication. It has an intermediate onset of action (2 hours) and duration (8 hours) compared to other stimulants. Pemoline is not considered first- or second-line therapy for ADHD due to potentially serious adverse hepatic effects and the need for routine liver function testing. If clinicians choose to use this medication, they are advised to discuss the potential risks and obtain signed informed consent (consent forms are available through the manufacturer). Pemoline should not be started in patients with abnormal baseline liver tests. Therapy should be discontinued if serum alanine aminotransferase (ALT) increases to 2 times or greater the upper limit of normal or if the patient develops signs and symptoms of liver failure. Therapy should also be discontinued if no significant clinical benefit is seen within 3 weeks.

The limitations that are associated with the traditional stimulant medications, such as acute tolerance, worsening symptoms as the stimulant wears off, and thus the need for multiple daily dosing, led to the development of newer, longer-acting stimulant preparations. The newer stimulants include Focalin (dexmethylphenidate HCL), Concerta (methylphenidate), Metadate CD (methylphenidate) and Adderall XR (dextroamphetamine/amphetamine mix).

Focalin (dexmethylphenidate HCL) is a new formulation of Ritalin that contains only the active d-enantiomer instead of both the d- and l-enantiomers of methylphenidate. Currently there are no published data to support the use of this medication over generic methylphenidate. However, it appears to be as efficacious as the racemic form of methylphenidate but at half the dosage. Side effects and dosing intervals are identical to the original preparations.

Concerta is an extended-release methylphenidate preparation that can be dosed once daily. The extended-release property of Concerta is based on its OROS delivery system (an osmotically active trilayer core surrounded by a semipermeable membrane with an immediate-release drug overcoat). The outer layer of medication provides an immediate release of methylphenidate within 1 hour, while the remainder of the medication is gradually released over 12 hours. In clinical trials, Concerta once daily was comparable to immediate-release methylphenidate administered 3 times daily every 4 hours. Concerta offers the benefits of immediate- and sustained-release methylphenidate in the convenience of one tablet.

Metadate CD, another once-daily extended-release methylphenidate preparation, is dosed as a capsule containing both immediate- and extended-release drug beads in a ratio of 30% to 70%, respectively. In a 4-week, double-blind, placebo-controlled crossover study, Metadate CD 20 mg once daily was comparable in effectiveness to immediate-release methylphenidate 10 mg administered twice daily, 4 hours apart.

Adderall XR is the once daily extended-release formulation of dextroamphetamine and amphetamine salts. Similar to Metadate CD, Adderall XR capsules contain two types of drug beads designed to give a double-pulsed delivery of amphetamines. Once daily Adderall XR is comparable to the same total daily dose of immediate-release Adderall administered twice daily, 4 hours apart.

While stimulants remain the first-line treatment of ADHD, there are disadvantages to their use. Young children commonly experience decreased appetite and may even lose weight associated with the use of these medications. Even if children do not actually lose weight, deceleration on their growth curve may become apparent. Weight should be routinely monitored and diets may require additional caloric supplementation, for example, by adding a snack before bedtime. Parents should be reassured that by the age of 18, the weight of children treated with stimulants should equal their peers. Other common side effects of stimulant medications may include delayed sleep onset, stomachaches, headaches, and jitteriness, while more severe complications may include motor tics, cognitive restriction, depression, tearfulness, psychosis, and mania. Early work suggested that children with tics should not be treated with stimulants due to the risk of tic exacerbation. However, more recent research suggests that stimulants may be used with such youths without worsening their tics. The reported stimulant-induced psychosis predominantly includes visual hallucinations and generally quickly resolves when the stimulant is discontinued. Some children may experience "rebound," a condition with transient behavioral disturbances and/or affective lability, as the medication wears off. When "rebound" occurs, it is usually most evident in the later afternoon and evening. As this is the time that children are at home with their parents, they may assume that the child is not experiencing any benefit from the medication. In some children, "rebound" may also occur during the daytime as doses of short-acting stimulant medication wear off. "Rebound" is generally managed by a later afternoon dose of a short-acting preparation to prevent this occurrence in the evening and by dosing more frequently during the daytime. However, the development of the long- acting preparations has helped to decrease the occurrence of "rebound" for most children.

The use of stimulant medication is poorly studied in children under 6 years of age. While the FDA has approved the use of dextroamphetamine, magnesium pemoline, and Adderall in children as young as 3 years of age, there are only six published controlled studies that include preschoolers aged 4 to 6 years. Methylphenidate is not approved for use in children less than 6 years of age and its use in this age group is considered "off-label." Patient selection for stimulant therapy is left to the discretion of the provider. Information relevant to the use of the stimulant medications in clinical practice is summarized in Table 22.3.

Antidepressant Medications

Antidepressant medications act on central pre- and postsynaptic receptors, affecting the release and reuptake of neurotransmitters including serotonin, norepinephrine, and dopamine which are thought to be related to their therapeutic effects. Antidepressant therapy is composed of four main drug classes: monoamine oxidase inhibitors (MAOIs), tricyclic antidepressants (TCAs), selective serotonin reuptake inhibitors (SSRIs), and newer atypical antidepressants. The older MAOIs are associated with a number of dietary and therapeutic restrictions that have made this antidepressant drug class very unpopular. This section will focus on the other three categories of antidepressants.

Several factors should be taken into consideration prior to the initiation of antidepressant therapy. Physical parameters that may be affected by pharmacologic treatment should be evaluated. Baseline assessments that may be of value include heart rate (HR), blood pressure (BP), weight, and possibly an ECG. Once antidepressant therapy has started, patients should be monitored regularly for the presence of drug-induced side effects. Early in antidepressant therapy, treatment duration should be established and discussed with the patient and his or her caregivers. Among younger patients, the average length of a depressive episode is about 7 to 9 months. The duration of antidepressant therapy is reflective of this timeline. The clinician should recognize that antidepressant effectiveness is not immediately apparent. Initial improvement can be expected after 4 to 6 weeks of pharmacotherapy. Substantial improvement may not be apparent for 8 to 12 weeks. Once the patient has achieved a remission of symptoms, the antidepressant

TABLE 22.3. STIMULANT MEDICATIONS

Drug	Chemical Effect	Average Daily Dose Range	Pharmacokinetic Parameters	Monitoring
AMPHETAMINE MIXTURES				
Adderall	Blocks reuptake of DA and NE, inhibits MAO	2.5–40 mg 1–3 div doses	4–6 h duration	Blood pressure, height, weight
Adderall XR		10–30 mg QAM	12 h duration	
DEXTROAMPHETAMINE				
Dexedrine	Blocks reuptake of DA and NE, inhibits MAO	5–40 mg 1–3 div doses	4–6 h duration	Blood pressure, height, weight
Dexedrine Spansules		5–40 mg QD	6–8 h duration	
METHYLPHENIDATE				
Concerta	Blocks reuptake of DA	18–54 mg QAM	12 h duration	CBC with differential, platelet count, blood pressure, height, weight
Metadate CD		20–60 mg QAM	9 h duration	
Focalin		5–20 mg 2 div doses	3–5 h duration	
Ritalin IR		5–60 mg 2–3 div doses	3–5 h duration	
Ritalin SR		20 mg QD	8 h duration	
OTHER				
Cylert (pemoline)	Blocks reuptake of DA	37.5–112.5 mg QD	6–8 h duration	Liver enzymes, height, weight

DA, dopamine; NE, norepinephrine; MAO, monoamine oxidase; CBC, complete blood count.

should be continued for a duration of 9 months to 2 years in order to prevent relapse. Patients with three or more episodes of depression and those whose first episode was unusually severe are at a high risk of recurrence and should be considered for long-term maintenance therapy. Discontinuation of antidepressant therapy requires careful attention and will be discussed later.

Antidepressant medications are not limited to the treatment of depressive disorders. In addition to major depressive disorder, certain antidepressants have been used effectively in the treatment of insomnia, ADHD, tic disorders, enuresis, obsessive–compulsive disorder, and other anxiety disorders. Each antidepressant class has a unique mechanism of action and side-effect profile.

TRICYCLIC ANTIDEPRESSANTS

TCAs were the first antidepressants to be used to treat depressive, obsessive–compulsive, and other anxiety disorders in children and adolescents. Other potential uses for this drug class include enuresis, ADHD, and disorders of sleep, including narcolepsy and cataplexy.

Double-blind placebo-controlled studies of the TCAs (e.g., imipramine, desipramine, nortriptyline) for the treatment of major depression in children and adolescents have found them to be no more effective than placebo. Use in anxiety disorders has had limited effectiveness as well. Studies examining the effects of TCAs on children with ADHD have been more successful. Eighteen controlled studies involving 953 children demonstrated at least moderate benefit compared to placebo controls. TCAs are considered second-line medications for the treatment of children with ADHD due to their adverse effects and narrow margin of safety.

The mechanism of action for the TCAs, as for all antidepressants, has not been fully elucidated. It is believed that they work by blocking the presynaptic reuptake of both norepinephrine and serotonin. The degree to which this blockade occurs varies by the chemical structure of the TCA. Tertiary amines (e.g., amitriptyline, imipramine, doxepin) primarily block serotonin reuptake, and secondary amines (e.g., desipramine, nortriptyline, protriptyline) principally block norepinephrine reuptake.

TCAs are well absorbed, readily distributed, and highly bound to plasma proteins. Of particular note, TCAs are hepatically metabolized substrates for several cytochrome P450 isoenzymes (e.g., 1A2, 2C9, 2C19, 2D6, 3A3/4) and subject to many drug interactions. Drugs that either inhibit or induce the same hepatic enzymes will influence the serum concentration of the TCAs. The rate of metabolism can be patient variable. Patients who are considered "slow hydroxylators" should receive lower doses.

TCAs have a wide range of receptor affinities including muscarinic, histaminic, and α-adrenergic receptors. Blockade of these receptors is associated with a variety of adverse effects. Common treatment-emergent side effects include dry mouth, constipation, blurry vision, orthostasis, and urinary retention. Further information is available in Table 22.4. TCAs have a narrow therapeutic window. Higher doses, drug interactions, and slow metabolism can lead to cardiotoxicity and lethality. The risks associated with overdose have significantly reduced the popularity of these drugs. In particular, in the 1980s, a series of sudden deaths were reported in children prescribed desipramine. This apparent risk of cardiotoxicity along with the development of safer classes of antidepressant medications led most prescribers to discontinue the routine use of all TCAs in children and adolescents. Treatment with TCAs should typically be preceded by an ECG, with follow-up ECGs performed at appropriate intervals during therapy, such as with changes in dosage or the addition or elimination of another medication. Accompanying serum levels may also be useful to avoid toxicity. TCAs should never be accessible to young children for self-administration due to their lethality in overdose.

TABLE 22.4. ANTIDEPRESSANT MEDICATIONS

Drug	Chemical Effect	Average Daily Dose Range	Side Effects	Monitoring
TRICYCLIC ANTIDEPRESSANTS				
Amitriptyline (Elavil) (tertiary TCA)	5HT, ±NE	Children: 1–3 mg/kg/d in 3 div doses Adolescents: 25–300 mg/d	Anticholinergic side effects, orthostatic hypotension, sedation, GI intolerance, weight gain, sexual dysfunction	ECG, CBC, blood pressure, heart rate, weight, plasma concentrations
Imipramine (Tofranil) (tertiary TCA)		Children: 1.5–5 mg/kg/d in 1–4 div doses Adolescents: 25–300 mg/d		
Nortriptyline (Pamelor) (secondary TCA)	NE, ±5HT	Children: 1–3 mg/kg/d in 3–4 div doses Adolescents: 30–150 mg/d in 3–4 div doses	Same as above; less anticholinergic and sedative effects	
SELECTIVE SEROTONIN REUPTAKE INHIBITORS				
Citalopram (Celexa)	5HT	No dosing information available for children	GI intolerance, sexual dysfunction, activation, mania, sleep disturbance	Weight, liver function, drug interactions
Escitalopram (Lexapro)	5HT			
Fluoxetine (Prozac)	5HT	5–20 mg/d (can be given 3 times a wk)		
Fluvoxamine (Luvox)	5HT	50–200 mg/d (may need multiple daily dosing)		
Paroxetine (Paxil)	5HT	5–20 mg/d (limited data)		
Sertraline (Zoloft)	5HT	Children: 25–100 mg/d Adolescents: 50–100 mg/d		
ATYPICAL ANTIDEPRESSANTS				
Bupropion (Wellbutrin, Wellbutrin SR, Wellbutrin XL)	NE, DA	Limited data with pediatric patients; typical adult dose is 100 mg tid.	Agitation, insomnia, GI intolerance	Weight, blood pressure, seizure threshold
Venlafaxine (Effexor, Effexor XR)	5HT, NE	No dosing information available for children	GI intolerance, sexual dysfunction, activation, mania, sleep disturbance, hypertension	Weight, blood pressure, drug interactions
Mirtazapine (Remeron)	5HT, NE	No dosing information available for children	Somnolence, weight gain	Lipids, weight, agranulocytosis
Nefazodone (Serzone)	5HT	No dosing information available for children	GI intolerance, insomnia, agitation	Liver function, drug interactions

TCA, tricyclic antidepressants; GI, gastrointestinal; 5HT, serotonin; NE, norepinephrine; DA, dopamine; ECG, electrocardiogram; CBC, complete blood count.

SELECTIVE SEROTONIN REUPTAKE INHIBITORS

The SSRIs are now the most frequently prescribed antidepressants for children and adolescents with depression and anxiety disorders. Currently available SSRIs include citalopram, escitalopram, fluoxetine, fluvoxamine, paroxetine, and sertraline. The FDA has established pediatric indications for sertraline (obsessive–compulsive disorder), fluvoxamine (obsessive–compulsive disorder), and fluoxetine (depression and obsessive–compulsive disorder). While these drugs have been extensively studied in adult populations, their long-term effects on children and brain development are not well defined. The SSRIs are structurally dissimilar, yet they share many pharmacologic properties due to their relatively selective serotonin reuptake inhibition. Their exact mechanism of clinical effectiveness is unknown. Their selectivity for serotonin and potency of reuptake inhibition differ, however, this has limited impact on their therapeutic efficacy. Further factors of differentiation between the SSRIs include their degree of cytochrome P450 isoenzyme inhibition, protein binding, and half-lives.

All of the SSRIs are metabolized by the liver, but their cytochrome P450 isoenzyme profiles set them apart. Fluoxetine and fluvoxamine are the two SSRIs associated with the most drug interactions. They inhibit many of the common P450 isoenzymes including 1A2, 2C9, 2C19, 2D6, and 3A3/4. Paroxetine inhibits the 2D6 isoenzyme, and sertraline has the potential to inhibit the 2C19 and 3A3/4 isoenzymes. Citalopram and escitalopram are associated with the least number of drug interactions as they are not potent inhibitors of any of the P450 isoenzymes. In addition, they are less influenced by protein binding. Therefore, citalopram and escitalopram are good choices when drug–drug interactions need to be minimized, such as for children and adolescents with serious medical illness who are receiving multiple other medications. Generally, the SSRIs are dosed once daily based on a long half-life. The presence of an active metabolite is partially responsible for longer half-lives. Fluoxetine has the longest half-life at 2 to 3 days. The other SSRIs have half-lives ranging from 15 to 35 hours. However, half-lives of the SSRIs are not well established for children. Their higher rate of metabolism may lead to shorter half-lives and may necessitate twice daily dosing.

SSRIs have been studied and prescribed for a variety of disorders including depression, anxiety, panic disorder, obsessive–compulsive disorder, and eating disorders. Their effectiveness in the adult population has been well established. Double-blind placebo-controlled studies of fluoxetine and citalopram with depressed children and adolescents and of paroxetine and sertraline with depressed adolescents have demonstrated efficacy superior to placebo. However, there are only a few such systematic SSRI studies with youths, and efficacy in these studies is not as robust as has been repeatedly demonstrated with depressed adults. To further cloud understanding of the SSRIs' applicability to youths, selected drug companies have allegedly withheld results of clinical trials that did not support efficacy of their specific SSRI, suggesting that efficacy may be even lower than currently reported in the literature. At this writing, data are being reexamined and debate is ongoing.

Because of their pharmacologic profiles, the SSRIs cause fewer anticholinergic, cardiovascular, and hyperphagic side effects than the older antidepressants. However, while the SSRIs have fewer and less severe adverse effects compared to the TCAs, they are not benign. Common side effects include headache, nausea, vomiting, diarrhea, nervousness, sleep disturbance, and sexual dysfunction. The use of SSRIs at high doses or with other serotonergic agents (e.g., MAOIs, certain cold preparations) may also result in a hyperserotonergic state known as the serotonin syndrome. This syndrome is characterized by clinical features such as mental status changes, agitation, diaphoresis, fever, hyperreflexia, incoordination, myoclonus, shivering, and tremor. Treatment should include the immediate discontinuation of the offending agents. In more serious cases, the patient may require hospitalization and supportive care.

SSRIs, like all antidepressants (TCAs, MAOIs, venlafaxine, trazodone), can be associated with withdrawal symptoms if abruptly discontinued, likely associated with anticholinergic withdrawal. The signs and symptoms of this syndrome include dizziness, headache, nausea, vomiting, diarrhea, movement disorders, insomnia, irritability, visual disturbances, lethargy, anorexia, tremor, electric shock sensations, and lowered mood. Generally, patients experiencing withdrawal from SSRIs will describe these symptoms as "flulike." The occurrence of withdrawal side effects is least frequent with fluoxetine, most likely due to its longer half-life; and most frequent with paroxetine, due to its shorter half-life. The discontinuation syndrome is best avoided with a slow taper of the medication.

The most important adverse effects of these drugs relate to their reported association with mania, disinhibition, and "activation" in young children. Such activation has received considerable coverage in the professional and lay media due to the associated emergence of suicidal thinking and behaviors in approximately 3% of youths with no prior suicidality. The SSRI first so identified was paroxetine. The FDA issued an advisory against using it with children. The pharmaceutical maker of venlafaxine issued a similar warning. However, it should be realized that all of the SSRIs, as well as other antidepressants with predominant serotonergic effects, carry the risk of such activation. In December 2003, increasing recognition of this issue led the Committee on Safety of Medicines (CSM) in the United Kingdom to state that paroxetine, venlafaxine, sertraline, citalopram, and escitalopram are actually contraindicated in the treatment of pediatric major depression. They also recommended that because of the lack of safety and efficacy data on fluvoxamine that it not be used with children or adolescents. The CSM did support fluoxetine for pediatric major depression, stating that the balance of risks and benefits of fluoxetine appears favorable. In March 2004, the FDA issued a public advisory on antidepressant medication that included bupropion, nefazodone, and mirtazapine in addition to the SSRIs. The FDA did not ban the use of these medications with youths, but advised health care providers to monitor both adults and children carefully for the emergence of suicidal ideation or worsening of depression. They now require drug companies to include a warning on bottles of these medications advising patients of the associated risks.

By contrast, the American College of Neuropsychopharmacology (ACNP) Task Force and the American Academy of Child and Adolescent psychiatry (AACAP) note that the evidence for the benefits of the SSRIs outweigh their risks in treating juvenile depression. The ACNP cites a review of clinical trials of over 2,000 youths treated with SSRIs in which there were no deaths nor significant increases in suicidal behavior or thoughts. These findings have recently been supported by a new controlled study from Pittsburgh of depressed adolescents undergoing psychotherapy but not receiving any antidepressant or other medication. This study found that over several weeks of psychotherapy, 12% of youths developed new suicidal thinking. This study underscores common clinical knowledge, that suicidality is a common manifestation of depression and that suicidality may become most problematic as individuals enter the early stages of recovery from depression. Another recent study, *Treatment for Adolescents with Depression Study* (TADS), suggests a more complex relationship between SSRI medication and suicidality. This study evaluated fluoxetine alone, cognitive-behavioral therapy (CBT) alone, combined fluoxetine with CBT, and placebo. Combined therapy was superior to other interventions in reducing depression and suicidal ideation but also had the highest number of suicide attempts. Post hoc analyses indicated some imbalance across the four treatment groups regarding baseline suicidality. Clearly, further study of this complex issue is needed. The FDA is monitoring the use of antidepressants with youths and will update their advisory as new information is available. For now, careful consent with families and close monitoring are needed when prescribing an SSRI for any purpose.

ATYPICAL ANTIDEPRESSANTS

Atypical antidepressants, so called based on unique mechanisms of action, include ven- lafaxine, mirtazapine, nefazodone, and bupropion. These medications will only be men- tioned briefly. Although widely used in youth and adult populations, there is a lack of evidence regarding their use in childhood psychiatric disorders.

Bupropion (Wellbutrin, Wellbutrin SR, Wellbutrin XL) has a unique and poorly under- stood mechanism of action. In addition to the inhibition of norepinephrine reuptake, bupropion appears to have an indirect dopamine agonist effect. Structurally, bupropion is similar to psychostimulants, including amphetamine. Bupropion has been successfully used in the treatment of depression, smoking cessation, and ADHD. Clinical lore posits that bupropion may be less likely to induce mania, and many clinicians prefer it for the treatment of bipolar depression. Depending on the dosage form, it may need to be dosed once, twice, or three times daily. Side effects may include headache, increased sweating, ir- ritability, insomnia, and gastrointestinal (GI) intolerance. It is the least likely of all antide- pressants to cause adverse sexual side effects. Bupropion can lower the seizure threshold, and caution should be used when prescribing other medications that may also lower the seizure threshold (e.g., TCAs, clozapine). Bupropion is relatively contraindicated in pa- tients with seizure disorders or eating disorders that may be associated with a lower seizure threshold. However, preliminary evidence suggests that the newer long-acting preparation may be less likely to have this adverse effect.

Venlafaxine (Effexor, Effexor XR) is pharmacologically similar to the SSRI class but also includes norepinephric properties giving it TCA qualities without the apparent toxicity. Though conclusive studies are not available, venlafaxine may have a quicker onset of ther- apeutic effectiveness in adults compared to other antidepressants and may be considered more effective in treatment-resistant depression. Treatment-emergent side effects associ- ated with venlafaxine are common and similar to the SSRIs, including hyperstimulation and sexual dysfunction. However, venlafaxine appears to minimally inhibit the P450 en- zymes, similar to citalopram and escitalopram, and fewer drug–drug side effects may occur. Also, similar to the SSRIs, withdrawal effects may occur upon medication discon- tinuation after only 1 week of therapy.

Mirtazapine (Remeron) also enhances both serotonergic and noradrenergic neurotrans- mission. It is a potent histamine antagonist, a moderate α-adrenergic antagonist, and a moderate muscarinic receptor antagonist. Mirtazapine is indicated for the treatment of de- pression in adults. Adverse effects associated with the use of mirtazapine include somno- lence, dry mouth, constipation, and rare increases in liver function tests and triglycerides. Due to high affinity for histamine receptors, mirtazapine is also associated with significant weight gain.

Nefazodone (Serzone) is a serotonin (5HT2) receptor antagonist. Its use has greatly fallen out of favor after the FDA required the drug's manufacturer to include a black-box warning in the package insert regarding the potential for life-threatening liver damage. Information regarding the use of antidepressants with young people is summarized in Table 22.4.

Mood Stabilizers

There are three commonly used and well-studied mood stabilizers: lithium, valproate, and carbamazepine. Of the three, only lithium is FDA approved for the treatment of bipolar disorder in adolescents (over the age of 12). Lithium, discovered in 1817, is the oldest and best-studied mood stabilizer. It is effective for the treatment of both manic and depressive episodes in bipolar patients. Lithium's exact mechanism of action is unknown. Lithium has effects on intracellular processes, which lead to decreased cellular response to neurotransmitters. Typically, onset of action occurs between 5 and 14 days (at therapeutic serum levels of 1.0 to 1.2 mEq per L) with full efficacy taking up to 6 to 8 weeks in children and adolescents. During the interim, concurrent medications, such as antipsychotics or benzodiazepines, may be required to control endangering symptoms and provide relief for patients.

Common side effects of lithium include fluid retention, weight gain, acne, increased thirst, drowsiness, nausea, diarrhea, polyuria, polydipsia, headaches, fine hand tremors, and more importantly, memory impairment. Furthermore, lithium toxicity can relatively easily occur, for example, with excess fluid loss during exercise or with the use of diuretics or nonsteroidal antiinflammatory agents. The long-term side effects of lithium on the thyroid require routine monitoring of thyroid function (T4, free T4 and T3), though true hypothyroidism is rare. For stabilized patients with hypothyroidism, the clinician is advised to consider the use of thyroid supplementation rather than switching to a different mood stabilizer that might lead to a loss of medication effectiveness and reemergence of life-threatening symptoms of bipolar disorder. Renal functioning is also routinely monitored. Though the significance is unclear, it is also important to note that lithium can affect bone metabolism, and adequate calcium intake should be encouraged.

Lithium is available in tablets, capsules, and liquid. Extended-release preparations are available for patients who experience intolerable GI side effects with the immediate-release products. The elimination half-life of lithium is typically 18 to 24 hours. Blood plasma levels should be checked once the drug has reached steady state and should be drawn 12 hours after the last dose is given. Lithium is almost entirely excreted through the kidneys and is reabsorbed with water and sodium. Poor kidney function and sodium depletion can lead to lithium toxicity.

Valproate and carbamazepine are both classified as anticonvulsants. While there have been several studies of their anticonvulsant effects in pediatric patients, currently there are no randomized controlled trials of their mood stabilization effects in this population. Studies with adult patients suggest that valproate and carbamazepine may be more effective than lithium in patients with rapid cycling, dysphoric, or mixed mania as well as those with co-morbid substance abuse. As children and adolescents with bipolar disorder frequently present with mixed states, these mood stabilizers have become the preferred mood stabilizers with young people. However, it should also be noted that mixed states at all ages are difficult to treat and may require more than one mood stabilizer.

Valproate preparations (divalproex, valproic acid, or sodium valproate) are becoming increasingly popular as thymoleptics in children and adolescents. Although less well studied than lithium in the treatment of mania in adults, valproate appears to be as effective as lithium for the acute treatment of mania and may be better tolerated in some patients. Its mechanism of action is unknown, but it does appear to inhibit the degradation and enhance the release of γ-aminobutyric acid (GABA), an inhibitory neurotransmitter.

Valproate is easily dosed and has a fairly rapid onset of action. Its half-life ranges from 8 to 17 hours. Therapeutic serum levels (50 to 120 mg per mL) should be checked once the drug has reached steady state, typically after 3 to 4 days. Common side effects include sedation, alopecia, nausea, weight gain, tremor, and GI upset. Thrombocytopenia and agranulocytosis are less common, but they are major complications. Valproate is metabolized hepatically, and drug interactions are common (valproate is a CYP2C9, 2D6, and weak 3A3/4 enzyme inhibitor). Though typically clinically insignificant, transient increases in hepatic enzymes are common. Fatal hepatotoxicity, though rare, has been reported in a small number of children under the age of 10. Children under 2 years of age are reported to be at increased risk of hepatotoxicity, particularly if prescribed more than one anticonvulsant. Polycystic ovary disease has been associated with valproate, particularly with women who are mentally retarded. However, this issue has never been satisfactorily clarified or resolved. Thus, with women, other mood stabilizers may be preferable. Careful review of this complication and an informed consent is important to obtain from the youth and family.

Carbamazepine is structurally related to the TCAs. In adults, carbamazepine is effective for the treatment of bipolar mania; however, due to marked intolerability and the potential for rare but serious side effects, carbamazepine should not be used first line. Common side effects include dizziness, impaired coordination, slurred speech, ataxia, drowsiness, nausea, vomiting, rash, and blurred vision. Rare, but potentially lethal idiosyncratic reactions include bone marrow suppression, liver toxicity, and skin disorders including Stevens-Johnson syndrome. Carbamazepine is metabolized by the liver. Its half-life initially ranges from 25 to 65 hours. After time, the half-life ranges from 8 to 14 hours in children. Half-life decreases over time because carbamazepine is an autoinducer. During the period of autoinduction (4–17 days) serum levels can be misinterpreted. Carbamazepine is a 1A2, 2C, 3A3/4 isoenzyme inducer. Information regarding the clinical use of these three major mood stabilizers is summarized in Table 22.5.

Other anticonvulsants, including gabapentin (Neurontin), lamotrigine (Lamictal), carbazepine (Trileptal), and topiramate (Topamax), have been tried as possible mood stabilizers, but there is limited evidence of their effectiveness or adverse effects with young people. Nevertheless, in clinical practice they are increasingly used for several reasons, including no need for laboratory monitoring that requires phlebotomy, which can be traumatizing to children; lack of hyperphagic effects, which are common with the other mood stabilizers; and the frequent need for dual therapy for bipolar disorder. Gabapentin has recently fallen from favor, even as a second-line or adjunctive medication, due to reported lack of effectiveness.

Antianxiety Medications

Anxiolytic medications, despite a lack of evidence, have been used in the pediatric population for many years. Drugs with anxiolytic activity include benzodiazepines, buspirone, TCAs, SSRIs, β-blockers and α-2a agonists such as clonidine or guanfacine. Of these, only benzodiazepines and buspirone are considered anxiolytics. Antihistamines, barbiturates, neuroleptics, and propanediols are no longer favored in the treatment of anxiety for reasons of safety, lack of specific anxiolytic activity, or the availability of more effective and safer medications.

Benzodiazepines (e.g., diazepam, alprazolam, clonazepam, lorazepam, oxazepam) have a long history of use in adult patients. These drugs are frequently used in the treatment of anxiety and panic disorders. Other indications include the treatment of sleep disturbances, musculoskeletal disorders, seizure disorders, alcohol withdrawal, and the acute treatment of neuroleptic-induced akathisia. Benzodiazepines potentiate the inhibitory effects of GABA and thereby open the chloride ion channel. Through the potentiation of GABA, benzodiazepines are thought to have a direct anxiolytic effect on the limbic system.

There are many intragroup differences among the benzodiazepines. Drugs within this class vary in potency, time to onset, duration of action, side effects, route of metabolism, and potential for withdrawal. Typically, benzodiazepines are classified clinically

TABLE 22.5. MOOD STABILIZER MEDICATIONS

Drug	Chemical Effect	Average Daily Dose Range	Side Effects	Monitoring

Lithium carbonate (Lithobid, Eskalith)	5HT, ±NE	Children: 15–60 mg/kg/d in 3–4 div doses
		Adolescents: 600–1800 mg/d in 3–4 div doses or 2 div doses for sustained release products
			Sedation, thirst, polyuria, polydipsia, weight gain, GI intolerance, tremor, hypothyroidism, seizures, acne	ECG, CBC, electrolytes, renal function tests, thyroid function tests, weight, plasma concentrations
				Serum levels:
				  Acute mania: 0.8–1.5 mEq/L
				  Maintenance: 0.6–1 mEq/L

Valproate, valproic acid (Depakote, Depakene)	GABA	30–60 mg/kg/d in 2–3 div doses	Sedation, thrombocytopenia, alopecia, nausea, weight gain, tremor, GI upset, hepatotoxicity, agranulocytosis, neutropenia	CBC with platelets, liver function tests, weight, menses, plasma concentrations Serum level: 50–125 µg/mL
Carbamazepine (Tegretol, Carbatrol)	Multiple CNS effects	Children: 10–20 mg/kg/d in 3–4 div doses Adolescents: 400–800 mg/d in 2–3 div doses	Dizziness, rash, impaired coordination, slurred speech, ataxia, drowsiness, nausea, vomiting, agranulocytosis, hepatotoxicity	CBC, ECG, weight, plasma concentrations Serum level: 8–12 µg/mL

5HT, serotonin; NE, norepinephrine; GI, gastrointestinal; GABA, γ-aminobutyric acid; ECG, electrocardiogram; CBC, complete blood count; CNS, central nervous system.

by their rate of onset and duration of action. Those agents with a rapid onset of action (highly lipophilic) are more likely to induce initial euphoric effects. Compounds with a long half-life are associated with an increased risk of drug accumulation. Benzodiazepines with short and intermediate half-lives are more likely to cause rebound or withdrawal effects.

Side effects associated with benzodiazepines are plentiful. The most common short-term adverse effects noted in adult patients are sedation, drowsiness, incoordination, confusion, and memory impairment, including anterograde amnesia, and disinhibition. Disinhibition is more problematic with children than with adolescents or adults. More serious adverse effects include respiratory depression, drug-induced delirium, hypotension, encephalopathy, and psychological and physical dependence. Certain benzodiazepines are associated with distinct withdrawal symptoms such as nervousness, anxiety, irritability, and insomnia. Benzodiazepines are generally recommended for short-term use.

The metabolism of benzodiazepines is an important clinical difference. Some benzodiazepines undergo hepatic metabolism via oxidation (e.g., diazepam, flurazepam), while others are processed through glucuronide conjugation (e.g., lorazepam, oxazepam). Because most benzodiazepines are metabolized hepatically, it has been suggested that pediatric patients may require higher doses to account for increased rapidity of metabolic processes. This has not proven to be true. Lower doses are recommended to minimize adverse effects.

Buspirone (BuSpar) is an azapirone anxiolytic without anticonvulsant, sedative, or muscle-relaxant properties. Its effectiveness may be related to a reduction in serotonergic neurotransmission. Clinically, buspirone appears to have minimal anxiolytic effects. Buspirone is metabolized hepatically and is a substrate for the cytochrome P450 3A4 isoenzyme. Its half-life is typically short (2–11 hours in adults) and is increased in renal or hepatic dysfunction. Unlike benzodiazepines, the anxiolytic effect of buspirone is not immediate and can take up to 2 to 3 weeks. Buspirone offers several important advantages over benzodiazepines: it is not potentiated by alcohol, it is not associated with dependence or withdrawal reactions, it does not cause memory or psychomotor disturbances, and it has no demonstrated potential for abuse. As an anxiolytic, buspirone has a comparatively benign side-effect profile. The side effects reported with greatest frequency include dizziness, headache, lightheadedness, and nausea. Information regarding the use of anxiolytics in clinical practice is summarized in Table 22.6.

TABLE 22.6. ANTIANXIETY MEDICATIONS

Drug	Chemical Effect	Average Daily Dose Range	Side Effects	Monitoring
BENZODIAZEPINES				
Alprazolam (Xanax)	GABA	0.375–3 mg/d in 3 div doses	Sedation, disinhibition, drowsiness, incoordination, confusion, memory impairment	HR, RR, BP, CBC, liver function
Clonazepam (Klonopin)	GABA	0.1–0.2 mg/kg/d in 3 div doses		
Diazepam (Valium)	GABA	0.12–0.8 mg/kg/d in 3–4 div doses		
Lorazepam (Ativan)	GABA	0.02–0.1 mg/kg every 4–8 h		
NONBENZODIAZEPINES				
Buspirone (BuSpar)	5HT	0.3–0.6 mg/kg/d in 2 div doses	Dizziness, headache, lightheadedness, nausea	Liver function, renal function

GABA, γ-aminobutyric acid; 5HT, serotonin; HR, heart rate; RR, respiratory rate; BP, blood pressure; CBC, complete blood count.

Antipsychotic Medications

The diagnosis of schizophrenia is rare in children but frequently has an onset in mid to late adolescence. Despite this, antipsychotic medications, or neuroleptics, are used with increasing frequency with children with serious psychopathology including other psychotic disorders, psychotic depression, mania, autism spectrum disorders, Tourette disorder, self-injurious behaviors in developmentally impaired children, and severe aggressive behaviors associated with central nervous system (CNS) insults such as fetal alcohol exposure. It is recommended that patients with diagnosable primary disorders (e.g., ADHD, anxiety) receive an adequate trial of at least one first-line agent (e.g., stimulants, SSRIs) prior to the initiation of antipsychotic therapy. Knowledge of both the safety and efficacy of the antipsychotics comes from clinical studies in adult patients. Studies of antipsychotics in pediatric patients are in progress, but only open label studies have been published to date. These reports generally support safety of the antipsychotics with youths.

There are two general classes of antipsychotics used in clinical practice: the traditional antipsychotics and the atypical antipsychotics. Both categories of antipsychotics effectively treat the hallmarks of psychosis, that is, the positive or active symptoms including hallucinations, delusions, bizarre behavior, disordered thinking, and severe agitation. The newer atypical antipsychotics are more successful at ameliorating the negative symptoms of schizophrenia such as apathy and avolition. It is this latter action plus their less severe side effect profile that has led to the atypical antipsychotics replacing the traditional antipsychotics as first-line antipsychotic medications.

The major chemical classes of traditional antipsychotics include phenothiazines (e.g., chlorpromazine and thioridazine), butyrophenones (e.g., haloperidol), and thioxanthines (e.g., thiothixene). The efficacy of traditional antipsychotics is thought to be related to their dopamine-2 receptor antagonist properties. Other mechanisms of actions may help explain why some patients will preferentially respond to one traditional agent over another. Generally, traditional antipsychotics are metabolized in the liver and are substrates for the cytochrome P450 2D6 isoenzyme. Their half-lives are typically 24 hours or longer. Depot formulations have even longer elimination half-lives. Depot injections are available for both haloperidol and fluphenazine. They are especially useful for noncompliant patients.

The side effects associated with traditional antipsychotics are plentiful, the severity of which depends on the drug's potency (affinity for the dopamine-2 receptor) and affinity for other receptors (e.g., α-adrenergic receptors, histamine receptors). Acute side effects include sedation, orthostatic hypotension, anticholinergic effects, and extrapyramidal symptoms (EPS) such as parkinsonism, dystonia, and akathisia. EPS can be treated by lowering the antipsychotic dosage or by the use of anticholinergic agents such as benztropine. Akathisia is a restlessness and agitation that may be more subjectively distressing than objectively evident, as patients often describe feeling like they are going to "jump out of their skin." It can be mistaken for the reemergence of psychosis. Neuroleptic malignant syndrome (NMS) is a potentially fatal complication of antipsychotic medications that is related to malignant hyperthermia. It is characterized by muscle rigidity, autonomic instability, increased white count, increased creatine phosphate kinase (CPK), and changes in mental status, such as delirium. The long-term use of these drugs can cause tardive dyskinesia, a writhing athetoid movement predominantly in the face, mouth, and hands. Abrupt discontinuation of antipsychotics can cause withdrawal dyskinesias such as blepharospasm.

Newer atypical antipsychotics (including clozapine, risperidone, olanzapine, quetiapine, ziprasidone, and aripiprazole) are mechanistically dissimilar from traditional agents. Atypical agents have low affinity for blocking dopamine-2 receptors but often are potent serotonin type 2A receptor antagonists. They differ in their ratios of dopamine to serotonin effects, probably accounting for their differential effects in individual patients. Aripiprazole, a partial agonist at the dopamine-2 receptors, is pharmacologically different from all other atypical antipsychotics. In general, atypical antipsychotics are equally effective to traditional antipsychotics in treating active symptoms of psychosis, but they are more effective in treating the negative symptoms and are associated with safer side effect profiles (due to decreased affinity for dopamine receptors). For these reasons, atypical antipsychotics are now used as first-line medications.

No data are available regarding the relative superiority of one atypical antipsychotic over another, except that clozapine is the preferred drug for schizophrenia refractory to other medication trials. Antipsychotic choice is, therefore, based on comorbid medical and psychiatric conditions, side-effect profiles, long-term treatment complications, individual patient characteristics, and medication cost.

All atypical antipsychotics are associated with considerable adverse effects. Clozapine is associated with glucose intolerance, severe weight gain, sedation, hypersalivation, and an increased risk of seizures. In early adult studies, approximately 1% of patients treated with clozapine developed agranulocytosis, a potentially life-threatening adverse effect. Thus, frequent laboratory testing is required to ensure adequate white cell counts during treatment. On the basis of the seriousness of these complications, clozapine is reserved for treatment-resistant patients. At higher doses, risperidone can cause EPS similar to traditional agents. While not usually clinically significant, ziprasidone has the greatest potential of all atypical antipsychotics to prolong the QTc interval. Some clinicians obtain baseline and follow-up ECGs to monitor for cardiotoxicity in children. Aripiprazole has the potential to exacerbate psychosis due to its partial dopamine agonist activity.

Potential long-term complications of most atypical antipsychotics include hyperprolactinemia, EPS, and tardive dyskinesia, although this last risk may be more potential than real. Nevertheless, youth should be monitored for the development of abnormal motor movements. The Abnormal Involuntary Movements Scale (AIMS) is commonly used to monitor for the development of tardive dyskinesia, and the Simpson-Angus Scale (SAS) for Extrapyramidal Symptoms is commonly used to monitor symptoms of EPS. These scales are provided in appendices I and II respectively.

The most common serious complication is the development of metabolic syndrome characterized by hypertriglyceridemia, hyperglycemia, and hyperleptinemia due to severe weight gain that may develop in response to the hyperphagia associated with most of the atypical antipsychotics. Additionally, the FDA has issued a warning that all of the atypical antipsychotics carry a risk of precipitating type-2 diabetes. Olanzapine and clozapine are associated with the greatest weight gain and glucose intolerance. Ziprasidone has the fewest metabolic side effects, including lower hyperphagic effects. The newest atypical antipsychotic, aripiprazole, reportedly causes the least hyperphagia and therefore should have a decreased risk of metabolic syndrome. However, experience with this medication with children is limited. Because these side effects can be physically, mentally, and socially detrimental, the American Diabetes Association (ADA) recommends that weight be actively managed and the development of metabolic syndrome monitored. Specifically, the ADA recommends measurement of fasting glucose, lipids, and BP at baseline, then again after 3 months of treatment, and then yearly. If problems develop, more aggressive monitoring and intervention may be needed. Additionally, waist circumference and body mass index (BMI) should be measured at baseline, then monthly for 3 months, and then quarterly. Information regarding the use of antipsychotics in clinical practice is summarized in Table 22.7.

TABLE 22.7. ANTIPSYCHOTIC MEDICATIONS

Drug	Chemical Effect	Average Daily Dose Range	Side Effects	Monitoring
TRADITIONAL ANTIPSYCHOTICS—LOWER POTENCY AGENT				
Chlorpromazine (Thorazine)	DA	0.5–1 mg/kg every 4–6 h	Anticholinergic effects, orthostasis, sedation, EPS, NMS	CBC, BP, AIMS, SAS
TRADITIONAL ANTIPSYCHOTICS—HIGHER POTENCY AGENT				
Haloperidol (Haldol)	DA	0.01–0.15 mg/kg/d in 2–3 div doses	EPS, NMS hyperprolactinemia	ECG, BP, CBC, electrolytes, AIMS, SAS
ATYPICAL ANTIPSYCHOTICS				
Aripiprazole (Abilify)	DA	No data in children. Adult dose: 10–15 mg/d	Headache, akathisia, sleep disturbance, orthostasis	Weight, BMI, glucose, fasting lipids, BP, AIMS, SAS
Risperidone (Risperdal)	5HT, DA	Adult dose: 2–6 mg/d	Orthostasis, hyperprolactinemia, weight gain, EPS	
Olanzapine (Zyprexa)	5HT, DA	Adult dose: 10–20 mg/d	Sedation, weight gain, hyperglycemia, hyperlipidemia	
Quetiapine (Seroquel)	5HT, DA	Adult dose: 150–800 mg/d	Sedation, orthostasis, weight gain	
Ziprasidone (Geodon)	5HT, DA	Adult dose: 80–160 mg/d	Sedation, akathisia	
Clozapine (Clozaril)	5HT, DA	Adult dose: 200–900 mg/d	Orthostasis, weight gain, hyperglycemia, hyperlipidemia	

DA, dopamine; 5HT, serotonin; EPS, extrapyramidal symptoms; NMS, neuroleptic malignant syndrome; CBC, complete blood count; BP, blood pressure; ECG, electrocardiogram; BMI, body mass index; AIMS, abnormal involuntary movement scale; SAS, Simpson–Angus scale.

Other Agents

A variety of other agents have been frequently used in the treatment of child and adolescent psychiatric disorders that do not fit into the aforementioned drug classes. A few of these agents will be briefly discussed.

Atomoxetine (Strattera) is the newest addition to the nonstimulant medication class. It is the first nonstimulant medication approved for the treatment of ADHD. Though its true mechanism of action is unknown, it is thought to be related to the selective inhibition of the presynaptic norepinephrine transporter. Atomoxetine is rapidly absorbed and reaches a maximal plasma concentration within 1 to 2 hours. It is eliminated primarily by oxidative metabolism through the cytochrome P450 2D6 isoenzyme. Its half-life is about 5 hours but may be extended substantially in patients who are poor 2D6 metabolizers. Side effects include dyspepsia, nausea, vomiting, fatigue, decreased appetite, dizziness, and mood swings. It may induce mild increases in BP and pulse, but no ECG changes. The superior effectiveness of atomoxetine compared to first-line stimulant medications has not been demonstrated in blinded head-to-head randomized controlled clinical trials. A target dose for the treatment of ADHD is 1.2 mg per kg administered as a single daily dose in the morning or in two divided doses in the morning and late afternoon/early evening. Atomoxetine may find a special niche for youths with ADHD and tics.

Clonidine, an α-adrenergic agonist, has been widely used in child and adolescent psychiatry. It is widely used to treat tics. It has also been used with some success in the treatment of ADHD and anxiety disorders. The α agonists are especially helpful for the hyperactivity and impulsivity of ADHD and for anxiety disorders, such as posttraumatic stress disorder, in which there is physiologic arousal with increased sympathetic outflow. It is especially helpful in settling such youths at night so that they can fall asleep. Other uses have included the control of aggression toward self and others in youths with developmental disorders.

Clonidine stimulates α-2-adrenoreceptors in the brain stem, resulting in reduced sympathetic outflow. This is thought to account for its therapeutic effects. It is metabolized hepatically to inactive metabolites and has a half-life of 8 to 12 hours in children. Clonidine should be used with caution in combination with methylphenidate (may increase likelihood of ECG abnormalities) and other drugs that may potentiate the hypotensive effects. Side effects include hypotension, headache, drowsiness, dry mouth, and constipation. Both BP and pulse should be monitored regularly. Clonidine should not be withdrawn abruptly, as doing so may cause rebound hypertension. A typical dose for the treatment of ADHD is 3 to 5 μg/kg/day given in three to four divided doses throughout the day. For patients who are too sedated with clonidine, a second α-2a agonist, guanfacine (Tenex), offers both less sedation and longer duration of action. Guanfacine is a more selective α-2 agonist affecting the α-2a receptor that may account for its lower occurrence of sedation.

Diphenhydramine (Benadryl) and hydroxyzine (Atarax, Vistaril) are antihistamines used for a variety of psychiatric disorders and side effects of psychiatric medications. Diphenhydramine has been used to effectively treat sleep disturbances (short term), anxiety, and EPS. Hydroxyzine is commonly used for the treatment of anxiety. Both drugs have a quick (15 minute) onset of action and half-lives of 2 to 8 hours. Side effects include sedation, dizziness, and dry mouth. Commonly, diphenhydramine is dosed 5 mg/kg/day in divided doses every 6 to 8 hours. Hydroxyzine is dosed 2 mg/kg/day in divided doses every 6 to 8 hours. These medications may cause frightening visual hallucinations in young children due to a central anticholinergic-type effect.

Conclusions

Research in pediatric psychopharmacology has made considerable strides over the past 2 decades. We have learned that both the effectiveness and side effects of psychiatric medications may differ with youths compared to adults. At the same time, the specificity of pharmacotherapy is being better defined. The FDA has called for more investigation of the use of psychiatric medications with youths. Thus, the future should clarify the indications for psychopharmacotherapy, bring new treatment options, and possibly provide prevention strategies to interrupt the evolution of disorders that adversely effect our young patients' well being.

BIBLIOGRAPHY

American Academy of Pediatrics. Clinical practice guideline: treatment of the school-aged child with attention-deficit/hyperactivity disorder. *Pediatrics* 2001;108:1033–1044.

Bradley C. The behavior of children receiving Benzedrine. *Am J Psychiatry* 1937;94:577–585.

Emslie GJ, Mayes TL. Mood disorders in children and adolescents: psychopharmacological treatment. *Biol Psychiatry* 2001;49:1082–1090.

Greenhill LL, Pliszka S, Dulcan MK, et al. American Academy of Child and Adolescent Psychiatry. Practice parameter for the use of stimulant medications in the treatment of children, adolescents, and adults. *J Am Acad Child Adolesc Psychiatry* 2002;41(Suppl.):26–49.

Martin A, Scahill L, Anderson GM, et al. Weight and leptin changes among risperidone-treated youths with autism: 6-month prospective data. *Am J Psychiatry* 2004;161:1125–1127.

Pappadopulos E, MacIntyre JC, Crismon ML, et al. Treatment recommendations for the use of antipsychotics for aggressive youth (TRAAY). Part II. *J Am Acad Child Adolesc Psychiatry* 2003;42:145–161.

Schur SB, Sikich L, Findling RL, et al. Treatment recommendations for the use of antipsychotics for aggressive youth (TRAAY). Part I. *J Am Acad Child Adolesc Psychiatry* 2003;42:132–144.

Treatment for Adolescents with Depression Study (TADS) Team. Fluoxetine, cognitive-behavioral therapy, and their combination for adolescents with depression: Treatment for Adolescents with Depression Study (TADS) randomized controlled trial. *JAMA-Express* 2004;292:807–820.

Wolraich ML. Annotation: The use of psychotropic medications in children: an American view. *J Child Psychol Psychiatry* 2003;44:159–168.

Zito JM, Safer DJ, dosReis S, et al. Psychotropic practice patterns for youth: a 10-year perspective. *Arch Pediatr Adolesc Med* 2003;157:17–25.

SUGGESTED READINGS

American Academy of Child and Adolescent Psychiatry. http://www.aacap.org
(*A good resource for clinicians interested in pediatric psychiatry*), 2005.

Medications. NIH Publication No. 02-3929 Revised April 2002, reprinted September 2002.
(*Information for families about psychotropic medications. It is free by downloading at* http://www.nimh. nih.gov/publicat/medicate.cfm.)

Stanley P, Kutcher MD. *Practical child and adolescent psychopharmacology*. New York: Cambridge University Press, 2002.
(*A good basic text of pediatric psychopharmacology for clinicians.*)

Timothy Wilens MD. *Straight talk about psychiatric medications for kids*. New York: Guilford Press, 2002.
(*An easy to understand and informative text written for parents.*)

APPENDIX I Abnormal Involuntary Movement Scale (AIMS)

Name of Patient: _____   Name of Rater: _____

Date: _____

Instructions:

Either before or after completing the examination procedure, observe the person unobtrusively at rest (e.g., in waiting room). The chair to be used in this examination should be a hard, firm one without arms. Ask the person whether there is anything in his/her mouth (i.e., gum, candy, etc.), and, if there is, to remove it. Ask the person about the *current* condition of his/her teeth. Ask the person if he/she wears dentures. Do teeth or dentures bother him/her *now*? Ask whether he/she notices any movement in mouth, face, hands, or feet. If yes, ask to describe and to what extent they *currently* bother the person or interfere with his/her activities. After observing the person, he/she may be rated on a scale of 0 (none), 1 (minimal), 2 (mild), 3 (moderate), and 4 (severe) according to the severity of symptoms (e.g., involuntary body movements).

0	1	2	3	4	Have patient sit in chair with hands on knees, legs slightly apart, and feet flat on floor. (Look at entire body for movements while in this position.)
0	1	2	3	4	Ask patient to sit with hands hanging unsupported. If men, between legs, if women and wearing a dress, hanging over knees. (Observe hands and other body areas.)
0	1	2	3	4	Ask patient to open mouth. (Observe tongue at rest within mouth.) Do this twice.
0	1	2	3	4	Ask patient to protrude tongue. (Observe abnormalities of tongue movement.) Do this twice.
0	1	2	3	4	Ask the patient to tap the thumb with each finger, as rapidly as possible for 10–15 seconds; separately with right hand, then with left hand. (Observe facial and leg movements.)
0	1	2	3	4	Flex and extend patient's left and right arms (one at a time).
0	1	2	3	4	Ask patient to stand up. (Observe in profile. Observe all body areas again, hips included.)
0	1	2	3	4	# Activated movements—Ask patient to extend both arms outstretched in front with palms down. (Observe trunk, legs, and mouth.)
0	1	2	3	4	# Activated movements—Have patient walk a few paces, turn, and walk back to chair. (Observe hands and gait.) Do this twice.

APPENDIX II   Simpson-Angus Scale (SAS) for Extrapyramidal Symptoms

Patient Name: _____

Rater Name: _____

Date: _____

1. Gait	0	1	2	3	4
2. Arm dropping	0	1	2	3	4
3. Shoulder shaking	0	1	2	3	4
4. Elbow rigidity	0	1	2	3	4
5. Fixation of position or wrist rigidity	0	1	2	3	4
6. Leg pendulousness	0	1	2	3	4
7. Head dropping	0	1	2	3	4
8. Glabella tap	0	1	2	3	4
9. Tremor	0	1	2	3	4
10. Salivation	0	1	2	3	4

0-least severe; 4-most severe.

CHAPTER 23

Behavioral Interventions

TIM CATLOW

Introduction

Treatment of childhood psychiatric disorders can be greatly augmented with the use of behaviorally oriented interventions. Rather than targeting internal states such as thoughts and feelings, behavioral interventions target observable behavior through the intentional manipulation of contingencies. A contingency is a rule-based pairing of stimuli and behavior, and manipulation of a contingency is known as *conditioning*. There have been two primary schools of behavioral conditioning: classic, or Pavlovian, and conditioning and operant, or Skinnerian, conditioning.

Classical Conditioning Versus Operant Conditioning

CLASSICAL CONDITIONING

Behaviorists distinguish between *classical* and *operant conditioning* based on the timing of the intervention. In classical conditioning, the controlling stimulus *precedes* the behavior in question. An alarm clock blaring at 7:00 AM would be an example of a stimulus in a classical conditioning paradigm, and waking up would be the resulting behavioral response. Because a blaring alarm clock will awaken anyone without any conditioning trials, it would be described more accurately as an *unconditioned stimulus,* and waking would be considered an *unconditioned response*. If a neutral stimulus is paired with an unconditioned stimulus (i.e., occurs right before the unconditioned stimulus), at some point the neutral stimulus will also start to elicit the same response from the individual. For example, the quiet little click that occurs right before some alarm clocks sound can, after a while, elicit wakefulness just as effectively as the blaring alarm, even if the click initially was too quiet to do so. In these instances, the click has become paired with the loud alarm that follows. No longer neutral in regard to waking behavior, the click is now described as a *conditioned stimulus*, and the waking behavior is a *conditioned response*, even though it looks essentially the same as the unconditioned response, that is, the waking behavior that results from the alarm.

OPERANT CONDITIONING

Operant conditioning, on the other hand, focuses on stimuli that occur after a behavioral event. In other words, in operant conditioning it is the consequence of a behavior that is described as the controlling stimulus. Fumbling around in the dark to turn off the alarm clock at 7:01 AM would be an example of operant conditioning. The alarm is not eliciting the fumbling in the same way that it elicited wakefulness; rather, fumbling is due to the fact that in the past an individual was eventually able to find the button that successfully turns off the alarm. If hitting that button did not result in a cessation of the alarm, some other behavior would be elicited to turn off the alarm, like pulling the plug. Similarly, a teenager's postalarm clock behavior is affected more by the consequences the teenager has experienced in the past as the result of his or her postalarm clock behavior than with the nature of the alarm itself. In other words, just because a teenager wakes up to the sound of his or her alarm does not determine whether that teenager will actually get out of bed, get ready for school, and make it to class on time. This is true for many children. For example, parents may connect their teenager's alarm clock to a high-decibel fire alarm, only to have their child continue to be late to school. Because the teenager's behavior after waking is determined by consequences rather than by the nature of the alarm, it is described more effectively by operant conditioning than by classical conditioning.

The essential features of classical conditioning and operant conditioning are summarized in Table 23.1. The types of behaviors governed by these principles are summarized below.

TYPES OF BEHAVIORS GOVERNED BY CLASSICAL CONDITIONING PRINCIPLES

Classical conditioning is used when the goal is to get a neutral stimulus to elicit a hard-wired behavior. These are behaviors that already occur naturally and automatically in the individual as the result of an unconditioned stimulus. The behaviors relevant to classical conditioning tend to have more to do with the internal homeostasis of an individual (e.g., sleep,

TABLE 23.1. ESSENTIALS OF CLASSICAL CONDITIONING VERSUS OPERANT CONDITIONING

Classical conditioning

- The controlling stimulus occurs *before* the individual exhibits a behavioral response.
- Behaviors are reflexive, hardwired, and help an individual maintain internal homeostatic balance.
- Behaviors occur naturally and automatically in the individual's species given the appropriate unconditioned stimulus.
- Behaviors are simple, unvarying, and limited in number.
- Only one contingency choice to make: conditioning a neutral stimulus or neutralizing a conditioned stimulus (extinction).

Operant conditioning

- The controlling stimulus occurs *after* the individual exhibits a behavior (consequence, reward, and punishment are all terms from operant conditioning).
- Targets nonreflexive behaviors that facilitate an individual's adaptation to the external environment.
- Behaviors do not occur naturally in the individual's species without training.
- Behaviors can be chained together to form increasingly complex routines of behavior.
- Wide variety of contingency choices to make: punishment vs. reward, continuous schedule vs. variable schedule, ratio vs. frequency, negative consequence vs. positive consequence, primary reinforcement vs. secondary reinforcement.

digestion, and elimination). Because classical conditioning behaviors are hardwired, the behaviors are unvarying in their nature, and there are a limited number of them.

TYPES OF BEHAVIORS GOVERNED BY OPERANT CONDITIONING PRINCIPLES

Operant conditioning addresses behaviors that help individuals to adapt to their external environment in increasingly complex and sophisticated ways. Operant behaviors are not hardwired and are not produced naturally or automatically by an individual. Instead, operant behaviors are comprised of increasingly complex chains of behavior built up over time as a result of the consequences of exhibiting those behaviors. A child learning to play the piano would be an example of operant behavior. Piano playing does not occur naturally in children. No stimulus will automatically elicit piano playing in a child. Even the initial pounding on the keys is not due to the visual stimulus of the keyboard. Rather, the pounding on the keys is repeated because doing so initially (perhaps by chance, perhaps with some encouragement by parents) resulted in a stimulus that encouraged more key pounding. Over time, the child learns to play increasingly complex pieces of music as a way of adapting to an external environment that encourages this behavior. Because operant conditioning behaviors help an individual adapt to ever-changing environments, the behaviors governed by operant principles are virtually limitless and vary widely. Even chickens can learn to play the piano if conditioned properly. However, operant conditioning also tends to be a lot more complicated than classical conditioning paradigms because many more variables must be specified in operant conditioning. The next section describes a number of the most important variables operating in operant conditioning paradigms.

Operant Conditioning

INCREASING BEHAVIOR

Any consequence of a behavior that results in an increase in the frequency of a behavior is called *reinforcement*. Giving a teenager extra privileges for getting to school on time or withholding privileges for arriving late could both conceivably result in an increase in the teenager's on-time behavior, and, in fact, both are examples of reinforcement. When reinforcement consists of presenting a stimulus to the subject, it is known as *positive reinforcement*. When reinforcement involves withholding a stimulus from a subject, it is known as *negative reinforcement*.

One of the reasons operant conditioning can result in so many different types of behaviors is that the person who controls the consequence of a behavior also chooses what behavior will trigger the consequence. Now, in the case of a parent trying to affect a child's behavior, the parent may complain, with justification, that the child is not exhibiting a desired behavior frequently enough for reinforcement to occur. If this is the case, the parent may need to reinforce behaviors that may not be perfect but that at least take the child in the right direction. After these initial steps in the right direction have increased in frequency, the parent can raise the bar by reinforcing behaviors that are even closer to the desired outcome. This process of bringing a child's behavior along in a stepwise fashion until the child is exhibiting the desired outcome is called *shaping*, or *successive approximation*.

In deciding on what to use as a reinforcer, it is important for parents to understand that a consequence is only reinforcing if it actually results in a future increase in the behavior that precedes it. It does not matter if the parent intends for a consequence to be reinforcing. If the consequence does not result in an increase in behavior, then it is not a reinforcer. If the teenager who is frequently late to school is given candy when he or she arrives on time, but the frequency of being late remains constant, then candy is a neutral stimulus in regards to on-time school behavior.

Interestingly, the properties of a stimulus can change over time. For example, it may lose its potency as a reinforcing stimulus and become a neutral stimulus if it is presented too frequently, a process known as *satiation*. Consider that candy tends to have less reward potency on the day after Halloween. Similarly, the potency of a stimulus can be increased by restricting the availability of a stimulus, a process called *potentiation*. For example, television is potentiated as a reinforcing stimulus if a child is restricted from it for a while.

Parents may at times find it inconvenient to allow a child to have a reinforcer at the time the child earns it. As a result, *secondary reinforcers* are sometimes necessary. A secondary reinforcer is something that symbolizes for the child that he or she has earned what would be called the *primary reinforcer*, something that has intrinsic value to the child. Secondary reinforcement is the key concept behind token economies, which will be discussed later in the chapter.

DECREASING BEHAVIOR

A consequence that results in a decrease in the frequency of a preceding behavior is called an *aversive stimulus*, or *punishment*. Once again, if a consequence does not result in a decrease in behavior, then by definition it is not a punishment. If the teenager gets extra chores for playing video games instead of getting ready for school, and continues to play video games, then the extra chores are not accurately described as punishment.

DECIDING WHEN TO PRESENT CONSEQUENCES

Another variable a parent must choose in setting up an operant conditioning paradigm is how often to present consequences, known as a *schedule*. Presenting a reward each time a child exhibits the target behavior is called *continuous reinforcement*. But there are times when it is more effective for stimulus presentation to be intermittent, not to mention being more convenient and less costly. If consequences occur only after a period of time, it is called an *interval schedule of intermittent reinforcement*. If consequences occur only after the child has exhibited the specified behavior a certain number of times, it is called a *ratio schedule of intermittent reinforcement*. Both interval and ratio intermittent schedules can be *fixed*, in which case the interval and ratio is always the same. The intermittent schedules also can be *variable*, in which case the interval or ratio varies around some average number determined by the parent.

Each of the possible schedules in an operant contingency has a different impact on the future probability of the target behavior reoccurring. As a result, different situations call for different schedules, depending on the impact needed. For example, continuously reinforcing a behavior quickly results in an increase in that behavior. However, if the reinforcement remains continuous, the rate of behavior does not become as high as it could be, and interrupting reinforcement causes the behavior to return quickly to the original rate of behavior frequency, or *baseline*. Also, it is simply more difficult for a parent to sustain a continuous reinforcement schedule. *Intermittent schedules* of reinforcement take longer to affect a behavior, but once it does, removal of the reinforcement takes longer to lead to a decrease in the behavior. Combining these two observations, if a parent wants to increase a child's behavior in some area and then have the child sustain that increase, the parent would begin with a continuous reinforcement and then gradually switch to an intermittent schedule so that the behavior increase is greater and lasts longer. This technique of switching from continuous to intermittent reinforcement is called *thinning* the schedule.

Theoretically, thinning can be carried to its logical conclusion in which reinforcement is stopped altogether. If a previously reinforced behavior stops receiving reinforcement, the frequency of the behavior eventually will decrease, or cease altogether, a process called *extinction*. This process takes some time and can even result in an initial increase in the behavior, a phenomenon known as an *extinction burst*. However, if the behavior does not eventually decrease in frequency, then extinction is not occurring, regardless of the intentions of the parent implementing the procedure. If a behavior persists in spite of attempts at extinction, it may be that the behavior is being inadvertently reinforced in some way.

Now, a parent likely will not want his or her teenager to prepare for school all the time. For example, it would be inappropriate for the teenager to get ready for school at 2:00 AM. As a result, the parent will likely put some restrictions on when a reward is given to the teenager for getting ready for school. For example, reinforcement may occur only between 7:00 AM and 8:30 AM. This time period then becomes what is called a *discriminative stimulus*, or S^d. It is also called an *antecedent stimulus*. The combination of antecedent stimuli, behavioral response, and consequence is called a *three-term contingency*. In operant conditioning, the S^d does not control future probability of the behavior recurring. Remember, in operant conditioning it is only the consequence of a behavior that does this, not a stimulus that precedes the behavior. Rather, the S^d lets the child know that a contingency for a given behavior is now operative, whereas the absence of the S^d indicates that the contingency is not operative. A telephone ringing is a good example from everyday life of a discriminative stimulus. The ringing occurs before we engage in phone-answering behavior, so the ring would not be described as a reinforcing stimulus. Recall that in operant conditioning the controlling stimulus occurs after the behavior, not before. Instead, the ringing of the telephone is an S^d that signals that a reward is likely to occur if the subject picks up the phone. The reward, of course, is the opportunity to speak with a person on the other end. Take away this reinforcing consequence and eventually people would stop answering ringing phones. With regard to affecting a child's behavior, utilizing an S^d can help a parent get the attention of a child to communicate a contingency more effectively. For example, a parent turning off the television before giving a directive can be a powerful S^d that signals to the child that the parent is more serious this time.

Clinical Examples

Behavioral interventions can be very effective in treating children and adolescents with behavioral problems. The aforementioned types of interventions are summarized in Table 23.2. Examples of these interventions are demonstrated through descriptions of their use in elimination disorders, anxiety disorders, and disruptive disorders.

TABLE 23.2. SUMMARY OF BEHAVIOR INTERVENTIONS

Aversive stimulus: Any consequence of a behavior that results in a decrease of that behavior when presented or an increase in behavior when withdrawn.

Baseline: The stable frequency of behavior that occurs naturally as a matter of course prior to intervention.

Classical conditioning: The intentional manipulation of an individual's behavior by presenting a neutral stimulus slightly before or at the same time as a stimulus that already elicits species-specific behavior, thereby giving the heretofore neutral stimulus the ability to elicit the species-specific behavior as well.

Conditioned stimulus and response: A conditioned stimulus is a stimulus that previously was neutral in regard to some behavior but now elicits that behavior as the result of being paired with an unconditioned stimulus. A conditioned response is the behavioral response to a conditioned stimulus. Usually the conditioned response looks virtually identical to the unconditioned response. It is called a conditioned response because it occurs as a result of a conditioned stimulus rather than as a result of the unconditioned stimulus.

Discriminative stimulus (S^d): An antecedent stimulus in an operant conditioning paradigm that signals to the subject that a particular contingency is operative at that time.

DRA (differential reinforcement of alternative behaviors): A strategy of rewarding appropriate behaviors that are incompatible with unwanted behaviors, thereby decreasing the frequency of undesired behaviors.

Exposure and response prevention: A procedure for reducing avoidance behaviors associated with anxiety disorders in which an aversive stimulus is presented at a time when the subject can inhibit or be prevented from escaping the aversive stimulus.

Extinction: The process in which the frequency of a behavior eventually decreases as the result of the removal of a reinforcing stimulus.

Extinction burst: The temporary increase of an unwanted behavior that sometimes occurs before the desired decrease in the frequency of that behavior during an extinction procedure.

Fixed: Used to describe an intermittent schedule that has a constant interval or ratio between stimulus presentations.

Interval schedule: The intermittent presentation of a behavioral consequence that occurs only after a certain amount of time has passed since the last instance of the target behavior.

Negative punishment: Any withdrawal of a stimulus that happens as a consequence of a behavior and that decreases the future likelihood of that behavior occurring.

Negative reinforcement: Any withdrawal of a stimulus that happens as a consequence of a behavior and that increases the future likelihood of that behavior occurring.

Operant conditioning: Behavior changes that occur as the result of presenting a stimulus in a systematic fashion after a behavior occurs.

Positive reinforcement: Any presentation of a stimulus that happens as a consequence of a behavior and that increases the future likelihood of that behavior occurring.

Positive punishment: Any presentation of a stimulus that happens as a consequence of a behavior and that decreases the future likelihood of that behavior occurring.

Potentiation: When the rewarding properties of a stimulus are enhanced by withdrawing the stimulus for a while.

Primary reinforcement: A stimulus that is inherently reinforcing, like candy or a toy.

Punishment: Any consequence of a behavior that decreases the future likelihood of that behavior occurring.

(Continued)

TABLE 23.2. Continued

Ratio schedule: The intermittent presentation of a behavioral consequence that occurs as a function of how many instances of a target behavior have occurred since the last consequence.

Reinforcement or reward: Any consequence of a behavior that increases the likelihood of that behavior occurring in the future.

Response cost: The removal of a previously reinforcing stimulus as the consequence of an unwanted behavior, with the hope that negative punishment will occur.

Satiation: When a stimulus loses its potency as a reward due to repeated presentations of the stimulus to the subject.

Schedule of reinforcement: The planned intermittent rate at which a target behavior is to be rewarded.

Secondary reinforcement: Reinforcement that is not inherently reinforcing but that, because it can be exchanged for primary reinforcement, comes to have reinforcing properties.

Shaping and successive approximation: An operant conditioning intervention in which an individual learns a complex behavior in stages, each stage more closely resembling (i.e., approximating) the final desired outcome.

Thinning: A planned gradual reduction in the amount of reward presented as the consequence of a subject exhibiting a behavior without resulting in extinction of the desired behavior.

Three-term contingency: Antecedent stimuli, behavioral response, and consequence combined in one contingency schedule.

Threshold behavior: The minimally sufficient behavior that will trigger a consequence.

Time-out: Moving a child from a high-reinforcement environment to a low-reinforcement environment in order to decrease an unwanted behavior or increase a wanted behavior.

Token economy: The planned use of secondary reinforcers, such as check marks, stickers, or poker chips, that can be turned in for primary reinforcers, such as candy, TV time, an activity, baseball cards, etc.

Unconditioned stimulus and unconditioned response: The unconditioned stimulus is an environmental factor that elicits a behavioral response from an individual without training. The unconditioned response is the automatic behavior exhibited by an individual after experiencing a particular stimulus from the environment.

Variable: Used to describe an intermittent schedule that presents consequences based on an interval or ratio. The interval or ratio may vary from instance to instance of stimulus presentation, but overall the interval and ratio are based on a set average.

ELIMINATION DISORDERS

Before using behavioral approaches for treating elimination disorders, it is recommended that medical causes of the problems be ruled out first.

Nocturnal Enuresis

Nocturnal enuresis can be treated with an intervention based on classical conditioning principles. Classical conditioning principles are appropriate here because the behavior is an automatic, naturally occurring, hardwired behavior, that is, waking behavior. The goal is to change the stimulus that elicits the child's waking, which is a classical conditioning paradigm. We are not really trying to eliminate or increase any behavior, which would call for an operant conditioning paradigm. After all, the child must urinate at some point, and the child will eventually wake up.

Ordinarily, a child's waking is elicited by the sensations of a full bladder. In the case of nocturnal enuresis, the sensations of a full bladder have become a neutral stimulus with regards to waking behavior. The sensations do not elicit the behavior of waking. Instead, the child wakes as a result of the unconditioned stimulus of a cold, wet bed if he or she wakes up at all. The neutral stimulus of full-bladder sensation occurs too long before the unconditioned stimulus of the wet bed occurs for the neutral stimulus to become a conditioned stimulus of the waking behavior. An effective intervention, therefore, requires the introduction of a new unconditioned stimulus to be placed closer in time to the neutral stimulus so that the full-bladder sensations become conditioned. A nighttime moisture alarm has been shown to work well for this situation. This device is a pad that is placed under the child. An alarm built into the pad senses moisture and sounds an alarm. The alarm is loud enough to wake the child as the child is urinating, well before the child would wake as a result of the cold, wet bed. Eventually, the sensations of a full bladder elicit the waking behavior due to being paired with the alarm stimulus, and the alarm is no longer needed as an unconditioned stimulus for waking behavior. It is important to explain to children that the pad is not going to shock them, and that the purpose of the pad is to help them regain control of their bladder functioning. Children are generally able to understand the process when it is explained that the device simply helps to retrain their brains to know when their bladder is full and that as soon as their brains are retrained, the pad can be discontinued.

Encopresis

When encopresis is accompanied by constipation, a painful bowel movement has generally caused the child to retain normal bowel movements. Overflow incontinence does not constitute a full bowel movement but rather the leakage of feces around the larger impacted fecal blockage. Because encopresis is associated with constipation, the first step is to relieve the constipation medically. Sometimes, even after the constipation has been relieved, however, the child has difficulty regaining control of the muscles that facilitate normal bowel movements. Retraining these muscles then must occur so that they function only when the child is sitting on the toilet. In behavioral terms, the toilet has become a neutral stimulus in regard to bowel movement muscle relaxation. Once again, this is a classical conditioning situation focused on reflexive behavior that has lost its association with a stimulus. The desired result is that the muscle relaxation needed to produce a bowel movement becomes conditioned to occur on the presentation of the toilet stimulus. In order to accomplish this, parents can take advantage of the fact that the consumption of food is an unconditioned stimulus for bowel movement a short time later. To take advantage of this biologic tendency, the parent should schedule some time for the child to sit on the toilet for 10 or 15 minutes after each meal, perhaps reading a book or being read to by the parent. The desired response is more likely to occur if the child is relaxed, since it is the parasympathetic nervous system that controls this function. After a while, the toilet should become a conditioned stimulus for bowel movement function. It may be necessary for the parent to adjust the timing of the toilet sessions. It should also be made as positive an experience as possible. If it is an aversive experience, it may trigger avoidance behavior.

ANXIETY DISORDERS

Although behavioral interventions do not target anxiety *per se*, they can target the avoidance behaviors that often accompany anxiety disorders. Avoidance behaviors are those behaviors that an individual exhibits in order to avoid anxiety associated with some stimulus. Avoidance behaviors have a broad range, but there are some common ones that give children particular difficulty, such as school avoidance in school phobia, avoidance of social interactions in social phobia, avoidance of traumatic memory triggers in posttraumatic stress disorder (PTSD), and compulsive washing and counting in obsessive–compulsive disorder (OCD).

Avoidance behavior can be understood as an instance of negative reinforcement. Recall that negative reinforcement occurs when the future probability of a behavior increases if the behavior is followed by the removal of an aversive stimulus. If a child is able to avoid an aversive stimulus through some avoidance behavior he or she exhibits, then the avoidance behavior will be self-reinforcing. For example, if the process of going to school is aversive to a child, and the child is allowed to stay home from school as a result of school avoidance behavior such as having a tantrum, then the school avoidance behavior has been successful and reinforcement has occurred. Likewise, if the act of touching a doorknob is aversive to a child, and the child is allowed to avoid the aversive stimulus of touching doorknobs, then the avoidance behavior has been successful and reinforcement has occurred. In the case of PTSD, situations that the child has come to associate with past trauma are avoided. Because such triggers of traumatic memories can be everyday experiences, avoidance responses involved in PTSD can seriously undermine a child's successful adaptation.

In order to disrupt the reinforcement of avoidance behaviors, exposure to the aversive stimulus must occur while the child's avoidance response is prevented from successfully removing the aversive stimulus. This is called exposure and response prevention (E/RP). For the purposes of this chapter, the underlying behavioral principles of E/RP are explained. When actually used in clinical practice, E/RP is typically supported with cognitive interventions that help the child tolerate the stress of E/RP. John March and Karen Mulle discuss the procedure extensively in their 1998 book, *OCD in Children and Adolescents: A Cognitive-Behavioral Treatment Manual*.

When using E/RP, it is important to correctly identify the aversive stimulus and the avoidance response. For example, a child who verbalizes a fear of deadly disease while washing his hands repeatedly and avoiding doorknobs does not need to be exposed to deadly disease to overcome the avoidance behavior. In this instance, the aversive stimuli are unwashed hands and doorknobs. It is exposure to unwashed hands and doorknobs that is indicated. The child's verbalization of a fear of deadly disease is an instance of the child's avoidance behaviors. In other words, it is a behavior that was rewarded in the past by making it possible for the child to avoid an aversive stimulus. We might not be able to determine exactly how the aversive stimulus became aversive, but, for a behavioral intervention to be successful, determining the history of a contingency is not important. In the case of PTSD, how the stimuli became aversive is known, that is, through association with past trauma. But the past trauma *per se* is not the aversive stimulus. E/RP works through exposure to the aversive stimulus, and it is obviously not necessary to reexpose someone to traumatic situations. Rather, the aversive stimuli are the traumatic memories and triggers of traumatic memories that occur in the individual's *current* experience. Similarly, in school phobia and separation anxiety disorder, the child's imagined fears of what might happen if he or she is separated from the parents are not the aversive stimuli. The aversive stimulus is the act of going to school or the act of separating from the parent. The verbalized fears the child uses to explain his or her fears are instances of verbal avoidance behavior that are rewarded when they lead to successful avoidance of the actual aversive stimuli.

Essentially, E/RP is an extinction model. The individual's avoidance behaviors are no longer reinforced through the removal of an aversive stimulus and so eventually become extinguished. The basic model of E/RP is simple, but there are some special considerations when using E/RP with children. Motivation is perhaps the most important of these. Most people, regardless of age, have difficulty tolerating discomfort in the here and now for the sake of some benefit down the road; but at least adults are more prepared in terms of cognitive development to do so. Children, on the other hand, have difficulty delaying gratification now for future gain. As a result, the younger the child the more important it is to move slowly and to avoid overwhelming the child with goals that are too ambitious. One strategy March and Mulle recommend is to show the child how to measure his or her anxiety using a drawing of a thermometer for rating various anxiety-provoking activities. It may be argued that this is not a behavioral intervention. However, this strategy is not part of the behavior-changing intervention. It is a rapport-building strategy that allows implementation of the behavior-changing intervention. The strategy calls for the child to rate a variety of situations with regard to their anxiety-inducing properties. Some situations will not be very "hot" on the thermometer and do not offer much of a challenge for the child. Other aversive situations will be too "hot" and would be, therefore, more likely to overwhelm the child. However, some situations will be in the "work zone," and these are the situations to tackle with E/RP. Soon work-zone situations will become "cold" and the focus can shift to the hotter situations, until the child has eliminated all the avoidance behaviors.

The exception to this step-by-step procedure is school phobia. In the case of school phobia, it is necessary to do the procedure in one step, with more of a "Band-Aid off" method. The reason is that school is a black-and-white stimulus that is either present or not. Any step short of getting the child back into the school will be reinforcing for the avoidance behaviors because the result is successful avoidance of the aversive stimulus. Nevertheless, there are some ways to ease the transition with school phobia. For example, the child can be given some change to make a call home. Forcing the child to use a pay phone allows the parent to limit the number of calls the child makes. The child can also be given a tape recorder with a parent's voice making reassuring statements on it. However, the procedure works best if these transitional strategies are not utilized.

DISRUPTIVE BEHAVIOR DISORDERS

Disruptive behavior disorders (DBDs) include attention deficit hyperactivity disorder, oppositional defiant disorder, and conduct disorder. Operant conditioning strategies for these disorders vary greatly in regard to how involved and complicated they get. This is an important dimension to consider because behavioral interventions can become aversive to parents if they get too complicated, eliciting the parents' own avoidance behaviors! The strategies that are discussed here are *extinction, satiation, differential reinforcement of alternative (DRA) behaviors, token economies, response cost,* and *time-out from positive reinforcement.*

Extinction occurs when a behavior that has been reinforced is no longer reinforced and the behavior eventually reduces or disappears. Extinction is called for in DBDs when a child has learned to emit a disruptive behavior because a parent has responded to the misbehavior by giving in to the child's demand. In essence, there are two contingencies at play. The child's misbehavior is positively reinforced because it increases as a result of the presentation of a reinforcing stimulus, that is, the parent provides what the child wants. The parent's behavior is negatively reinforced because it increases as a result of the removal of an aversive stimulus, that is, the child stops the misbehavior, at least for the time being. Thus, the parent's behavior is in reality an instance of avoidance behavior! Like any avoidance behavior, the parent's avoidance can be treated with E/RP by having the parent expose him- or herself to the aversive stimulus of the child's misbehavior without capitulating to the child's demands.

One common mistake parents make in using extinction is to rely on it exclusively to bring about behavior change. Extinction is a reductive technique that by itself does not produce desired behaviors. As a result, while the parent ignores his or her child's misbehavior, the child may try increasingly disruptive behaviors to elicit the reward. If the parent now gives in after the child has found an even more disruptive behavior, then an even more powerful intermittent reinforcement schedule has been established that will be even more difficult to extinguish. Setting up a *differential reinforcement of an appropriate behavior* (see below) may be necessary. Another common problem with extinction occurs when the actual reinforcement has not been removed. Sometimes, children are not reinforced by what the parent believes is rewarding the behavior. It may be necessary to shift gears and consider withholding a different stimulus if the initial extinction fails.

Satiation can be used to treat some behaviors that are self-reinforcing, like playing with matches. Recall that satiation occurs when the reinforcing properties of a stimulus are undermined by repeatedly presenting the stimulus. If a child who has a problem playing with matches is required to strike and extinguish matches until he or she gets bored with it, sometimes satiation will occur and match play is no longer self-reinforcing.

DRA behaviors, differential reinforcement of incompatible behaviors (DRI), and *differential reinforcement of other behaviors* (DRO) are slight variations of the same basic strategy. The strategy will be referred to here as DRA for convenience. Essentially, a child's disruptive behavior is reduced by increasing the frequency of a competing behavior that is more desired. The idea behind DRA is fairly straightforward, but there are some elements to consider for maximal effectiveness. First, some thought should be put into choosing which new behavior is to be differentially reinforced. The procedure works best if the behavior is one that is already in the child's repertoire, that benefits the child in some way, and that will elicit reinforcement from the environment naturally even after the artificial reinforcement is removed. Second, an equally important consideration is choosing an effective reinforcer. The reward chosen to reinforce the DRA must actually be reinforcing to the child. Frequently a behavioral intervention will not work because the stimulus chosen as a reinforcer is not reinforcing for that particular child. A simple test of the reinforcer can be conducted by asking the child to do a specific task that is undesirable. If the child does not comply, indicating that the task is indeed undesirable, then ask the child again if he or she will do the task if given the reinforcer. If the child does, then there is some confidence that this reinforcer will be effective. A third issue to consider is which schedule of reinforcement to use. DRA works best if it is begun with a continuous schedule of reinforcement to get the contingency established. Then, the schedule can be *thinned* to an intermittent schedule gradually over time. This is important because intermittent schedules are much more resilient and powerful than continuous schedules at maintaining behavioral changes, not to mention that they are easier on the parent to maintain. A disrupted continuous reinforcement schedule will result in a quicker return to baseline levels of behavior than a disrupted intermittent schedule.

In deciding how to implement a DRA program, a parent may find that it is difficult to maintain a high enough frequency of primary reinforcers to maintain the desired behavior. In this case, the parent may want to try a *token economy*. A token economy allows the parent to use secondary reinforcers, such as check marks, stickers, or tokens, that can be turned in for the primary reinforcer, such as candy, TV time, an activity, baseball cards, and so on. The child earns the secondary reinforcers by successfully completing tasks that have been difficult or by behaving well during a period of time that has been difficult. The components of a token economy are summarized in Table 23.3.

Token economies can vary in how involved they are. The simplest token economy is the check mark on an index card. In this procedure, the parent identifies a limited period of time during which the child is having difficulty and tells the child that he or she needs to earn five check marks on an index card during that time period to earn a small reward. Every so often during the specified period of time, the parent takes out the index card and without speaking shows the card to the child and adds a check mark to the

TABLE 23.3. ESSENTIALS OF A TOKEN ECONOMY

Token economies require the following components:
- Identified behaviors that will earn secondary reinforcement, such as chores completed, respectful behavior for specified period of time, homework completed, etc.
- Method of tracking secondary reinforcement, such as check marks on an index card, stickers on a poster, coupons, poker chips, etc.
- Supply of primary reinforcers, such as candy, playing time on video games, computer time, TV time, extra one-on-one time with parent, toys, large-ticket items such as skateboard, etc.
- Rules about how the token economy will be applied specifically in a particular household, such as when secondary reinforcements can be exchanged for primary reinforcements, who will be keeping track of secondary reinforcements, a decision on whether or not it will be possible to lose secondary reinforcements for misbehavior, etc.

General considerations when implementing a token economy:
- Complexity of token economy should be geared to the motivation and skill level of the parent. Overly complex or demanding token economies ultimately fail because the parent cannot sustain them. It is better to start simple and build in complexity as needed.
- It is important that the primary reinforcers in the token economy (i.e., the items the child buys with the secondary reinforcers) are actually reinforcing.
- Use a mixture of bigger, more costly reinforcers and smaller, more affordable reinforcers.
- Use response cost (subtracting points, check marks, etc.) sparingly as a powerful but limited intervention. Subtracting points too often can be demoralizing.
- Parents should adjust the prices of the primary reinforcers as they gain experience with the token economy.
- Warn the parents not to overreact if a child tries to cheat (e.g., tries to add unearned checkmarks). Cheating at least means the incentive is working.

card. The period between check marks should be variable to take advantage of the most powerful of reinforcement schedules, which is the *variable intermittent schedule*. Misbehavior results in one of the check marks being erased, again without speaking but in view of the child. This removal of a secondary reinforcer is a type of punishment called *response cost*, which will be discussed later.

One of the benefits of the index card strategy is that the parent engages in less verbal discussion with the child. Frequently, the well-meaning parent will spend too much time trying to convince the child to behave, with endless discussions unintentionally rewarding the child's attempts to avoid the desired behavioral response. The parent's intention is for the lecturing to constitute a punishment of the misbehavior, thereby reducing it, and a negative reinforcement of positive behavior, with the hope that the child will behave to stop the parent's lecturing. However, what often happens is that the parent's verbal behavior allows the child to avoid some unwanted task. The lecturing, therefore, actually results in reinforcement of the misbehavior. By making the punishment of the misbehavior nonverbal, no unintentional reinforcement of misbehavior occurs.

More complex token economies involve identifying desired behaviors, assigning a value to each of the behaviors in terms of a token amount (often checkers are used, but a "checkbook" style token economy can also work), and reinforcers that can be purchased for a preset amount of tokens. Once again, the basic idea is simple, but the implementation can be difficult, particularly in the beginning when it is not so clear how much each reinforcer should cost. For the token economy to work, the parent must have sufficient energy, organizational skills, and motivation to get the system up and running. The realities of each family's situation will dictate the details of a token economy to a large extent.

There are some specific issues, however, that tend to make or break a token economy. First, start simple and build on success. Picking too many behaviors to target can be frustrating for both the parent and the child. Second, start generously to get the child into the system; then thin the reinforcement schedule by raising the price of items. Third, be conservative about subtracting points already earned for misbehavior, a strategy called "*response cost*." This is a legitimate intervention but can backfire if overused. Children will already be suspicious of a token economy when it is introduced. They know it is an attempt to control their behavior and may be extra sensitive to issues of fairness. If every time the child misbehaves the parent takes the tokens away, the child may become demoralized and stop trying. Charging the child for an egregious violation can be a powerful intervention, but once the token deduction has been made, the parent must be cautious about getting into a power struggle. When the child says, "I don't care about those stupid tokens," this is a good time for the parent to allow the child to have the last word. After all, if the child really did not care, he or she would not be so angry. Fourth, when starting out, the parent should alert the child that prices are temporary and will need to be adjusted when the parent has had time to determine how well the system is working. Fifth, encourage the parent to vary reinforcers between smaller short-term reinforcers and some larger long-term prizes. Having only smaller rewards get boring and having only larger long-term prizes get frustrating.

A common intervention strategy with children with DBDs is the *time-out from positive reinforcement*. This involves sending the child to his or her room or requiring the child to sit in a chair or stay in a limited area for a specified amount of time. Most parents are aware of this intervention, but it is described here in behavioral terms in order to illustrate why this intervention sometimes fails. Often when a parent finds this intervention ineffective it is because the actual execution of the time-out subtly violates some important behavioral principle. Time-outs work by moving a misbehaving child from a high-reinforcement environment in which unintended reinforcement of unwanted behavior may be occurring to a low-reinforcement environment in which the parent has more control over what behaviors are or are not reinforced. This is why it is called a "time-out from positive reinforcement." Because it is a time-out from positive reinforcement, the presence of alternative reinforcers in the room, such as video games, a telephone for calling friends, toys, candy, and so on, can make the time-out ineffective. In these cases, either clearing out the room or changing the time-out location to a chair at the end of a hallway may work to increase the strategy's effectiveness. Another way in which the effectiveness of time-outs can be undermined is when the child comes out of the room for bathroom breaks several times or finds other ways to draw the parent into a reinforcing interaction. It is important to remember that social interaction, even seemingly negative interactions, can be reinforcing for some children. In these cases, the time-out should not begin until the child has stopped interacting with the adult. Another way time-outs may be undermined occurs when the child complies with the letter of the time-out without getting the intended message the parent is trying to send. The parent may end the time-out, only to have the child mumble disrespectfully under his or her breath, slam the bedroom door, or continue arguing about the issue that resulted in the time-out in the first place. From a behavioral perspective, the child is still exhibiting the undesired behavior when allowed to return to the high-reinforcement environment. As a result, the misbehavior is reinforced, but now on a much more potent variable reinforcement schedule! In these cases it may be necessary for the parent to start the time-out over until it is completed properly so that no unintended reinforcement occurs.

Overall, the behavioral strategies reviewed here are rooted in solid scientific theory. However, in practice they do not comprise inflexible laboratory experiments. Rather, their successful implementation relies on the treating clinician's full repertoire of theoretic and clinical skills. The essentials of implementation are summarized in Table 23.4.

TABLE 23.4. ESSENTIALS OF EFFECTIVE BEHAVIORAL INTERVENTIONS

- Developing behavioral interventions requires a somewhat cold, scientific, unbiased stance, but selling the ideas to parents and children requires warmth, engagement, and the ability to establish rapport.
- In making recommendations about behavior interventions to parents, consider the effects of punishment and reinforcement on the parents. If enacting an intervention is aversive to the parents (e.g., it is too complicated or too demanding on them), the intervention may never be used. If the parents are being rewarded by the presence of a behavioral problem (e.g., through SSI disability payments), they may undermine the effectiveness of the intervention.
- A child who feels unfairly manipulated and excluded from treatment decisions may pit his or her will power against the success of the program.
- A parent who perceives the suggested intervention as dismissive of their attempts to solve the problem or as an implied criticism of their abilities as a parent may also undermine the success of the program. The ideal manner to adopt with parents and children is that of collaborating scientists, members of the same team working toward a common goal.
- Exposure and response prevention are especially effective in the treatment of agoraphobia, social phobia, simple phobias, and obsessive–compulsive disorder.
- For disruptive behavior problems, it is generally more effective in the long run to focus on increasing desired behaviors than it is to focus on decreasing unwanted behaviors.
- Reinforcement models should always be part of a behavioral intervention for disruptive behaviors, whether or not there is a punishment component. At times a punishment component is called for, but punishment should always be accompanied by reinforcement of positive replacement behaviors.
- Behavioral intervention should be reviewed for effectiveness and revised if the intervention is not having the desired effect. If an intervention is not effective, there are several possibilities that should be considered.
    - The intended reinforcement may not really be reinforcing for the particular child.
    - The intended punishment may not really be aversive for the particular child.
    - There may be unintended reinforcement of the unwanted behavior.
    - There may be unintended punishment occurring.
    - The child may be more highly reinforced by aspects of the unwanted behavior than he or she is by the reinforcement intervention. Therefore, it may be necessary to increase the intensity of the consequences of the behavior by increasing the rewarding consequences or aversive consequences.
- Reinforcement programs should be thinned from continuous to intermittent as the child's targeted behavior improves over time.

Conclusions

Behavioral interventions often serve as the cornerstone of treatment planning for many child and adolescent psychiatric disorders. Both *classical conditioning* and *operant conditioning* are appealing in that they target observable behaviors and their effectiveness can be empirically tested quite easily in the clinical setting. Progress, or lack thereof, can be readily determined and the behavior program can be modified accordingly. Thus, behavioral interventions are incorporated into inpatient, residential, school, community, and outpatient settings. Perhaps, their applicability and success are best evidenced by the increasing number of such therapies in treating serious psychiatric disorders among youths. The next decade will likely witness an increasing array of behavioral interventions focused on other types of problems, such as internalizing disorders.

BIBLIOGRAPHY

Barkley RA. *Taking charge of ADHD: the complete, authoritative guide for parents*, 2nd ed. New York: Guilford Press, 2000.

Barkley RA, Benton CM. *Your defiant child: 8 steps to better behavior*. New York: Guilford Press, 1998.

Cooper JO, Heron TE, Heward WL. *Applied behavior analysis*. New York: Macmillan, 1987.

Ferster CB, Culbertson SA. *Behavior principles*, 3rd ed. Englewood Cliffs, NJ: Prentice Hall, 1982.

Heflin AH, Deblinger E. Treatment of an adolescent survivor of child sexual abuse. In: Reinecke MA, Dattilio FM, Freeman A, eds. *Cognitive therapy with children and adolescents*. New York: Guilford Press, 1996:199–226.

March JS, Mulle K. *OCD in children and adolescents: a cognitive-behavioral treatment manual*. New York: Guilford Press, 1998.

Pavlov IP. *Conditioned reflexes: an investigation of the physiological activity of the cerebral cortex*. London: Oxford University Press, 1927.

Skinner BF. *The behavior of organisms: an experimental analysis*. New York: Appleton-Century Co, 1938.

SUGGESTED READINGS

Barkley R. *Taking charge of ADHD: the complete authoritative guide for parents*. New York: Guilford Press, 2000.
(*Packed with information and advice for parents either trying to determine if their child is ADHD or struggling to manage a child who is ADHD.*)

Barkley R, Benton C. *Your defiant child: eight steps to better behavior*, New York, NY: Guilford Press, 1998.
(*A parent-friendly step-by-step manual for improving a child's behavior that can be read in an afternoon.*)

Cooper J, Heron T, Heward W. *Applied behavior analysis*, New York, NY: Prentice Hall College Division, 1987.
(*Classic textbook that provides a comprehensive introduction to the principles, research methods, applications and techniques of applied behavior analysis.*)

Kazdin A. *Behavior modification in applied settings*, Belmont, CA: Wadsworth Publishing, 2000.
(*Introduces underlying principles of behavior modification as well as real-world applications in a variety of settings, using case studies, charts, and tables.*)

Zirpoli T, Melloy K. *Behavior management: applications for teachers and parents*: Prentice Hall College Division, New York: Macmillan, 1993.
(*A comprehensive volume for teachers and parents that contains many examples of behavioral plans for specific behaviors.*)

CHAPTER 24

Psychotherapeutic Interventions

KEITH CHENG

Introduction

According to the American Academy of Child and Adolescent Psychiatry, "*Psychotherapy* refers to a variety of techniques and methods used to help children and adolescents who are experiencing difficulties with emotion and behavior. Although there are different types of psychotherapy, most rely on communication as the basic tool for bringing about change in a youth's thoughts, feelings, and behaviors. Psychotherapy may involve an individual child, group, or family. With children and adolescents, playing, drawing, building, and pretending, as well as talking, are important ways of sharing feelings and resolving problems." In essence then, for this chapter, *psychotherapy* can be defined as "an interaction between a psychotherapist and a child that leads to changes—from a less adaptive state to a more adaptive state—in the youth's thoughts, feelings, and behaviors." This definition is limited to psychosocial interventions such as learning, persuasion, social support, discussion, and communication directly or indirectly through play. Excluded from the definition of psychotherapy are any interventions that use pharmacologic, biologic, or medical means of bringing about change.

Overview

Psychotherapeutic interventions are indicated for the majority of psychiatric disorders diagnosed in youths. A wide range of chief complaints brings children and adolescents into psychotherapy, and there are numerous types of psychotherapies for these situations. Many of these therapies have an evolving evidence base. For example, *short-term crisis intervention* sessions are used for teenagers who become situationally depressed and suicidal after breaking up with a girlfriend or boyfriend. *Desensitization* techniques help fearful youths, for example, youths with fear of needles develop skills to cooperate with medical procedures while those with specific phobias become tolerant of the feared object. *Cognitive-behavioral therapies* (CBTs) have been developed for several specific clinical problems. The best developed and utilized are CBT for adolescent depression that can be delivered in either an individual or group setting and CBT for obsessive–compulsive disorder (OCD) that focuses on decreasing compulsive behaviors by increasing tolerance for the anxiety that drives these compulsions. A variant of CBT, called *dialectical behavior therapy* (DBT), is used for youths with character pathology suggestive of borderline personality disorder and involving self-harm behaviors. Another variant is *exposure and response prevention* (E/RP) for phobic symptoms. For more common disorders, such as adolescent depression, there is more than one evidence-based treatment. For example *interpersonal psychotherapy* and *psychoeducational* approaches in group or individual settings are effective alternative treatments for depressed youths not amenable to CBT. Long-term *supportive* and *psychodynamic* therapies are often necessary in treating children who are victims of abuse or who are showing early signs of character pathology. *Behavioral therapies* such as *behavior modification* help autistic and other youths in residential settings. *Family therapy* is frequently needed to address dysfunctional dynamics that are exacerbated by a youth with a newly diagnosed psychiatric illness or for families with "high expressed emotion" that can worsen the course of a major mental illness, such as schizophrenia or depression. Finally, *parental guidance and counseling* is a therapist-driven intervention developed to guide parents in managing the difficult behaviors of their difficult or mentally ill children.

Many psychotherapeutic interventions for children and adolescents are derived from adult treatments. CBT was first created for adults by Aaron Beck and now has been adapted for use with children and adolescents. Marsha Linehan's DBT for adults with borderline personality disorder is now used with adolescents. There are, however, several aspects of psychotherapy with children that are distinctly different from therapy with adults. The developmental perspective forms the cornerstone of psychiatric assessment and intervention with children and adolescents, taking into account the cognitive, social, academic, emotional, and physical domains that change as they mature. Consequently, psychotherapeutic techniques change over the life span to address children's and adolescents' mastery or deficits at each developmental stage.

Another difference in child and adolescent therapy is the importance of working with parents. Parents, or the primary parental figures, need to be educated about their child's problems and share a vision with the therapist regarding the goals of treatment and the therapeutic interventions. Parents are often at a loss regarding how to provide for their children's special needs. The effectiveness of *parenting skills training* in treating externalizing problems is well established.

Historic Antecedents

The roots of child psychotherapy are often traced to Sigmund Freud. Though he never directly treated a child, the case of "Little Hans" showed Freud that children could be treated for psychiatric symptoms using nonmedical interventions. Little Hans was able to overcome his fear of horses after being indirectly treated by Freud. Through conversations between Hans' father and Freud, an understanding of Hans' psychological problem was developed. With this dynamic formulation, Freud was able to advise Little Hans' father on how to intervene. After a 4-month "psychoanalysis," Hans was freed from his horse phobia. In 1921, Hermine von Hug Hellmuth authored the first record of children treated directly with psychoanalytic theory. She used toys with children 7 years and younger to elicit their inner conflicts. Anna Freud and Melanie Klein went on to refine the practice of childhood psychoanalysis. Their continued use of play as a core technique to help children express their psychological problems helped solidify the term "*play therapy.*" Much of their theories persist, although their developmental focus has yielded to ecologic models of childhood psychopathology. As therapists became dissatisfied with the outcomes of individual psychotherapy, psychoanalysts explored family interventions and found them to be effective in cases where individual therapy had failed. Family therapies use concepts from ecologic models, such as the nonlinear or cyclic nature of family interactions, to treat behavioral disturbances.

In the 1950s, mental health professionals began using *behavioral therapies* to treat the emotional and behavioral problems of youths. These behavioral interventions, based on the theories of Thorndike, Watson, and Bandura, emphasized the use of operant and classical conditioning to ameliorate infant and childhood behavioral problems. Their seminal work persists as the basis of behavior interventions taught in *parent skills training* curricula.

During the 1970s clinicians such as Aaron Beck laid the foundation for cognitive therapies. Based on the premise that thinking style and expectations drive behavior, *cognitive therapy*, or *CBT*, attempts to change how individuals think about themselves and their world. Most CBTs for children and adolescents were introduced in the 1980s. The work of Kendall for anxiety disorders, Clarke and Lewinsohn for depressive disorders, Kazdin for conduct disorder, and Webster-Stratton for early onset conduct disorders are examples of how cognitive-behavioral theory can be successfully applied to the treatment of various pediatric psychopathologies.

Over the past 10 to 20 years, more complex "multimodal" and "eclectic" therapies have evolved. Rather than using just one type of therapy, these treatments choose different psychotherapeutic techniques to address specific components of a youth's treatment plan. For example, the National Institute of Mental Health (NIMH) Multimodal Treatment Study (MTA) of attention deficit hyperactivity disorder (ADHD) has shown that children with comorbid ADHD and other psychiatric disorders fare better when pharmacologic, behavior, education, and parent training interventions are integrated into a systematic approach. *Multisystemic therapy* (MST) goes beyond the traditional individual and family therapy paradigm to include case management and coordination of community services to treat youths with conduct disorders. *DBT* for borderline personality disorder incorporates individual and group psychotherapies, as well as relaxation techniques and assertiveness training, to help individuals to manage their affective dysregulation and interpersonal conflicts. All these treatment interventions are based on cognitive and behavioral approaches, psychoeducation of the parents, skills training, and coordination and collaboration with community agencies, that is, multimodal, multidisciplinary, and multiagency interventions, as well as innovative thinking.

Research on the efficacy of psychotherapy for children began in the 1960s. One of the first reviews concluded that these treatments did not seem more effective than "tincture of time." These findings have spurred research on the efficacy of child and adolescent therapies, and the establishment of "evidence-based practice" (EBP). Some states, such as Oregon, now legislatively mandate that Medicaid-funded residential treatment facilities and clinics base their treatment on EBPs. Increasing emphasis on EBP represents an important advance in psychotherapeutic treatment of pediatric psychopathology.

Categories of Psychotherapies

Psychotherapies have been traditionally categorized in two main ways: (a) who participates in treatment or (b) theoretic construct.

PARTICIPANT-BASED APPROACHES

Therapies based on participation refer to individual, group, and family therapies. Modeled after adult psychotherapeutic interventions, individual therapy usually denotes a child meeting with a therapist on an individual basis without the presence of a parent, although additional psychotherapeutic sessions with the parent may be needed. This form of therapy assumes that a child or adolescent alone with his therapist will be able to self-disclose without the assistance of a parent and without fear of retribution by a parental figure. Because younger children cannot adequately conceptualize and verbalize their problems, play is employed to access the inner life of a child. The child enacts, or acts out, his conflicts. Through interpretation of the enactment, the child gains insight or psychological understanding. Mastery over emotional disturbance ensues, allowing the child to develop more adaptive behaviors. The term *play therapy* describes this form of psychotherapy, but the goal is not to simply engage the child in play and games. *Play therapy* is hard work. It is a process by which children learn to express, understand, regulate, and alter their life experiences. Lewis emphasizes that there is no indication for individual psychotherapy with younger children without concomitant parental interventions, such as *parental guidance and counseling, parent skills training,* or *family therapy*. Sometimes parental interventions may be limited to simple support to ensure that parents continue to involve their child in treatment. The type of parental involvement is individualized to the child's treatment needs. In adolescence, the role for parental intervention and involvement is more variable. The available research base has supported the involvement of parents in some therapies, such as *interpersonal therapy for adolescents*, but not for others, such as *cognitive-behavior therapy,* which is conducted in a group setting. Therefore, parents' participation in adolescents' treatment varies.

During the past 10 years, several hundred publications have presented an evidence base for *group psychotherapy*. Participants in *group psychotherapy* may be similar or diverse diagnostically but usually are of the same developmental stage. *Group psychotherapy* has become an integral part of inpatient and outpatient treatment planning. A meta-analysis by Hoag and Burlingame in 1997 examined 56 outcome studies on the effects of group treatment for children and adolescents. The results showed that *group psychotherapy* was more effective than placebo controls or being placed on a wait-list. *Group psychotherapies* for children and adolescents are frequently constructed around specific problems. For example, *group therapy* is a mainstay of treatment for substance use disorders and often incorporated into treatment for depression, anxiety, bereavement, poor social skills, and impulse dyscontrol. In most problem-oriented groups, group membership consists of youths in the same developmental phase so that they share similar challenges and so that core techniques are applicable to the entire group. However, in some group treatments, groups of families are formed, and, in this case, ages of youths may vary. *Group therapy* is increasingly difficult to find for privately insured individuals due to poor financial reimbursement. Ironically, in some public agencies, group treatments are used to reduce individual treatments that are considered more costly.

Family psychotherapy refers to interventions that are aimed at changing maladaptive or harmful interactions among family members so as to improve the functioning of individuals as well as the family as a whole. *Parental skills training* and *psychoeducation* should not be considered a form of *family therapy* because they do not focus on family relationships. *Family therapy* is especially indicated for families whose parents have already received skills training but are unsuccessful because of their individual resistance or family dysfunction. Family interventions have an evidence base for treating pediatric depression, anxiety, substance abuse, ADHD, and even psychosis. Contemporary approaches to child treatment stress the integration of *family therapy* into the comprehensive treatment plan. For example, *family therapy* is an integral intervention in multimodal treatment of ADHD and anxiety disorders. *Family psychotherapies* may include many different constellations of family members. In its most traditional format, *family therapy* includes members of the nuclear family. The constellation of family members included in treatment may change as therapy progresses. *Family therapy* may start with parental sessions that may include one or both parents. *Family sibling therapy* may include two or more siblings together in session. *Intergenerational therapy* may include family members from several generations of a family. Psychotherapy research and community-based interventions place a premium on family psychotherapies. Family interventions are empirically supported for successfully treating children with conduct disorders or substance use disorders. Chapter 25 discusses the specific types of family interventions.

THEORY-BASED APPROACHES

Psychotherapies are frequently categorized according to a theoretic perspective. The Surgeon General's Report of 1999 states that the major types of psychotherapeutic interventions for children are *psychodynamic psychotherapy, supportive psychotherapy, cognitive-behavioral psychotherapy, interpersonal psychotherapy,* and *family systemic interventions*. With the exception of the last, these therapies originally were developed for adults and then adapted for children. Detailed descriptions of *family therapies* and *behavioral interventions* are discussed in chapters 25 and 23 respectively.

Psychodynamic psychotherapies, also termed *insight-oriented psychotherapies*, rely on theories of intrapsychic development and functioning. There are several such theories with different foci. The most traditional and older therapies posit that children show maladaptive behaviors because of overwhelming or unresolved intrapsychic conflicts. These conflicts can be caused by multiple sources ranging from mother–child relationship problems to frank environmental trauma. For example, a 6-year-old boy who witnessed his mother robbed at gunpoint on a bus may develop transient hysteric blindness anytime he sees a bus. A young boy may become anxious about his anger at his mother for not gratifying his wishes because his anger conflicts with his need for her love. *Psychodynamic therapy* for older children or adolescents requires a level of psychological development that allows conscious awareness of conflict and the ability to tolerate anxiety-provoking interpretations that connect feelings and behaviors during therapy. This higher level of psychological development is also needed in order for the youth to maintain a helpful relationship with his therapist during difficult times of the treatment process and to not act out in a self-destructive or socially harmful manner. For example, a teenaged girl whose parents have had a contentious divorce may enter treatment because she feels uncomfortable in dating and has started cutting herself. After connecting her psychological discomfort with her guilty distortions that she caused her parents' divorce, such a youth may be able to better tolerate a romantic relationship. In psychodynamic approaches with younger children, often referred to as *play therapy*, conscious insight into troubled feelings may not be gained. However, unconscious conflicts may be resolved in the metaphor of the play themes acted out in treatment sessions. Mastery over a psychic insult (a perception of danger to the ego) may be gained through the expression of internal experiences during play and appropriate interpretations. This mastery over a threatened ego and confusing emotions may then generalize to a youth's outer world, evidenced by movement from a regressed position of self-protection to an adaptive position of meeting developmental challenges.

Supportive psychotherapy originated in psychoanalytic theory. However, in contrast to psychoanalytic therapies, *supportive psychotherapy* focuses on supporting the individual's psychological strengths and defenses, not uncovering unconscious conflicts or exploring the meaning of maladaptive behaviors, which is anxiety provoking for the patient. The focus is on containing the individual's anxiety. For example, in *supportive therapy*, a therapist may help a child to better understand his or her parents' divorce and maintain positive relationships using statements such as "Your parents say you did not cause their divorce; it is nobody's fault" and then helping the child to develop coping strategies. A depressed teen might be gently confronted about her overreaction to breaking up with a boyfriend with supportive statements such as "It is difficult now, but you have shown the ability to cope with a previous breakup; this does not have to affect your other relationships and school work." A child therapist will encourage a child to use verbal skills in dealing with a school bully and help him or her to develop strategies for that situation based on the child's demonstrated abilities in other areas, for example, "You are good at using words, so let's think about some statements you can use in these situations." *Supportive therapy* emphasizes the identification of strengths and the appropriate use of these abilities to resolve difficult situations. The therapist may also provide limited advice, such as when to involve adults when being bullied. In addition, *supportive psychotherapy* utilizes direct environmental interventions. The therapist may suggest to children and parents specific ways of changing their physical environment to meet the challenges of perceived problems. In the bullying example, a therapist might suggest that the child avoid being alone while walking home after school, having the parent pick up the child directly from school, speaking to the principal, confronting the parents of the bully, or even enrolling the child in martial arts training.

Cognitive therapies are based on social learning theory and also integrate several psychotherapeutic techniques based on operant and classical conditioning. According to Aaron Beck, cognitive therapy describes five major interrelated elements that contribute to psychological difficulties: interpersonal-environmental context, an individual's unique physiology, emotional functioning, behavior, and cognition. These elements form the complex system that is addressed by *cognitive therapy*. Depressed children and adolescents, similar to depressed adults, display Beck's proposed "triad," that is negative attitudes (or distortions) regarding themselves, their environment, and the future. "Catastrophizing" and perceiving situations only in "black and white" are other maladaptive attributional styles used by depressed youths. Cognitive therapists consider a youth's particular circumstances and intervene at both cognitive and behavioral levels to influence thinking, acting, feeling, and somatic reaction patterns. According to McClure and Friedberg, the framework for *cognitive therapy* sessions includes the following six components: (a) mood or symptom check-in, (b) homework review, (c) agenda setting, (d) addressing session content, (e) homework assignments, and (f) eliciting feedback. Successfully integrating each of these elements in a cognitive therapy session facilitates effective and efficient interventions. Through cognitive treatments, a child learns the relationships between his cognitions (thoughts or thinking style), feelings (emotions), and behaviors. Ultimately, changing underlying cognitions can reduce depressed or anxious emotions and maladaptive or inappropriate behaviors. Thus, the structured cognitive therapies do not rely on exploration of underlying conflicts, intrapsychic origins of the depressed or anxious feelings, or the youth's self-expression through verbal or play interaction.

Behavior therapies are now widely accepted in the mainstream practice of various psychotherapies. They have an evidence base in treating various psychiatric disorders from the self-harming behaviors that occur in autism to the avoidant behaviors characteristic of anxiety. *Behavioral therapies*, most notably implemented as *behavior modification*, are based on the behavioral concepts of classical conditioning and operant conditioning. *Classical conditioning* is the type of learning made famous by Pavlov's experiments with dogs. An example of *behavior modification* using classical conditioning is the use of the bell and pad for training an enuretic child. The major theorists in the development of *operant conditioning* are Edward Thorndike, John Watson, and Burrhus F. Skinner. Positive reinforcement or the use of "rewards" is an example of *operant conditioning* used to shape behaviors. A *token economy* is a system in which a child is positively reinforced, or "receives tokens," for demonstrating specific adaptive behaviors. Teaching parents about such behavioral interventions is a major part of *parenting skills training*. Because *behavioral therapies* have a strong evidence base for treating children, they should be part of a clinician's approach to caring for children with disturbed behavior.

Developmental Considerations

One of the challenges to working with children is that their cognitive, social, and emotional development is constantly changing. A child's developmental level plays a major role in determining the effectiveness of a treatment intervention and should guide a clinician in choosing an intervention.

Developmental sensitivity has led to the use of play in treating younger children who do not have the ability to conceptualize their problems verbally. In order to understand children's fantasy worlds, therapists develop a dialogue through the use of drawings, storytelling, and playacting. For example, children may not be able to tolerate the conscious awareness and discussion of their violent homes. They may be able to displace their distress onto a set of family figures or puppets to enact their terror and reveal aspects of their family life. These figures become representations of their own lives without the threat of real physical danger or threat to their egos. Younger or more immature youths are less able to tolerate the emotions that arise during therapy. Extra time is often needed in the first stage of the psychotherapeutic process for younger children to become comfortable with the play therapy paradigm. Feeling safe in therapy makes it easier for young children to tolerate and express intense feelings.

According to Piaget's Theory of Cognitive Development, during the first year of life, when the *sensorimotor* stage of cognitive development occurs, infants try to coordinate their five senses and muscles (motor function) to master their environment. Cognitive function is focused on sensing environmental stimuli and responding in motor activity. Clearly, infants in this stage of development cannot make use of insight-oriented or cognitive interventions as they lack skills in conceptualization, metaphoric thinking, language, or even the motor control to use puppets or dolls. However, behavioral interventions can be useful for reshaping problem behaviors in infancy. For example, behavioral methods are commonly used to treat dysregulated sleep or feeding patterns.

As a child's brain develops, the capacity for symbolic thinking and language at around 12 months becomes evident. Toddlers rapidly develop vocabularies to symbolize objects in their environment during the *preoperational* stage of cognitive development. However, their cognitive abilities, conceptualization of their affective states, and vocabulary are not developed enough to use cognitive psychotherapies. They lack the ability to organize and categorize their thoughts and feelings despite their increasingly rich vocabularies.

Preschoolers still cannot use these words to adequately represent their feelings or to "self-talk" in order to delay gratification. Thus, behavioral therapies are still the interventions of choice during this stage of development as they rely on an adult to implement strategies that help the toddler gain mastery.

According to Piaget, the stage of *concrete operations* typically starts when children enter school. Piaget notes that during this stage of cognitive development children develop the ability to identify, organize, and categorize their experiences and thoughts. Furthermore, they are able to make simple connections between cause and effect, as evidenced in their ability to tell when they have done something wrong, to show embarrassment, or to show shame. CBTs are usually considered effective for children beginning at age 6 or 7. By first or second grade, most children have a rudimentary awareness of their emotions and the capacity to follow directions. Hence, with guidance from their therapists, school-aged children are able to utilize cognitive interventions, and they become capable of creating some of their own solutions.

By adolescence, most children enter the stage of *formal operations*, the last stage of Piaget's theory of cognitive development. During formal operations, adolescents develop the ability to conceptualize issues from different points of view, in contrast to the typical "egocentric" perspective of school-aged children. Youths with "formal operational" thinking are more aware of the origins of specific feelings, are able to assess their thinking processes, are able to reflect on the decisions they make, and are able evaluate the outcomes. The relationship between cognitive development and the psychotherapeutic process is summarized in Table 24.1.

Most psychodynamic or *insight-oriented psychotherapies* require capacity for abstract thinking, optimally at a level of *formal operations*. Cognitive therapies require *concrete operations* at a minimum. Children in the preoperational level of cognitive development cannot

TABLE 24.1. COGNITIVE DEVELOPMENT AND THERAPEUTIC INTERVENTIONS

Piaget Stage of Development	Level of Cognitive Functioning	Effective Psychotherapeutic Interventions
Sensorimotor operations	• Connecting sensations from five senses • Yoking them with motor function • Developing motor responses to things that are seen, heard, felt, tasted, and smelled	Behavioral
Preoperational	• Developing symbols for objects • Developing language • Naming objects and feelings • Very egocentric	Behavioral
Concrete operations	• Categorizing objects and feelings • Figuring out cause and effect, how things are connected to each other; still considerably egocentric	Behavioral Cognitive
Formal operations	• Abstract thinking • Thinking about one's thinking, being able to reflect about the quality of one's ideas and thoughts • Understanding the origins of feelings • Development of psychological self-awareness • Understanding mixed emotional states	Behavioral Cognitive Insight-oriented

use cognitive interventions. Thus, treatment focuses on behavioral and parental approaches to preoperational children. The ages associated with Piaget's cognitive developmental stages can be somewhat fluid depending on individual development and life events. For example, an 8- or 9-year-old child with a life-threatening cancer may be able to develop an abstract adultlike understanding. So, while *insight-oriented psychotherapy* would seem more optimal for an older child in this situation, it may be as effective as cognitive approaches for a latency-aged child facing external events that catapult him into early maturity.

Often, *group psychotherapies* appear more effective than individual interventions for older children. From a social development perspective, as a child enters adolescence, his or her peer group becomes increasingly influential. *Group psychotherapies* for adolescents make use of this developmental factor by promoting change through the adolescent's identification with the therapeutic group. However, the change can be negative too. Groups for preadolescent and early adolescent youths with conduct disorders and substance use disorders may result in identification with deviant peers and thus more maladaptive behaviors in middle school-aged children. Early adolescents experimenting with various identities are more likely to adopt the mores of same aged peers and older adolescents who may model drug-using lifestyles.

The Psychotherapeutic Process

While there are many forms of psychotherapy, all of them follow a basic psychotherapeutic process, which has been well described in a 1982 publication by the Group for the Advancement of Psychiatry Committee on Child Psychiatry. The committee outlines a five-stage process, as outlined in Table 24.2.

TABLE 24.2. THE STAGES OF THE PSYCHOTHERAPEUTIC PROCESS

Stage of Psychotherapy	Tasks of the Stage
Establishing the working relationship	• Engaging with the child and parents • Identifying any transference or countertransference problems • Developing trust in treatment relationship
Analysis of the problem and its cause	• Examination of the child's life • Assist the patient in developing a problem list • Assist the parents in developing a problem list • Integrate the problem list for next stage
Developing an explanation of the problem	• Describe the possible reasons for the identified problems • Outline the work needed to be done • Define the rules for the working relationship (appointment times, billing, cancellations, etc.) • Agree on a treatment plan
Establishing and implementing the formula for change	• Implement the treatment plan ("prescription for change") • Readjust formula for change as indicated • If there is now progress, review and adjust initial problem list and selected formula for change
Termination	• Review the reasons for entering treatment • Summarize what was helpful and not helpful in solving presenting problems • Consolidate therapeutic gains with praise • Address any loss issues • Review any needed follow-up • Review indications for return to treatment

From Group for the Advancement of Psychiatry (GAP) Committee on Child Psychiatry. *The Process of Child Therapy.* New York: Brunner/Mazel, 1982, with permission.

Establishing the working relationship, or engagement period, is the first stage of any psychotherapy. Gaining a patient's trust and drawing him or her into a therapeutic relationship are the primary goals of this stage of treatment. This process begins while taking an initial history. The therapist must understand the patient's conceptualization of how the therapy will unfold and develop a sense of how the patient experiences the therapeutic relationship. Engagement in treatment may not happen if the patient or parents perceive their therapist in a negative manner. The therapist must be aware of the relationship distortions, or "transferences," or other impediments to establish a working relationship. Furthermore, retaining children and families in treatment is perhaps the biggest challenge. Wierzbicki and Pekarik report that 40% to 60% of children who begin treatment drop out before their treatments are finished. Furthermore, premature termination may be more common for the most severely ill youths and families. Suicidal youths are at unexpectedly high risk, perhaps due to the dysfunctional family environment that contributes to both their suicidality and termination of treatment.

During this *engagement period,* the therapist assesses his own attitudes, or "countertransference," elicited by the relationship with the patient. Intense negative feelings may exist. Self-monitoring ensures that these attitudes are understood in the context of the patient's dynamics and treatment needs. If problematic countertransference persists, either consultation with professional peers or a supervising clinician is indicated. In exceptional cases, care may need to be transferred to another caregiver.

Therapists develop therapeutic relationships through the use of empathy, an intrapsychic process in which the therapist recognizes and identifies with the persona and feelings that the patient projects onto the therapist. However, therapists must also maintain appropriate therapeutic distance. Patients and parents will have more positive regard for the treatment process if they believe their therapist understands their problems. Parents are likely to disrupt treatment if they do not perceive a shared view with the therapist regarding their children's problems. Without a strong collaborative relationship with parents, there is a high risk that parents will pull their children out of treatment or that their children will not complete treatment due to unconscious collusion with their parents' dissatisfaction. In some situations, a parent forms a negative view of treatment if his own needs are not being met by his child's therapist. Some parents feel threatened if they perceive that the therapist is taking sides with the child against the parent or that the therapist is supplanting the parent. In cases with prominent parental dysfunction, many neophyte therapists do in fact find themselves aligned with the child against the parent. A vision of the presenting problems and indicated treatments prevents this situation.

In the second stage of the psychotherapeutic process, *problem analysis,* the therapist and child or family identify the problems that will be addressed in therapy. The analysis of the problem may be narrowly focused or broad, depending on the conceptual framework of the therapist. The task of identifying dysfunction usually focuses on distinguishing developmental derailment from normative functioning. This stage of treatment may take several sessions for psychodynamic approaches. In behavioral and cognitive interventions, this stage is commonly addressed in a single session or during the clinical assessment. In psychodynamic approaches, this stage of treatment is nondirective, and problem identification and analysis unfolds according to the child's ability. In cognitive interventions, therapists are directive and more active in focusing on specific problems and helping a patient to identify these problems.

The third stage, *problem explanation,* consists of an explanation of the problems that were presented at the time of referral and what treatments are needed. After an initial assessment, it is common practice for clinicians to meet with parents, with or without the identified child patient, to review the assessment. During this "evaluation feedback," an explanation of the presenting problems and associated developmental dysfunction are discussed, along with specific treatment recommendations. Here again, the time spent in this stage of treatment varies. Agreement on what problems are going to be addressed in treatment, what are the likely causes of these problems, and what interventions should be utilized, needs to occur for treatment to go forward. In manualized treatments, such as the various *cognitive therapies,* this stage is usually allotted no more than one or two sessions, which are part of scheduled topics that are to be covered in the intervention. In psychodynamic or insight-oriented treatments, this may take several sessions. Whatever the intervention, goals for treatment should be agreed upon by the end of this stage.

The fourth stage, *formula implementation,* consists of implementing the formula for change. For example, in *parenting skills training* an outline of interventions is presented and then administered. A child with severe oppositional behaviors may be given a token economy intervention. The details of the plan and its administration need to be reviewed with the child and his parents. Once the plan is set, the child and family implement the plan and the therapist monitors adherence to the plan and addresses challenges as they arise. In cognitive approaches, the therapist presents the cognitive techniques that the child will use. Subsequent sessions follow a schedule of techniques to teach during therapy sessions and homework to complete between sessions. *Psychodynamic therapy* may have more open ended and less concrete sets of instructions or interventions. However, the therapist is still guided by the treatment goals set in the previous stage. The length of the fourth stage of treatment, *formula implementation,* varies. The *Coping Cat* treatment program for anxiety disorders is administered over 16 sessions. *Interpersonal Psychotherapy for Depression in Adolescents* schedules 12 sessions to complete treatment objectives. Russell Barkley's *Parent Training Curriculum for ADHD* is to be completed in 10 sessions. *Psychodynamic psychotherapies* do not generally have a standard length of treatment. Although several time-limited psychodynamic therapies have been developed for adults, there are no time-limited psychodynamic therapies developed for youths. The problem being addressed, the resistance encountered during treatment, and the youth's progress determine the length of psychodynamic interventions.

The fifth stage, or *termination stage,* of treatment signals that the end of the therapeutic process is near. However, there are still several issues to address before treatment ends. A review of problems that brought the child or adolescent into treatment is a critical part of this stage. An understanding of the presenting complaints along with the subsequent treatment and explanation should be reviewed. Therapy gains should be noted, praised, and consolidated. Interventions or techniques that were the most helpful are identified for continued implementation by the youth and his or her family. Worries about termination or feelings of abandonment are explored. Finally, indications for returning for treatment are delineated in case more treatment is needed in the future. Here again, nonpsychodynamic psychotherapies usually allot one to two sessions for termination, while psychodynamic interventions often have an indeterminate number of sessions for this last phase of treatment.

Practical Aspects of Psychotherapeutic Applications

Choosing a psychotherapy for a clinical problem is predicated on the available evidence base for treating specific problems, as well as a therapist's training and experience. For some presenting problems, the choice of interventions is obvious. For example, enuresis is best treated with parent education and behavioral interventions because physiologic problems respond well to operant and classical conditioning. The types of psychotherapies chosen and the timing with which they are applied may unfold in a naturalistic fashion or may be more planned by the treating clinician. In the enuresis case, parental guidance and a simple behavior plan may be the first intervention. Treatment failure, however, may prompt the therapist to work individually with the enuretic child to reduce resistance to using the behavioral plan. Further psychological treatment may require facilitating change in family dynamics through family therapy. Psychological approaches may be augmented with pharmacologic interventions.

Other situations may present in a complex way at the time of assessment. A child with dysfunctional family relationships, social phobia, and major depression, presenting with refusal to attend school, challenges a therapist to implement a sequence of different psychotherapies. Safety considerations usually determine which symptom cluster to address first. If the child in this example is depressed with suicidal ideation and outpatient services are not sufficient to contain the suicide risk, hospitalization will be indicated. Sometimes pharmacologic interventions can make a child more available to psychotherapeutic interventions. For example, treatment with an anxiolytic may allow the child to leave home to receive supportive psychotherapy in concert with parental guidance and counseling. Once the risk of self-harm is minimized, treating depressive symptoms with *interpersonal therapy for adolescents* or *structural family therapy* may reduce the recurrent use of suicidal behavior to escape intolerable psychic distress and/or to manipulate the family relationships. Finally, systematic desensitization may be used to treat the social phobia and school refusal and thus improve social integration. With a reduction in social isolation and psychic distress, the youths will be able to develop coping skills that lead to new relationships and academic success.

Therapists' initial training and subsequent experience usually determine their repertoire of psychotherapeutic interventions. Therapists trained only in the use of individual psychodynamic approaches are not likely to use cognitive and family approaches. This may limit the ability to treat certain types of psychiatric illnesses. Team approaches usually can provide a larger number of effective treatments, particularly for the most disturbed youths. In team approaches, two or more clinicians provide treatment. For example, one therapist might provide individual therapy to the child while another provides family therapy. In particular, adolescents may prefer that their individual therapist not be shared with their parents. Individual practitioners may choose to provide both individual therapy and other therapeutic interventions. However, it is also common for such practitioners to "share" patients with other clinicians for selected interventions. Psychopharmacologic interventions are frequently used concurrently with psychotherapy. Such medical therapies may be provided by a psychiatrist who is also conducting the psychotherapy; or alternatively, medications and psychotherapy may be provided by different clinicians. Two recent studies have shown that youths do better with combined psychotherapeutic and pharmacologic treatments. The MTA study of youths with ADHD comorbid with other disorders supports combined stimulant and behavioral treatment; and NIMH's investigation, the Treatment of Adolescent Depression Study (TADS), supports combined selective serotonin reuptake inhibitor (SSRI) and psychotherapy. This evidence base supporting combined treatment will increasingly lead to more than one clinician involved in a youth's mental health care.

Consent and Confidentiality Caveats

Consent may be defined as the process in which a patient formally agrees to an evaluation or treatment. In most states by legal definition, consent can only be provided by adults as minors lack the cognitive ability to enter such an agreement. Minors can provide *assent. Assent* differs from *consent* in that it is not part of a legally binding contract and does not imply a full and complete understanding of the indications, risks, alternatives, and goals of treatment.

In psychotherapy practice, the consent process for children is more complex than for adults. Rather than obtaining consent from the patient, consent is obtained from a parent. If a parent consents to treatment for the child, but the child does not provide assent, the therapy is set up for possible failure as the child may never engage during the first stage of psychotherapy. This problem does not appear in the adult psychotherapeutic process, unless treatment is court ordered or coerced by significant others, for example, employers. This is usually more problematic for adolescents who are establishing their autonomy. Clinicians can often defuse this problem by including the adolescent in the decision making, especially in determining their parents' involvement. The reverse situation occurs when an adolescent provides his own consent for treatment. Many states have provisions for youths under the age of 18 years to consent for medical and psychiatric treatments. In this situation, some youths do not want their parents to know about their participation in psychotherapy. Usually, therapy with minors works better when there is parental support, and a clinician has to carefully consider the pros and cons of proceeding without parental support. If an adolescent stays engaged in treatment, the clinician can help the youth to allow parental involvement at a later date.

Divorced parents often cannot agree on their child's best interest. Clinicians risk further disrupting a youth's life by providing therapy with the consent of only one parent. The same conflict occurs if a child in state custody is treated against the will of the parents. Without the support of the important adults in the child's life, any therapeutic benefit is jeopardized, in addition to legal risk for the therapist. Clinicians should address the lack of shared consent before providing treatment.

Another complication to the consent process is the clinician's responsibility to provide confidentiality. Confidentiality is usually implied or overtly stated in the psychotherapeutic situation. Breaking confidentiality compromises the therapeutic relationship. For example, in most states, therapists are required to report suspected child abuse. A child who reports, accurately or inaccurately, that a parent is abusive alters the course of therapy. Once the clinician reports the case to Child Protective Services, trust is broken. The child may feel violated. Even if treatment continues, the youth may be less engaged. Another challenge to therapy is a youth's revelation of the use of life-threatening drugs, placing the clinician in an awkward position. In most situations, it would be important for the parents to be aware of such drug use. To avoid these binds, some clinicians inform youths and their parents during the consent process of what will be kept confidential and when confidentiality will need to be broken.

Evidence-based Psychotherapies

EBPs refer to psychosocial treatments for which systematic controlled studies have established efficacy. The Cochrane Collaboration and the American Psychological Association (APA) have developed definitions of EBP. The Cochrane Collaboration requirements for evidence-based treatments include: (a) randomized controlled research, (b) research designs with adequate sample size and defined study populations, and (c) independent replication. The APA Task Force in 1995 expanded these requirements in defining evidence-based effectiveness to take into account feasibility, generalizability, cost, and benefit.

As noted earlier, there are many types of evidence-based psychotherapies including: *CBTs, interpersonal therapy, DBT, parenting skills training,* and *MST.* These are summarized in Table 24.3. Currently, CBTs enjoy the best empiric support, including interventions for children and adolescents. These include CBT for depression, CBT for OCD, and CBT for impulsive children. CBT is also effective for the anxiety disorders including specific phobias, separation anxiety disorders, and generalized anxiety disorder. CBTs have been shown to be superior to nondirective therapy for reducing symptoms in sexually and physically abused youths with posttraumatic stress disorder (PTSD). However, what is *efficacious*

TABLE 24.3. EXAMPLES OF EVIDENCE-BASED PSYCHOTHERAPIES

Psychiatric Problem	Evidence-based Psychotherapies	Developers
Anxiety	Coping cat	Kendall
	Coping koala	Barrett
	Family anxiety management	Dadds
OCD	CBT for OCD	March
Depression	CBT for depression	Asarnow, Stark
	IPT-A	Mufso et al.
	Primary and secondary control enhancement training	Weisz
	Adolescent coping with depression	Clarke
ADHD	DCP	Barkley
	STP	Pelham
Conduct disorder	PSST and PMT for conduct disorder	Kazdin
	MST	Henggeler
	Anger control training with stress inoculation	Feindler
	Anger coping program	Lochman
	Behavior parent training for youth with conduct problems	Patterson
	Incredible years BASIC parent training program	Webster-Stratton
ODD	Parent–child interaction therapy for oppositional children	Hood
	DCP	Barkley
Borderline personality disorder	DBT	Linehan (see Katz in bibliography)
SUD	MST	Henggeler

OCD, obsessive–compulsive disorder; CBT, cognitive-behavioral therapy; IPT-A, interpersonal psychotherapy for depressed adolescents; ADHD, attention deficit hyperactivity disorder; DCP, defiant children program; STP, summer treatment program; PSST, problem-solving skills training; PMT, parent management training; MST, multisystemic therapy; ODD, oppositional defiant disorder; DBT, dialectical behavior therapy; SUD, substance use disorders.

in controlled studies may not be *effective* in clinical practice, and, ideally, EBPs examined in research settings would also be examined in clinical settings. The next decade should bring the development of more EBPs, with more diverse examination of their effectiveness, and the ability to better individualize youths' treatment.

Conclusion

Psychotherapeutic interventions are an integral part of any comprehensive treatment plan for youths with psychiatric disorders. Although EBPs are available to treat several disorders of childhood and adolescence, such therapies are often only available at academic centers. This will likely change over the next decade and therapists in all settings should emphasize EBPs in order to assure their patients of optimal care and increase their accountability in practice. The availability of relevant EBPs and a child's developmental level should guide clinicians in determining the most appropriate interventions for a particular child. Whatever intervention is chosen, a close working relationship with their patients' parents is necessary to ensure successful treatment. Increasingly, treatment will be shared by two or more clinicians. In these cases, close collaboration among clinicians will ensure optimal care for our young patients.

Case Vignettes

Case vignette #1

Darlene is an 11-year-old girl who looks older than her chronologic age with Tanner stage 4 development. She has a longstanding history of mild disruptive behaviors since kindergarten. She has an "individualized education plan" (IEP) for speech and language delays. Despite her learning problems, Darlene appeared to do well socially. Her teacher noted that she was able to conceal her learning problems. Darlene comes from a difficult family situation. Her father is in prison for physically abusing her. For the past year her disruptive behaviors were becoming impossible to manage in her mainstream classroom. This increase in disruptive behaviors corresponded with the increase in her father's physical discipline and violence. A black eye noted at school led to the arrest of her father. She was referred for PTSD treatment with a local psychotherapist. The therapist reasoned that Darlene's behavior problems related to her trauma and conflict with her father. She began intensive insight-oriented therapy with the goal of Darlene connecting her disruptive behavior with her anger toward her father and with reactivation of this trauma when her teacher looked sternly at her. However, after several months of psychotherapy, Darlene's behavior problems increased at school and home. Her therapist sought consultation with a senior clinician.

The consulting clinician noted that the therapist treated Darlene more like a 15-year-old than a latency-aged child. Darlene appeared more mature by dressing like a high-school student and acting as if she understood her therapist's interpretations. The therapist tested this hypothesis and discovered that Darlene did not understand her therapy due to her delayed language skills. A reevaluation of her cognitive and emotional development found Darlene to be functioning at a level lower than the average 5th grader. Darlene found it very difficult to verbalize her feelings and perceptions, particularly the intense emotional states that led to her disruptive behavior. Thus, she was also unable to problem solve or create strategies to deal with these emotional explosions. Her therapist decided to reorient Darlene's treatment by limiting her insight-oriented therapy and collaborating with the school in employing a token economy that rewarded Darlene for small incremental positive behavioral changes. Darlene's behavior improved and she was able to stay in her mainstream classroom while receiving supplemental language services.

Case vignette #2

Jackson is a 15-year-old teen, well known for being the neighborhood troublemaker. Raising him in a single parent home has been overwhelming at times for his harried mother. He was diagnosed with ADHD when he was 7 years old and has been prescribed various stimulant and nonstimulant medications; currently he is prescribed Strattera. His mother laments, "all these medications seem to help him a little bit, but they never get him to stop his really naughty ways." He has stolen from homes on his street. At school, he is a bully and has been suspended from school for threatening another child with a hunting knife. Jackson has been banned from the local stores for shoplifting. More recently, he has started smoking "pot," after he started hanging out with some older "street" kids. Jackson has been to several individual psychotherapists. None has been able to form a therapeutic alliance. Family therapy has also been unsuccessful. His mother cannot set any limits and gives excuses for Jackson's behavior, "if only his father were around he would behave." One therapist warned his mother that Jackson's lack of remorse was worrisome and that she should consider sending him to a residential treatment facility. Now things have worsened. Jackson stole his mother's credit card and with the help of his new street friends ran up a bill of $2,000. Friends, relatives, and even his therapist urged Jackson's mother to press charges. But she was afraid that a police record would ruin his future. "He really is a smart boy. I'm sure he'll grow out of this phase or they'll find a medication that really works." Finally, he and his friends burned down an abandoned building and he was arrested.

This might be considered fortunate as Jackson was assigned a probation officer who recommended that Jackson be placed in MST within the Juvenile Justice System. With an emphasis on providing a coordinated multimodal approach, Jackson's MST therapist was able organize the various agencies already involved in his life. His mother's denial was challenged when a joint meeting was held with Jackson's school principal, therapist, and probation officer. Structural family therapy helped his mother to return to her leadership role in the family and to enforce rules. The MST emphasis on eliminating contact with deviant peers eliminated Jackson's supply of drugs. A year later, Jackson still had problems getting along with classmates at school and lying to his mother, but he had not run away again, stopped using drugs, stayed in school, and, most surprisingly, improved his grades.

Case vignette #3

Julie is a 13-year-old girl who excels in school. She was shocked when her parents announced they were divorcing the month before she was to start high school. Within a week of the divorce announcement, Julie's mother had moved out of the house and was living across town. Julie continued to live with her father. However, Julie's father was distraught and would not talk to anyone. Julie's older sister was already in college and not available to provide her any emotional support. Despite her request for more time with her mother, Julie only received a weekly phone call. Relationships with both her family and friends began to deteriorate. After the first 2 months of school, Julie was failing all her classes and refused to talk to any of her family members. She began to lose weight and was unable to sleep.

A school counselor referred Julie to a psychiatric nurse practitioner after Julie said she did not care if she lived or died. Julie was diagnosed with major depression and an antidepressant was prescribed. Within 2 months her sleeping improved, her appetite increased, and she no longer had thoughts of death. However, she was still disinterested in her schoolwork or socializing with her friends. Despite two increases in her antidepressant dose over 6 months, Julie was still anhedonic and listless. Therefore, Julie's nurse practitioner referred her to a local psychologist for psychotherapy. The psychologist started interpersonal psychotherapy because Julie complained that while she felt less depressed, she did not know what to do with the damaged relationships between herself and her family and her friends. After completing this manualized treatment, Julie was able to socialize more with her friends, but the problems with her parents persisted. Bolstered by her social successes with her peers, Julie gained enough strength to ask her parents to participate in family therapy. They grudgingly agreed to treatment.

BIBLIOGRAPHY

American Academy of Child and Adolescent Psychiatry (2001), What is Psychotherapy for Children and Adolescents? Available at: http://www.aacap.org/publications/factsfam/therapy.htm. Accessed March 6, 2005.

American Psychological Association, Task Force on Promotion and Dissemination of Psychological Procedures. Training in and dissemination of empirically validated psychological treatments. *Clin Psychologist* 1995;48:3–23.

Arnold LE, Chuang S, Davies M, et al. Nine months of multicomponent behavioral treatment for ADHD and effectiveness of MTA fading procedures. *J Abnorm Child Psychol* 2004;32:39–51.

Asarnow JR, Carlson GA. Childhood depression: five-year outcome following combined cognitive behavioral therapy and pharmacotherapy. *Am J Psychother* 1988;42:456–464.

Barkley RA. Psychosocial treatments for attention-deficit hyperactivity disorder in children. *J Clin Psychiatry* 2002;63(Suppl. 12):36–43.

Barrett PM, Duffy AL, Dadds MR, et al. Cognitive-behavioral treatment of anxiety disorders in children: long-term (6-year) follow-up. *J Consult Clin Psychol* 2001;69:135–141.

Beck AT, Rush AJ, Shaw BF, et al. *Cognitive behavioral therapy of depression.* New York: Guilford Press, 1987.

Brent DA, Kolko DJ, Birhamer B, et al. Predictors of treatment efficacy in a clinical trial of three psychosocial treatments for adolescent depression. *J Am Acad Child Adolesc Psych* 1998;42:12.

Clarke GN, Rohde P, Lewinsohn PM, et al. Cognitive behavioral group treatment of adolescent depression: efficacy of acute treatment and booster sessions. *J Am Acad Child Adolesc Psychiatry* 1999;38: 272–279.

The Cochrane Collaboration. Preparing maintaining and promoting the accessibility of systematic reviews of the effects of healthcare interventions. www.cochrane.org, 2002.

Dadds MR, Holland DE, Laurens KR, et al. Early intervention and prevention of anxiety disorders in children: results at 2-year follow-up. *J Consult Clin Psychol* 1999;67:145–150.

Feindler EL, Ecton RB, Kingsley D, et al. Group anger-control training for institutionalized psychiatric male adolescents. *Behav Ther* 1986;17:109–123.

Group for the Advancement of Psychiatry (GAP) Committee on Child Psychiatry. *The process of child therapy.* New York: Brunner/Mazel, 1982.

Henggeler SW, Cunningham PB, Pickrel SG, et al. Multisystemic therapy: an effective violence prevention approach for serious juvenile offenders. *J Adolesc* 1996;19:47–61.

Hoag MJ, Burlingame GM. Evaluating the effectiveness of child and adolescent group treatment: a meta-analytic review. *J Clin Child Psychol* 1997;26:234–246.

Hood KK, Eyberg SM. Outcomes of parent-child interaction therapy: mother's reports of maintenance three to six years after treatment. *J Clin Child Adolesc Psychol* 2003;32:419–429.

Katz LY, Cox BJ, Gunasekara S, et al. Feasibility of dialectical behavior therapy for suicidal adolescent inpatients. *J Am Acad Child Adolesc Psych* 2004; 43:276–282.

Kazdin AE, Stolar MJ, Marciano PL. Risk factors for dropping out of treatment among white and black families. *J Fam Psychol* 1995;9:402–417.

Kazdin AE, Esveldt-Dawson K, French NH, et al. Problem-solving skills training and relationship therapy in the treatment of antisocial child behavior. *J Am Acad Child Adolesc Psych* 1987;26:416–424.

Kendall PC, Howard BL, Epps J. The anxious child. Cognitive-behavioral treatment strategies. *Behav Modif* 1988;12:281–310.

Lewis, M. Intensive individual psychodynamic psychotherapy: the therapeutic relationship and the technique of interpretation. *Child and adolescent psychiatry a comprehensive textbook.* Baltimore, MD: Williams & Wilkins, 1991:796–805.

Linehan MM, Heard HL, Armstrong HE. Naturalistic follow-up of a behavioral treatment for chronically parasuicidal borderline patients. *Arch Gen Psychiatry* 1993;50:971–974.

Lochman JE, Nelson WM, Sims JP. A cognitive-behavioral program for use with aggressive children. *Clin Child Psychol* 1981;10:146–148.

March JS, Franklin M, Nelson A, et al. Cognitive-behavioral psychotherapy for pediatric obsessive-compulsive disorder. *J Clin Child Psychol* 2001; 30:8–18.

McClellan JM, Werry JS. Evidence-based treatments in child and adolescent psychiatry: an inventory. *J Am Acad Child Adolesc Psych* 2003;42:12.

Mufson L, Weissman MM, Moreau D, et al. Efficacy of interpersonal psychotherapy for depressed adolescents. *Arch Gen Psychiatry* 1999;56:573–579.

Nixon RD, Sweeney L, Erickson DB, et al. Parent-child interaction therapy: a comparison of standard and abbreviated treatments for oppositional preschoolers. *J Consult Clin Psychol* 2003;71:251–260.

Patterson GR, Ray RS, Shaw DA. Direct intervention in families of deviant children. *Oregon Res Inst Res Bull* 1968;8:1–11.

Pelham WE, Gnagy EM, Greiner AR, et al. Behavioral versus behavioral and pharmacological treatment in ADHD children attending a summer treatment program. *J Abnorm Child Psychol* 2000;28:507–525.

Piaget, J. *The psychology of the child.* New York: Basic Books, 1972.

US Department of Health and Human Services. *Mental health: a report of the surgeon general.* Washington, DC: US Government Printing Office, 1999.

Webster-Stratton C, Hammond M. Treating children with early-onset conduct problems: a comparison of parent and child training interventions. *J Consult Clin Psychol* 1997;65:93–109.

Weisz JR, Thurber CA, Sweeney L, et al. Brief treatment of mild to moderate child depression using primary and secondary control enhancement training. *J Consult Clin Psychol* 1997;65:703–707.

Wierzbicki M, Pekarik G. A meta-analysis of treatment outcome dropout. *Prof Psychol Res Pract* 1993;24:190–195.

SUGGESTED READINGS

Gabel S, Oster G, Pfeffer C, eds. *Difficult moments in child psychotherapy.* New York: Plenum Publishing, 1988.
(*A highly entertaining and informative collections of case vignettes from well-known senior child psychiatrists.*)

Kazdin A, Weisz J, eds. *Evidence-based psychotherapies for children & adolescents.* New York: Guilford Press, 2003.
(*A good review for clinicians of several evidence-based psychotherapies used in children and adolescents.*)

McClure J, Friedberg R. *Clinical practice of cognitive therapy for children and adolescents: nuts and bolts.* New York: Guilford Press, 2002.

(*For clinicians who want a concise and user friendly summary of cognitive therapy techniques for youths.*)

Mufson L, Moreau D, Weissman M, Dorta K. *Interpersonal psychotherapy for depressed adolescents,* 2nd ed. New York : Guilford Press, 2004.
(*For clinicians who want an example of a manualized evidence based psychotherapy.*)

Weisz J. *Psychotherapy for children & adolescents: evidence-based treatments & case examples.* New York: Cambridge University Press, 2004.
(*For clinicians who want specifics about the implementation of evidence-based psychotherapies.*)

CHAPTER 25

Family Process and Interventions

KEITH CHENG

Introduction

Accurate psychiatric assessment and effective treatment of an individual child must involve an examination of family process. Family process refers to the repetitive patterns of interaction between members. Contemporary pressures upon youths and families, and the ever-broadening definition of what constitutes "family," only serve to underscore the importance of family process. Failure to recognize the importance of family process may prevent the initiation of appropriate treatment interventions and may place a psychiatric clinician in the role of unwitting participant in an unhealthy family system. The challenge to keeping family process in the forefront of assessment and treatment is partly based on the evolution of psychiatric practice. Psychiatrists, pediatricians, nurses, and family practitioners are increasingly thought of as prescribers of medication rather than clinicians who are able to see cases in a multidimensional fashion. This focus often obscures the more salient effects of the family system upon the patient. A classic example of this process is when treatment of a child reinforces a family's belief that only the identified patient is dysfunctional, which may prevent the treating clinician or psychiatrist from hearing about the real locus of symptomatology. For instance, medications may be prescribed for disruptive behaviors or signs of anxiety when the presenting symptoms are secondary to physical or sexual abuse, parental alcoholism, or other family stresses.

The primary goals of this chapter are to provide a broad-based understanding of family process and outline specific family therapy techniques used to ameliorate dysfunctional family structure and process, which contribute to the identified patient's problem behaviors. Specific attention is also given to the problem of the treating clinician becoming an unwitting participant in an unhealthy family system.

THEORETIC UNDERPINNINGS AND HISTORIC BACKGROUND

Prior to the 1940s, the treatment of children was based on psychoanalytic techniques. The prevailing practice was to treat children separately from their parents and families. Dissatisfaction with treating the child individually led to the technique of meeting with the family as a whole. The formal development of family therapy can be traced back to the 1950s. During this time pioneers such as Ackerman, Bowen, Bateson, Haley, Satir, and Lidz began to develop their techniques to ameliorate dysfunctional family dynamics. In the 1960s, charismatic therapists such as Whitaker and Minuchin further enhanced and refined the practice of family therapy. These family therapy theorists agree that the treatment of individual patients always and inevitably involves family process, and this process is often hard to discern and difficult to manage. Furthermore, they focus on clinician involvement in the family process and how to use this involvement as part of the treatment.

Two of the most influential approaches to family interventions stem from systems and structural theories. Much of family systems theory is based on the work of Murray Bowen. This influential family therapist based his conclusions about family process not only on observations of families, but also on his study of universal biologic processes. In both situations there is a continual tug-of-war between being a part of a whole on one hand and an individual entity on the other. This tension naturally but inexorably generates anxiety in individuals and their families. Bowen conceptualizes this anxiety not as a symptom or an example of neurosis, but a natural and systemic phenomenon, which flows from one generation to the next. This anxiety also plays out in a continuum of "self-differentiation," which is defined on the one end by unhealthy togetherness or "fusion," and on the other, unhealthy self-differentiation or a "cutoff" from family, that is, an emotional removal of oneself from the family unit. The center of the continuum is the ideal balance of being appropriately independent and connected. A family member who no longer feels angry or exasperated at a meddling sibling or an overly authoritarian parent and refrains from becoming "caught" in the emotional anxiety triggered by these family members exemplifies an ideal level of self-differentiation. Self-differentiation represents a process of striving to maintain emotional balance despite the opposing forces of togetherness and separateness. Both structural and systems theory stress the importance of healthy boundaries. Clear and flexible boundaries promote healthy family relationships.

Nonverbal communication often "trumps" verbal communication in family units. Gregory Bateson et al. from the Palo Alto group examined this concept in families with schizophrenic children. Mothers of schizophrenic children were observed to give pleasant verbal greetings to their schizophrenic children and at the same time show contradictory stiffening body language and negative nonverbal communications. These observations confirmed the applicability of systems theory in human relationships and directed attention away from the verbal content of a patient's complaints toward interest in nonverbal communications. This systemic perspective is critical in becoming attuned to family process. The systemic perspective widens the range of communications to consider, from what is said or presented to what is being communicated nonverbally.

Perhaps the most fundamental property of a family system is its tendency to maintain a homeostasis or be impervious to change regardless of rational intervention and interpretation. A similar and related phenomenon is that of a closed feedback loop, in which outputted information circles back as input. These concepts are particularly applicable to

family interactions. Families and individual family members often seek to solve their problems and "change." These efforts, however, genuinely intended, essentially constitute
minor adjustments to the system but do not transform it. In order to transform the family,
a therapist must decipher unspoken rules, discover family myths, and understand
metamechanisms, which define and maintain the family system. An example of such a
"rule" is the unspoken but nonetheless powerful delegation of one family member to be
the sick or dysfunctional one. Medical treatment of such an individual therefore serves primarily to maintain the unhealthy system rather than effect symptom amelioration. Structural family therapists make it their goal to change unhealthy homeostasis. They join and
enter family systems to change and disrupt ingrained dysfunctional patterns of interaction.

Principles of Family Process

Principles of family process are based on common patterns of family interactions. While the
following principles are designed to provide a framework for clinicians to identify family
dysfunction, it is important to note that the accompanying patterns of family interaction
represent varying degrees of functioning. All families develop certain patterns of interaction
and they are usually adaptive in nature. The following principles provide a foundation for
understanding the impact of family interactions on the development of pathologic dynamics. These principles are derived mainly from systems and structural family theories.

COMMUNICATIONS INCLUDE NONVERBAL AS WELL AS VERBAL COMPONENTS

One cannot "not" communicate. Communication patterns include nonverbal as well as verbal components. Sometimes, what is not said is more powerful than what is spoken. Body
language communications may convey more information than verbalizations. For example,
a family's failure to talk when members are angry at each other often leads to misunderstandings or disagreements. A family therapist who observes this process may choose to create a family therapy goal of improving communication skills.

FAMILIES TEND TO MAINTAIN A HOMEOSTATIC POSITION

Repetitive patterns of interaction are characteristic of all families. These patterns tend
to become resistant to change even when they are dysfunctional. Typically, a state of
"disequilibrium" occurs when family members exhibit normal developmental changes.
As children get older they place pressure on the family system to adjust relationship
patterns. Because of the tendency to maintain homeostatic patterns, parents may not
allow a rebellious teenager more autonomy than when the child was in grade school.
Parents may say they want to change, but they may not implement therapeutic recommendations. A family therapist might use this example of homeostasis as a demonstration to the family of how patterns of interaction persist despite attempts at change.

SELF-DIFFERENTIATION IS AN INDIVIDUAL'S ABILITY TO FUNCTION IN AN AUTONOMOUS, BALANCED, AND SELF-DIRECTED MANNER WITHOUT BEING CONTROLLED, IMPAIRED, OR FEELING OVERLY RESPONSIBLE FOR OTHER FAMILY MEMBERS

Self-differentiation is manifested by the extent that a family member is able to think,
plan, and decide on his or her own goals and values without being unduly influenced

automatically by emotional cues of others in the family. For example, a teen who decides to take a job working at a gas station without consulting his family on the effect of this decision may find intense levels of conflict at home. The conflict arising out of an adolescent's desire to be more independent may lead family therapy to focus on how the family may allow autonomous decision-making without a breakdown in family relationships.

ENMESHMENT OCCURS WHEN THE EMOTIONAL BOUNDARIES ARE TOO DIFFUSE

Enmeshment refers to intense family interactions in which members are overconcerned and overinvolved in each other's lives. In families with diffuse boundaries, children may act like adults and adults may treat children as equals. In extreme cases, the lack of individual member identities makes separation from the family an act of betrayal. In a family where both parents are doctors, a child who wants to become a lawyer and not take over the family practice may be labeled a traitor. The goal in family therapy would be to clarify boundaries. Clearly defined boundaries between family members help maintain separateness and at the same time emphasize belongingness to the overall family system.

OVERLY RIGID BOUNDARIES LEADS TO DISENGAGEMENT

Disengaged families have members who are likely to function autonomously but with little sense of family loyalty. In this situation, family members, when in need, lack the capacity to ask for support from each other. Communication in these families is often strained and guarded. A child who is being bullied at school may avoid asking his parents or siblings for help. He or she would rather get suspended from school for fighting than get rejected by family members when asking for help. In this situation, family therapy would focus on changing the inflexible or rigid boundaries that lead to alienation between members.

THE CHILD AS THE IDENTIFIED PROBLEM MAY BE SERVING A COMPLEMENTARY FUNCTION

Identified patients may have symptoms and act out not necessarily because they are "sick," but because their condition and behaviors reinforce the family's pathologic homeostasis. This may occur in a family that delegates a child as a scapegoat to cover up tension in the marriage. A family therapist can use this pattern of interaction to make overt to the family how promulgation of one maladaptive pattern is secondary to another pathologic dynamic.

FUSION RESULTS IN FAMILY MEMBERS WHO ARE POORLY DIFFERENTIATED

The greatest amount of fusion tends to occur between the lowest functioning members of a family. The thoughts and feelings of these members tend to be automatic or involuntary in nature. These members tend to become dysfunctional when experiencing minimal amounts of anxiety. Bowen notes that intensely fused individuals with few independent views of their own are likely to be become "stuck" in the position they occupied in their family of origin. For example, the son of a highly anxious mother becomes extremely quarrelsome with his father every time his mother worries that her husband is having an affair. In this case, family therapy may focus on the worries of the mother and not include the child in any part of the treatment.

EMOTIONAL CUTOFFS DEVELOP IN RESPONSE TO HIGH LEVELS OF FUSION

Emotionally cutting oneself off from one's family of origin may frequently represent a desperate attempt to deal with either unresolved or overwhelming fusion between a child and one or both parents. These cutoffs may range from emotionally distancing ("I don't care what you say") to physical distancing (moving to another country). Emotional cutoffs tend to occur in families where there is a high level of rigidity, anxiety, and emotional immaturity. For example, despite their desire to go to college, adolescents may run away from home and drop out of school to live with friends on the street to escape from parents who cannot tolerate the fact that their children are not getting straight "A"s.

FAMILY DYSFUNCTION MAY BE TRANSMITTED OVER SEVERAL GENERATIONS THROUGH THE MULTIGENERATIONAL TRANSMISSION PROCESS

To the degree there is fusion or a cutoff in one or more relationships in a single generation, there is a correlative likelihood that these processes will take place in another generation. For example an overinvolved parent may find his or her child becoming an emotionally distant parent when he or she starts a family. Intergenerational family therapy techniques, such as genogram analysis, use identification of these patterns to help families avoid extremes in relationship boundaries.

TRIANGULAR RELATIONSHIPS ARE USED TO REDUCE TENSION OR ANXIETY

When two family members are under stress or upset with each other, they may attempt to reduce the tension in their two-party relationship by engaging a third person. This results in a relationship triangle. These triangular relationship patterns represent subsets of the family system, which may either work in concert with or against other such triangles. The most common examples are a parent and a child versus another parent or child, or parents versus children. Extramarital affairs and issues regarding in-laws represent other examples of relationship triangles. Identifying and avoiding "triangulation" and its maladaptive consequences are common goals for family therapy sessions with triangulation problems.

FAMILIES WILL TRY AND INCLUDE TREATING CLINICIANS IN THEIR FAMILY "DANCE"

From a family systems point of view, a physician simply cannot not become a part of the family process. In analyzing this phenomenon, it is important for clinicians to be aware of their own family history, transferences, and projections. For example, a physician who is working with a family with a coercive parent may be pressured into prescribing antidepressants or attention deficit hyperactivity disorder (ADHD) medications for a troublesome child. In this situation it is likely that coercive parenting is contributing to disruptive behavior seen in the identified child patient. The physician in this situation, using his or her feeling of being coerced to prescribe, may generate a goal for helping parents feel empowered to have influence over their child's symptoms without use of coercion. Rather than coercing individuals outside of the family to address their child's problems, the parents can be coached to use other methods of responding to their child's disruptive behaviors.

Family Assessment

The assessment of family process varies according to a family therapist's theoretic preferences. Psychoeducational, cognitive-behavioral, and solution-focused therapists use a prepared approach to assessing families. In these types of therapy approaches, the role of the therapist is to function as a teacher. Assessment is guided by formal standardized outlines or schemas. Structural, strategic, and systemic therapists rely on an unstructured approach to family assessment. During an assessment, these types of therapists purposely avoid structuring the interview and concentrate on observing the family for maladaptive patterns of interaction. These patterns of interaction then guide therapists in their choice of intervention. During the assessment, structural and systemic therapists will carefully observe for the patterns of interaction that have been described previously (in the Principles of Family Process section), including dysfunctional communication patterns, distorted relationship boundaries, entrenched homeostatic interaction patterns, family member triangulation, and the inability to manage stressful emotions. Genograms and family rating scales are also used in the assessment process.

The construction of the family tree or genogram is a common technique for assessing family function. Family therapists typically use this technique, but there is no inherent reason to proscribe its utilization by other clinicians or in non–family therapy settings. A genogram, as presented by McGoldrick, is a practical and useful framework for understanding family patterns, and through a series of squares, circles, lines, and symbols, maps out how family members are biologically and legally related one to another from one generation to the next. The symbols reflect such items as marriages, adoptions, deaths, divorces, sibling position, and informal kinship relationships. Genograms may also include other information such as histories of physical and mental illnesses, suicides and attempted suicides, psychiatric hospitalizations, school difficulties, or other relevant historic events. The history of family dislocation, drug or alcohol problems, physical or sexual abuse, and legal problems related to the family or mental illness in previous generations, should if present, be included in construction of the family genogram. The occurrence of the aforementioned family events in more than one generation provides data indicating the presence of systemic multigenerational processes mediated by family scripts, legacies, and myths.

A variety of ratings scales are available to help the clinicians assess family functioning. These scales measure parameters such as overall family functioning and problem solving abilities, intrafamily communications, behavioral control, affective processes, and family cohesion and adaptability. Examples of family rating scales include the Family Environment Scale (FES), the Family Adaptability Cohesion Evaluation Scale (FACES III), and the Family Assessment Device (FAD). The FES by Moos and Moos measures family cohesion, expressiveness, conflict, independence, and achievement. This scale is also widely used as a research instrument. The third edition of the FACES by Olson et al. is a self-report instrument that describes family processes such as negotiation, family roles, boundaries, coalitions, decision making, assertiveness, and discipline. The FAD described by Miller is based on a problem-centered model of family therapy and examines the structure of families regarding problem-solving abilities, communication, roles, and general functioning.

Family Therapy Techniques

It is beyond the scope of this chapter to provide an in-depth examination of the practice of family therapy, but in order to provide some background, Table 25.1 outlines a number of commonly used family therapy approaches.

TABLE 25.1. COMPARISON OF FAMILY THERAPIES

Family Therapy Perspective	Basic Tenets of Perspective	Role of Therapist	An Example
Structural	1. Often invisible and idiosyncratic "rules" based on power and affiliations organize into family boundaries. 2. If boundaries are too rigid, family members are disengaged, lack intimacy. 3. If boundaries are too diffuse, family members experience lack of autonomy and are enmeshed.	Active—Action precedes insight. The therapist is like a movie producer, attempting to discern and reframe the structure or hierarchy within the family, such as who speaks and who remains silent, or sibling versus parental groups in order to encourage flexibility.	The therapist notices the parents sit on opposite sides of the room and the mother is between the two kids. The therapist will use this grouping in making an initial assessment about the family hierarchy and may, for example, have the parents sit together.
Strategic	1. Communications are the focus, including both verbal and nonverbal. 2. Family has already tried "first-order" solutions which did not threaten the family homeostasis. 3. Induce "second-order" change by focusing on process.	Active—The therapist develops a strategy, which may include a symbolic act such as prescribing the symptom, or a task or ritual which focuses attention on nonverbal communication. It is not important to determine "why" a family operates as it does.	Parents and their adolescent daughter/son are struggling with issues of autonomy and closeness by engaging in frequent verbal exchanges. The therapist may "prescribe" that they make plans to have a fight or schedule at least one fight a day.
Systemic	1. Although to an outsider family behavior may seem maladaptive, it should be viewed as positive to the extent it preserves the cohesion of the family group. 2. There are alliances and subgroups within families. 3. There are similarities between the systemic and strategic models.	Neutral but not uninvolved—Through "circular" questioning similar to feedback, the therapist seeks to uncover family history. Other techniques include strategic methods such as symptom prescription.	Two families have come together as a result of divorce and remarriage but each comes with its own family culture. Other interests and alliances within the family come to light through therapy, such as the children versus the parents or the younger siblings versus the older.
Cognitive behavioral	1. Emphasis upon empiric scrutiny. 2. Identification of problem behaviors through functional analysis. 3. Utilization of operant reinforcement techniques.	Active—Therapy includes education, communications skills, and problem-solving training.	It is determined that the single-parent father is often overwhelmed by two children. The therapist will determine what he does well and encourage it and/or set up a family contract regarding expectations, duties, and rewards.

(Continued)

463

TABLE 25.1. (CONTINUED)

Family Therapy Perspective	Basic Tenets of Perspective	Role of Therapist	An Example
Solution focused	1. Each family has strengths which should be encouraged in order to assist them through "stuck" spots. 2. Forget the problem and target the solution. 3. The process of acknowledging and encouraging family competence generates longer term solutions.	Active but as cocreator of solutions – The focus here is to ask questions which assist families in identifying and expanding the use of strengths that all families have. After all, therapy is inherently time limited and the therapist cannot be with the family all the time.	A child has a number of emotional and neuro-cognitive deficits, but the mother is found to be very effective in advocating for this child to receive needed treatment. The father realizes he can restructure his work schedule to be with his child and help his wife pursue her personal goals.
Psychoeducational	1. Family members need to understand the nature of an illness or problem they are facing in order to cope with it. 2. If possible, use of many mental health and other specialties is helpful. 3. Need to establish boundaries between identified patient and family.	Active—Therapist(s) need to allow family to process meaning of an illness, provide information from mental health/medical professionals about the illness, and help with coping skills.	A son has schizophrenia. A multifamily group is formed. The various family members share the down-to-earth, often emotional meaning of schizophrenia. A day-long workshop from mental health/medical professionals educates about schizophrenia. The group continues, with professional support, including job training, etc.
Symbolic experiential	1. Intergenerational processes are important, and different generations have different tasks and roles. 2. All families have problems but unhealthy families view them disproportionately. 3. This approach is not viewed from a structural standpoint so much as an emotional one.	Cotherapy preferred. Active but not directive role, much as a coach. The therapists look for codependencies, family legacies, and attempt to increase the family's sense of cohesion and support in order to allow family members to complete developmental tasks. Focus is on emotional "sweatbox" of therapy.	A wife had a rejecting and/or absent father, so when her husband is late from work she feels he does not care. This emotional history and the resulting meaning of the husband's behaviors to the wife must be explored.

Family therapy models rely on specific techniques. These techniques may be as simple as listening carefully and giving advice to troubled families or as complicated as using paradoxical statements to catalyze change in families entrenched in pathologic patterns of interaction. Psychoeducational interventions rely on traditional relationship models between therapists and patients, in which an authority figure gives information and advice to troubled families. Structural therapists use the techniques of unbalancing, enactment, and reframing to bring about changes in family hierarchies and homeostatic mechanisms. Family systems therapists make use of Bowen's "cerebral" coaching approach in helping family members develop healthy boundaries—"self-differentiation." Therapists frequently find that the therapeutic use of the double bind in the strategic interventions, such as prescribing the symptom and relabeling, is more effective in emotionally primitive families. Solution-focused therapy emphasizes the use of possibility acknowledgement, being open-minded and keeping alive the prospect for change despite past failures to resolve conflicts. Behavior and functional analysis along with contingency contracts are mainstays of cognitive-behavioral interventions.

The aforementioned techniques represent commonly used interventions by family therapists. The following descriptions should give clinicians an idea of how family therapy techniques catalyze change in dysfunctional families, leading to healthier family process.

Psychoeducational family therapy interventions are indicated when mental illness affects a family system. Psychoeducational approaches are aimed at educating families in how to effectively cope with mental or physical disabilities and the dysfunctional family interactions, which frequently result from the stress imposed by the illness of a family member. In addition to providing general information about mental illness, specific coping plans are furnished to families including problem-solving skills training, crisis management, and parenting skills training. For example, families with a newly diagnosed child with schizophrenia benefit from psychoeducation focused on lowering "expressed emotion" in the home. Multiple studies have shown that lowering expressed emotion is linked to reduced relapse rates for schizophrenia.

Unbalancing is a technique used to change the customary positions or roles taken by family members. In a family where a father's role is minimized by an enmeshed relationship between mother and an adolescent daughter, a therapist may "unbalance" the usual patterns of interaction by focusing more session time on the father, emphasizing his points of view, and finding similar viewpoints between father and daughter. In this way, the unhealthy closeness between mother and daughter can be weakened and the daughter can be allowed to have more autonomy.

Reframing is a very useful technique for helping families see themselves in a more adaptive fashion. It is typical for dysfunctional families to blame a specific child for the troubles in the family rather than look at the family as a whole and see how each member may be contributing to the problem. The basic idea is to provide an alternate way of understanding the causes of troubled family interactions. By changing the family perspective, a change in family behaviors becomes possible, leading to new options and alternatives for all members.

In families who minimize the presence of dysfunction, the technique of enactment can allow the therapist not only to observe family conflict but also help modify the dysfunctional patterns of interaction. A therapist using this technique actively identifies or creates a scenario during the session in which family members manifest maladaptive interactions. For example, a therapist may ask an indulgent mother to not give a begging and whiny son a breath mint. As the boy begins to have a screaming, yelling, breath-holding tantrum, the mother shows signs of giving in. The therapist encourages the mother not to give in. When discovering that her son eventually stops his tantrum, the mother realizes she has some control over her ill-tempered child, which results in the cessation of daily tantrums at home.

One of Bowen's favorite images for systemic family therapists is the *coaching* metaphor. In contrast to structural family therapists who are to become part of the family process, Bowen prefers that the therapist serve as a cerebral teacher or coach. The therapist serves as an expert consultant who provides calm assistance in the form of low-key questioning and objective points of view. For example, coaching parents to avoid highly charged interchanges with their children and to focus on identifying and avoiding triangular relationship patterns results in an eventual change from overly emotional outbursts to calmer and more thoughtful interactions with healthier boundaries between family members.

Strategic family therapy models emphasize the use of the therapeutic double bind. This term describes a variety of paradoxical techniques used to change entrenched family patterns. The therapeutic double bind is intended to force families into "no lose" situations. Prescribing the symptom is a specific form of the therapeutic bind. An example of prescribing the symptom for a mother and adolescent daughter who fight all the time about unsupervised teen socializing would be to instruct them to fight 3 times a day, after every meal. In the past, former therapists had advised the mother to stop being "overly controlling" and allow her daughter more freedom. This resulted in more intense fights as the mother struggled to keep her daughter from growing up. The directive prescribing fights 3 times a day places this mother–daughter dyad in a win–win situation. They now have permission to fight all the time or they will stop fighting. Since the fighting no longer serves the purpose of keeping mother and daughter together, they will now find new ways of interacting.

Another form of the therapeutic double bind is relabeling. The relabeling process consists of changing the label attached to a person or problem from negative to positive. In the above example, the overprotective mother would be labeled as trying to be "helpful." This label removes a pejorative connotation and replaces it with a positive spin. This places pressure on the family to change the structure of their relationships, which is the goal of therapeutic double-bind techniques.

The cornerstone of cognitive-behavioral techniques is the use of behavioral or functional analysis. Since cognitive-behavioral interventions are based on specific cognitive distortions or negative behaviors, an evaluation is required to identify these symptoms. A behavioral analysis seeks to pinpoint specific behaviors to be corrected; a functional analysis focuses on understanding the connections between behavioral deficits and the interpersonal relationships of the family members involved. For example, this could include a focus upon the family's structure of rewards or incentives and punishments. It may be that a family focuses only upon punishments and does not focus sufficient time on rewarding positive behavior, or one parent punishes behavior that the other parent rewards or at least tolerates.

Contingency contracts are based on operant conditioning theory. Usually used to decrease parent–child conflict, these contracts are formal in nature. These agreements are typically in written form and spell out specific rewards or consequences for specific behaviors. Chronic bickering between parents and teens can be ameliorated with contingency contracts. Nagging and threats from parents are replaced with rules spelled out on paper. Without these negative parental behaviors, a teen has no authority to oppose.

THE PHYSICIAN AS PART OF THE SYSTEMIC FAMILY PROCESS

As stated earlier, from a family systems point of view, a physician simply cannot "not" become a part of the family process. Another way of looking at this statement is through the analysis of transference and countertransference reactions. Transference refers to the psychological phenomenon in which patients experience and treat their caregivers as if the clinician were another person. For example, a patient might experience a physician as a good parent or relative or be perceived as a critical parent. Positive transference often presents as a useful, healthy, and mutually rewarding doctor–patient relationship, but negative transference can undermine treatment. Negative transference can stimulate countertransference in the treating clinician. Countertransference may be defined as a psychological phenomenon in which the clinician experiences the patient in a distorted fashion that usually prevents the provision of optimal care. From a systemic perspective, countertransference reactions to challenging transference phenomenon may become fodder for circular feedback loops and unsuccessful outcomes.

Determining when a clinician has been inducted into a family system is not an easy task. Evidence that this is taking place may be as simple as experiencing a sense of discomfort with the family or a hesitance to pursue certain lines of inquiry. Clinicians themselves may also need to recognize their tendency to want a "quick fix" for the presenting problem. A clinician who hears a frantic request to "do something, anything" when the circumstances do not necessarily warrant such urgency may be wise to consider other options. Another example that indicates induction into the family "dance" is when the treating clinician finds no matter what is done, the problem never seems to be taken care of, or new symptoms repeatedly surface. On the other end of the spectrum, there is the patient or parents who consistently minimize symptoms. Unexplained medical symptoms and psychosomatic complaints also raise suspicions to the presence of underlying family system dysfunction. There are an infinite number of situations that may result in the induction of the treating clinician into the family process. The clinician's own intuition, professional experience, and ability to keenly attend not only to a patient's words but nonverbal communications are key in identifying these situations. Ultimately, consultation with colleagues may be needed to recognize the extent of unhealthy involvement in family process. All clinicians need to have colleagues they can consult when difficult cases arise.

Multiple Health Care Providers Also Constitute a System

Clinicians should be aware that issues arising from health care organizations apply not only with an individual clinician dealing with a family unit, but can arise with multiple health care providers and insurance providers. In such cases, conflicting opinions regarding health care choices may be given to different family members. Family members, as well as health care providers and managed care staff, may support one opinion or treatment option against another, to "split" what might otherwise be a viable health care alliance. Dysfunction within the health care system, therefore, may arise from within the treatment team or reflect the family system inducing a particular transactional pattern among the treatment team. In both circumstances, the underlying process needs to be addressed before effective treatment can develop.

Indications for Family Evaluation and Intervention

Common indications for family evaluation and intervention are the presence or identification of serious medical conditions or psychiatric disorders (see Table 25.2), the passing of important life-cycle transitions and events, and failure of non–family therapy oriented psychological or medical treatments. Families in these situations are more vulnerable to environmental stresses, and youths with medical or psychiatric disorders are more likely to aggravate existing family pathology. Any family-oriented approach to these issues require the treating clinician to recognize that it is virtually impossible to separate an identified patient's complaints and symptoms from a larger systemic and family context. With this recognition, the clinician is ready to develop an effective treatment plan.

TABLE 25.2. CHILD OR ADOLESCENT MEDICAL CONDITIONS THAT SHOULD TRIGGER A FAMILY FOCUS

- Severe mental illness such as bipolar illness, psychotic disorders, or schizophrenia
- Alcohol and drug abuse
- Chronic illness, such as diabetes or cystic fibrosis
- Disabling or disfiguring illnesses, such as paralysis or burns
- Rapidly deteriorating or frightening illnesses such as cancer or HIV
- Domestic violence

HIV, human immunodeficiency virus.

PRESENCE OF MEDICAL OR PSYCHIATRIC CONDITIONS

Serious medical conditions such as asthma and diabetes are known for associated maladaptive family dynamics. These medical conditions unquestionably have an effect upon family functioning and even in the context of a time-pressed medical practice should automatically trigger a focus on family dynamics. From a family process standpoint, medical conditions do not simply generate symptoms but exist within a larger family context. Within this context, these conditions can evoke special meaning for the patient and the family. For example, a divorced and remarried mother may resent the increased caretaking role she is thrust into by having to care for step or adopted children from her new husband's first marriage. Another example would be a parent too ashamed to seek assistance from other family members because of a perception that he or she is at fault for a child's disability. Two studies, one by Miller and the other by Yuen, have shown that a cohesive family unit correlates with better mental and physical health outcomes for children with human immunodeficiency virus (HIV) or cystic fibrosis. Parents need to be given an opportunity to deal with their feelings of guilt, shame, remorse, and anger, which can complicate relationships with the identified patient as well as between spouses and partners, and other members of the family. Two studies, one by Wilson and another by Aldridge, have described children who have been prematurely thrust into a caretaking role and therefore require extra practical and emotional support on both individual and family levels.

In treating families that have a member with a medical condition or psychiatric disorder, two key concepts have emerged: the need for boundaries clarification between and among the identified patient and other family members, and the importance of family wide psychoeducation. The needs of an identified patient can place considerable strain upon a family from many standpoints, including increased time pressures and financial and emotional stresses. Such illnesses also occur within extended family processes and include adolescents attempting to leave home and decisions of how to care for aging parents. The needs of the identified patient need to be honored, but at the same time the medical condition should not take over the family unit and its members. From the systemic approach, it is critical to recognize that medical conditions often carry with them important nonverbal meanings. Sometimes nonverbal communication takes on mythologic proportions for families and subsequent generations. A patient who refuses treatment because his or her parent died after going to the hospital or who perceives illness as a sinful condition exemplifies this situation. In such circumstances, treatment will be thwarted for the patient as well as the family until the underlying family story or myth is addressed.

Another clinical need for patients with medical or psychiatric conditions is the necessity to provide education not only to the patient, spouse, or partner, but, when indicated, to the nuclear and extended family. Such education might, for example, include information about the disease, its process, and its effect on family life. Once educated about a member's medical or psychiatric condition, it is necessary for the family to discuss the meaning and ramifications for the family and its individual members. Family therapy may be needed to facilitate this process. An example of these considerations can be found in a McFarlane's model for families with schizophrenic patients, which includes multiple family group therapy, medical management, and a psychoeducational intervention. Use of this model has resulted in reducing patient's relapse rates and increasing job retention.

LIFE CYCLE EVENTS AND TRANSITIONS

Important life cycle transitions and events frequently trigger the need for family assessment. These events are summarized in Table 25.3. Families and their respective members must respond to a variety of life cycle events. These include starting and graduating from school, bar mitzvahs, and first communions. How families and family members navigate through these transitions are subject to cultural differences and familial resources. While one family may avoid transition complications, another may experience substantial difficulties. For example, entry into kindergarten, junior, and senior high school are transition points that commonly aggravate family dysfunction. School refusal or truancy are common problems that arise in these transitions. Family dysfunction is frequently part of school transition difficulties. Family assessment and treatment in these cases may warrant inclusion of extended family. For example, it may be that having the child remain at home serves the needs of the extended family members, or school attendance may result in parenting conflicts between family members providing after-school supervision and working parents. Instead of being considered a welcome resource, the presence of extended family members in the home may be experienced as a burden or an extension of an unhealthy family process.

Another common example of a critical life cycle transition is when a child's or adolescent's parents are in the midst of a separation, divorce, or living in separate residences. In these situations, simple communications regarding basic child care, medication dosages, discipline, or medical conditions can become enormously complicated. In this example, indications for family treatment include the inability of parents to coparent or agree on the nature of their child's special needs.

WHEN PATIENT-FOCUSED MEDICAL TREATMENT HAS FAILED

When a number of medical or psychiatric treatment options have been tried with marginal success or failure, consideration should be given to family assessment and intervention. These failures often highlight the resistance of the system to "perturbation" or change. The following case example demonstrates this point.

TABLE 25.3. EXAMPLES OF LIFE CYCLE EVENTS AND TRANSITIONS

- Birth or miscarriage
- Diagnosis of a chronic or severe illness
- Move from one home or geographic location to another
- Death or significant loss
- Starting or graduating from elementary/middle/high school or college
- Job loss or career change
- Moving into a senior or residential center or being the child of a parent who is moving
- Retirement
- Certain milestone birthdays such as becoming 16, 21, or 50
- Onset of menses, puberty/adolescence
- Menopause and midlife "crises"
- Divorce, separation, or end of long-term relationship
- Celebratory events such as first birthday, first communion, or bar mitzvah

Norman, a 44-year-old manager, and Cathy, a 43-year-old high school teacher, have two children, Sam, who is 11 years old, and Amy, who is 9 years old. Sam missed a lot of school because of anxiety, rage attacks, and tics, and he is aggressive at home. The parents have been very supportive of Sam, although Cathy has been the primary parent dealing with Sam's treatment. The parents attended a parenting skills class and attempted to put these skills into practice. However, the disruption at home did not get better. Sam continued to be impulsive and easily distracted. Stimulants helped somewhat but problems with concentration and school fears continued, and when at home Sam had frequent "meltdowns." A brief hospitalization resulted in the addition of a mood stabilizer. Intelligence testing revealed a full-scale intelligence quotient (IQ) in the average range; the subtests were consistent and failed to reflect a clearly defined learning deficit. After discharge from the hospital, the patient's behavior initially seemed to improve, but his disruptive symptoms returned. A referral for neuropsychological testing revealed problems with planning, organizing, and sequencing information, accounting for why Sam tended to get "stuck," particularly when a language component was involved. In addition, testing showed a tendency for rigid thinking and to become illogical when under stress. An occupational therapy evaluation confirmed this data.

A treatment plan was developed which focused upon different medication trials, occupational therapy, and behavioral management. Arrangements were made to have professionals come into the family home to provide more parenting skills coaching and obtain more information about family interactions. Once again, there was minimal progress and eventually the patient was admitted into therapeutic foster care where his behavior stabilized.

In this case there were clear indications for a variety of medical and behavioral interventions, but the patient failed to improve. As this process unfolded, it became increasingly clear that these interventions served to focus attention on Sam and not on the family process. Family therapy was indicated and an initial family history was taken along with the completion of a genogram. The history identified the presence of numerous health problems, depression, and obsessive–compulsive traits in the mother, and possible obsessive–compulsive disorder (OCD) in the maternal grandmother. The father realized that he, too, had problems with anxiety and inattention. As a result of this insight, Sam's father had a better understanding of what his son was experiencing. Preparation of a genogram highlighted family discord in previous generations, which helped clarify the family diagnostic picture and continued to influence family functioning. Salient family issues identified included school failures and anxiety on both sides of the family, a series of divorces and deaths in the father's family, and affairs, divorces, and the death of a child on the maternal side of the family.

As family therapy began, it became clear that the couple's relationship had become very distant and their only tangible interactions centered on caring for Sam. Therapy proceeded to focus on the marital unit. As the therapy progressed, it was discovered that as Norman became more competent, Cathy evidenced more anxiety and obsessive-compulsive symptoms. Cathy realized that she had used her relationship with her mother to "gang up" on Norman. This prevented healthy interactions from developing between Norman, herself, and her mother. Medications were prescribed for Cathy's anxiety and OCD symptoms. As mother and father began to work on their relationship as a husband and wife, they began to communicate about past and present issues. They realized that most of their conversations focused upon Sam, which was not helpful for them as individuals, as a couple, or for Sam. As the couple's communications improved, Sam was better able to state what was wrong with him. It was also discovered that Sam was frequently sleeping in the parents' bedroom because of fears of the dark, which had repercussions for martial intimacy. Another factor which surfaced was that Norman's father, who was close to the entire family, was ill and this situation was taking its toll on the family. While it was a difficult transition for everyone, the entire family worked on obtaining for the grandfather an apartment closer to the family. This was a great success for all, including the grandfather who could now come to visit and be a significant support for Sam. As these issues were addressed, Sam made home visits and his behaviors significantly improved. He was able to leave his foster home and return to the home of his parents.

This case illustrates the interplay between medical and family interventions. When care was focused primarily on medical interventions, treatment was unsuccessful. Once the salient family processes were identified, effective treatment planning was possible. Family therapy was indicated in this situation and proved to be instrumental in treating Sam and his family's dysfunctional dynamics.

Effectiveness of Family Therapy

Sprenkel found that family and marriage therapies produce clinically significant results in 40% to 50% of those treated and therefore are clearly more effective than no treatment. It is unclear whether one treatment approach or technique is more effective than another. Sandberg et al. state that numerous studies show behavioral family therapy to be highly efficacious and, in particular, effective in reducing depressive symptoms, marital distress, and family substance abuse. A review by Charles in 2001 of eight empirical research articles published in the last decade provided support for Bowen's concepts, including self-differentiation, triangulation, and fusion. A meta-analysis presented by Shadish and Baldwin in 2002 found that the desire to identify empirically supported treatments (ESTs) or evidence-based practices (EBPs) had resulted in an emphasis upon the compilation of protocols and therapeutic techniques through manuals. One group referred to such ESTs as "EMPSTs," or "effective, manualized, population-specific treatments." Miller et al. have concluded that while important, technique is outweighed by such factors as the relationship quality between patient and therapist and processes which occur outside the therapeutic hour. These processes include the pretreatment decision to seek treatment, improvement between sessions, and extratherapeutic efforts to seek support for positive change. These conclusions, however, serve more to highlight areas that contemporary family therapists need to attend to and encourage rather than disproving the efficacy of family therapy and family process. Clearly, family therapists use a variety of techniques in meeting the needs of their patients. Indeed, as recognized by Sandberg et al. in 1997, 68% of therapists perceive themselves as having an eclectic practice.

Family Therapy Referral

Before a family is referred to a family therapist, particularly when dealing with disruptive behaviors and lack of parenting skills, a behaviorally based assessment and interventions are usually indicated. A broad behavior based assessment as suggested by Faloon should examine the following: (a) a functional analysis of the problem behaviors; (b) identification of what responses directly or indirectly reinforce the problem, which include both negative and positive attention, support, and/or sympathy; (c) when the problem is reduced in intensity; and (d) how family members cope, including identification of the family's assets and deficits. Armed with this information, a skills trainer or primary care clinician can provide brief coaching in basic communications skills, problem solving, and use of time-outs, reward systems, and behavioral contracts. If these interventions fail, referral to a family therapist may be in order.

A most useful tool for locating an experienced family therapist is the American Association for Marriage and Family Therapy. Its website is http://www.aamft.org. As described in this website, marriage and family therapists have graduate training in marriage and family therapy and at least 2 years of clinical experience. There is also a division of the American Psychological Association regarding family psychology. Many psychiatrists, and particularly child and adolescent psychiatrists, provide family therapy for their patients. It may, in fact, be important to make the referral to a psychiatrist when medical management is also needed. Such a referral may be the most efficient choice since it avoids the complications attendant with interprofessional communications and/or the "splitting" of the treatment processes. The psychiatrist should also be able to determine whether an additional referral is needed.

Conclusion

Psychiatric treatment of children and adolescents requires an understanding of family process. Behaviorally disturbed children have an impact on family systems and aggravate existing family pathology. Failure to recognize the importance of family process may place a psychiatric or primary care clinician in the role of unwitting participant in an unhealthy family system. Prescribing clinicians, in particular, are at risk for becoming part of a dysfunctional family system. There are many family techniques available for clinicians to use. Whatever intervention is utilized, the goal is the same, catalyzing families to a more adaptive homeostasis.

Case Vignette

Case vignette #1: Intergenerational transmission of anxiety and family roles

Presenting complaint: The 6-year-old daughter is oppositional.

Description of family: The father is an only child and the product of a divorce when he was 5. He was primarily raised by his emotionally unavailable father and stepmother. He is now intensely attentive to the point of being overprotective. The mother is the youngest of 3 children and runs a business in the home.

Analysis/recommendations: The father experienced a "cutoff" during his parents divorce and is overcompensating by becoming "fused" with his children. This fusion engenders anxiety throughout the family system. It is to be noted that the divorce occurred when the father was 5 and the daughter is now 6.

Family process concepts: The intergenerational transmission of anxiety and family roles are central to this case. Cutoff and fusion processes represent maladaptive efforts by the father to deal with anxiety and the effort to self-differentiate.

Intervention: The father is assigned the task to reconnect or at least make contact with his emotionally absent father and perhaps discover the "story" behind the divorce. This may result in a less anxious and more normalized view of the "cutoff" by the father and result in less emotional anxiety within the family. Attention should be given to the mother/wife's situation and uncovering any similar issues within her family.

Case vignette #2: Fusions and cutoffs

Presenting complaint: The 19-year-old son is depressed and wants to move across the country to attend college. He is the oldest of four children.

Description of family: The father is very busy with his profession and is an alcoholic. The mother in this family is a homemaker whose job is to take care of the children. The mother's uncle committed suicide when she was 21 years old; this uncle and the father were good friends. A few months after the suicide, the mother's mother was hospitalized, and the couple married 6 months later.

Analysis/recommendations: The 19-year-old son who wishes to leave home has been serving in a caretaking role for his mother and his siblings; this fusion of mother and son reflects emotional anxiety within the family. It is suspected that the son's desire to move away from home may result in a cutoff.

Family process concepts: Parent–child fusions frequently result in cutoff reactions. In this family, the past suicide by the mother's uncle, the impending move of the son, and the hospitalization of the maternal grandmother can all be experienced as emotional cutoffs. Persons tend to marry and/or have relationships with persons who have the same level of self-differentiation. In this family, both parents reflect competence as well as emotional difficulties.

Intervention: It is unlikely that the parents have sufficiently dealt with the death of the mother's uncle and the subsequent hospitalization of the grandmother. It would be important to examine both family histories to determine whether other "stories" might have evoked similar emotional distress and how the families dealt with the events.

Case vignette #3: Systemic homeostasis

Presenting complaint: A 10-year-old child is anxious and depressed and frequently comes in for treatment of respiratory and gastrointestinal complaints. He is on antidepressant medications. The parents are wondering whether they should engage in family therapy or examine additional medication interventions.

Description of family: This blended family has been formed through the marriage of two previously divorced parents. The mother/stepmother has two children, including the identified patient, and the father/stepfather has two children. Both parents attempt to spend "quality" time with the entire family. The mother is the primary disciplinarian. The father is not permissive but is more casual regarding expectations.

Analysis/recommendations: There are two separate family systems or cultures in this situation. Even though both parents could benefit from each other's example, they cling to their own view of how to parent. These parents recognize that they have a problem with poor parental teamwork. They focus primarily upon the anxious child's physical complaints, which is one of the few areas of parental agreement.

Family process concepts: This family thinks they are trying to solve "the" problem and sincerely seek treatment, but the "solution," more medical interventions, essentially feeds into the dysfunctional homeostatic system. This family tends to recognize only those experiences and values that are congruent with the family's view of the anxious child.

Intervention: A focus upon the family, as opposed to the anxious child, may result in positive change. This focus may include discussion of the differences and similarities between the families, including, for example, styles of emotional connection and when and how the children are disciplined. Another way to catalyze the formation of a new equilibrium is to focus upon and strengthen commonalities within subunits of the families, such as the teenagers or the younger children.

Case vignette #4: Enmeshment

Presenting complaint: An adolescent son with diabetes does not adequately monitor his blood sugar. He has had a behavioral problem since birth, but his grades recently have become worse than usual.

Description of family: This family is composed of two parents, who are in their 50s and have been married for over 30 years, the identified patient, and an adult daughter. The adult daughter is in an excellent college and doing quite well.

Analysis/recommendations: Both mother and father have genuine concerns about their son's casual attitude about diet and blood testing, but the mother "nags" and the father chooses not to worry about the situation. The family picture held by all the members is that the son is the "bad" kid and the daughter is all "good." His mother feels it is her fault that her son has diabetes. Diabetes runs in her family.

Family process concepts: There is a clear enmeshment between the diabetic son and his mother. Medical symptoms need to be treated, but unless family process is addressed, such treatment essentially represents feedback and reinforces the system. It may therefore be dangerously ineffective.

Interventions: Encouraging the mother to back out of dealing with her son's diabetic issues and have the father take over may move the family into a healthier homeostatic state. A focus upon the son's positive attributes as an individual and a family member may also help.

BIBLIOGRAPHY

Ahn H, Wampold B. Where oh where are the specific ingredients? *J Couns Psychol* 2001;48:251–257.

Aldridge J, Becker S. Children as careers: the impact of parental illness and disability on children's caring roles. *J Fam Ther* 1999;21:303–320.

Bateson G, Jackson DD, Haley J, et al. Toward a theory of schizophrenia. *Behav Sci* 1956;1:251–264.

Borkan J, Reis S, Medalie J. Narratives in family medicine: tales of transformation, points of breakthrough for family physicians. *Fam Syst Health* 2001;19:121–134.

Broderick CB, Schrader SS. The history of professional marriage and family therapy. *Handbook of family therapy*, Vol. II. Bristol, PA: Brunner Mazel, 1991:3–40.

Brown RT, Lambert R. Family functioning and children's adjustment in the presence of a chronic illness: Concordance between children with sickle cell disease and caretakers. *Fam Syst Health* 1999;17:165–179.

Carr A. Evidence-based practice in family therapy and the systemic consultation I: child focused therapies. *J Fam Ther* 2000a;22:29–60.

Carr A. Evidence-based practice in family therapy and the systemic consultation II: adult focused therapies. *J Fam Ther* 2000b;22:273–295.

Charles R. Is there any empirical support for Bowen's concepts of differentiation of self, triangulation, and fusion? *Am J Fam Ther* 2001;29:279–292.

Drumm M, Carr A, Fitzgerald M. The Beavers, McMaster and circumplex clinical rating scales: a study of their sensitivity, specificity and discriminant validity. *J Fam Ther* 2000;22: 225–228.

Faloon IRH. Behavioral family therapy. *Handbook of family therapy*, Vol. II. Bristol, PA: Brunner/Mazel, 1991:65–97.

Feldman MD, Christensen JF. *Behavioral medicine in primary care: a practical guide*, 1st ed. Stamford, CT: Appleton & Lange, 1997.

Friedman EH. Bowen theory and therapy. *Handbook of Family Therapy*, Vol. II. Bristol, PA: Brunner/Mazel, 1991:134–170.

Garrity CB, Baris MD. *Caught in the middle: protecting the children of high-conflict divorce*. San Francisco, CA: Jossey-Bass, 1994.

Guerin PJ, Fogarty TF, Fay LF, et al. *Working with relationship triangles: the one-two-three of psychotherapy*. New York: Guilford Press, 1996.

Guttman H. Systems theory, cybernetics, and epistemology. *Handbook of Family Therapy*, Vol. II. Bristol, PA: Brunner/Mazel, 1991:41–64.

Johnson P, Waldo M. Integrating Minuchin's boundary continuum and Bowen's differentiation scale: a curvilinear representation. *Contemp Fam Ther* 1998;20:403–413.

Kaslow FW. Continued evolution of family therapy: the last twenty years. *Contemp Fam Ther* 2000; 22:357–386.

Kerr ME, Bowen M. *Family evaluation: an approach based on bowen theory*. New York: Norton, 1988.

McFarlane WR. Multiple family groups and psychoeducation in treatment of schizophrenia. *Arch Gen Psychiatry* 1995;52:679–687.

McGoldrick M, ed. *Re-visioning family therapy: race, culture, and gender in clinical practice*. New York: Guilford Press, 1998.

McGoldrick M, Gerson R, Shellenberger S. *Genograms: assessment and intervention*. New York: W.W. Norton, 1999.

Miller SD, Duncan BL, Hubble MA. *Escape from Babel: toward a unifying language for psychotherapy practice*. New York: W.W. Norton, 1997.

Miller I, Kabacoff R, Epstein N. Development of a clinical rating scale for the McMaster model of family functioning. *Fam Process* 1994;33:53–69.

Miller R, Murray R. The impact of HIV illness on parents and children, with particular reference to African families. *J Fam Ther* 1999;21: 284–302.

Miller RB, Johnson LN, Sandberg JG. An addendum to the 1997 outcome research chart. *Am J Fam Ther* 2000;28:347–354.

Monk G, Winslade J, Crocket K, , eds. *Narrative therapy in practice: the archaeology of hope*. San Francisco, CA: Jossey-Bass, 1997.

Moos R, Moos B. *Family environment scale manual*. Palo Alto, CA: Consulting Psychologists Press, 1980.

Napier AY, Whitaker CA. *The family crucible*. New York: Harper & Row, 1978.

The National Advisory Mental Health Council Workgroup on Child and Adolescent Mental Health Intervention Development and Deployment. *Blueprint for change: research on child and adolescent mental health*. Washington, DC: The National Institutes of Mental Health, 2001.

Olson DH, McCubbin HI, Barnes H. *FACES III: family adaptibility and cohesion evaluation scales*. St. Paul, MN: University of Minnesota, Family Social Science, 1982.

Roberto LG. Symbolic-experiential family therapy. In: Gurman AS, Kniskern DP, eds. *Handbook of family therapy*, Vol. II. Bristol, PA: Brunner/Mazel, 1991:444–476.

Sandberg JG, Johnson LN, Dermer SB. Demonstrated efficacy of models of marriage and family therapy: an update of Gurman, Kniskern, and Pinsof's chart. *Am J Fam Ther* 1997;25:121–137.

Shadish WR, Baldwin SA. Meta-analysis of MFT Interventions. In: Sprenkle DH, ed. *Effectiveness research in marriage and family therapy*. Alexandria, VA: American Association for Marriage and Family Therapy, 2002:339–370. pp

Sprenkle DH, ed. *Effectiveness research in marriage and family therapy*. Alexandria, VA: American Association for Marriage and Family Therapy, 2002.

Titelman P. *Clinical applications of Bowen family systems theory*. New York: Haworth Press, 1998.

Watzlawick P, Beavin JH, Jackson DD. *Pragmatics of human communication: a study of interactional patterns, pathologies and paradoxes*. New York: W.W. Norton, 1967.

Watzlawick P, Weakland JH, Fisch R. *Change: principles of problem formation and problem resolution*. New York: W. W. Norton, 1974.

Wilkinson I. The darlington family assessment system: clinical guidelines for practitioners. *J Fam Ther* 2000;22:211–224.

Wilson J, Fosson A, Kanga JF, et al. Homeostatic interactions: a longitudinal study of biological, psychosocial and family variables in children with cystic fibrosis. *J Fam Ther* 1996;18:123–139.

Yuen EJ, Gerdes JL, Waldfogel S. Linkages between PCP's and mental health specialists. *Fam Syst Health* 1999;17:295–307.

SUGGESTED READINGS

Friedman EH. Bowen theory and therapy. In: Gurman AS, Kniskern DP, eds. *Handbook of family therapy*, Vol. II. Bristol, PA: Brunner/Mazel, 1991:134–170.

(This article provides an intriguing analysis of Bowen theory, and for those with a knowledge of biology, a unique reference point for understanding family

process. *The entire edited book also provides a veritable wealth of related information.*)

Guerin PJ Jr, Fogarty TF, Fay LF, et al. *Working with relationship triangles: the one-two-three of psychotherapy.* New York: Guilford Press, 1996.
(*This book focuses upon couples, families, and relationship triangles.*)

Goldenberg I, Goldenberg H. *Family therapy an overview*, 6th ed. Pacific Grove, CA: Thomson Brooks Cole, 2004.
(*This volume provides a very complete overview of a comprehensive list of family therapies for all clinicians.*)

Napier AY, Whitaker CA. *The family crucible.* New York: Harper & Row, 1978.
(*This book reads like a novel but provides an excellent foundation for understanding family process.*)

The author also recommends the following journals for those interested in the practice of family therapy.

- Journal of Marital and Family Therapy
- Family Process
- The American Journal of Family Therapy
- Contemporary Family Therapy
- The Family Psychologist
- Journal of Family Psychotherapy

The Individuals with Disabilities Education Act Serving Infants, Children, and Adolescents with Special Needs

ANN M. CHILDERS

Introduction

Public school systems hold a key place in communities as centers that provide the education, training, and socialization required for children to become contributing members of society. To participate fully in the educational process and progress alongside their peers, children must develop cognitive abilities, emotional maturity, social skills, physical abilities, and communication skills appropriate to age. Deficiencies in one or more of these areas place infants, children, and adolescents at risk of dropping out of school, and even society. The Individuals with Disabilities Education Act (IDEA) was established to safeguard the rights of at-risk children to a *Free Appropriate Public Education* (FAPE).

The evolution of laws and policies culminating in the IDEA began with *Brown versus Board of Education* in 1954. Addressing this case, the Supreme Court of the United States stated, "In these days, it is doubtful that any child may reasonably be expected to succeed in life if he is denied the opportunity of an education. Such an opportunity... is a right which must be made available to all on equal terms," and declared "all children must be guaranteed an equal educational opportunity."

Although the Supreme Court's decision paved the way to educational access for a large and previously underserved population of African American and other ethnic minority children, the two decades that followed showed that not all would benefit. Children with physical, cognitive, developmental, and emotional disabilities and differences continued to be systematically excluded from public education. Approximately 90% of developmentally disabled adults were not skilled enough to care for themselves, and so were housed in state institutions where they received long-term care under suboptimal conditions at a cost of billions of federal dollars.

The population of educationally excluded children with disabilities expanded unchecked, and in 1975 a report to Congress from the Bureau of Education for the Handicapped showed that in a population of approximately 8 million disabled children only 3.9 million received an appropriate education, 2.5 million received an inappropriate education, and 1.75 million received no educational services whatsoever. Emotionally disturbed children were among the most poorly served segment of this population, with 82% receiving inadequate educational services.

To address this situation, Congress enacted the *Education for All Handicapped Children Act* (EAHCA) in 1975, also known as Public Law 94-142. With this act, Congress intended that all children with disabilities should receive "a free appropriate public education," emphasizing, "special education and related services designed to meet their unique needs."

With the EAHCA, educational access for disabled children improved, but progress over the next decade and a half was slow. Congress concluded, "Implementation of this Act has been impeded by low expectations." In addition to retitling the EAHCA to IDEA in 1990, Congress intentionally raised educational expectations for children with disabilities, once again affirming the entitlement of all children to a FAPE. By promoting increased family support and involvement in early intervention and preschool programs, this early version of IDEA intended to prepare young children to receive an education.

In 1997, Congress once more confronted an educational system in which the status of children with disabilities continued to fall short of expectations. Many children with disabilities were excluded from the curriculum and assessments used with their nondisabled classmates, limiting their possibilities of performing to higher standards. Twice as many of these disabled children dropped out of school as compared to regular students. Once they dropped out, they did not return to school, had difficulty finding jobs, and often ended up in the criminal justice system. Girls who dropped out became unwed teen mothers at a much higher rate than their nondisabled peers. Lacking education, resources, and personal skills, young disabled girls with high-risk pregnancies brought forth a new generation of children at risk.

To address these issues, IDEA was amended and reauthorized in 1997, and continues to be reauthorized periodically. It is undergoing review at this writing. The consistent objectives of the amendments have been to raise educational expectations for children with disabilities and facilitate their participation in mainstream society. Children with disabilities are to be included in assessments, performance goals, and reports to the public. In recognition of the vital role of parents in the education of their disabled children and their responsibilities under IDEA, the amendments expand opportunities for involvement of parents in *special education*. The amendments promote successful mainstreaming of children into regular classrooms by integrating all facets of a child's education into his or her *individual education plan* (IEP). They provide for professional support and development of regular education teachers in addition to *special education* staff, including them in educational planning and assessment of progress for their disabled students.

IDEA is a public law that provides a federal statutory structure by which federal money is distributed to assist state educational agencies (SEAs) and local educational agencies (LEAs) to educate children with disabilities. It helps pay for additional costs incurred by states, school districts, and schools while providing services to special needs infants, children, adolescents, and their families. IDEA addresses a wide range of conditions and is unique in its role of providing services for individuals ages 0 to 21 with disabilities. No health care plan in the United States provides special education, occupational therapy, physical therapy, speech pathology services, psychology services, audiology, community nursing, and medical services (limited to diagnostic evaluations), provided at no charge to parents, and delivered in multiple settings, including homes, hospitals, and schools. IDEA is divided into sections that serve different age groups. Included are sections for infants and toddlers, preschool children, elementary school children, and adolescents in secondary education.

This chapter is an introduction to the IDEA, last amended in 1997, as it applies to infants, children, and adolescents with mental health and developmental needs. Its purpose is to present an overview of IDEA, along with some practical advice for health care providers and the families they serve.

Definitions under Individuals with Disabilities Education Act

For the purposes of the IDEA, the definition of a "child with a disability" means a child evaluated (*via* an individualized evaluation examining all aspects of potential disability, as performed by a multidisciplinary team that includes the parent) and determined to meet legal definitions under specifically defined categories as summarized in Table 26.1.

IDEA further defines *related services* as "transportation and such developmental, corrective, and other supportive services as are required to assist a child with a disability to benefit from special education...." These *related services* are broad and individualized to the child's needs, as summarized in Table 26.2. The section goes on to say, "if it is determined,

---

TABLE 26.1. IDEA CATEGORIES OF DISABILITIES

- Autism
- Deaf-blindness
- Deafness
- Emotional disturbance
- Hearing impairment
- Mental retardation
- Multiple disabilities
- Orthopedic impairment
- Other health impairment
- Specific learning disability
- Speech or language impairment
- Traumatic brain injury
- Visual impairment

IDEA, Individuals with Disabilities Education Act.

TABLE 26.2. RELATED SERVICES SUPPORTED BY IDEA

- Early identification and assessment of disabilities in children
- Medical services for diagnostic or evaluation purposes only, provided by a licensed physician to determine a child's medically related disability resulting in the child's need for special education and related services
- School health services provided by a qualified school nurse or other qualified personnel
- Psychological services
- Counseling services provided by qualified social workers, psychologists, guidance counselors, or other qualified personnel
- Occupational therapy
- Speech-language pathology and audiology services
- Physical therapy
- Rehabilitation counseling services
- Orientation and mobility services for children with visual impairments
- Recreation, including assessment of leisure function, therapeutic recreation services, leisure education, and recreation programs in schools and community agencies
- Parent training and counseling aimed at assisting parents in understanding the needs of their child, providing parents with information about child development, and helping them acquire skills to allow them to support implementation of their child's IEP
- Social work services in school, including group and individual counseling with the child and family; working with problems in a child's home, school, or community that affect his or her adjustment in school; and mobilizing school and community resources to enable the child to receive maximum benefit from his or her educational program

IDEA, Individuals with Disabilities Education Act; IEP, individualized education plan.

through an appropriate evaluation… that a child has one of the disabilities identified in… this section, but only needs a *related service and not special education*, the child is not a child with a disability…." In other words, a child must be found to have a handicapping condition requiring special education, and not just related services, in order to be eligible for programs and services under IDEA.

IDEA also states that, to qualify for *special education*, the child must have a handicapping condition that interferes with *educational performance*. Here it is important to note the term *educational performance* is not limited to school activities. Most courts and educators, consistent with what constitutes education, have broadly interpreted *educational performance* to encompass most life activities, well beyond the scope of basic academics.

The requirement that a handicapping condition interfere with a child's *educational performance* to qualify as a disability under IDEA is advantageous in a number of important respects. It makes *educational performance* the bellwether of a child's educational function. Since *educational performance* is measured objectively, the requirement that a handicapping condition interfere with a child's *educational performance* suggests the use of objective measures to evaluate children and measure their progress. Also, it broadens the field of conditions that may qualify as handicapping, an important feature for providers serving children with mental disorders, considering the vast overlap of disabling conditions endemic to child psychiatric populations.

There are exceptions to this requirement that the child have a *handicapping condition* to be qualified under IDEA. Exceptions include children ages 3 through 9 (or a subset of this population, such as ages 3 to 5) who qualify under individual state interpretations of IDEA as having *developmental delays*, and infants and toddlers from birth through age 2 eligible for early intervention services, as delivered in accordance with an *individualized family service plan* (IFSP). State and local education agencies that adopt the term *developmental delay* are not obligated to determine that a child in the designated age group has a specific disability to qualify the child for services. Rather, IDEA allows these states to define *developmental delays* and to establish appropriate diagnostic instruments and procedures to measure these delays. For children aged 3 through 9, the SEA and LEA may choose to include as an eligible *child with a disability* a child who is experiencing *developmental delays* in one or more of the following areas:

- Physical development
- Cognitive development
- Communication development
- Social or emotional development
- Adaptive development
- "… and who, by reason of *developmental delays*, requires *special education* and *related services.* "

The IDEA also provides for services to *at-risk infants and toddlers*. The term *at-risk infant or toddler* refers to an individual less than 3 years of age who would be at risk for a substantial developmental delay if early intervention services were not provided. Identification of a disability or developmental delay is not necessary to qualify an infant for services. Parents, physicians, and others may refer infants and toddlers who appear to be at risk to school districts for evaluation. A broad range of services is available to infants and toddlers who qualify. The IDEA specifies that such services be provided in the most natural setting for this population, usually in the family home.

Providing services to infants *at risk* and children with *developmental delays* focuses on the importance of early developmental interventions and on providing special education services to children at risk for, but not identified as having, disabilities. In recognition of the risk involved when developmental delays and risk factors in infants are not addressed, substantiation of risk factors in infants and, optionally, developmental delays in children ages 3 to 9 is all that is required for SEAs to qualify these children for services.

Individuals with Disabilities Education Act and Mental Health Populations

Between 70% and 80% of children who receive mental health services receive them in schools. For many of these children, school is their only mental health resource.

Under IDEA, the primary category under which children disabled by mental illness qualify for services is *severe emotional disturbance (SED)*, referred to as *emotional disturbance (ED)* throughout most of the IDEA. Federal regulations define *ED* as a condition that exhibits one or more of the following characteristics over a long period of time and to a marked degree and that adversely affects a child's *educational performance*:

- An inability to learn that cannot be explained by intellectual, sensory, or health factors
- An inability to build or maintain satisfactory interpersonal relationships with peers and teachers
- Inappropriate types of behaviors or feelings under normal circumstances
- A general pervasive mood of unhappiness or depression
- A tendency to develop physical symptoms or fears associated with personal or school problems.

Given these broad criteria, characteristics of children and adolescents qualifying for services under the category of *severe emotional disturbance* (sometimes referred to as SED, or ED) are wide ranging. Furthermore, they are often not well recognized by schools.

Prevalence of Developmental Disabilities and Service Utilization

The Centers for Disease Control and Prevention (CDCP) defines *developmental disabilities* as "a diverse group of physical, cognitive, psychological, sensory, and speech impairments that begin anytime during development up to 18 years of age." According to the CDCP, "About 17% of U.S. children under 18 years of age have a developmental disability." Given this broad definition, the vast majority of children receiving services under IDEA have one or more *developmental disabilities*, and developmental disabilities are endemic to child psychiatric populations.

Determining the numbers of children receiving services for *developmental delays* and for being at risk for *developmental delays and disabilities* is difficult, due to the variability in definitions and service utilization across states. However, since implementation of the IDEA 1997 amendment that allowed services to be provided to infants at risk and children 3 to 9 years old with developmental delays, the utilization of preventive services under IDEA has been increasing. As parents become better informed about developmental milestones and health care providers grow increasingly skilled at identifying significant delays, demands for corrective intervention services under IDEA have surged. In its 23rd annual report to Congress, the Department of Education, Office of Special Education Programs (OSEP) reports that during the 1999 to 2000 school year the numbers of children qualifying for services in the *developmental delay* category increased by 62.1% over the previous year.

Identifying Children with Disabilities: Child Find and Referrals

Identifying infants, children, and adolescents with *disabilities*, with *developmental delays*, and those *at risk for developmental delays* is central to the IDEA. Under Part C, states receiving funds under IDEA must actively search for, identify, and refer these individuals for services. This process of search and identification is referred to as *child find*.

Under Part C, the governor of each state that receives federal funds under IDEA is responsible to appoint or establish a lead agency for the establishment and operation of a comprehensive *child find* system making referrals to early intervention providers of IDEA services. The lead agency must collaborate with families to identify the individual needs of their infants and toddlers for the purpose of creating IFSPs. The lead agency is also responsible for creating a central directory detailing these services and resources.

The state's *child find* program must proactively reach families with children between the ages of 0 and 21 who may qualify for services and programs under IDEA. To achieve this, states must advertise widely, creating public awareness programs to disseminate information to parents regarding the early identification and referral of infants and toddlers with disabilities, "especially" through hospitals and physicians. The goal is to ensure "a timely, comprehensive, multidisciplinary evaluation of the functioning of each infant or toddler with a disability in the respective State." States must also locate, identify, and evaluate children who may be eligible for services, even those attending private schools (although public school districts are not required to provide services in private school settings).

State and LEAs receive referrals from parents, teachers, and less often from community sources. Unfortunately, relatively few IDEA referrals are made by primary health care providers serving children and families, despite their developmental expertise and familiarity with concerns of families seen in health care settings. While not obligated to evaluate children referred by health care professionals, school districts find their referrals compelling. Most parents whose children struggle socially and academically in schools are pleased when their doctors offer to write letters of referral, and children undergoing IEP evaluations benefit significantly from them. Letters highlighting pertinent diagnoses and physical findings increase the likelihood that a child will receive necessary services.

Concerned parents, who may or may not know how to initiate the evaluation process, represent the largest referral source. But most parents are unfamiliar with IDEA protocols and safeguards and are frustrated when their requests to schools do not result in evaluations. The most efficient request parents can submit is the *parent referral and consent letter*. For best effect, this letter should be legible; address its recipient by name (preferably the school principal or the chairperson of the IEP team); identify the child by first name, last name, and birth date; clearly describe concerns regarding the child's school performance and related complaints received from the school; request that the child be evaluated "in accordance with the Individuals with Disabilities Education Act (IDEA)," and identify itself as a document providing parental consent to the school and/or school district to initiate the evaluation.

To expedite the process, parents provide convenient contact information: work, home, and cellular telephone numbers, for example, and request that the school contact them to discuss the child within a finite period of time, usually 7 calendar days. The letter should be signed by the parent and duplicated, with an indication at the foot of the letter that the parent has retained a copy.

To establish a well-defined IDEA paper trail, it is important that receipt by the school be documented as to date and time received. This can be accomplished in a number of ways. The request letter can be sent via mail, either with "delivery confirmation requested" or as registered mail. The parent's copy documents the exact time the school received written parent consent and establishes a point of contact in the event the school's copy of the request is lost or misplaced.

Since evaluations must consider all available information and pertinent sources, referring parents are encouraged to collect collateral documents from persons and professionals familiar with their child. Questions about the child from the child's school can guide the parent's information gathering activities.

Schools that identify children for evaluations must inform parents in writing of their intent to evaluate, and obtain parental consent prior to the evaluation. Parents who agree to the school's proposal to evaluate may wish to engage in a process similar to that of the *parent referral and consent letter* to initiate a paper trail.

With rare exception, from written parental consent to completion of a child's evaluation, schools are permitted *a reasonable period of time*. IDEA leaves *a reasonable period of time* open to interpretation by individual states. Individual states commonly interpret *a reasonable period of time* in terms of *calendar days*, with periods ranging from 30 to 60 days. The term *calendar days* indicates consecutive days throughout the calendar year. States that incorporate this unit provide a dependable measure of time to parents and schools.

Defining *a reasonable period of time* in terms of *business days*, and particularly *school days*, creates significant variability. *Business days* are influenced by definitions of holidays, and the number of *school days* in any time period fluctuates with teacher workshops, school holidays, and vacations. Depending on the time of year that written parental consent is submitted, states allowing 60 *school days* to complete an evaluation can take 3 months, 5 months, or longer. By contrast, once the evaluation is complete, IDEA grants schools 30 *calendar days* from the time a child is determined eligible for services to conduct the first IEP meeting. Parents must be invited to this meeting and participate as members of the IEP team.

IDEA empowers parents to be full and equal participants in the special education process because parents know their children best. Another reason is the responsibility IDEA places on parents to monitor the process and address irregularities. Along with the U.S. Department of Education's OSEP, parents provide oversight to ensure the process is in their child's best interest. This role creates a significant impetus for IDEA to make provisions to empower parents. But child advocacy is an emotional journey that places a burden

TABLE 26.3. ESSENTIAL ELEMENTS OF AN INDIVIDUALIZED EDUCATION PLAN

- An IEP meeting includes the presence of guardians/parents, at least one regular teacher if the child is mainstreamed; at least one special education specialist; one school administration representative qualified to coordinate, oversee, and access special education resources; one school representative qualified to interpret evaluation testing; and the child when appropriate
- Documentation on the IEP includes:
  - Present levels of the child's performance, as measured objectively
  - Measurable educational goals and objectives
  - A plan adequate to enable the child to reach the educational goals
  - Adequate funding to provide the necessary educational services
  - Annual goals
  - Documentation of special and related services to be provided
  - Documentation of the level of participation with nondisabled children
  - Participation in state and district wide assessments
  - Dates, durations, and location(s) of services
  - Transition service needs (to be determined by age 14, younger as indicated)
  - Transition service needs (at least by age 16 yr; required for children 16 yr and older)
  - How the team will measure progress (note: objective measures, e.g., standardized tests, are most accurate)
  - How and when parents will be informed of progress

IEP, individualized education plan.

on parents of disabled children as these parents often shoulder considerable family and work responsibilities, frequently have more than one disabled child, and may struggle with disabilities of their own.

Once the evaluation begins, parents encounter a steep learning curve and a brisk pace. As their child's advocate, parents become students of IDEA. When they are not studying, they take notes at meetings, generate and receive e-mails, and document phone calls. They arrange IEP meetings, seek outside consultations, and organize a growing accumulation of documents. During the IEP meeting there are specific items that should be addressed and specific individuals who should be at the meeting. Essential elements of an IEP meeting are summarized in Table 26.3.

Establishing a clear and organized paper trail is the key to success in every aspect of the special education process. Parents must organize and dedicate a set of special education files for their child and become accustomed to documenting each step in the process, including telephone calls and casual conversations. In his advice to parents, Robert K. Crabtree, Esq., an attorney practicing special education and disability law, has proposed a practical and inclusive format for special education files, as shown in Table 26.4.

TABLE 26.4. SUGGESTED FORMAT FOR PARENTAL SPECIAL EDUCATION FILES

- Individualized educational programs (IEPs) and other official service plans
- Evaluations by the school system and by independent evaluators
- Medical records
- Progress reports and report cards
- Standardized test results
- Notes on the child's behavior or progress
- Correspondence
- Notes from conversations and meetings
- Documents relating to discipline and/or behavioral concerns
- Formal notices of meetings scheduled to discuss the child
- Samples of schoolwork
- Invoices and canceled checks
- Public documents

TABLE 26.5. IDEA PROCEDURAL SAFEGUARDS

- Independent educational evaluations
- Prior written notice
- Parental consent
- Access to educational records
- Opportunity to present complaints
- The child's school placement pending due process proceedings
- Procedures for students who are placed in an interim alternative educational setting
- Requirements for unilateral placement by parents of children in private schools at public expense
- Mediation
- Due process hearings, including requirements for disclosure of evaluation results and recommendations
- State-level appeals (if applicable in that specific state)
- Civil actions attorneys' fees. Section 615 (d) (2)].

IDEA, Individuals with Disabilities Education Act.

Establishing this type of filing format from the outset greatly enhances organization and ensures documents are available when needed.

State and LEA are required to assist parents in the enforcement of IDEA on behalf of their children. School districts are responsible for providing parents with written copies of the IDEA's procedural safeguards, in a form they can understand, at key points in the special education process. Safeguards must be written in the native language of the parents, unless it clearly not feasible to do so, written in a manner that is easy to understand, and must cover specific topics. These safeguards are summarized in Table 26.5.

The safeguard termed *prior written notice* deserves special mention as an important means by which due process rights are protected, as summarized in Table 26.6. In *prior written notice*, IDEA requires school districts to provide parents essential information in writing and in clearly understood language prior to taking action regarding their child.

Actions requiring *prior written notice* include initiation of special education services and denial of such services. Because of its influence on due process and the accountability of schools, courts take failures of school districts to provide prior written notice very seriously. Parents whose children receive evaluations under IDEA should ensure they receive every copy of prior written notice they are entitled to, whether or not the school district agrees to evaluate their child and irrespective of an evaluation's outcome.

IDEA provides for another resource parents may utilize in their advocacy efforts: the *Parent Information and Training Center* (PITC). The mission of PITCs is to provide training and information to parents of infants, toddlers, children, and youths with disabilities and to professionals and others who assist them. The purpose of PITCs is to enable parents to participate more fully and effectively with professionals in meeting the educational needs

TABLE 26.6. IDEA PRIOR WRITTEN NOTICE SAFEGUARDS

- A description of the action proposed or refused by the agency
- An explanation of why the agency proposes or refuses to take the action
- A description of any other options that the agency considered and the reasons why those options were rejected
- A description of each evaluation procedure, test, record, or report the agency used as a basis for the proposed, or refused, action
- A description of any other factors that are relevant to the agency's proposal or refusal
- A statement that the parents of a child with a disability have protection under procedural safeguards of IDEA; and if this prior written notice is not an initial referral for evaluation, the means for obtaining a description of the procedural safeguards; and sources for parents to contact to obtain assistance in understanding these safeguards

IDEA, Individuals with Disabilities Education Act.

of their children with disabilities. These federally funded centers do not provide legal assistance but furnish information regarding IDEA, especially as it is interpreted by laws in the states they serve, and make advocacy resources available to parents. Currently, PITCs can be found in every state in the United States and in the territories of American Samoa, American Virgin Islands, and Puerto Rico.

Parents of Infants, Children, and Adolescents Served in Department of Defense Schools

As with the states, the Department of Defense (DoD) is held to the standards of the IDEA for families stationed in the continental U.S. (CONUS) and overseas (OS). DoD Instruction 1342.12 is part of the DoD's interpretation of IDEA. This Instruction provides definitions and outlines *related services* (termed *medically related services* by DoD) provided through the DoD. DoD Instruction 1342.12 is subject to updates, and military parents are encouraged to obtain the most current copy.

A PITC exists to guide military families through the DoD educational system. Specialized Training of Military Parents (STOMP) answers questions, furnishes documents, and offers guidance for military parents with special needs children. Established in 1985, STOMP is a project of Washington PAVE (Parents are Vital in Education). Located in the State of Washington, STOMP receives funding through a grant from the U.S. Department of Education.

Individuals with Disabilities Education Act Services for Mental Health Populations

Teachers, administrators, and other school personnel generally receive insufficient training in the identification and placement of children with psychiatric disorders, and misconceptions about emotionally and behaviorally disturbed children are common. Emotionally fragile children and adolescents whose behaviors are disruptive often qualify for services under this category. Because these children are not well understood, disruptive conduct may be attributed to a child's ED without further inquiry into its etiology. The combination of emotional fragility and disruptive behavior carries special social risks. Disruptive behavior that interferes with educational performance of the child and those around him or her attracts negative attention from school personnel, increasing the risk of lost school days due to suspensions and expulsions, and negatively affecting the child's self-esteem.

Under IDEA, suspensions for children with IEPs are managed differently from those of their nondisabled peers. Within 10 business days after removing a student with disabilities from school, a school district is required to convene an IEP meeting to look at the student's functional behavior, his or her disability, and whether the current education program is appropriate. The IEP team must determine whether there had ever been a *functional behavioral assessment* (FBA) or a *behavior intervention plan* (BIP) for the student. If not, the IEP team must develop one. When a student faces suspension or expulsion for more than 10 days, the IEP team must meet to determine whether there is a relationship between the child's disability and the behavior. If a relationship exists, the student cannot be punished. But if, for any reason, a decision is made to remove a special education student from the school to an alternate setting, the student maintains eligibility for a FAPE and must continue to receive educational services in that setting.

The FBA and BIP were introduced with the 1997 reauthorization of the IDEA as procedures to assist children with disruptive behaviors. The FBA was instituted in recognition of the fact that failure to base any intervention on a specific cause (function) most often results in ineffective and unnecessarily restrictive procedures, for example, suspension. School districts are now required to conduct FBAs for children with problem behaviors under some circumstances, but whether it will survive reauthorization remains to be seen. It is currently intended that children who receive FBAs be thoroughly evaluated for the root causes of disruptive behavior, with positive contingencies to manage these behaviors (BIPs) made part of their IEPs. Child and adolescent health care providers with concerns as to behavior management at school may refer children who qualify as disabled under IDEA for an FBA through their school district.

Significant overlap exists between child mental health populations and populations qualifying for services under IDEA. Practitioners who diagnose and treat child and adolescent psychiatric conditions routinely encounter youths with at least one mental health condition that requires the unique evaluations, services, and educational support provided under IDEA. Additionally, comorbidities are prevalent in child mental health suggesting multiple roads to IDEA qualification.

As a category, *specific learning disabilities* represents roughly half of students served under IDEA. In this population, as in other special education populations, language and learning disabilities are common. A number of studies have demonstrated considerable overlap of language and learning disabilities with the *Diagnostic and Statistical Manual of Mental Disorders,* Fourth Edition (DSM-IV)-defined Axis I psychiatric conditions, that is, major mental health disorders. In its Practice Parameters for the Assessment and Treatment of Children and Adolescents With Language and Learning Disorders (LLDs), the American Academy of Child and Adolescent Psychiatry (AACAP) describes LLDs as "among the most common developmental disorders," and "the largest group of disorders requiring special services in the schools, accounting together for more than three quarters of all children or adolescents in special education." Drawing a correlation between LLDs and mental health, the authors go on to say, "Approximately 50% of children with LLDs have a clinically significant comorbid Axis I psychiatric diagnosis. Furthermore, the presence of LLDs contributes to persistence of symptoms of comorbid disorders and complicates their treatment."

The treatment for language and learning disabilities is *special education*, such as provided under IDEA, and the AACAP emphasizes the importance of referring children with DSM-IV-defined Axis I disorders who are suspected of having an underlying specific learning disability for psychoeducational evaluations through their schools.

Another important service provided under IDEA that is seldom utilized in child and adolescent mental health care settings is the evaluation of language with support from speech pathology and audiology services. Research over the past decade and a half indicates a strong role for developmental language disorders (DLD) in child and adolescent psychiatric morbidity. DLD, especially receptive language disorder (with little or no expressive component, contrary to language criteria listed in the DSM-IV), affects as much as 30% to 50% of the child and adolescent outpatient psychiatric population. Largely undiagnosed, DLD contributes to marked psychiatric morbidity, including significantly higher internalizing and externalizing characteristics in affected children. Perhaps the developmental disability/disruptive behavior disorder with the highest profile in both educational and mental health settings is attention deficit hyperactivity disorder (ADHD). Comorbid language disorders play key roles in this disorder as well. Pragmatic (social) speech disorder, a communication disorder that engenders low self-esteem, anxiety, and depression alongside impairment in social and vocational adaptations, is considered pervasive in this population. Along with language-related specific learning disabilities, other language-related comorbidities common to children and adolescents with ADHD are receptive language disorder and auditory processing disorder. Because the vast majority of psychiatric settings do not feature language evaluation services for children and adolescents, and these services are not routinely covered by medical insurance, evaluations and interventions provided under IDEA by schools become increasingly important to infant, child, and adolescent mental health.

Conclusions

Despite its vast offerings of services and interventions, the IDEA is unfamiliar to, and underutilized by, health care providers serving infants, children, and adolescents in medical settings. This is unfortunate as, under IDEA, referral of a patient to the schools will usually lead to appropriate educational evaluation and remedial services. Services provided under IDEA are necessary to promote adequate functioning in adulthood of *at-risk*, *developmentally delayed*, and *developmentally disabled* infants, toddlers, children, and adolescents. Health care providers serving children with mental and developmental disabilities can easily assist parents in obtaining these services, thereby improving the quality of life for children, families, and communities.

BIBLIOGRAPHY

Federal Register March 12, 1999 volume 64, no 48: Final IDEA Regulations The paper chase: managing your child's documents under IDEA by Robert K, Crabtree, B Esq. Document provided on the Wright's Law website, at http://www.wrightslaw.com/info/advo.paperchase.crabtree.htm

Toppelberg CO, Shapiro T. Language disorders: a 10-year research update review. *J Am Acad Child Adolesc Psychiatry* 2000;39:143–152.

The Work Group on Quality Issues. Practice parameters for the assessment and treatment of children and adolescents with language and learning disorders. *J Am Acad Child Adolesc Psychiatry* 1998;37(Suppl):46S–62S.

SUGGESTED READINGS

Levine M. *A mind at a time*, New York: Simon & Schuster, 2002.
 (*Provides a paradigm for understanding children with learning disabilities for clinicians and parents.*)

Wright PWD, Wright PD. *Wrightslaw: special education law*. Hartifield, VA: Harbor House Law Press, 1999.
 (*Excellent reference for informing parents of the legal rights for their children with disabilities, CD-ROM included.*)

CHAPTER 27

Levels of Mental Health Care in Community Settings

LARRY MARX

Introduction

According to the 2000 Surgeon General's Conference on Children's Mental Health, the nation is facing a public crisis in mental health care for infants, children, and adolescents. Many children and adolescents have mental health problems that interfere with normal development and functioning. In the United States, one in 10 youths has a mental illness severe enough to cause some level of impairment. Yet, in any given year, it is estimated that only about one in five of these youths is receiving specialty mental health services for his or her illness. There are many reasons why so few of these children actually receive mental health care. Lack of access to appropriate mental health services is one contributing factor. Too often, these troubled children and their families either do not receive mental health services when they need them or are offered no services at all.

Communities in the United States provide different types of treatment programs and services for children and adolescents with mental illnesses. Most urban areas have a variety of such mental health resources while rural areas may have few or none at all. A community that has a complete range of mental health services has a "continuum of mental health care for children and adolescents." This continuum includes primary prevention and early intervention, family self-help and support services, treatments that maximize a child's or adolescent's development within his or her home and community, as well as services requiring placement in more secure settings such as acute inpatient psychiatric hospitalization or residential care.

Not every community has every type of service or program on this continuum. Rapid changes in the behavioral health care systems, particularly in how mental health services are funded, have had dramatic impacts on decision making about the setting and intensity of mental health treatment. In general, this continuum of mental health care is now broadly conceptualized as mental health "level of care." Each level of care is defined by several factors including the setting where treatment is provided (e.g., outpatient mental health clinics, an inpatient psychiatric unit, emergency room, residential setting); the types of services offered in that setting (e.g., individual psychotherapy, group therapy, family therapy, medication administration, medical monitoring); and the frequency that the services are offered (e.g., 24 hours 7 days a week, 3 days a week, weekly, or monthly).

Influence of Managed Care on the Development of Mental Health Level of Care

Level of care definitions and the determination as to which child or adolescent would benefit from each level has been historically tied to the application of managed care principles to both the delivery and financing of mental health services. The early methodology of managed care set arbitrary mental health benefit levels based on large populations of generally healthy adults and children who were infrequent users of mental health services. This application of arbitrary benefit levels was particularly true in the late 1980s, which had seen an increase in the cost of mental health services with the development of free-standing for-profit psychiatric facilities and coverage for long-term individual psychotherapy. As well, the success of managed care organizations in controlling general health care costs led to the development of Behavioral Health Organizations (BHO) that used cost-containment strategies similar to those used by managed care entities for physical health care. These strategies include discounted fees to providers, preauthorization, and concurrent reviews primarily for high cost services such as inpatient treatment, retrospective denial of payment for services, and restricted provider networks. However, managed care also stimulated providers to redesign their services to be more accommodating to the demands of the BHO. To manage subgroups of children and adolescents with more serious mental illnesses, traditional providers of inpatient services and residential treatment began to develop new and less expensive alternatives, including mobile crisis services, partial hospital programs, or day treatment.

Another approach to utilization management in BHOs was the development of criteria that were specific to a given child or adolescent mental health program. BHOs have tended to group services or programs of similar intensity together within a level of care. Standardized and specific selection criteria for children and adolescents who might benefit from this level of care were also developed along with the level of care definitions.

The outcome of the application of these fiscal management controls, both in the private and public mental health care sectors, have affected the different levels of care that can be found in a community. As well, the types of financial strategies to control the cost of mental health care have affected the access, utilization, and quality of the mental health services that are offered to children, adolescents, and their families.

Level of Care Definitions within a Managed Care System

CRISIS ASSESSMENT

Mental health crisis assessment services are performed in two major ways: (a) in a separate identifiable organized mental health crisis unit within a mental health or general hospital facility; or (b) by a mobile crisis team either in the community or in a secure setting such as a general hospital emergency room. The goal of crisis assessment services is to evaluate and/or resolve behavioral health emergencies without hospitalizing a child or adolescent in an acute inpatient psychiatric setting. Crisis assessment services are most frequently utilized when there is evidence of an imminent or current mental health emergency that may require inpatient hospitalization. Children and adolescents who present with active suicidal or homicidal ideation, severe behavioral problems that put themselves or others at serious physical risk, or onset of acute psychotic symptoms should be considered in need of crisis assessment. This service may be linked to programs that provide temporary in-home or out-of-home respite for children and families in order to divert the need for inpatient placement. Arrangements are made for the child or adolescent to be evaluated at the appropriate level of care the following day.

23-HOUR CRISIS STABILIZATION BED

This service is a specialized form of crisis assessment and stabilization provided by a general or psychiatric hospital which offers acute psychiatric care management 24 hours a day, 7 days a week. The patient most likely is displaying acute and serious functional deterioration. Although this level of care is more commonly utilized for adults, a child's or adolescent's mental health treatment history might suggest that the patient is likely to respond to rapid initiation of medication or acute titration of current medications. Typically, youths evaluated in this level of care are experiencing an acute exacerbation of a previously diagnosed mental health condition, are receiving ongoing mental health service in another level of care, and do not require an intensive diagnostic assessment for their mental health condition. Acute care nursing, medication management, and monitoring are essential components of this level of care. If the patient responds and hospitalization is not warranted, the patient is given a next day appointment to begin services at the appropriate level of care.

ACUTE PSYCHIATRIC INPATIENT UNIT

This level of care is most appropriate for children and adolescents who present with serious and imminent risk of harm to self or others due to a psychiatric illness. Serious and imminent risk includes: (a) recent and serious suicide attempt as indicated by the degree of intent, impulsivity, impairment of judgment, and/or inability to contract for safety; (b) current suicidal ideation with intent, realistic plan, and/or available means; (c) recent self-mutilation that is medically significant and dangerous; (d) an active and realistic plan, intent, and available means intended to seriously injure another person; (e) recent assaultive behaviors that indicate a high risk for recurrence and serious injury to others; and (f) recent and serious physically destructive acts that indicate a high risk for recurrence and serious injuries to others. These patients exhibit serious and acute deterioration in functioning due to a psychiatric illness with a severe disturbance in affect, behavior, thought process, or judgment that cannot be safely managed in a less restrictive environment. As a result of their psychiatric disorder, these children and adolescents require 24-hour monitoring by nursing staff. The use of a seclusion room and physical restraints may be warranted. These patients are reevaluated daily by a physician for acute detoxification, medication management, or the management of a concomitant medical condition. Individual, family, group, and milieu therapies are generally provided. Aftercare plans are typically developed with the child or adolescent referred to the next most appropriate level of care after discharge.

RESIDENTIAL FACILITY/SUBACUTE UNITS

These programs provide active mental health and/or substance abuse treatment through specialized programming with observation and supervision 24 hours per day. These programs are typically offered in freestanding facilities that are not hospital based. Although these patients may require medical and nursing monitoring, their mental health condition does not warrant daily medical monitoring as would occur on an acute inpatient unit. However, patients in subacute units require more frequent monitoring by a physician than those patients placed in a residential program. These programs may utilize a seclusion room and use of physical restraints. They are appropriate for clinical situations in which the patient's support system is nonexistent or so severely affects the patient's ability to recover that treatment in a less acute or community-based setting is likely to be unsuccessful. Typically, these children and adolescents have a history of multiple out-of-home placements in either acute psychiatric inpatient units or foster homes. Individual, group, family, and milieu treatments are offered. Given that these patients are typically placed in these programs for long periods of time, an educational component is provided.

PARTIAL HOSPITAL AND/OR DAY TREATMENT SERVICES

These programs are typically freestanding or hospital based and provide services for at least 5 hours per day and at least 4 days per week. Patients for this level of care have significant impairment in psychosocial functioning due to a mental health condition. This mental health condition is associated with a likelihood of requiring acute inpatient hospitalization or placement in a residential facility. Patients in both of these programs are capable of being maintained in their home environment at the end of the treatment day and on weekends. Although these patients may require frequent monitoring of behavior and/or medication, they usually do not require a 24-hour structure, monitoring, or intensive nursing care. Partial hospitalization provides all the treatment services of a psychiatric hospital. Day treatment programs typically provide mental health treatment with special education. Pharmacotherapy may be offered to youths in day treatment either as a component of the program or by a physician in the community. Individual, family, group, and milieu therapies are provided.

HOME HEALTH

These are a specialized group of services designed to aid in the evaluation and management of high-risk patients with a multitude of medical as well as mental health treatment requirements. Typically, the patient is homebound secondary to either a medical condition or circumstances that temporarily prevent an office- or facility-based treatment. Also, these services are utilized for children and adolescents who have recently been discharged from a more restrictive level of care and are at significant risk of decompensation without home health. Nurses almost always provide these services with immediate access to a physician.

TABLE 27.1. ESSENTIALS OF LEVELS OF CARE IN MANAGED CARE

- Crisis assessment services
- 23-hr crisis stabilization bed
- Acute inpatient psychiatric unit
- Residential facility/ subacute unit
- Partial hospitalization and/or day treatment programs
- Home health services
- Outpatient mental health services

OUTPATIENT

Outpatient services are typically offered for clinical symptoms or behaviors caused by a mental illness that results in impairment or deterioration in psychosocial functioning. Usual services include initial diagnostic evaluations as well as individual, family, and group psychotherapies that are provided by a variety of mental health professionals. Medication evaluation and ongoing monitoring are also core medical services. The number of visits varies but is usually focused on achieving short-term goals with stabilization to previous level of functioning. This level of care is frequently utilized for child and adolescent mental health disorders (see Table 27.1).

Role of Assessment in Level of Care Determination

LEVEL OF CARE DETERMINATION BASED ON MEDICAL NECESSITY CRITERIA

In order to implement a managed care model, BHOs have relied on medical necessity criteria that are poorly defined and arbitrary across different payer systems. Medical necessity criteria have not been dependent on mental health diagnoses. These criteria have been dependent, however, on a child's or adolescent's previous history of service utilization and the perceived benefit derived from it. In theory, BHOs have implemented the principle of authorizing the "least restrictive" mental health treatment to meet the individualized needs of the patient. The concept of "least restrictive" mental health treatment has historically protected the rights of mentally ill individuals from being confined to long-term state institutions against their will. BHOs used this debatable and poorly understood concept as a rationale to restrict access to more expensive settings such as acute inpatient hospitalization, particularly if a child or adolescent had previous hospitalizations with little or no perceived benefit.

Although the mental health diagnosis may influence the different types of mental health treatment that are most appropriate (e.g., cognitive-behavioral therapy, medication, etc.), the diagnosis itself does not dictate the intensity, frequency, or setting of the treatment. Also, a child's or adolescent's past history of mental health service utilization does not necessarily dictate that the same service will be effective with the patient's current mental health needs. To the greatest extent possible, medical necessity criteria should include the individual child's or adolescent's strengths as well as his or her needs in determining the level of care to address the nature of his or her mental health condition. However, medical necessity criteria have defined the different types of mental health services that may exist in a community and provide a clinical rationale for the restrictiveness of the care.

LEVEL OF CARE BASED ON DIMENSIONAL ASSESSMENT

There have been a number of attempts to use clinical assessments as a method of determining level of care needs in children and adolescents. However, there has been no clearly defined method for linking the clinical assessment to the need for treatment or to the level of care best suited to deliver this treatment. The combination of these two concepts, the need for treatment and the optimal level of care, led the American Academy of Child and Adolescent Psychiatry Work Group on Systems of Care together with the American Association of Community Psychiatry to develop "dimensional" assessments for level of care determination. The Child and Adolescent Level of Care Utilization System (CALOCUS) combines a multidimensional assessment of a child's or adolescent's clinical needs, or functional status, with a clearly defined level of care based on discrete service components that vary in intensity and types of treatment. In CALOCUS, a mental health clinician assesses the child or adolescent and his family in six dimensions. Each dimension is scored and the total sum of the numeric values for each dimension guides the clinician toward a recommended level of service intensity. The algorithm for level of care determination is outlined in the CALOCUS manual. While the primary care clinician may not fully administer the CALOCUS, he or she may find the dimensions useful when evaluating a child or adolescent with a mental health problem by taking the information that is obtained for each dimension into consideration when collaborating with a mental health professional regarding level of care determination or appropriate interventions.

CALOCUS Dimensions for Mental Health Assessment

The dimensions of assessment covered by the CALOCUS are summarized in Table 27.2 and described below.

RISK OF HARM

This dimension is the measurement of a child's or adolescent's risk of harm to self or others by various means and an assessment of his or her potential for being a victim of physical or sexual abuse, neglect, or violence. Children and adolescents who appear to be at high risk of harm usually require highly structured and well-monitored settings, such as an inpatient hospital program for suicidal or homicidal ideation, intent, or plan.

FUNCTIONAL STATUS

This dimension measures the impact of a child's or adolescent's primary mental health condition on his or her daily life. Assessment of this dimension includes the child's or adolescent's ability to function in all age-appropriate roles: family member, friend, and student. A health professional would also assess the overall ability of the youth to meet basic daily activities such as eating, sleeping, and personal hygiene. A youth whose primary mental health condition dramatically affects his or her abilities in this dimension would frequently require more intensive supports than a youth whose mental health disorder has had limited impact on his or her overall functioning.

TABLE 27.2. ESSENTIAL DIMENSIONS FOR FUNCTIONAL ASSESSMENT: THE CALOCUS

- Safety/risk of harm
- Functional status
- Comorbidity
- Recovery environment
- Resiliency and treatment history
- Treatment acceptance and engagement

CALOCUS, Child and Adolescent Level of Care Utilization System.

COMORBIDITY

This dimension measures the coexistence of another disorder that might be complicating a child's or adolescent's mental health condition. The presence of a developmental disability, substance abuse problem, or an active or chronic medical condition may complicate a youth's mental health disorder as well as the other co-occuring problem. A patient with one or more comorbidities may require multiple interventions, in addition to mental health treatment, in order to stabilize him or her in the community without the use of institutional-based services.

RECOVERY ENVIRONMENT

The child's or adolescent's ability to benefit from mental health treatment directly relates to both the level of stress as well as level of support that the child or adolescent has in his or her immediate environment. An understanding of the strengths and weaknesses of the youth's family, as well as affect of the neighborhood and community's role in the process of a youth's recovery, may affect what level of services he or she may need in order to improve. For example, if a youth has a family with multiple problems and lives in a community that has a high rate of poverty and violence, this youth may require more intensive resources to support his or her recovery. Likewise, a youth in a family with few stresses and residing in a more stable community may require fewer resources to be maintained at home.

RESILIENCY AND TREATMENT HISTORY

Resiliency refers to a child's or adolescent's constitutional emotional strength to adapt to changing life circumstances with minimal disruption in his or her daily functioning. The concept of resiliency essentially addresses the ability of a youth with an emotional disability to self-regulate thoughts, feelings, and behavior when there are disruptions in his or her immediate environment. Children and adolescents who are highly resilient are able to use their own resources (e.g., intellectual capabilities, good verbal skills, capacity for empathy) to cope with major life changes and respond in a developmentally appropriate manner with minimal disruption in their functioning. A youth's mental health treatment history is usually a good indication of whether he or she is able to benefit successfully from formal mental health interventions. However, children and adolescents may respond well to some treatment situations but not to others. This may not only be related to the youth's internal capabilities but also to the characteristics, attractiveness, and/or cultural competency of the treatment provided. Thus, a previous failure to improve from one level of mental health service intensity does not automatically mean that the youth would not benefit from the same level of care at another time in his or her illness. What it does imply is that the health professional should review with the caregiver, as well as with the child or adolescent, whether the last mental health intervention was an appropriate fit with the youth's and family's strengths and needs. Also, youths who are highly resilient and have benefited from previous treatment may need a less intensive treatment environment in order to benefit from mental health care for their mental health problem.

TREATMENT ACCEPTANCE AND ENGAGEMENT

In order for a child or adolescent to benefit from mental health treatment, he or she must, within developmental constraints, be able to form a positive therapeutic relationship with the people providing his or her treatment. This includes the youth's ability to define the presenting mental health problem, to accept his or her role in the development or perpetuation of this problem, to accept his or her role in the treatment process, and to actively cooperate in treatment. This is equally true for the child's or adolescent's primary caregiver who must be willing and able to participate proactively in the intake, planning, implementation, and maintenance phase of the youth's mental health treatment. Youths and caregivers who have a clearer understanding of the nature of their mental health needs and a willingness to accept appropriate treatment tend to need less intensive mental health treatment. By contrast, those who have difficulty in accepting a mental health problem with a family that is resistant to treatment typically require services that are most intensive. It is critical, however, for a health professional to be aware of the cultural background of the primary caregiver and its effect on the caregiver's understanding and acceptance of the youth's mental health condition, as well as the choice of care options for solving it. It is also important to note barriers to proper assessment and treatment based on cultural differences between the youth and parent/caregiver and the health professional. If needed, consultation with culturally congruent staff may eliminate cultural barriers to effective mental health assessment and treatment.

Influence of Community-based System of Care on Level of Care Determination

The community-based system of care concept and philosophy has provided a framework for system reform in the children's mental health system since the mid-1980s. Stroul and Friedman were the first to define *system of care*: "A comprehensive spectrum of mental health and other necessary services which are organized into a coordinated network to meet the multiple and changing needs of children and adolescents with serious emotional disturbances and their families." The system of care concept represents a philosophy about the way in which services should be delivered to children and their families. The essential core values and guiding principles of a system of care are listed in Table 27.3.

Thus, level of care determination within a community-based system of care approach is similar to a managed care system in that both involve traditional clinical interventions such as mental health outpatient, inpatient, and residential treatment. Community-based systems of care, however, emphasize more flexible and individualized service approaches utilizing nontraditional service modalities such as home-based services, therapeutic foster care, and mentoring. In addition, systems of care involve highly trained clinicians of all disciplines, as well as paraprofessionals, families as providers, and other creative staffing strategies to meet different needs. This is usually not true in a typical BHO.

A primary goal of CALOCUS' multidimensional assessment is to customize the level of resource or service intensity as defined by a combination of service variables, such as physical facilities, clinical services, support services, crisis stabilization, and prevention services. With higher levels of care, a greater number and variety of these types of services are utilized. The requirement for active case management is needed at these higher levels of care.

One way to think about levels of care is to compare them with the difference between services in a primary care office (the lower level of care) versus a major medical center (higher levels of care). For well-baby checks and most common medical conditions, a child or adolescent can be treated in the pediatrician's office. For more complex problems, especially those that are disabling or life threatening, treatment at a major medical center would be appropriate due to the wider array of services and the availability of specialists.

TABLE 27.3. ESSENTIALS FOR A SYSTEM OF CARE

Core values
- The system of care should be child centered and family focused.
- The system of care should be community based with the locus of services, management, and decision-making responsibility resting at the community level.
- The system of care should be culturally competent, with agencies, programs, and services responsive to the cultural, racial, and ethnic differences of the population they serve.

Guiding principles
- Children with emotional disturbance should have access to a comprehensive array of services that address their physical, emotional, social, and educational needs.
- Children with emotional disturbance should receive individualized services in accordance with their unique needs and potential, and guided by an individualized service plan.
- Services should be provided within the least restrictive, most normative environment that is clinically appropriate.
- The families or surrogate families of these children should be full participants in all aspects of planning and delivery of services.
- Services for children with emotional disturbance should be integrated with linkages between child-serving agencies and programs and with mechanisms for planning, developing, and coordinating services.
- Children with emotional disturbance should be provided with case management to ensure that services are delivered in a coordinated and therapeutic manner and that they can move through the system of care based on their changing needs.
- Early identification and prevention of emotional disturbance should be promoted by the system of care in order to enhance the likelihood of positive outcomes.
- Children with emotional disturbance should be ensured smooth transitions to the adult service systems when they reach the age of maturity.
- The rights of children with emotional disturbance should be protected, and effective advocacy efforts should be promoted.
- Children with emotional disturbance should receive services without regard to race, religion, national origin, sex, physical disability, or other characteristics; and services should be sensitive and responsive to cultural differences and special needs.

Levels of Care within a Community-based System of Care

The fragmentation or duplication of mental health services, particularly for multiproblem youths involved in two or more child-serving systems, has led to the development of a "system of care" for mental health and related services in over 67 local jurisdictions in the United States. The $92 million federal program, the "Comprehensive Community Mental Health Services for Children and Their Families," has supported these local jurisdictions in establishing a coordinated system of care for high-risk children and adolescents. In addition to these 67 sites, there has been greater investment by states and local communities in creating services consistent with the system of care philosophy. The development of system of care in states and local communities has given rise to the reformulation of how mental health and related services are delivered to children and adolescents with serious emotional disturbance in a community.

CALOCUS has provided a framework for how the types and intensity of mental health and related services are organized in a community-based system of care. The CALOCUS' levels of care include the following services.

BASIC SERVICES FOR PREVENTION AND MAINTENANCE

Basic services are designed to prevent the onset of illness and/or limit the magnitude of morbidity associated with individual, family, or social risk factors, developmental delays, and existing emotional disorders in various stages of improvement or remission. An example of this type of service would be depression screening in a primary care office with referral to outpatient mental health services, if needed.

RECOVERY MAINTENANCE AND HEALTH MANAGEMENT

These services typically provide follow-up care to mobilize family strengths and reinforce linkages to natural supports. Individuals appropriate for this level of service either may be substantially recovered from an emotional disorder or have an emotional disorder that is sufficiently manageable within their families. Children with emotional disorders who benefit from this level of care are those for whom it is determined that their emotional disorder is no longer threatening to expected growth and development. Services in this level of care could be provided within an outpatient mental health center, family resource center, or primary care clinic. These services would include medication monitoring, after-school programming, and family support services such as respite care.

OUTPATIENT SERVICES

These services are usually for children, adolescents, and their families who have an active mental health disorder interfering with their functioning at home, school, or in the community. These services are frequently provided in mental health clinics or clinician offices. They may also be provided within a juvenile justice facility school, child welfare office, or other community setting. Children and adolescents most appropriate for outpatient services typically do not require extensive system coordination and case management as their families are able to use community supports with minimal assistance. The continuity of the child's or adolescent's treatment relationship with an outpatient mental health provider often is essential in maintaining the youth at higher levels of functioning. Clinicians offering follow-up outpatient services to children and adolescents transitioning from higher levels of care must be able to provide ongoing individual and family assessment as well as medication monitoring with the capacity to add services as needed.

INTENSIVE OUTPATIENT SERVICES

This level of care generally is appropriate for children and adolescents who need more intensive outpatient treatment and who are living either in their families with support or in alternative families or group facilities in the community. Typically, the child's or adolescent's family demonstrates significant strengths that allow the youth to remain at home. Treatment may be needed several times per week with daily supervision provided by the family or facility staff. Service coordination is essential for maintaining the youth in the community. Children or adolescents in this level of care frequently have comorbid mental health and physical health conditions that require medical care from a pediatrician or family physician in the community.

INTENSIVE INTEGRATED SERVICES WITHOUT 24-HOUR PSYCHIATRIC MONITORING

These services are provided to children and adolescents with a serious behavioral or emotional disorder but who are capable of living in the community with support, either in their families or in placement such as group homes, foster care, homeless or domestic violence shelters, or transitional housing. Typically, children or adolescents and their families in this level of care require services from multiple agencies in order to maintain them outside of a facility. For example, an adolescent with significant delinquency and school failure may require the involvement of a probation officer, a mental health clinician, a child and adolescent psychiatrist, and a special education teacher. These children and adolescents require a highly coordinated treatment plan that is monitored through a clinically informed case manager who can assist in the collaboration or coordination between service providers on the youth's or family's behalf. Services in this level of care include partial hospitalization, intensive day treatment, and home-based wraparound care.

NONSECURE, 24-HOUR SERVICES WITH PSYCHIATRIC MONITORING

This level of care refers to treatment in which the essential element is the maintenance of a milieu in which the therapeutic needs of the child or adolescent and family can be addressed intensively. This level of care traditionally has been provided in nonhospital settings such as residential treatment facilities or therapeutic foster homes. Equivalent services have been provided in juvenile justice and specialized residential schools. A highly coordinated clinically informed case manager is needed in preparing the children or adolescents and their families for reintegration back into the family and community systems.

SECURE 24-HOUR SERVICES WITH PSYCHIATRIC MANAGEMENT

These services are the most restrictive and often, but not necessarily, the most intensive in the community-based level of care continuum. Traditionally these services have been provided in a secure facility such as an acute inpatient hospital unit or locked residential program. This level of care may be provided through the intensive application of mental health and medical services in a juvenile detention and/or educational facility, provided that these facilities are able to adhere to medical and psychiatric care standards. Although high levels of restrictiveness are typically required for effective intervention, emphasis is on reducing the duration and pervasiveness of restrictiveness to minimize negative effects on youths. The services offered within a community-based system of care are shown in Table 27.4.

Mental Health Services in Other Child-serving Systems

The goal of clinicians who are treating children and adolescents who need mental health services is to provide appropriate treatment that will return these youths to their optimal level of functioning while decreasing their degree of distress. The goal of community-based interventions is to enable youths to function optimally in their environment while reducing the emotional or behavioral distress as much as possible. One method of

TABLE 27.4. ESSENTIAL MENTAL HEALTH SERVICES WITHIN A COMMUNITY-BASED SYSTEM OF CARE

Nonresidential Services	Residential Services
Prevention	Therapeutic foster care
Early identification and intervention	Therapeutic group home
Assessment	Therapeutic camp services
Outpatient treatment	Independent living services
Home-based services	Residential treatment services
Day treatment	Crisis residential treatment
Crisis services	Inpatient hospitalization

achieving this has been the integration of mental health services within the other child-serving systems in which children and adolescents with emotional or behavioral disturbance may be placed. The array and intensity of mental health services within these other child-serving systems vary from one community to the next. As well, each system may offer a set of mental health services, driven partially by the legal mandates that each system is expected to achieve. Thus, youths with special education needs may be offered a specific set of services that will enable them to improve in their academic achievement, while the same child may be given a different set of mental health services if placed within the child welfare system. For youths who are served by more than one system, this may even create fragmented or duplicative mental health care. The concept of a community-based system of care approach is needed to ensure that children and adolescents with mental health needs receive appropriate, coordinated care that is not dependent on which child-serving system the youth is currently placed. However, children and adolescents with mental health needs may receive services within other child-serving systems, often in unique and innovative ways. It is important for clinicians to know what types of mental health services are offered within school, child welfare, or juvenile justice systems in order to support and advocate that the youth's and family's unique mental health needs are well met by each system.

SCHOOL-BASED MENTAL HEALTH SERVICE DELIVERY MODELS

Consultation

One of the most widely used school-based interventions for a student with a mental health disorder is the mental health consultation model. Psychotherapists, psychologists, and/or child and adolescent psychiatrists, usually from outpatient mental health clinics or universities, meet with teachers to discuss a child's behavioral and academic performance problem and to plan appropriate interventions. Often, the mental health professional will evaluate the student in the school setting and participate in the formulation of the intervention plan. Mental health consultants often provide teachers with didactic information about various learning and emotional disorders and strategies on how the educator may meet the student's need in the classroom. Also, principals may also participate in the consultation in addressing administrative issues that affect the school's ability to manage problematic emotional or behavioral disorders that interfere with a student's ability to learn.

School-based health clinics

For over 25 years in the United States, school-based clinics have provided acute and referral physical health services to students primarily in middle and high schools. Many of these school-based clinics also provide some level of outpatient mental health services. These services typically include individual, family, and group psychotherapy as well as medication evaluation and monitoring services either by primary care providers or consulting child and adolescent psychiatrists. A multidisciplinary team, composed of primary care and mental health providers, often develops an individualized treatment plan for each student. Coordination with teachers and principals usually occurs on an individualized basis.

School-based family resource centers

In numerous cities, especially in poor and minority communities, school districts have established family service centers that offer a variety of services ranging from violence prevention, health promotion, social services, day care, after school recreation, and other community programming. These services may also include traditional outpatient mental health services not only for students in that particular school but to the neighborhood as a whole. Providers within these family resource centers typically collaborate with school staff and school district personnel in the development of effective, well-coordinated programs that meet both the school's and neighborhood's needs.

School mental health centers

These programs combine coordinated clinical services for children, adolescents, and families with mental health needs; consultative services for teachers and school staff; and preventative mental health educational curricula and enrichment programs for the general school population. These centers have evolved from the collaboration between the school district and a mental health entity, at times in collaboration with other child-serving entities. There are also school-based programs that have mental health promotion and prevention orientation and focus. These programs have strong mental health components and often combine clinical services with parent training, tutoring, and day care that foster parent participation in school activities. These programs may also focus on student alcohol and other drug abuse prevention efforts.

MENTAL HEALTH SERVICES WITHIN THE CHILD WELFARE SYSTEM

State and community child welfare agencies differ in their abilities to meet the mental health needs of children and adolescents who have been removed from their homes due to suspected abuse and/or neglect. Ideally, mental health treatment goals for youths who have been removed from their homes are consistent with expediting permanency through family reunification or adoption and reducing the time youths spend in foster care. Child welfare agencies are typically able to purchase mental health related services, in addition to traditional mental health services that are provided in the community, for children and adolescents in their custody.

Therapeutic foster care

Therapeutic foster care differs from regular foster care in that the foster parents are trained to deal with youths with emotional and behavioral problems. Care is delivered in a home setting using a family-based model to provide youths with a nurturing environment. Common features of therapeutic foster care include foster parents who are well trained in dealing with the mental health needs of youths in foster care, low number of children per foster parent (typically one child), and child welfare service workers with low caseloads, allowing them to provide more oversight, training, and care coordination to the therapeutic foster parents. Therapeutic foster care is usually combined with outpatient mental health services, crisis services, and in-home interventions.

Agency-based mental health consultation

Mental health services are incorporated into the social service system with the assignment of mental health clinicians to assist the child welfare staff in formulating and attaining permanency goals. This mental health clinician functions as a consultant and is available to meet with the child, biologic parents, and foster parents to assist the case planner and handle crises or conflicts that may arise in the implementation of the permanency goals. The mental health consultant works with the case planner to assess the youth's and family's needs, develop treatment and service plans, and design interventions. In conjunction with the social service team, the consultant helps determine referrals to specialized mental health services.

Therapeutic visitation

Therapeutic visitation is a mental health intervention that focuses on improving the quality of the visit between the youth and his or her biologic family. These visits provide an opportunity to assess the timing of the youth's return home and to facilitate the transition. The mental health care provider assists in identifying therapeutic objectives for the visit, modeling appropriate parenting skills, and supporting the biologic parents in interacting in an age-appropriate manner with the youth. These visits enable the mental health clinician and social service case planner to identify and resolve any parent-child conflict by giving the parent specific feedback about interactions observed.

Mental health screening and evaluation

Early screening and evaluation of children and adolescents entering the foster care system can increase the stability and quality of the youth's relationship with the foster care provider, reduce the risk of multiple foster home placements, and shorten the amount of time the youth spends out of the home. The benefits of screening include more timely referrals for comprehensive psychiatric, psychological, and educational evaluations; early identification of youths requiring higher levels of care such as therapeutic foster home or residential care; and early identification of and enhanced support services for difficult-to-manage youths, resulting in fewer disrupted foster home placements. Screenings and evaluations can be combined with psychoeducational training of foster parents that prepare the caregiver to deal with the needs of each youth as well as to educate the foster parent in common mental health issues that arise in youths who are placed in out-of-home care.

MENTAL HEALTH SERVICES WITHIN THE JUVENILE JUSTICE SYSTEM

Addressing the mental health needs of children and adolescents in the juvenile justice system requires an understanding of the goals of each respective system. Juvenile justice is primarily interested in reducing juvenile delinquency and recidivism rates and promoting public safety. Juvenile justice services are usually not voluntary as juvenile court is a civil system that adjudicates youths into services reflecting the court's view of the best mental health, substance abuse, or other interventions for addressing the juvenile's needs. The mental health system, on the other hand, focuses on the youth and family and aims to address emotional and behavioral needs through a voluntary process. Thus, the circumstances of youths receiving mental health services within the juvenile justice system differ from youths receiving mental health services within other community settings. Mental health services can be found in detention services, residential facilities, or in community-based systems.

Juvenile detention

Juvenile detention is a term that has traditionally been defined as maintaining a youth who has been adjudicated into a secure facility. The youth is usually held in a detention facility for temporary and safe custody in order to guarantee his or her appearance in court or in other instances to provide short-term sanctions for illegal behavior. A detention center may or may not have access to mental health professionals who can provide evaluation and treatment of mental health conditions in the youth. Some detention centers have integrated physical and mental health clinics within their setting. Some juvenile detention facilities may provide mental health consultation to detention staff about mental health issues. This type of consultation focuses on helping the detention staff to find appropriate ways to intervene with youths demonstrating behavioral problems based on their underlying mental health problems.

Residential programs

Long-term residential programs can vary in both size and settings but are designed specifically for youths in the juvenile justice system. Typically, these programs occur in locked facilities. Ideally, these programs provide educational and vocational training, individual and group counseling, health care, and psychiatric services. Youths in these programs are considered to pose serious community safety risks, and the programs aim to protect the public and rehabilitate the youths. Thus, these programs vary in the availability, as well as intensity, of formal mental health services. The quality of these mental health services varies from adequate to minimal in many communities and states.

Community-based treatment

The majority of youths in the juvenile justice system reside in their local community, and the most effective interventions to prevent delinquency are usually not delivered in a facility but rather in the community in which the youth resides. Evidence-based interventions include intensive home-based family therapy, mental health screening of first or second time juvenile offenders with the provision of intensive mental health treatment for those deemed at high risk for chronic delinquency, short-term foster care combined with individual counseling and parent management training, social competence promotion through such activities as participation in community service activities, as well as social skills training and the use of behavioral modification to address disruptive behavioral problems in group settings such as school.

Wraparound Services

Out of the system of care movement came the development of more strength-based, family focused care. Given the complexity of the child, adolescent, and family with multiple needs, flexible services have been developed that assist these youths and families in strengthening their natural support systems while addressing social issues that impacted the youth's ability to benefit from more formal mental health services. Intensive case management is the cornerstone of wraparound service models. A case manager is a specially trained individual who coordinates or provides psychiatric, financial, legal, and medical services to help the child or adolescent live successfully at home and in the community. In addition, family support services to help the families care for their child or adolescent include such interventions as parent training and parent support groups. Respite care services are usually part of the service array in a wraparound approach in which the child or adolescent can stay briefly away from the home with specially trained individuals. Nontraditional services such as tutoring, mentoring, recreational, or vocational services are often offered.

Wraparound services require interagency collaboration to provide appropriate services such as crisis intervention, education advocacy, individual and family therapy, psychological evaluation, medication evaluation and management, and social service interventions, among others. Services may be provided in various locations, including the youth's home, school, or community. The goal of the intervention is to provide appropriate interventions while preventing the youth from progressing into more restrictive levels of mental health care.

Wraparound services connote a philosophy that includes the youth and family in defining an individualized set of community services and natural supports aimed at achieving

TABLE 27.5. ESSENTIALS OF WRAPAROUND SERVICES

- Wraparound services must be based in the community.
- Services and supports must be individualized, built on strengths, and meet the needs of children, adolescents, and families across the life domains in order to promote success, safety, and permanency in home, school, and the community.
- The wraparound process must be culturally competent.
- Families must be full and active partners in every level of the wraparound process.
- The wraparound approach must be a team-driven process involving the family, youth, natural supports, agencies, and community services working together to develop, implement, and evaluate the individualized service plan.
- Wraparound teams must have flexible approaches with adequate and flexible funding.
- Wraparound plans must have a balance of formal services and informal community and family resources.
- The community agencies and teams must make an unconditional commitment to serve their youths and families.
- A service-support plan should be developed and implemented based on an interagency, community-neighborhood collaborative process.
- Outcomes must be determined and measured for each goal established with the youth and family, as well as for those goals established at the program and system level.

positive outcomes. Because professionals tend to view wraparound services as simply a group of services that address the various problems of a youth and family, it is essential to clearly define these services. Table 27.5 summarizes the essential elements of wraparound services.

Wraparound services are widely disseminated, with 88% of states reporting their use. Most wraparound programs are based in mental health systems, although many other service systems participate in these programs.

The Role of the Primary Care Provider in System of Care

The primary care provider offers a unique role in supporting youths and families in receiving services within a system of care model. Obviously, the primary care provider must be available to participate in service planning for children and adolescents with mental health needs, particularly if there is coexisting medical illness that is complicated by the youth's emotional functioning. Children and adolescents with emotional disturbances, particularly those placed in the child welfare or juvenile justice system, commonly have an unidentified or undertreated medical illness that requires physical health services. One strategy to achieve comprehensive health care is through the establishment of a "medical home." The medical home can provide the full range of care that addresses the comprehensive needs of the child or adolescent. Services within the medical home can either be directly provided by the primary care clinician or coordinated by ancillary personnel. As well, the primary care provider may be the central point to consolidate medical, mental health, educational, and social services information into a unified clinical record. In this role, the primary care provider may be central in asking for the other professionals within other child-serving agencies to develop a common treatment plan that addresses the youth's unique needs based on a comprehensive physical and developmental assessment. If this type of health care management cannot be met through the primary care provider, the provider may collaborate with the other child-serving agencies in developing a service plan that meets the youth's mental health, physical health, and developmental needs. Children and adolescents with multiple challenges affecting their functioning at home, school, and in the community require comprehensive treatments and can benefit from receiving services within a wraparound, community-based model.

Conclusion

Each state and community will vary in the types of mental health services available to children, adolescents, and their families. The array of services available to an individual is dependent both on third-party reimbursement and a youth's eligibility to receive services in other child-serving systems. Ideally, mental health services would be individualized and would meet the youth's needs in the least restrictive setting. Primary care providers can play a central role by either performing or ensuring a culturally sensitive assessment of the youth and his or her family. This assessment should direct, in partnership with the caregiver, the mental health services the child or adolescent receives in the settings that optimize individualized outcomes. Further research is needed to better define the type, intensity, and location of such mental health services.

Case Vignette

Case vignette #1

The following case illustrates the use of mental health and wraparound services within a community-based system of care.

Ashley, an 8-year-old girl in a third grade general education placement, was evaluated by a mental health professional after an incident in which she stabbed a classmate with a pencil and threatened to harm her teacher with a pair of scissors. Ashley has a history of disruptive behavioral problems since age 3. These behavioral problems have included a short attention and concentration span, distractibility in the classroom, hyperactivity as noted by an inability to stay seated in class, and a history of marked impulsivity and low frustration tolerance. Ashley's behavioral problems frequently result in temper tantrums when she is not given her own way both at home and at school. In addition, over the past year, Ashley had become increasingly argumentative with adults, been getting into physical altercations with her brother and sister, and recently set a fire at home. She also had an incident of hurting the family cat. Prior to this incident, Ashley had stabbed the classmate and had been suspended twice for fighting with classmates at recess.

Ashley has experienced numerous psychosocial stressors. Ashley's biologic parents divorced when she was 2 years old. Her mother remarried shortly after the divorce. Ashley has no contact with her biologic father. Her stepfather was incarcerated approximately 6 months ago after being physically violent toward Ashley's mother. Ashley was a witness to this domestic violence. She denied a history of physical or sexual abuse. Her mother lost her job 2 months ago after missing many days of work secondary to the abuse. She is currently unemployed. In addition, the mother had been reported to Child Welfare services after it was noted that Ashley frequently came to school complaining of being hungry and with unexplained bruises on her arms.

Ashley has a history of poorly controlled asthma that has resulted in numerous visits to the emergency room. In addition, Ashley was receiving Ritalin from her primary care provider, but her mother was inconsistent in giving her the medication, stating that Ashley "did not need it." Her teacher reported, however, that Ashley is better able to do her schoolwork when she has taken her Ritalin. Although the mother has been encouraged to attend meetings with the school social worker, she has claimed that child care and transportation problems prevent her from attending these meetings.

During the interview with the mental health clinician, Ashley stated that meeting with a therapist was "stupid" and that she "didn't have any problems." She was able to talk about missing her stepfather and worrying about family finances. She did state that she was "bored" at home and had "nothing to do" when she came home from school and on the weekends.

Clearly, Ashley has demonstrated serious functional impairment in her daily activities, which has been perpetuated by high environmental stress in her home environment with little emotional support from her mother. In addition, Ashley has chronic asthma that requires close medical supervision, which she is not obtaining. Both Ashley and her mother have been somewhat obstructive in forming a therapeutic relationship with both the mental health clinician and school social worker. Her serious disruptive behavioral problems put her in moderate risk for harm to others.

After the mental health assessment, it was obvious that Ashley and her family needed intensive wraparound services from a multidisciplinary team as Ashley displayed impairments in all the dimensions of the CALOCUS. Thus, her plan of care needed to contain elements that are found in each CALOCUS level of service intensity. The mental health clinician was able to convince Ashley's mother that Ashley was a potential danger to others and that Ashley would be at risk of placement into a therapeutic foster home or a residential treatment center. The mental health clinician also stated that Ashley might require psychiatric inpatient hospitalization if she continued to pose a threat to classmates or her teacher. The mental health clinician, school social worker, and child welfare worker were able to develop a plan of care with Ashley's mother to address Ashley's and her family's multiple needs. The child welfare worker was designated as a case manager to coordinate the activities of daily living, including food, transportation, child care, and necessary financial assistance. The case manager also assisted the mother in making regular follow-up appointments with the primary care provider to stabilize Ashley's asthma and to restart her Ritalin. The mental health clinician agreed to see Ashley on a weekly basis for individual therapy and to work with Ashley's mother on improving her parenting skills. The school social worker was able to develop a behavioral management plan with Ashley's teacher and arranged for Ashley to go to the local Boys & Girls Club after school. Ashley now has a Big Sister from this club to take her on activities on the weekend. This plan has allowed Ashley to remain in her general education classroom as well as at home with her family.

BIBLIOGRAPHY

American Academy of Child and Adolescent Psychiatry Work Group on Systems of Care and American Association of Community Psychiatry Psychiatrists. *Child and Adolescent Level of Care Utilization System (CALOCUS) user's manual, version 1.3.* Washington, DC: American Academy of Child and Adolescent Psychiatry Work Group on Systems of Care and American Association of Community Psychiatry Psychiatrists, 2003.

Rogers K. Evidence-based community-based interventions. In: Pumariega AJ, Winters NC, eds. *The handbook of community-based systems of care: the new community psychiatry.* San Francisco, CA: Jossey Bass Publishers, 2003:149–170.

Stroul BA. Systems of care—a framework for children's mental health care. In: Pumariega AJ, Stroul B, Friedman R. *A system of care for children and youth with severe emotional disturbance,* Rev ed. Washington, DC: Georgetown University Child Development Center, National Technical Assistance Center for Children's Mental Health, 1986.

Stroul BA. Systems of care: a framework for children's mental health. In: Pumariega AJ, Winters NC, eds. *Handbook of community-based systems of care: the new child and adolescent community psychiatry.* San Francisco, CA: Jossey Bass Publishers, 2003:17–34.

Task Force on Healthcare for Children in Foster Care. *Fostering Health: Health Care for Children in Foster Care.* New York: American Academy of Pediatrics, District II, New York State, 2001; www.aapdistrictii.org/committeecorner/foster.htm.

U.S. Department of Health and Human Services (2000), *Report of the surgeon general's conference on children's mental health: a national action agenda.* Rockville, MD: U.S. Department of Health and Human Services.

Winters NC, eds. *Handbook of community-based systems of care: the new child and adolescent community psychiatry.* San Francisco, CA: Jossey Bass Publishers, 2003:17–34.

SUGGESTED READINGS

Burns B, Hoagwood K. *Community treatment for youth: evidence-based interventions for severe emotional and behavioral disorders (Innovations in Practice and Service Delivery With Vulnerable Populations).* London: Oxford University Press, 2002. *(A good resource for clinicians, researchers, and consumers.)*

Pumariega AJ, Winters NC, eds. *Handbook of community-based systems of care: the new child and adolescent community psychiatry.* San Francisco, CA: Jossey Bass Publishers, 2003. *(A comprehensive overview and history for clinicians working within systems of care.)*

Index

Tables are indicated by page numbers followed by *t*